Palliative Care Nursing
Quality Care
to the End of Life

Second Edition

Marianne LaPorte Matzo, PhD, APRN, GNP-BC, FAAN

Dr. Matzo is a Professor and the Frances E. and A. Earl Ziegler Chair in Palliative Care Nursing at The University of Oklahoma Health Sciences Center College of Nursing in Oklahoma City, Oklahoma. She is also a member of the Doctoral Faculty at The Union Institute and University in Cincinnati, Ohio and a Soros Scholar for the Project on Death in America. She was awarded a doctorate in Gerontology from the University of Massachusetts–Boston and a master's degree in Nursing from the Gerontological Nurse Practitioner Program at the University of Massachusetts–Lowell. Her work for the Project on Death in America has included undergraduate curriculum development on the care of the dying patient and family, work as a hospice nurse, and continuing education programs related to death, dying and bereavement. Her research has included nurse's practices of assisted suicide and a quantitative study of health care providers' responses to the death of their patients. Dr. Matzo has presented educational programs both regionally and nationally on many topics related to care of the dying person, gerontological nursing, and curriculum development. Her work has been published in *Nurse Practitioner, Nurse Educator, Geriatric Nursing, Nursing Homes, Geriatric Psychiatry, The Journal of Gerontological Nursing, Gerontology and Geriatrics Education, Applied Nursing Research, Heart and Lung, Nursing Education Perspectives* and the *Geriatric Clinics of North America.*

Deborah Witt Sherman, PhD, APRN, ANP-BC, FAAN

Dr. Sherman is Associate Professor, Director of the Doctoral Program at New York University College of Nursing, and faculty of the Advanced Practice Palliative Care Master's and Post-Master's Programs. She is also Co-Director and faculty for the Bronx Veterans Medical Center Interdisciplinary Palliative Care Fellowship Program. Dr. Sherman's education includes a BSN from Mount St. Mary College in Newburgh, New York, a master's degree from Pace University in Tarrytown, New York, a doctorate from New York University, and post-master's certificate in adult health from New York University. Dr. Sherman's background in critical care nursing and hospice nursing and her certification as an adult nurse practitioner, as well as her research focus on populations with life-threatening and terminal illness, are foundational to her expertise and commitment to palliative care, for which she developed the first nurse practitioner palliative care master's and post-master's programs in the United States.

In 1998, Dr. Sherman was awarded the prestigious Project on Death in America Faculty Scholars Fellowship, funded by the Soros Foundation, to implement the Advanced Practice Palliative Care Master's Program at New York University and to participate as a nurse practitioner on the palliative care team of Mount Sinai Medical Center in New York. Dr. Sherman was also awarded an advanced nursing practice training grant by the Department of Health and Human Services to fund the Advanced Practice Palliative Care Master's Program at New York University.

Dr. Sherman has been funded by the National Institute of Health for a two-year pilot study entitled "Interventions and Quality of Life for Patients with Advanced Cancer or AIDS and their Family Caregivers." She is also a co-investigator on a four-year randomized control trial funded by the National Cancer Institute to examine the effects of psychoeducation and telephone counseling on the adjustment of women and partners experiencing early stage breast cancer.

She is a member of several editorial boards and professional nursing organizations including the National Hospice Organization, Hospice and Palliative Care Nurses Association, The Association of Death Educators and Grief Counselors, Oncology Nursing Society, and the Association for Nurses in AIDS Care. Dr. Sherman serves on the advisory board and as faculty on the End of Life Nursing Education Consortium, whose aim is to educate nurses in palliative care across the country. Dr. Sherman has served as a member of an Interdisciplinary Steering Committee of a National Consensus Project, which developed national guidelines for quality palliative care. She has led the initiative to develop the Scope and Standards for Advance Practice Palliative Care Nursing approved by the ANA. Dr. Sherman secured funding to develop the first national Advance Practice Palliative Care Credentialing Examination, which was completed in May 2003.

Palliative Care Nursing
Quality Care to the End of Life

Second Edition

Marianne LaPorte Matzo, PhD, APRN, GNP-BC, FAAN
Deborah Witt Sherman, PhD, APRN, ANP-BC, FAAN

Editors

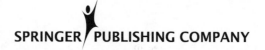

SPRINGER PUBLISHING COMPANY

Springer Publishing Company, Inc.
11 West 42nd Street, 15th Floor
New York, NY 10036-8002

Editor: Sally Barhydt
Production: Print Matters, Inc.
Cover design: Mimi Flow
Composition: Compset, Inc.

Library of Congress Cataloging-in-Publication Data

Palliative care nursing : quality care to the end of life/Marianne LaPorte Matzo, Deborah Witt Sherman [editors].—2nd ed.
　　p.; cm.
　Includes bibliographical references and index.
　ISBN 0-8261-5794-7 (hc)
　　1. Terminal care. 2. Palliative treatment.
　　[DNLM: 1. Terminal Care. 2. Hospice Care—psychology. 3. Palliative Care. WY 152 P1677 2005] I. Matzo, Marianne. II. Sherman, Deborah Witt.

RT87.T45P343 2005
616.02′9—dc22   2005051706

Printed in the United States by Bang Printing

For LeaRose and Giuliana, the most precious gifts of my life, and to Roland, who shares and supports my life. I love and treasure all of you.

—MLM

With deep love for my children, Ben, Rachael, and Joe, who are the joy and the pride of my life, and to my mother, Mary; my sisters, Kathy and Diane; brother, Jim, and dearest of friends, Heloise, Fran, Esther, and Chris, who share in my happiness and are always there with love and support in times of need. I thank God for blessing me with an incredible family and friends whom I adore.

—DWS

Contents

List of Education Plans for Achieving Competencies

Contributors

Marilyn Bookbinder, RN, PhD
Director of Nursing
Department of Pain Medicine and
　Palliative Care
Beth Israel Medical Center
New York, New York

Nessa Coyle, NP, PhD, FAAN
Pain and Palliative Care Service
Memorial Sloan-Kettering Cancer Center
New York, New York

Suzanne K. Goetschius, MSN, APRN, BC
Clinical Specialist, Gerontology
Department of Nursing Research and
　Education
Fletcher Allen Health Care
Burlington, Vermont

Mary Layman-Goldstein, RN, MS, OCN
Pain and Pain and Palliative Care Service
Memorial Sloan-Kettering Cancer Center
New York, New York

Mary Jo Jacobs, RN, MN
Consultant
Chicago, Illinois

Mary K. Kazanowski, APRN, BC,
　PHD, CHPN
VNA Hospice of Manchester and
　Southern New Hampshire
Saint Anselm College Department of
　Nursing
Manchester, New Hampshire

Margaret Kiss, RN, MSN, AOCN
Quality Improvement
Memorial Sloan-Kettering Cancer Center
New York, New York

Lisa M. Krammer, RN, MSN, ANP,
　AOCN, BC-PCM
Northwestern Memorial Hospital
Palliative Care and Home Hospice Program
Chicago, Illinois

Judy Lentz, RN, MSN, NHA
CEO
Hospice and Palliative Nurses Association
Pittsburgh, Pennsylvania

Carla Mariano, EdD, RN, AHN-BC, FAAIM
Adjunct Professor
New York University College of Nursing
New York, New York

Jeanne Martinez, RN, MPH, CHPN
Quality and Education Specialist
Northwestern Memorial Home Health Care
Chicago, Illinois

Kathleen O. Perrin, PhD, RN, CCRN
Professor, Nursing
Saint Anselm College
Manchester, New Hampshire

Mertie L. Potter, ND, APRN, BC
Associate Professor of Nursing
Saint Anselm College
Manchester, New Hampshire

Gloria C. Ramsey, RN, BSN, JD
Consultant
New York University College of Nursing
New York, New York

Eileen A. Ring, RN, MN
Northwestern Memorial Hospital
Department of Emergency Medicine
Chicago, Illinois

Judith Kennedy Schwarz, RN, PhD
Consultant in Ethics and End-of-life Care
Patient Support Coordinator, Compassion
    and Choices of New York
Adjunct Faculty
Hunter College, City University of New York
New York, New York

Mary Beth Williams, RN, MN
Consultant
Chicago, Illinois

Foreword

Betty Rolling Ferrell

Imagine that someone you love is dying, perhaps a grandparent, a spouse, or even a child. Who will be with your loved one? The answer is, a nurse. Nurses are the presence for patients and families facing the end of life regardless of the setting of care, the time of life in which such a horrendous event can occur, or the cause. It is nurses who support parents as they watch their beloved infant die in a neonatal intensive care unit. And it is nurses who comfort the elderly spouse outside a cardiac care unit. It is nurses who stand by to support families in the emergency room as they learn that the best technology available was not enough to sustain the life of the one they love. It is the nurse on the night shift in the long-term-care setting who holds vigil with the dying elder who has no family available. And it is the nurse who supports the parents in an intensive care unit when their adolescent son has died in a tragic automobile accident after having left home only hours earlier as a healthy child.

If you were to stand by as someone you love dies, what would you want those nurses to know? With certainty, anyone reading this page would immediately come to the same conclusions: We would expect nursing competence in relief of pain, attention to other distressing symptoms, assurance that the most advanced care is provided, and clear communication about what is happening in the chaotic world of health care. You would want to know that your cultural beliefs are respected, that spiritual care is provided without hesitation; that nurses, along with their interdisciplinary colleagues, would deal with the ethical dilemmas common in each of these settings; and that your family was helped with the complex array of decisions faced in life-threatening disease. Along with all of those areas of competence, you would hope for compassion.

How will nurses know these things and have the skills to provide the kind of care you would want if it were you or someone you love? There is only one way, and that is if they are taught the essentials of palliative nursing care. Nursing as a profession has been dedicated to these ideals since its inception. In many ways, the principles of comfort, pain relief, support, and respect for human dignity probably had a stronger foundation earlier in our course of history, before the advent of high-tech, curative care. But now, as our society ages and our health care system is burdened financially beyond the brink, we are returning to our foundation and recognize that care focused on the comfort of patients and families is at the heart of nursing. Over the past three decades, the hospice movement in the United States has brought us back to the traditions that have evolved into palliative nursing care. Nursing has been fortunate to have as leaders Florence Wald, Jeanne Quint-Benoliel, and Dame Cecily Saunders (nurse, social worker, and physician, who died during the production of this text) who began the formation of what would become palliative nursing care. The editors of this text, Dr. Marianne Matzo and Dr. Deborah Sherman, have made their contributions over the past decade by leading the transformation of nursing education in palliative care. Building upon the work of previous nursing leaders, these editors and the authors of this text have worked diligently to create new models of nursing education so that each of the aspects of care cited above are in fact being integrated into nursing programs across all levels of nursing education. These authors and the pages of this text will create the blueprint for building the kind of care system we all wish for our loved ones.

The first edition of this book appeared in 2001. Since that time, this text has been recognized as an invaluable resource for educators throughout the country. It has been used as a resource in the End of Life Nursing Education Consortium (ELNEC), which is supported by the Robert Wood Johnson Foundation, and the National Cancer Institute, which has successfully trained thousands of nurse educators to join this cadre of nursing professionals in transforming care.

In the 4 years since the text was originally published, much has happened in the field of palliative care and within the nursing profession. The National Consensus Project for Quality Palliative Care has released consensus guidelines to define and establish the domains of palliative care (www.nationalconsensusproject.org). Nursing programs across the United States are evolving significant models of education by developing separate courses addressing end-of-life care, creating of palliative care tracks within graduate education, promoting nursing research in the field, and starting model programs to ensure that basic nursing education provides the essential elements of palliative care.

This second edition keeps pace with the evolving world around it by updating available knowledge in the field and also by sharing many trusted strategies for the most effective education. It too will become a handbook for nurse educators and will be one of the essential elements to guide practice.

What if it were you or someone you loved on the other side of the bedrails looking up to the nurse who will provide the care experience in the last days and hours of life?

Preface

Deborah Witt Sherman and Marianne LaPorte Matzo

Palliative care is a philosophy of care that provides a combination of disease-modifying and supportive, compassionate therapies intended to alleviate pain and other symptoms while addressing the emotional, social, cultural, and spiritual needs of patients and families who are experiencing life-threatening progressive illness [National Consensus Project, 2004, (www. nationalconsensusproject.org)]. The current trend is toward the integration of hospice and palliative care and the inclusion not only of individuals with cancer or AIDS, but also of patients with end-stage organ diseases, neurodegenerative diseases, and dementia. Palliative care is offered from the time of diagnosis with advanced disease until death, and continues for families during the bereavement period.

Research has indicated that the education of health professionals in end-of-life care has been limited or nonexistent in nursing and in medicine. Given that competent and compassionate end-of-life care is a responsibility of all health professions, each discipline must determine strategies to educate its students and professionals in palliative care. As Project on Death in America Faculty Scholars, the editors have assumed the responsibility in their roles as nurse practitioners, educators, and researchers to work collaboratively with nursing colleagues in developing, implementing, and evaluating nursing initiatives in palliative care within the United States, and developing the knowledge base of palliative care through related research studies.

Palliative Care Nursing: Quality Care to the End of Life, in both the first and second editions, has been written as a contribution to the initiatives of the nursing profession regarding palliative care. These initiatives began in 1998 when the American Association of Colleges of Nursing (AACN) brought together palliative care experts and health care ethicists to develop undergraduate competency statements and curricular guidelines for end-of-life nursing care. The document entitled "Peaceful Death" outlines 15 end-of-life competencies and serves as the organizing framework for this book. Along with the Toolkit for Nursing Excellence at the End of Life (TNEEL) and the End of Life Nursing Education Consortium (ELNEC), this text provides the essential information to achieve best practices in palliative care nursing.

This second edition of *Palliative Care Nursing* addresses the content, knowledge, attitudes, skills, undergraduate and graduate behavioral outcomes, and appropriate teaching and learning strategies to achieve the AACN End-of-Life nursing competencies. It is expected that the graduate-level nurse will have already mastered the undergraduate behavioral outcomes that reflect the integration of his or her knowledge, attitudes, and skills. As such, this text is applicable to students, to educators, and to practicing nurses. Nursing students enrolled in advanced practice palliative care master's programs, including nurse practitioner, post-master's certificate, and clinical nurse specialist programs will find this book an asset in providing care to patients with complex physical, emotional, social, and spiritual needs across health care settings. With knowledge of advanced pathophysiology, pharmacology, and physical assessment, advanced practice palliative care nurses can prescribe a vast array of pharmacological and nonpharmacological interventions that are discussed in this book. Throughout the illness and dying trajectory, graduate nurses also assume leadership roles as members of interdisciplinary palliative-care teams, develop standards of care, clinical guidelines, and health care policies, and they serve as consultants in the development of clinical practice, education, and research initiatives. Advanced practice palliative care nurses also educate and mentor undergraduate-prepared nursing colleagues and participate in or develop research proposals to support evidence-based practice. The information presented in this text therefore will serve as a foundation to advanced palliative care competencies.

This text is organized to emphasize the importance of a holistic perspective and an understanding of the patient and family as individuals with diverse spiritual and cultural needs and expectations. Part I addresses these more abstract needs of patients, families, and health care providers, with an emphasis on the value of complementary holistic modalities in promoting health, wholeness, and wellness even as death approaches. In Part II, societal aspects of end-of-life care are discussed, followed by the psychological aspects of dying in Part III. The four chapters in Part IV cover the physical aspects of death and dying, specifically pain and symptom management and the needs and experiences of individuals who are actively dying. The authors believe that decisions regarding physical interventions at the end of life must be addressed based on knowledge of the spiritual, social, and psychological beliefs, values, expectations, and wishes of the patient and family.

As the largest number of health care professional in the country, nurses have a tremendous potential to change the care of the dying and their families. Nursing professionals can capitalize on the individual's desire for autonomy and control of his or her life by reinforcing the importance and value of actively participating in the decisions at the end of life through advanced care planning. As nurses frame the discussion of dying and death within the context of hope and meaning and as an opportunity for choices and continued achievement of goals, uncertainty is replaced with certainty, hopelessness with faith, and despair with empowerment. The possibility exists that dying and death then will become one of the most meaningful and significant acts of life.

Palliative care nursing therefore offers an exquisite blend of holistic, humanistic caring coupled with aggressive management of pain and symptoms associated with advanced disease. Educational and research initiatives will transform the care offered to patients and families at the end of life and improve their quality of life until death. Through collaborative interdisciplinary care, patients and families can regain a sense of trust and security in knowing that a peaceful, respectful death is their right. Society may come to acknowledge dying and death without fear. The envisioned possibilities are of dying as an opportunity for continued growth and transcendence. Palliative care nursing promotes quality of life for patients and families who are experiencing life-threatening illness throughout the illness/dying trajectory, and thereby has changed the experience of dying in America.

Section I

Looking at the Whole Person in Palliative Care

April 12

Today, I admitted Candy Harris to our home-care agency. Candy is a 42-year-old woman who up until a month ago worked as a nurse with developmentally delayed children. She has been married to Ron for the last 20 years; a picture taken of them at their Senior Prom sits on a bookshelf. They have two children ages five and eight and live in a new neighborhood development. She seemed so sad when I arrived, but I would be, too, if I were in her situation. I find admissions like this so difficult; she is close to my age and we are so similar in other ways.

She tells me the history of her disease in a very matter-of-fact way. For the nine months prior to her diagnosis, Candy had noticed increased flatus that had not gotten better, despite alterations in her diet. For the two months prior she said that she had little appetite, but still had gained 5 pounds. She felt bloated all of the time and the waistbands of her clothes were tight. Her mother started menopause in her early 40's and died at age 56 of breast/ovarian cancer. Candy thought that her symptoms were related to the early start of menopause and so decided to visit her nurse practitioner for a physical exam and pap smear.

Given Candy's symptoms and her positive family history of cancer, the nurse practitioner ordered an abdominal CT scan in addition to a complete physical work-up. An ovarian mass was detected and Candy was scheduled for a laparotomy. Stage III ovarian cancer was diagnosed. The surgeon was able to use cytoreduction to decrease the tumor volume to <2 cm in diameter and the oncologist suggested platinum-based combination chemotherapy. She was in shock that all of this was happeneing to her so fast. The children were really too young to completely understand what was going on and her husband insisted that they were going to "fight this."

Candy had just finished her third cycle of chemotherapy. She is very weak and in need of home health care support. Candy was sitting in a chair in the living room when I arrived. Her hair had all fallen out and her eyes were red, as though she had been crying, and she was holding a rosary in her hand. One section of the wall was covered with get-well cards; she referred to this area as her "prayer wall." As I was assessing her, she burst into tears and told me that she thinks "God is punishing her for something" and that this is why she has cancer. This was not the first time that I have heard this from a patient. Believing in the importance of atoning for her sins, Candy has been attending mass whenever she has the strength, praying the rosary regularly, and asking the church congregation to pray for her. She has gone to confession and received the "Sacrament of the Sick." She also admitted that she wanted to "cover all of her bases" and that she has turned to holistic interventions in addition to her chemotherapy so that her body, mind, and soul will also heal. After her initial diagnosis she researched complimentary interventions for cancer and started on a macrobiotic diet with additional B12 and D vitamins.

Candy receives Reiki twice a week and is seeing a therapist weekly. She said that she and her husband use mental imagery and relaxation techniques to imagine her body defenses as a powerful source to annihilate the cancer cells. Candy said that she has so much to live for, that she has a lot of good friends, a loving husband, and great kids. She really doesn't know what she has "done wrong" but she asks for God's forgiveness and hopes to get on with her life.

As a nurse, I marvel at her will to live and her determination to beat this disease. She seems to draw her strenght from her religion and her relationships. Her strength is an inspiration to all who care for her.

1

Spirituality and Culture as Domains of Quality Palliative Care

Deborah Witt Sherman

AACN Competency

#4: Recognize one's own attitudes, feelings, values, and expectations about death and the individual, cultural, and spiritual diversity existing in these beliefs and customs.

> *Death is not the ultimate tragedy of life. The ultimate tragedy is depersonalization—dying in an alien and sterile environment, separated from the spiritual nourishment that comes from being able to reach out to a loving hand, separated from a desire to experience the things that make life worth living, separated from hope.*
>
> —Norman Cousins, 1979

Spirituality and culture are among the most important factors that structure human experience, values, behaviors, and illness patterns. Spirituality plays a vital role in times of crisis and illness as it provides a sense of connection to self, others, nature, and God and is a means to cope with loss, grief, and death (Weaver, Flannelly, & Flannelly, 2001). As a system of shared symbols and beliefs, culture supports a person's sense of security, integrity, and belonging and provides a prescription for how to conduct life and approach death (End of Life Nursing Education Consortium [ELNEC], 2001). Life-threatening illness is a crisis on many levels—physical, psychological, familial, social, and spiritual

(Doka & Morgan, 1993). Given the uniqueness and individuality of each person, even people of the same religion or culture may have different backgrounds, experiences, needs, concerns, and interpretation of illness. In addition to the individuality of the person, the nature of the life-threatening illness may be different and the person may be at different points in adapting to the reality of the disease. Spiritual and cultural concerns may permeate the illness experience or may arise at any point across the illness/dying trajectory. For patients and families who are experiencing life-threatening illness, the concerns may be of suffering that may take multiple forms relative to the mind-body-spirit.

It is now recognized that the uncertain and long-term nature of many life-threatening illnesses pose the potential for pain, alterations in body image, and confrontation with death, which may lead to spiritual distress. The renewed focus on incorporating spiritual care into nursing practice is congruent with nursing's commitment to holistic practice and the renewed valuing of human experiences that defy scientific description and explanation (O'Neill & Kenny, 1998). Within the past few years, research has shown that religious beliefs and spiritual practices affect the meaning of illness, physical and emotional well-being, coping with illness, and health care decisions, particularly for individuals facing life-threatening illness (Koenig, 1999).

Every culture has a worldview or construct of reality that defines the individual within that reality. Patients' cultural backgrounds are therefore fundamental in defining and creating their reality and determining their purpose in life (Ersek, Kagawa-Singer, Barnes, Blackhall, & Koenig, 1998). A transformation of identity begins when an individual is diagnosed with a terminal illness. Cultural rituals provide the sacred elements that support patients and families during times of illness and transition. Specific rituals assist individuals and families in coping with death, which is the final transition in life. The rituals of death change the identity of the patient from the living to the dead, and also the identity of the family member, for example, from spouse to widow or widower (Kagawa-Singer, 1998).

Spiritual and cultural competence are central tenets of palliative care. As a philosophy of care, palliative care combines active and compassionate therapies to support and comfort individuals and families who are living with life-threatening illness. Palliative care strives to meet the physical, psychological, social, and spiritual expectations and needs, while remaining sensitive to personal, cultural, and religious beliefs and practices (Ferris & Cummings, 1995). Undergraduate-prepared nurses and advanced practice nurses must become spiritually and culturally competent in the care they offer across the illness/dying trajectory. Such care is critical to enhancing the quality of life and quality of dying and to supporting the intrinsic dignity of patients and their families.

THE SPIRITUAL NATURE OF THE PERSON

Spirituality is often the lens through which people interpret their world, as they search to understand themselves, their needs, and their relationships to self, others, nature, and God. The word spirituality derives from the Latin *spiritus,* which refers to breath, air, and wind. "Spirit" connotes "whatever is at the center of all aspects of one's life or that which gives life to a person" (Dombeck, 1995, p. 38). Spirituality has also been described as our inner being (Carson, 1989), or as the integrating life force, which allows human beings to transcend their physical nature (Conrad, 1985). Moberg (1984) conceptualized spiritual well-being as encompassing both vertical and horizontal dimensions that involve transcendence. The vertical dimension refers to our sense of well-being in relation to God, while the horizontal dimension refers to a sense of purpose in life and life satisfaction.

Recognition of the spiritual nature of human beings was reflected in the early writings of Florence Nightingale, who viewed spirituality as a dimension of human nature and the highest level of human consciousness. Nightingale espoused that human beings must use God-given powers to discover and apply the universal laws to relieve pain and suffering on physical, emotional, social, and spiritual levels (Macrae, 1999). She felt that religion was a means of expressing and developing spirituality, but that it is possible to develop spirituality outside of organized religion (Macrae, 1999). Believing that God's plan is to raise mankind from imperfection to perfection, which cannot be completed in one lifetime, Nightingale viewed death as a new mode of existence that allows for continued development (Macrae, 1999).

The concept of spirituality includes references to the spirit, the soul, spiritual perspectives, spiritual needs, and spiritual well-being and is viewed as more basic than and different from religion (Burkhardt, 1989). Spirituality is a broader concept than religion, although religion is one form of expression of spirituality as is prayer or meditation (Puchalski,

1998a). The quest for meaning in life and transcendence has been typically conducted within the framework of organized religion. In recent years, the meaning of spirituality has changed as individuals searched for personal and transpersonal meaning outside the confines of organized religion (Wink, 1999). Moore (1992) identifies the spiritual quest as a process of "resacralization" of the self and the world surrounding us. The goal is to embark on a personal journey in discovering the transcendent in everyday life and in all human relationships. According to Moore, the outcome of the spiritual quest is not to find some higher, inner-order truth, but rather is the ability to inject magic, mystery, and sacredness into every moment of one's life and in everything one does.

Ryan (1997), a chaplain, proposes that every human being has five fundamental spiritual needs: (1) the need to find meaning in life, particularly at times of illness; (2) the need for a relationship with a transcendent other, through which we find meaning and purpose in life; (3) the need to change whatever causes us to suffer or be unhappy; (4) the need for hope no matter how difficult life can be; and (5) the need for others who will care for us and are willing to co-journey with us.

Individuals with life-threatening illness may ask, "Why did this happen to me?" "Why is God allowing me to suffer?" "What will happen after I die?" "Will I be remembered or missed?" or "Will I be able to finish my life's work?" (Puchalski, 2002). True healing requires an answer to these questions because healing can be experienced as acceptance of illness and peace with one's life (Puchalski, 2001). Furthermore, individuals may question the purpose of their lives as they suffer and seek to transcend their suffering. Arnold (1989) believes that spirituality embodies the ultimate virtues of life in the form of hope, courage, faith, love, acceptance, and a meaningful encounter with death. Understand-

ing the nourishment of the spirit by either prayer, religious commitment, personal faith, or relationships with others, health professionals can be a source of support or solace in achieving spiritual well-being and healing. The word "heal" comes from the Old English word *haelen*, which means not only to restore by way of cure, but also "to make whole or sound" (Urdang, 1972, p. 609). To heal can therefore mean to "restore a person to spiritual wholeness."

Fricchione (1999) believes that the crisis of physical illness leads to adaptive tasks and the testing of coping skills that will determine the outcome of the crisis. As a physician, he has learned from his patients that the worst part of illness is often the fear of separation and loss of attachment. Illness creates an intermediate area between separation and attachment, a point where spirituality in medicine and nursing may be examined and nurtured (Fricchione, 1999). Indeed, research indicates that 78% of Americans receive comfort and support from religious beliefs and perceive greater trust in health professionals who ask them about their spiritual or religious needs (Koenig, 2002).

For individuals who are dying, the task work often involves spiritual energy and hope. At this time, the task may be to find a source of spiritual energy or reaffirm one's spiritual focus (Corr, Nabe, & Corr, 1997). Spiritual energy may come from a personal God or from an individual value system. Doka (1993) identified three principal spiritual tasks for those who are dying: to find meaning in life; to die in a way that is consistent with one's self-identity; and to find hope that extends beyond the grave. This may go beyond the hope of cure to the hope of symbolic immortality, as one lives on genetically through one's children or is remembered through one's artwork, music, writing, or contributions to the community.

In caring for patients with life-threatening illness or those who are actively dying, nurses need to recognize that spiritual concern or distress can affect physical well-being. An individual's beliefs and values can significantly affect how they cope with illness and its treatment. In assessing patients' spiritual well-being, the questions explored may include the following:

- Are they suffering in physical, emotional, social, or spiritual ways?
- Do they see purpose in life as they suffer?
- Are they able to transcend their suffering and see something or someone beyond that?
- Are they at peace, hopeful, or do they despair?
- Do personal beliefs help them to cope with anxiety about death, their pain, and achieving peace? (Puchalski, 1998a)

People who are dying need to make peace not only with death, but also with life. Rather than encouraging people to fight death to the end, health professionals can provide an opportunity for them to bring closure to their lives; to complete unfinished goals; to forgive those they had conflicts with and be forgiven; to make peace with themselves and with God; to say goodbye, and to die with dignity. Therefore, "remembering, assessing, searching for meaning, forgiving, reconciling, loving, and hoping are all part of the spiritual journey especially active during the time of dying" (Puchalski, 1998a, p. 38). Spiritual care changes chaos to order, and seeks to discern what if any blessings might be revealed in spite of and even through tragedy (Purdy, 2002). As people are dying, they want to be listened to, to have someone share their fears, to be forgiven by God or by others, and they want to believe they will live on in the hearts of others or through their good works (Puchalski, 2002). According to McGregor

(1999), the healing work of the soul in illness, dying, and bereavement happens when illness becomes an opportunity for connection, personal growth, and the finding of meaning; and when dying becomes an opportunity for growth, resolution, and transcendence for oneself and others.

SUFFERING AS A HUMAN CONDITION

Suffering is a part of life and the human condition, with suffering either personally experienced in a physical, emotional, social, or spiritual way, or experienced as witnesses to another's suffering. Cassell (1982) defines suffering as "the state of severe distress associated with events that threaten the intactness of a person" (p. 639). Suffering can be defined as the endurance of, or submission to, affliction, pain, or loss. Suffering is usually psychological, as a result of distressing circumstances that arise in the process of living, but can also be the effects of physical pain. Cassell (1982) believes that many aspects of a person can be sources of, or be affected by, suffering, such as personality, character, the past, relationships, life experiences, roles, one's rights and responsibilities, family, and cultural background.

According to Kahn and Steeves (1996), suffering is a private lived experience of a whole person, unique to each individual. As such, suffering cannot be assumed present or absent in any given clinical condition or situation because suffering is dependent on the meaning of the event or loss. The experience of suffering is also both intrapersonal and interpersonal because it involves the person's own coping with suffering and the caring of others (Kahn & Steeves, 1996). Although we may not find answers about why we suffer, as a part of the human family, we build relationships, communities, and society to reach out to one another to relieve suffering and sustain us in our struggle (McGann, 1997).

Suffering varies with the type of disease, type of personality, and the relationship between these factors. "The loss of physical integrity and the impending destruction of the unity of one's person can cause profound suffering" (DeBellis et al., 1986, p. 6). Within the context of illness, suffering can occur because of unfavorable prognoses, loss of function, disability, the complexity of treatment, failure to achieve relief of symptoms, the expense of treatment, and the effects of disease on all social relationships and economic security (DeBellis et al., 1986).

Although suffering and pain often are referred to interchangeably, they are not identical. In some cases, they are mutually present; at times, one exists without the other. The transition from pain to suffering can occur when pain is unrelieved and out of control or when the source of pain is unknown. The persistence of pain and uncertainty therefore can increase suffering exponentially. Yet, suffering can continue even when pain is controlled. At the end of life, suffering may be exacerbated because of protracted or chronic illness, multiple simultaneous diseases and comorbid conditions, recurrent disease, and awareness of mortality. Because suffering has to do with a personal understanding of the physical, emotional, and spiritual self and their interrelationships, we learn about suffering only by the ways in which an individual expresses an awareness of the threats to their personal wholeness (Smith, 1996).

Coyle (1995) gives examples of suffering, such as when patients experience despair, loneliness, and vulnerability; feel trapped by fear and bewilderment; experience loss and worry about treatment decisions; worry about being a burden; have financial concerns; experience abandonment; or fear dying yet are weary of life, and experience pain or the loss of hope. Families suffer as they assume the responsibilities of caregiving; watch the patient's deterioration; become exhausted; neglect their own needs; experience uncertainty about goals of care and anxiety about the place of care. The suffering of family members also occurs because of fear of the dying process and the experience of the loss of life as it was, the person they knew, and of hope, as well as guilt in wanting death to come soon.

Reciprocal Suffering of Patients and Family

Within the context of life-threatening illness, suffering, in the form of physical, emotional, social, and spiritual distress, often becomes an experience not only of the patient, but also of the family caregivers, as the suffering of one amplifies the distress of the other (Foley, 1995). Family members, like patients themselves, are in transition from living with the disease to anticipating the death of their loved one from the disease (Davies, Reimer, & Marten, 1994). They fear that death will occur in their absence, and may therefore refuse to leave the patient's side for even a moment. There is also a strong compulsion to attend to the patient's every need with disregard for their own needs (Klein, 1998). As the patient's illness progresses, the needs of the family also intensify and change, with both patients and family caregivers potentially experiencing a significant compromise in the quality of their lives (Sherman, 1998).

Although family members may express the rewards of caring for terminally ill relatives, such care can have major psychosocial and physical effects, including heightened symptoms of depression, anxiety, psychosomatic symptoms, restrictions of roles and activities, strain in relationships, and poor physical health (Higginson, 1998). As witnesses to the patient's pain and suffering, family caregivers may also experience a sense of powerlessness, and are often frightened and confused by the dramatic physical and emotional changes they perceive in their loved one as the disease progresses (Loscalzo & Zabora, 1998).

There are also many conflicting emotions and adjustment tasks, including conflict among feelings of loss, sadness, guilt, difficulty in knowing how to talk with the person who is dying, and worry about dying and death (Beeney, Butow, & Dunn, 1997). Furthermore, the family caregiver must adapt to changes in family roles and responsibilities, while attempting to meet the increased emotional needs of other family members and performing standard family functions (Doyle, 1994). Given that 25% of caregivers lose their job due to caregiver responsibilities and nearly one third of families lose their major source of income or their savings, families also experience significant financial burdens (Lederberg, 1998). This may lead to feelings of anger, jealousy, and an increase in the family caregiver's own needs because of heightened psychological distress. In addition, there is often a loss of social mobility, as well as social abandonment by friends, which negatively impact on the quality of life of family caregivers (Lederberg, 1998).

From a spiritual perspective, family members may question the meaning of the illness and suffering. They often spend considerable time reviewing painful aspects of the past with feelings of regret for disagreements, conflicts, or failures and a wish that relationships with the patient and with each other were somehow different. With each family member's unique experience of the stress, families may find it difficult to come together to effectively cope with the imposed life changes (Sherman, 1998). In their search for meaning, patients and families affirm spiritual values, change life priorities, and examine how

the experience of illness has contributed to their personal growth. Like their dying loved one, they live day to day to make the most of the present as they prepare for death on practical, cognitive, emotional, and spiritual levels (Davies et al., 1994). The hope is that through palliative nursing care, both patients and family members can transcend their reciprocal suffering and experience growth as they face the challenges of life-threatening or terminal illness (Sherman, 1998).

The Care of Those Who Are Suffering

Cassell (1982) believes that the ways to relieve suffering are first, through the assignment of meaning to the injurious condition or event; and second, through transcendence, which is the most powerful way of restoring an individual's personhood to wholeness. Watson (1986) proposes four generic meanings of suffering, which include *correction* in which an individual is being corrected of their wrongdoing; *affirmation* in which a person is affirmed of their "rightdoing" and the ability to be a role model for others; *naturalism* in which the individual is experiencing general human destiny; and *altruism* in which an individual's suffering will have benefit to others. In caring for those who are suffering, health professionals may help individuals come to a healthy, maintainable higher meaning to their suffering. From a theological perspective, Smith (1996) discusses the religious response to suffering and the possibility of transcendence of suffering through intellectual, ethical, and experiential dimensions of religion. The intellectual dimension involves the realization of some transcendent meaning, which connects the suffering person with some greater reality and delivers the individual from the threat of meaninglessness that is raised by illness and pain. The ethical dimension of religious life provides a perspective regarding how to interpret and respond to suffering. Suffering may be seen as a test of one's virtue or fidelity to God, a test of the worth of religious commitment, or as an opportunity of personal transformation. Within the experiential dimension of religion, the life of oneself and others and of the relationship of these lives to each other and to God are contemplated. The religious experience of suffering may therefore enable an individual to provide redemptive relationships with others, including God, and experience transcendence.

In caring for the suffering, Spross (1996) believes that the role of the nurse is one of coaching. "Coaching is an interpersonal intervention that requires the therapeutic use of the self, involving one's mind, past experience, words, heart, and hand—to comfort those who suffer" (Spross, 1996, p. 201). In coaching, the nurse

- establishes a trusting partnership;
- assesses those who are at risk for suffering or who are vulnerable;
- reassures patients that although their suffering may not disappear, they will not be abandoned;
- identifies factors that may be eliminated or modified to alleviate suffering; and
- intervenes to facilitate expression of feelings, find meaning in suffering, and help patients and families redefine the quality of life.

Spross (1996) states that the ability to alleviate suffering or find meaning in the experiences of suffering depends on the intrapersonal and interpersonal qualities of the nurse. The nurse must be self-accepting, secure in his or her own self-concept, and feel confident in strengthening others. As coach, the nurse values others and communicates that the individual's feelings, goals, and opinions are respected, while conveying that the person is trustworthy, responsible, capable of self-direction, and able to identify relevant goals and find meaning in life.

Watson (1986) believes that nurses and other health professionals can relieve suffering in six ways: First, by being a companion to sufferers by identifying the pain of their losses, and exploring the circumstance and extent of the loss. Second, by listening for statements of meaning from sufferers and allowing the person's natural instincts and energy to surface the issue of higher meaning. Third, by valuing any self-disclosure on meaning that a sufferer offers, by analyzing the meaning of the statements and learning what the statement reveals about the sufferer's view of him- or herself. Fourth, by encouraging the sufferer's interpretation of their own experience. Fifth, by validating the sufferer's interpretation of their own experience while clarifying the meaning, seeking further definition of the meaning, and offering alternatives for reframing the meaning. Last, the nurse can identify supportive resources and hope for the sufferer to extend his or her identity and meaning in the future.

In alleviating the suffering of others, Bird (1986) offers seven principles to be considered within the context of nursing practice:

1. Remember that institutions don't dehumanize patients; staff members do.
2. Assume responsibility for morale whenever you are in the chain of command.
3. Be a whole person yourself, with a healthy sense of humor and attitude.
4. Do not add clinical ineptitude to the further suffering of patients.
5. Be empathetic rather than sympathetic to patient's needs; otherwise human suffering can emotionally devastate one.
6. Offer holistic care and well-chosen words to allay suffering.
7. Determine to touch the life of at least one patient daily with some depth.

Halifax (1999) believes that health care providers, patients, and families can go to the root of their own suffering and transform the suffering into inherent wisdom. As a Buddhist, she reminds health professionals to come to the caregiving relationship with loving kindness, compassion by being in touch with one's own and others' suffering, joy in the well-being of others, and equanimity.

SPIRITUAL AND RELIGIOUS PERSPECTIVES ON DEATH

Losses in life often challenge our faith and philosophical systems. Those who experience loss and grief may differ regarding religious and spiritual perspectives from which they seek answers, search for meaning, and to which they turn for ritual, comfort, and support (Doka & Davidson, 1998). Understanding the ways that spirituality or religiosity facilitates or complicates the adjustment to loss and grief is a critical task to those involved in palliative care.

Death from a Jewish Perspective

Judaism began when the descendants of Abraham's grandson Israel were enslaved in Egypt. Moses led them to Palestine. During this time, Jewish law, known as the Torah, was divinely revealed to Moses. The Sabbath is celebrated from sunset on Friday to sunset on Saturday evening. The Sabbath is the day of rest. The degree to which a Jew observes the Sabbath and other rituals depends on whether he or she is Orthodox, Conservative, or Reformed. (Sherman, 2004a). The focus of those of the Jewish faith is on life and its preservation and in fostering and establishing religion in the life of people on earth, rather than focusing on the world beyond. The Jewish faith offers consolation in death by affirmation of life. Sickness and death are viewed as neither punishment nor reward. Death is not considered evil but rather inevitable and natural, as it comes from God and should not be feared. Jewish teachings are that the soul exists before the body comes into existence and continues to live on after the body is dead. Although the Orthodox believe in resurrection, this belief may be figurative rather than literal (Grollman, 1993).

Jewish death practices help the bereaved to realize that the loved one is dead and to gradually fill the void in a constructive way. The memory of the deceased must be perpetuated. Although Jews are usually buried, cremations are also done. A religious rite is the rending of mourners' clothes, signified by the cutting of a black ribbon that is pinned to the mourners' clothing in the funeral chapel or cemetery. This signifies the loss of a loved one. The Jewish funeral is a rite of separation, in which the casket actualizes the experience. The rabbi recites prayers expressive of the spirit of Judaism and the memory of the deceased. Shiva refers to the 7 days of intensive mourning beginning right after the funeral. The bereaved remain at home and condolence calls are made to pay respects to the family. The shiva candle burns for 7 days and the family prepares the meal of consolation, known as seudat havra'ah. Following shiva comes the 30 days of sloshim. During this time normal activities are resumed but entertainment is avoided. If a parent dies, the mourning continues for an entire year. The mourner's prayer is called the Kaddish, which is recited during the weekly Sabbath as a pledge to dedicate one's life to God, acknowledge the reality of death, and affirm life. The anniversary of the death is called yahrzeit. The Kaddish prayer is recited and yahrzeit candles are again kindled (Grollman, 1993).

Death from the Roman Catholic Perspective

In Catholicism, it is believed that Jesus experienced suffering, grief, and death. Jesus' death and the death of all others are viewed as a part of God's divine providence. As sinners, human beings experience the tragedy of death, yet are beneficiaries of its forgiveness and liberation. In Catholicism, resurrection is integral to death. Catholics believe that Christ died and rose from the dead, and that faith will allow them to see death as an entry into life with God. Confession and Communion are important rituals conducted by priests. The sacrament of the anointing of the sick provides bodily and spiritual renewal and has replaced the term "the last rites," which was viewed as a harbinger of death.

Since the second Vatican Council, the Catholic contemporary view places emphasis on risen life. There is a move from a preoccupation with sin and death toward an orientation of blessing for a Christian life. Christians follow Jesus into the mystery of death in order to find a life like his own (Miller, 1993). The funeral becomes one of thanksgiving and consolation; the funeral mass is offered on behalf of the deceased, aiding them to the other side of death and giving the bereaved the consolation of hope. It is believed that Christ accompanies the dying person to heaven and that dying is an act of faith in God (Miller, 1993).

Death from the Protestant Perspective

In Protestantism, spirituality is viewed as a dimension of humanness, a process of interaction, and an awareness of relationship. Spirituality cannot be lived in the abstract but rather is lived through one's religion, which is regarded as a cultural institution (Klass, 1993). God is viewed as a single being, who spoke to his people through the Bible; God protects but also judges. Each Protestant has a direct and personal relationship with God, unmediated by priest or sacrament. The church is viewed as a voluntary association of believers. The Protestant community is the local congregation or particular denomina-

tion supporting interpersonal relationships, yet is often split along racial, ethnic, and social class lines (Klass, 1993). Anointing the sick is accepted by some groups. Although there are no last rites, prayers are given to offer support.

Death is a challenge because it raises the problem of evil and the problem of the meaningfulness of suffering. Suffering and overcoming evil are the core of Protestant teaching. For Protestants, the focus is salvation, which depends on the moral quality of life on earth. Heaven is known in hope, but not as a guarantee. The belief in an afterlife is through experiences of memory and sense of presence and shared community. Although Jesus is a model for physical, emotional, social, and spiritual suffering, the individual faces the cosmos alone. The issue is not how the individual can participate in Jesus' suffering, but rather the individual's accepting the gift of God's grace in Jesus' death (Klass, 1993).

Death from the Islamic Perspective

Islam means submission. *Muslim* means one who submits. A Muslim is one who submits to Allah, the Arabic word for God. Muslims, Jews, and Christians worship the same God. The founder of Islam is Mohammad, who received a vision while meditating, which later became the Koran. The five pillars of Islam are confession of faith daily in front of witnesses, prayer five times a day, fasting during the month of Ramadan, almsgiving, and a pilgrimage to Mecca. Fasting during Ramadan is not required of the sick. Second-degree male relatives (e.g., cousins or uncles) should be contacted when a person is sick. They determine if a person or family should be told the diagnosis or prognosis. Patients may choose to face Mecca (East) and the head should be elevated above the body. Discussions about death are not usually welcomed. Grief may be expressed by slapping or hitting the body. Same-sex Muslims should handle the body after death; otherwise the individual should wear gloves so as not to touch the body.

Death from Eastern Perspectives

Hinduism originated in India, with belief in the cycles of being born and dying in an infinite series of lives or successive creations. Hinduism teaches the belief in karma, which is that every act of a human being, even an internal act, such as desire, has an effect on who that person becomes. One becomes virtuous by good actions and bad by bad actions (Ryan, 1993). A Supreme Being exists in the individual's soul and is the ultimate all.

Originating in India, Buddhism teaches the belief in karma and rebirth. Buddhists believe that life changes and death occurs. Buddha taught that a way to overcome ignorance and attain truth is through the path to enlightenment or changed state of awareness called Nirvana. Buddhists believe that the way to Nirvana is through meditation, while others believe it can be attained through faith.

Yet another Eastern tradition is that of Confucianism, which has its origins in China and stresses the importance of improving human relationships. The proper relationship between the living and dead is one of continuous remembrance and affection, through which one attains social immortality. The value of rituals is that they relate the living with the dead. Memories of parents and ancestors are kept through regular remembrance rituals, which also provide a vehicle for the expression of the human emotions of grief and affection.

Taoism has its origins in China. In Taoism, the focus is on nature and remedying society's disorder and lack of harmony. One looks toward nature to discover the principles of life. Life is viewed as the companion of death, and death is viewed as the beginning of life and part of the living-dying process. Taoism offers a way of transcending the limits of the world, as there are ceaseless transformations where the person is not lost. The yin and yang are the basic principles for all natural change. The yang is the light half, which is characterized as masculine, active, hot, bright, dry, and hard. The yin is the dark half, which is characterized as feminine, passive, cold, dark, wet, and soft. They are viewed as complementary forces that transform into the other. There is no light without dark, evil without good, or life without death (Ryan, 1993).

Many Asian patients—Chinese, Japanese, Koreans—have an Eastern perspective in which formal behaviors are valued. It is believed that to rebel against death reveals a fundamental lack of understanding about life. Therefore, sadness and grief are kept private. Such behavior sets a good example and contributes to one's good reputation (Ryan, 1993). Patients may seek comfort in images, such as Buddha, Krishna or the Divine Mother, or in repeating holy mantras. Those from an Eastern perspective believe that a person's final dying thoughts may determine one's rebirth.

Spiritual Issues in Death and Dying for Those Who Have No Conventional Religious Beliefs

Religion traditionally has provided a context for understanding and interpreting death. However, individuals who are not religious can still find comfort and meaning through spirituality and by stepping back from the material world (Orion, 1993). Individuals with no conventional religious beliefs often interpret life based on a sense of being a part of a larger whole and from a scientific worldview. There is belief that an individual's life has a beginning and an ending, but the life process is indefinite. Whether the process is defined in terms of social or biological continuity, the brevity of life does not suggest insignificance. A particular life is short and seemingly inconsequential but assumes value and importance as a significant element in the entire ongoing process. Even brief life is viewed as a contribution to the life process.

Those without conventional religious beliefs often consider the present as the real world and take full responsibility for their decisions. There is the belief that immortality occurs by biological immortality such as living on in the genetic pool of one's descendants, or living on in the memories of others or one's contributions to the world (Orion, 1993). The focus is on actualizing human potential. From the naturalistic perspective, death is not avoided or denied. Death is viewed as real, final, and inevitable and a mark of humans' solidarity with nature and the evolutionary process. Naturalism leads an effort to place the death of an individual in a framework of the process of living and dying, emergence, and extinction. In this framework, death is

- a working out of the natural law by which all living things die;
- the absorption of the differentiated person in the natural process;
- a contribution to the evolutionary process;
- cessation of life's potential for negative and positive contributions; and
- reabsorption into new ways in nature. (Orion, 1993)

Fear of death can be overcome by remembering that everything dies, but existence goes on. When death is seen as part of the natural order or part of the universal condition, it can be tolerated more easily. Life and death are continuous parts of the whole (Orion, 1993).

RESEARCH REGARDING SPIRITUALITY

Over the last 10 years, there has been increasing interest in the relationship between spirituality, religion, and health care. A Gallup

Poll Survey (1990) showed that religion, an expression of spirituality, plays a central role in the life of Americans. Ninety-five percent of those Americans polled espoused a belief in God, with 57% praying daily, and 42% attending a weekly worship service. In 1997, a Gallup Poll indicated that people overwhelmingly want their spiritual needs addressed at the end of life and felt that health professionals, physicians, and nurses should speak with patients about their spiritual concerns. A national survey of 1,200 adults (Nathan Cummings Foundation, 1999) explored the relationships between the dying process and spiritual needs. Respondents expressed a need for companionship and spiritual support, particularly in the form of human contact, and to have the opportunity to pray alone or have someone pray for or with them. Eighty-one percent of the respondents stated the importance of receiving comfort, particularly from family and close friends, with only 36% finding comfort in the support of clergy or from doctors or nurses. Those who sought support from clergy were more often female, older than 65 years, having less than a college education, and incomes under $40,000.

The relationship between the frequency and characteristics of religious coping and depression was examined by Koenig et al. (1992). Based on a sample of 850 hospitalized elderly men, the results indicated that 20% reported the use of religion for coping, and 56% gave a rating of 7.5 or higher on a scale of 0–10 of the importance of religion as a method of coping. Religious coping was inversely but weakly related to depression scores ($r = 16, p < .001$).

The relationship between death anxiety, age, and intrinsic religiosity was examined by Thorson and Powell (1992), based on a sample of 345 individuals from diverse settings. The results indicated that intrinsic religiosity, or one's sense of personal connection, was positively related with age ($r = 27, p < .001$), while death anxiety was negatively correlated with age ($r = -27$, $p < .001$). There was no difference in religiosity by gender; however, females were slightly more death anxious than males ($r = 10$, $p < .05$).

Based on a sample of 600 severely ill hospitalized patients, age 55 and over, Koenig (1998) found that spiritual coping via connection with God and receiving religious support was associated with less depression, greater compliance with care, and better quality of life. Roberts (1997) reported that for women coping with gynecologic cancer, religion had a serious place in their lives (76%), helped them sustain their hopes (91%), and supported their sense of worth (41%). According to Kaldjian (1998), patients who are HIV-positive expressed less fear of death when they read the Bible frequently, attended church regularly, and saw God as playing a central role in their life.

Studies also indicate that those who are religious or spiritual have lower blood pressure, fewer cardiac events, better result following heart surgery, and longer survival in general (Koenig, 2002). Furthermore, spirituality counteracts stress-related physiologic states that impair healing and facilitates coping with chronic pain, disability, and serious illness by enhancing a sense of control that interrupts the cycle of anxiety and depression (Koenig, 2002). Those who participate in religious services express less loneliness and isolation as they receive support from others and believe that God is with them.

Poloma and Pendleton (1989) studied the effects of various types of prayer on quality of life by conducting a random telephone survey of 560 individuals. Using multiple regression analysis, prayer experience was positively related to quality of life, existential well-being, happiness, and religious satisfaction. Meditative prayer was positively associated with existential well-being and religious satisfaction.

Colloquial prayer of thanking God was positively associated with happiness, with both below the 0.5 level of statistical significance.

Based on a qualitative study, it was also reported that patients with cancer use prayer to cope with their illness. Participants described prayer as an active cognitive process involving talking to God, or beseeching God, while others described a passive process involving listening to God and accepting that "God's will be done" (Taylor & Outlaw, 2002).

In a phenomenological study of spirituality and life-threatening illness, Albaugh (2003) interviewed 7 participants who had either cancer or heart or lung disease for at least 1 month. Participants described a sense of comfort from aspects of spiritual life, such as belief in support from God, feelings of not being alone, and the power of prayer. The participants expressed a trust in God, believing that God would provide the means to get through the experience either by restoring their health or through death. The strength of their spiritual beliefs, feelings of being blessed despite or through the illness, and a deeper meaning to life after facing life-threatening illness were described. The study supports the need to acknowledge patients' spirituality and assist them in meeting their spiritual needs.

Through a qualitative study involving 28 African American and European American adult patients with cancer and their caregivers, Taylor (2003a) examined participants' expectations of nurses in meeting their spiritual needs. Participants identified six approaches of nurses in addressing spiritual needs: (1) showing kindness and respect; (2) talking and listening; (3) prayer, such as offering verbal prayer or saying, "You are in my thoughts and prayers"; (4) connecting with authenticity and genuineness; (5) quality temporal nursing care, such as coming back to check on the patient; and (6) mobilizing religious or spiritual resources. The authors concluded that nurses need to consider their role in spiritual care and educate the public about their role as holistic health care providers.

The effects of spirituality on well-being of people with lung cancer were studied by Meraviglia (2004). Based on a sample of 60 adults who were predominately Caucasian and female, it was found that higher meaning-in-life scores were associated with higher psychological well-being and lower symptom distress. Prayer was positively related to psychological well-being, explaining 10% of its variance. Regression analysis indicated that meaning in life mediated the relationship between functional status and physical responses to lung cancer and explained 9% of the variance in symptom distress. The author concluded that this study supports the importance of providing spiritual care for patients with cancer.

QUALITY NURSING CARE: ADDRESSING THE SPIRITUAL NEEDS OF PATIENTS AND THEIR FAMILIES

Spiritual Caregiving

Munley (1983) believes that spiritual caregiving is the human capacity to enter the world of others and respond with feeling, touching them at a level that is deeper than doctrinal differences. Spiritual care involves the nurse's presence, compassion, hopefulness, and recognition that although it may no longer be productive, life remains fruitful and an opportunity to connect with others in a very meaningful way. Being present to terminally ill patients and their families means listening in the broadest sense of the word and conveying unconditional acceptance and compassion. According to Puchalski (1998a), individuals with life-threatening illness often ask

questions such as: What gives meaning in my life? Why is this happening to me? How will I survive this loss? What will happen to me when life ends?

Although nurses may not be able to cure the disease and restore physical integrity, they can promote hope and promote patients' healing through compassionate care. As an ongoing process, healing continues within the context of a person's life pattern of religious beliefs and practices and provides the opportunity for renewal and rebirth in relationship to oneself and with a higher being. Patients may also enrich nurses' lives as they allow nurses to enter theirs and share in their journey at extremely intimate and vulnerable times.

Integrating religion and spirituality into nursing care is therefore important because (a) nursing is concerned with the whole person, body-mind-spirit; (b) many though not all patients are religious or spiritual; (c) many patients want to address spiritual issues; (d) and religious commitment is associated with relief from physical and emotional suffering and with enhanced quality of life (Matthews, 1999). Matthews also proposes that spirituality and religion are of benefit because they construct a coherent worldview to help individuals interpret life experiences and suffering and develop meaning and purpose in life and connectedness with others; and engender serenity and transcendence, thereby buffering stress.

According to Doka and Morgan (1993), the spiritual care offered to patients and families should be based on the following principles:

- Each person has a spiritual dimension that must be considered along with mental, emotional, and physical dimensions.
- A spiritual orientation influences mental, emotional, and physical responses to dying and bereavement.

- When facing a terminal illness, death and bereavement may be a stimulus for spiritual growth.
- No single approach to spiritual care is satisfactory for all individuals given the diversity of individuals from different cultures.
- Spirituality is expressed and enhanced in formal and informal, religious and secular ways, including symbols, rituals, practices, patterns, gestures, art forms, prayers, and meditation which should be accessible and available.
- Care should be taken to offer settings, which will accommodate individual preferences as well as communal experiences.
- Health care systems should support spiritual care in their written statements of philosophy, and resources of time, money, and staff.
- Patients and caregivers should feel free to express humor and to laugh as this provides medicine for the soul.
- A caring environment should be in place to promote spiritual work at any time.

Assessment of Spiritual Well-Being

An awareness and appreciation of a patient's and family's spiritual orientation is essential to holistic care. Although patients may have a strong religious affiliation, this may either support or hinder spiritual exploration and the acknowledgment of spiritual issues. It is important to know if the patient's and family's religious affiliation is a source of strength and support and was used to meet needs in the past. It is also important to understand if an individual's religious beliefs are a source of fear and distress, particularly if the individual fears judgment. The spiritual pain of an individual is often evident by the manifestation of sorrow and grief, isolation from self and

others, a sense of meaninglessness and emptiness, fear and avoidance of the future, hopelessness and despair, and anger and bitterness towards God (Matthews, 1999).

Although it is not the responsibility of nurses to solve all spiritual problems or provide the answers, a nurse can create an environment that nurtures the patients' exploration of spiritual needs and concerns and supports them in their search for answers. This can be done by asking basic questions like the following: How are your spirits? Can you share with me your spiritual journey? How do you define your spirit? or What nourishes your spirit? (O'Connor, 1993). These questions often reveal patients' spiritual orientation and validate their spiritual nature.

By taking a spiritual history, nurses learn about patients' beliefs or what is important to them. A nurse can ask questions during the history and address spirituality at each follow-up visit, as spirituality is an ongoing issue. In conducting such a history, it is important for the nurse not to impose his or her values, but to listen in a nonjudgmental way. However, nurses often recognize that awareness of one's own spiritual and religious values may assist in providing a supportive environment for the patient. With support, the patient is not isolated by pain but may be brought closer to the source of meaning and to the community that shares the meaning. This leads to transpersonal transcendence (O'Connor, 1993).

Assessment of valuable spiritual interventions that are preferred by the patient and family may range from religious rituals such as prayer, communion, and blessing of the sick to secular observances such as sunsets, music, or poetry (O'Connor, 1993). Nurses also may ask the question, "How did you relieve your spiritual pain in the past?" It must be recognized that spiritual pain, like physical pain, may change in intensity over time, and that the time of dying may raise spiritual issues though not necessarily spiritual pain (O'Connor, 1993). Nurses should also listen not only to verbal but also nonverbal messages that may indicate the patient's feelings, needs, or spiritual pain. In some circumstances, spiritual pain can be eased, yet in other circumstances, spiritual pain may be viewed by patients as a way to salvation, making them more worthy of heaven or the afterlife, or as a way of coming closer to God.

In taking a spiritual history, Puchalski (1998b) suggests that the acronym FICA be used: "F" standing for faith or beliefs; "I" referring to the importance and influence of spirituality or religiosity in one's life; "C" signifying participation in a spiritual or religious community; and "A" asking if they would like the health professional to address spiritual issues. Specific questions in the spiritual history therefore may include the following:

Faith: What is your faith or belief? Do you consider yourself spiritual or religious? Does religious faith or spirituality play an important part in your life? What things give you meaning in life?

Influence: How does your religious faith or spirituality influence the way you think about health or the way you take care of yourself?

Community: Are you a part of a spiritual or religious community or congregation? Does this support you?

Address: Would you like me to address any religious or spiritual issues and concerns with you? (Puchalski, 1998b)

As another approach, Highfield (2000) uses the word "SPIRIT" to remember questions appropriate to a spiritual interview, specifically

S Spiritual belief system (religious affiliation)

P Personal spirituality (beliefs and practices of affiliation that the patient and family accept)

I Integration with a spiritual community (role of the religious/spiritual group; individual's role in the group)

R Ritualized practices and restrictions (beliefs that health care providers should remember during care)

I Implications for medical care (beliefs that health care providers should remember during care)

T Terminal events planning (impact of beliefs on advance directives; contacting the clergy)

Spiritual Interventions and Care

"Spiritual care is so much more than religious care. Spiritual care discovers, reverences, and tends the spirit—that is the energy or place of meaning and values—of another human being" (Driscoll, 2001, p. 334). Nurses can alleviate spiritual distress by inquiring about religious beliefs and practices; encouraging such religious practices, traditions, and rituals; praying with or for the patient; providing spiritual support; or referring the patient to the clergy or chaplain. In the past, nurses often called exclusively on clergy to facilitate resolution of spiritual issues and crises, yet the emerging focus on holistic care has reinforced the role of nurses as providers of spiritual care (O'Neill & Kenny, 1998). However, collaborative relationship with the clergy, as members of the interdisciplinary team, can provide the best possible support for patients experiencing spiritual distress and lead to the development of a spiritual plan of care to help them cope with whatever is happening in their lives.

When a patient or family is praying for a miracle even in medically futile situations, the role of health professionals is to respect their beliefs and remain supportive by trying to understand their worldview and the role their beliefs have in coping. Criticism or confrontation will lead to distrust and close the dialogue between health care professionals and the patient. When patients and their families feel they can talk to health professionals about their religious or spiritual beliefs, there is a greater chance they will accept what the professional is saying. One response could be, "Sometimes God answers our prayers for healing in interpersonal ways that may ultimately be more important than physical healing" (Koenig, 2002, p. 492).

Direct spiritual care may involve crisis intervention, pastoral visitation, group facilitation, prayer and worship, ministry to families, ministry to staff, and ethical consultations (Driscoll, 1999). Ongoing spiritual care across health care settings may involve pastoral counseling and therapy, spiritual direction, parish or congregational connection, and linkages with community resources.

In providing spiritual care, all practitioners, whether health care practitioners or spiritual care practitioners, can provide a listening presence and assist people in articulating their spirituality in either religious or nonreligious language. Health professionals must not assume that spiritual care is being given just because a patient has expressed a religious affiliation. Active listening and presence, therefore, should be spiritual interventions for all patients. In addition to clarifying a patient's spiritual concerns and needs by following spiritual cues, and exploring emotions with emphatic support, health care professionals may also do the following:

- Make wish statements, such as "I also wish you were not ill."

- Identify common goals for care and reach agreement on clinical decisions.
- Mobilize support for the patient and family from family, church members, or the community. (Lo et al., 2002)

Patients should be encouraged to tell their life stories, with the possibility of recognizing the meaning and purpose of their lives. Spiritual care may also involve empowering people to draw upon their strengths to overcome feelings of isolation and loneliness and a sense of pain, suffering, and powerlessness. Matthews (1999) suggests that nurses can connect spiritually with patients by using the acronym "WEB":

Welcome by demonstrating acceptance that "you're welcome here" and providing reassurance and concern regardless of faith background or for those without a particular faith. It also involves inviting the patient to discuss important issues of faith and belief as exemplified by such statements as "Please feel free to talk about whatever is of most importance to you or of concern to you, including matters of faith."

Encouragement reinforces to persons of faith the value of continuing healthy religious beliefs and practices. A nurse may say, "I see that you joined the prayer group. I've noticed that patients who participate in these groups often feel less isolated and more at peace." Encouragement of others to consider spiritual practices can be discussed within the context of the scientific literature, which shows the benefits of spiritual and religious practices in promoting well-being and quality of life. The nurse may say, "Many studies now show the benefits of spiritual practices. Would this be something you would like to pursue?" If a patient expresses a wish to pray, the nurse may offer to pray with or for the patient.

*B*lessings refers to the expression of blessings in a faith-sensitive manner. The nurse may say "Blessings to you," "God bless you," or "Shalom."

Patients may also be asked if they would like someone to pray with or for them or have spiritual reading materials. Prayer has been identified as the most frequently reported alternative treatment modality of elders, with women and Blacks using prayer as a coping strategy significantly more than men and Whites do (Dunn & Horgas, 2000). Prayer is about encountering God, not only in creating thoughts to send to God, but also by being in the present moment, living in the presence of God simply by appreciating a smile or the sky (Taylor, 2003b). At times, if the patient is of the same faith background as the health professional, the patient may request prayer. However, prayer is appropriate only when the patient wants it and will be comforted by it (Koenig, 2002). Prayer should not be prescribed, as there is a risk that the intention may not be patient-centered but rather provider-centered. In that context, prayers offered by health professionals may be viewed as coercive (Koenig, 2002). "Respectful care requires that nurses follow the patient's expressed wishes regarding prayer with the patient" (Winslow & Winslow, 2003, p. 173). The existing religious or spiritual beliefs of patients should be supported and encouraged, yet this is not the appropriate time to introduce new or unfamiliar spiritual beliefs or practices (Koenig, 2002). Nurses should also use prayer that is consistent with their own beliefs. If a nurse is an atheist, it would be unethical to betray his or her personal beliefs to perform an act of prayer. Although most people prefer spontaneous, conversational prayer, ritual prayers may provide great comfort and insight during one's encounter with God Taylor, 2003b). Examples of ritual

prayer may be the 23rd Psalm ("The Lord is my shepherd") or the Jewish prayer Sh'ma.

To anoint patients with peace, nurses can also give the gift of music as they sing a gentle, loving song to their patients. The patient may also find comfort in speaking an audible mantra (Taylor, 2003b). As part of deathbed healing, music thanatologists play the harp, which is a contemplative practice, and the medicine of attunement. Music at the end of life can alleviate pain and suffering. The rhythm of the music mirrors the natural rhythms of the patient's body, breathing, or heart rate, allowing the person to unbind from the physical body. Music offered by others is another form of physical and spiritual presence, which supports dying persons as they begin their journey (Schroeder-Sheker, 1999).

As an element of spirituality and a coping method for spiritual growth and healing, humor can be transcendent, momentarily removing one from an isolated state to join in surprise at ludicrous human situations (Johnson, 2002). Based on a study of breast cancer patients, Johnson (2002) reported that the use of humor was a step to recovery because it healed and gave hope to survive the moment.

Patients may also be spiritually uplifted as they socialize with family, friends, and children and are encouraged to help others. Supporting others preserves a person's meaning and purpose in life and provides an opportunity to pass on their legacy by means of story telling and reminiscing about the past (Hermann, 2000).

If a person is isolated, the health practitioner can suggest watching spiritual or religious television programs (Hermann, 2000). Nurses may encourage opportunities for patients to experience nature in whatever ways they can, such as a walk or wheelchair ride in the garden or courtyard, as they sit outside feeling the air and warmth of the sun (Sherman, 2004a). In the present moment, spirits can be uplifted by focusing on realistic hopes, such as relief of pain and symptoms, hope for peace and comfort, and a life after death. Patients' spirits also can be lifted by reliving a pleasurable experience in the their past, while simultaneously making plans in the near future to experience a physical or emotional pleasure, such as having a favorite meal or a visit from a special person (Sherman, 2004a).

Spiritual care can also involve "making meaning" through forms of life review, such as looking at old photographs or personal memorabilia, reading old letters or diary entries, and talking about life experiences, including accomplishments, hopes, and dreams (Sherman, 2004a).

Educating Nurses and Physicians Regarding Spirituality

Puchalski and Larson (1998) have identified key components to educating nurses and physicians regarding spirituality. They include the following:

- Demonstrating the completion of a spiritual history/assessment as part of the routine history
- Role-playing as a way of learning to discuss spiritual/religious beliefs and values in a respectful, nonjudgmental way
- Critiquing the research regarding the role of spirituality in health care
- Discussing illustrative cases where patients' beliefs negatively affected their health and potential spiritual interventions
- Discussing the role of clergy as members of the interdisciplinary team in palliative care
- Conducting a value clarification exercise for students to identify their own spiritual values

- Role-playing compassionate and effective communication regarding spiritual issues and needs of patients from diverse cultures; or role-play conducting values clarification with patients and family members
- Reviewing religious traditions and aspects that may affect health care choices

LIFE AND DEATH ACROSS CULTURES

Increasing cultural diversity within American society challenges nurses and other health professionals to look through different eyes in providing holistic care (Showalter, 1998). Culture is defined as a way of life. While culture is often identified with ethnicity, it's a far broader concept that encompasses the components of gender, age, sexual orientation, differing abilities, educational level, employment, and place of residency (ELNEC, 2001). For example, cultures may value male children more than female; value the wisdom of the old or work productivity of the young; may accept or reject homosexuality, or devalue those who are less educated, unemployed, or homeless. A person's cultural background also relates to issues of power, decision making, communication, degree of community support, and sense of fatalism verses activism in controlling life, maintaining hope, and accepting death (ELNEC, 2001).

Culture also relates to the issue of patient autonomy, which emphasizes patients' rights to be informed about their condition, treatments, and right to choose or refuse life-prolonging therapies (Sherman, 2004a). For example, patients from Asian cultures may believe that the family rather than the individual should make decisions regarding treatment (Kagawa-Singer & Blackhall, 2001).

Culture can influence patients' feelings of mistrust regarding the intentions of health care providers and responses to the inequities in the health care system. Minority groups, such as African Americans, may perceive discussions of the costs of technology and the ineffectiveness of treatment as a devaluation of their life (Crawley, Marshall, Lo, & Koenig, 2002), and may be concerned that in signing advance directives they will be denied access to desired care at the end of life. Cultural mistrust, particularly of African Americans, also results in low hospice utilization. Born, Greiner, Sylvia, Butler, and Ahuwalia (2004) conducted a qualitative study to identify factors that affect the utilization of hospice care by African Americans and Latinos and found the following prevailing themes related to preferences for end of life care: (1) the practice of having families provide and direct care for loved ones; (2) the desire to reduce caretaker burden; (3) reliance on spirituality as the primary means of coping with suffering and death; (4) concern for the holistic well-being of the patient and family members, including freedom from pain and suffering; (5) lack of awareness of hospice service; (6) prohibitive cost of health care; (7) language barriers; and (8) mistrust of the health care system.

Communication and language barriers may lead to mistrust and conflict between patients and families and their health care providers. These barriers can be decreased by avoiding medical jargon, checking for understanding, and hiring trained interpreters because family or untrained interpreters may misinterpret communication or censor sensitive or taboo topics (Crawley et al., 2001). A related issue is truth telling in which individuals in certain cultures believe that information regarding diagnosis or prognosis may cause harm to the patient, and may ask the health care team not to tell the patient the truth regarding his or her condition. In these situations, the health care provider can ask patients in the presence of their families if they want to know everything and the truth about their illness; or providers can conduct a family meeting with the patient present to clarify issues and discuss the decisions and preferences of the patient (Sherman, 2004a).

When working with culturally diverse groups, conflicts can arise when health professionals automatically apply European American cultural concepts, inherent in the use of advance directives, to other sociocultural groups. The interrelated values that underlie end-of-life decision making and the use of advance directives include patient autonomy, informed decision-making, truth telling, and control over the dying process. In a review of the literature regarding multicultural considerations in the use of advance directives, Ersek and colleagues (1998) reported that in many non–European American cultures, interdependence among family and community members is valued more than autonomy, particularly with respect to decision making. Families plan, manage, and participate in all aspects of patient care as a basic duty. In many non–European American cultures full disclosure and truth telling is prohibited because the information is believed to burden the patient, while other cultures view full disclosure of information as disrespectful and rude. For non–European American cultures, controlling life and death is unnatural and inappropriate; the belief is that death is a part of the life cycle and natural.

Nurses must recognize that there are cultural differences between groups—based on treasured beliefs, shared teachings, norms, customs, language and meaning—that influence the individuals and families response to illness, treatment, death, and bereavement (Showalter, 1998); and they must also recognize that there may be individual or within-group variations attributed to acculturation differences, as well as to differences related to age, education, geographic location, and social context (Kagawa-Singer & Blackhall, 2001). It is important to inquire whether an individual patient adheres to the beliefs and practices of his or her cultural group, rather than assuming an adherence to the same values and beliefs (Crawley et al., 2002). Concepts of culture and ethnicity may be useful for making generalizations about populations; however if they limit appreciation of the unique differences of people and are used to predict individual behavior, they may lead to stereotyping (Koenig, 2002). It is therefore important to appreciate the cultural background of a patient and family and respect their feelings and perceptions, and it is equally important to recognize the unique perspectives of the patient to avoid stereotyping.

Members of the palliative care team bring their own cultural perspectives and life experiences to the caregiving setting. Hospice and palliative care nurses must be culturally sensitive and responsive, providing care in a culturally appropriate manner. Although nurses and other health professionals acknowledge death as a common human experience, they often fail to recognize that loss, grief, death, and bereavement occur within a cultural context. Across cultures, people differ in their beliefs and attitudes about life, illness, and death; in what they feel, what evokes emotions, the implications of those feelings, and the ways of expressing and dealing with emotions (Rosenblatt, 1993). With such acknowledgment comes the opportunity to support the bereaved and channel the grief through specific cultural rituals.

With a broad understanding of the meaning and function of cultural beliefs and practices, nurses are able to provide appropriate and culturally sensitive interventions to support patients and families in times of loss and transition. Ethnic and cultural differences are often influential in "the methods of coping with life-threatening illness, the perception of pain, the support of the dying, the behavioral manifestations of grief, mourning styles, and funeral customs" (DeSpelder & Strickland, 1999, p. 108). Various cultures have different beliefs about dying and the relationship of the deceased with their loved ones. Many cultures maintain a strong bond between the living and the dead, who are the voice of the ancestors. Most cultures do not shun their dead, but honor them and hold ceremonies to celebrate their lives. In some cultures, the dead perform services for the living as interpreters and intermediaries. Depending on the culture, calling the names of the dead may be avoided so as not to disturb them or may stem from a desire to minimize grief (DeSpelder & Strickland, 1999). However, in other cultures, names have special meaning and value in honoring the deceased.

In some cultures, there is a circular pattern of life and death with multiple deaths and rebirths. For Native Americans and some sects of Buddhism, in death there is a parallel world where the dead can affect the lives of the living. In many cultures, there is ancestor worship where the deceased communicate with the family through daily rituals. However, in some cultures there is an abrupt and final disengagement from the deceased, with sanctions against speaking the deceased person's name, which may keep them from moving to the land of the dead and maintain their ghostly presence on earth (Kagawa-Singer, 1998). In the majority of cultures, funeral rites help ensure the successful journey of the soul into the realm of the dead and are of benefit to the living.

Understanding the cultural backgrounds of individuals is fundamental to the development of a trusting and supportive relationship among patient, family, and health care professionals and is essential in developing a plan for health care that is consistent with their cultural expectations and health beliefs (Sherman, 2004a). The cultural perspectives regarding illness and death of Native Americans, African and African Americans, Hispanics, and Asians will be discussed to provide a framework for offering culturally competent palliative care.

CULTURAL PERSPECTIVES REGARDING ILLNESS AND DEATH

Native American Perspectives

For Native Americans, the tribe is the focus of their identity, with values and beliefs varying among tribes (Brokenleg & Middleton, 1993). Life and death are viewed as parts of a natural process. Time is not considered linear but a recurring cycle. Native Americans are interested mainly in how this cycle affects people in this life and only have a vague notion of another existence after death. Death is viewed as a motivation to treat people kindly and have a good life (Brokenleg & Middleton, 1993). In communicating, Native Americans tend to avoid eye contact and are stoic regarding the expression of pain and suffering. Traditional tribal medicines are used to treat conditions, and prayer is a means to accept the order of things and the outcomes of situations (Brokenleg & Middleton, 1993).

Given their reverence for the body in life and death, autopsies and cremation are not acceptable (Sherman, 2004a). Funerals are usually at home, with members of the community expected to stay with the mourners. A death song is sung that represents the summary of a person's life and acknowledgment of death. The dead are considered guardian spirits. After death, the spirit lingers near the site of the death for several days. Native Americans use a funeral pyre and adorn the corpse with flowers, feathers, and skins. For 6 months to a year, the name of the deceased is not called, in order to confirm their separation from the living. All material possessions of the deceased are given away so that the family can begin its new life without the presence of that person (Brokenleg & Middleton, 1993). In the Cocopa tribe, violent grief is expressed until cremation when they invite the spirits to join them in celebration. In the Hopi tribe, death is kept at a distance because it threatens order and control. The expression of grief remains limited and funerals are attended by few and held privately. For Native Americans, hallucinations in which they see and converse with the dead are regarded as a part of mourning (DeSpelder & Strickland, 1999).

Based on focus groups representing many Native American tribes and conducted by Native American nurses, Lowe and Struthers (2001) identified seven themes that represent core principles relevant to health care: (1) caring, which embodies characteristics of health, relationships, holism, and knowledge, and was characterized as a "partnership in healing"; (2) traditions, which refers to the characteristics of respect, wisdom, and values and refers to the valuing and connection with heritage; (3) respect, which includes characteristics of honor, identity, and strength and refers to the components of presence and compassion; (4) connection, which honors all people, the past, present, and future, harmony with nature, and explores differences and similarities; (5) holism, which includes balance and culture; (6) trust, which is characterized through relationship, presence, and respect; and (7) spirituality which includes unity, honor, balance, and healing and includes components of touching, learning, and utilizing traditions to recognize oneness and unity.

African and African American Perspectives

Within the African culture, death is integrated into the totality of life. Ancestor worship involves communion with the living dead through memories, and the deceased are remembered by name. When the deceased are no longer remembered by people who are alive, they becomes part of the anonymous dead, but by this time their spirit has been reborn in a new child. Within the African community, death elicits a response from all members. Funeral ceremonies serve three purposes: to separate the dead from the bereaved family; to serve as an opportunity to redistribute the roles of the deceased to living persons; and to acknowledge that the dead join the ancestors and the living return to the community in a way that reflects their changed status.

African Americans have their own perspectives that are informed by the oppression of slavery. The focus during the time of slavery was on a better life after death, and many African Americans converted to Christianity. Slavery and racism had an impact on the way suffering was perceived when compared to the White majority. Common themes of justice and respect have reinforced the importance of self-determination. Undesired deaths from cancer, AIDS, suicide, and violence are higher in African American communities than in general society. Given that African Americans do not benefit from modern medical technology to the same degree as the European American population, they have a lower life expectancy and higher death rate. This has created a distrust of the medical system and a lack of interest of African Americans in hospice care (DeSpelder & Strickland, 1999). There is also a low rate of organ donations after death.

For African Americans, the church has been important in maintaining their spirit, and Black preachers are viewed as the shepherds of their flock. There is a strong belief in family and the valuing of each other as brothers and sisters that is a source of mutual aid and support. Family is therefore central to the care of the terminally ill. Patients rely on family, friends, church associates, and neighbors

for support. Black families have a more adoptive, absorptive sense of community with an unfavorable response to outside help. Given a strong sense of family loyalty, they are reluctant to hospitalize family members and prefer keeping the ill person at home (DeSpelder & Strickland, 1999).

In a study of a small Black Baptist church, Abrums (2000) conducted life history interviews of 9 churchgoing women, ranging in age from 19 to 82, to explore the meaning of death and the experience of grieving. The findings indicated that the women had been taught to be strong in the face of death and to handle their grief "head on," believing that they would one day be reunited with their loved ones. They used the words "passed on," "passed away," or "died." The women described spirit visits for the purpose of offering warnings or as direct messages, which sustained their belief in an afterlife. They believed that God spoke to them in many ways through premonitions, perceived as the voice of God. There was strong perception of the journey of life in which there was a job to do on earth and a purpose to one's life. No life was in vain. Participants also described the importance of hope, acceptance, and responsibility to comfort the dying and the bereaved.

African Americans regard funerals as important and the number of people who attend the funeral and the appearance of the casket reflect the value of the deceased. In the African American culture, the deceased is touched but not kissed, and families are unlikely to visit the grave. Visits from family and friends are important to the bereaved with a strong expression of emotion and unrestrained grief (DeSpelder & Strickland, 1999).

Hispanic Perspectives

The cultural group referred to as Hispanic includes individuals who are Mexican, Puerto

Rican, and Latino. Given that cultural values profoundly influence the experience of health and illness for individuals, Martinez (1995) conducted a qualitative study of 14 Hispanic participants, ranging in age from 60 to 89, along with 6 health professionals and 2 clergy members who practice in the community. Participants held holistic views of self and emphasized the spiritual aspects of life in relation to health. Mental health was described as knowing what is right, living a life consistent with one's beliefs and values, trusting that life will work out, and maintaining faith in God. Caring for self was through caring for others for whom one had responsibility. In dealing with illness, there was a blending of modern medicine and traditional healing remedies. It was also appropriate to include family members in making health decisions.

Within the Mexican culture, it is believed that the dying should be protected from knowing their prognosis, as death is viewed as an adversity. Women show extreme grief or hysteria, while men show little or no grief. Death is often confronted with a humorous sarcasm and is viewed as an equalizer (DeSpelder & Strickland, 1999). Mexican Americans, as well as other Hispanics, are likely to call the priest for the sacrament of the sick, and the bereaved may take shifts being with the deceased person. There is strong support of family as a unit. The funeral is the single most important family ceremony and goes on for several days, as there is the belief that it takes time to grieve. Individuals are prohibited from speaking ill of the person who has died and the bereaved visit the grave frequently. The day of the dead is celebrated in November and coincides with All Saints' Day, the feast of the commemoration of the dead. It is a time of celebration with special foods, music, and the decoration of graves. It is believed that the dead return to the world of the living for this special celebration, and families are scorned if they neglect their re-

sponsibilities. The bereaved are discouraged from crying too many tears, as excessive grief may make the pathway traveled on by the dead slippery and burden them in the journey (DeSpelder & Strickland, 1999).

Asian Perspectives

In Asian cultures, family is essential to social structure. From the centrality of the family arise duty to family, manifested by respect and reverence for parents; conformance to family and societal norms and especially not bringing shame to the family; family recognition through achievement; emotional self-control manifested through reserved and formal public verbal and nonverbal communications with disagreement or demands kept to a minimum; collectivism, as evidenced by a focus on the family and community over self; and humility, manifested by a lack of striving for individual achievement except achievement that is related to the family (Kemp & Chang, 2002). Given the hierarchical and patriarchal family structure, the oldest adult male is the primary decision-maker, along with the significant influence of elders (Sherman, 2004a). Health care decisions are considered within the context of what is best not only for the individual, but also for the family. Symptom management may be complicated by the patient's and family's reluctance to complain and by respect for those in a position of authority. Concerns also center on fears of addiction, the desire to be a good patient, and fear of distracting the physician from treating the disease. In some cases, patients even deny symptoms when asked directly, although the use of the visual analog scale and numeric rating scale can be used to assess pain. Patients may want to keep warm during illness by wearing sweaters or socks in bed and drinking warm liquids and avoiding cold drinks. As death nears, the family may wish to call monks or nuns for ritual prayers (Kemp & Chang, 2002).

Families often believe that discussing end-of-life issues is like wishing death upon the person or may lead to hopelessness, especially because terminal illness is not socially accepted. As death approaches, it is believed that a person's final days should be characterized by calm and the patient should not be involved in decision making. The best way to handle the conspiracy of silence is to ask the patient whom the information should be given to and who should make decisions. Families often feel it is their cultural obligation to care for the person who is dying and therefore hospice services are often refused (Kemp & Chang, 2002).

In Asian cultures, there is great respect for the ancestors, as they are part of the biological and social past. Funeral and memorial rituals transform the ancestors into sources of blessings for the living (DeSpelder & Strickland, 1999). The dead share the joy of the achievements of the living and may be given credit for the success.

Although the primary religion in China is Buddhism, many Chinese follow the traditions of Confucianism and Taoism. Confucianism emphasizes the value of the familial relationships of parents and their children and living life according to strong ethical principles. Taoism stresses the balance of yin (female energies) and yang (male energies) and the relationship with the five elements of earth, water, wood, fire, and metal to achieve immortality (Klass & Goss, 1998). The Chinese culture believes that the most important obligation in life is to bury the dead and honor the ancestors with religious rites. Chinese Americans hold funerals in funeral homes and the women are more demonstrative in their grieving (Klass & Goss, 1998). Mourners pick up wrapped candy as they leave the funeral, which wards off bad luck

for those who have come in close proximity to the dead. White clothes are often worn, though brightly colored clothes are worn to celebrate the life of the elderly. Most Chinese Americans practice burial rather than cremation. The procession back from the grave symbolizes the movement of the bereaved back to life without the deceased. After the funeral, all mourners attend a banquet feast. Post-funeral ceremonies continue 3 days after death when the family burns paper money, and leaves food at the gravesite. These rituals occur again on the 21st, 35th, and 49th days after the death, which reinforces the bond between the living and the dead ancestors.

In the Japanese culture, there are strict funeral rituals and the family is not likely to touch the deceased person's body. Ancestors are venerated by installing an ancestral shrine in the home called a *budsudan* or household altar. On the 49th day after death, the deceased is transformed into a benevolent ancestor, the spirit having lingered in the home during this time. The rituals of the first 49 days accomplish what Western society would call grief work (Klass & Goss, 1998). The body is cremated, and ashes and bones are put in an urn and buried in the family grave (*haka*) following a funeral service. Buddhist scripture is read and the deceased is given a Buddhist name, indicating that the material aspect of the individual is gone. The name (*kaimyo*) is inscribed in the budsudan. Memorial ceremonies are held on the 100th day after death, on the first and third anniversaries, and at fixed intervals thereafter. The *O-bon* marks the annual celebration of the return of the ancestral spirits to their families. Japanese attitudes and practices support the idea that survivors seldom sever their bonds with deceased loved ones, but rather the inner representations of the dead continue to have an active role in the ongoing life of the bereaved (Klass & Goss, 1998).

Asian Indian Perspectives

Among Asian Indians, extended families are prevalent: elders are highly respected; a husband's parents often move in with the family after retirement, when the family decides to have children, or if there is an illness; and grandparents play a strong role in raising children. In Indian culture, independence and privacy are valued, yet family issues are discussed within the immediate family before outside help is sought and health decisions are made by the family (Bhungalia & Kemp, 2002). Many Indians are of the Hindu faith.

The caste system is part of Hinduism. In this system, society is divided into four social classes: the highest class are the priests, or Brahmans, and the lowest are the laborers, or Sudras. A person's class is inherited at birth based on his or her karma. Aspects of Hinduism that affects patient care include

- karma, or the consequences of one's actions or behaviors, that influences the circumstances of life and may have caused an illness;
- the importance of meditation and prayer; and
- the practice of vegetarianism in which Hindus pray a specific prayer before eating, asking forgiveness for eating a plant or vegetable in which a soul may dwell. (Bhungalia & Kemp, 2002)

The Indian system of medicine is known as *Ayurveda,* which means knowledge of life. In Ayurveda, the body comprises three primary forces, called *dosha,* specifically the *Vata, Pitta,* and *Kapha.* Each represents characteristics derived from the five elements of space, air, fire, water, and earth. These forces must be balanced in order to have health. In this system, disease may be related to the environment or other factors Herbal remedies

are used by more than 80% of people in India to cure or prevent illness. There are approximately 1,400 plants used in Ayurvedic medicine. Most Indians eat two to three meals a day, eating with the fingers of their right hand, and avoiding distractions while eating, such as watching television or excessive talking. Some foods are considered hot and others cold and should not be eaten in combination as it may affect bodily functions (Sherman, 2004a).

With respect to end-of-life care, it is important for elders to complete unfinished business and resolve relationships. Home is the preferred place of death, with many family members present. Symptoms may not be reported as it is believed that suffering is inevitable and the result of karma. Many seek a conscious dying process without mental clouding from medications. As death approaches, the following rituals are valued:

- A lamp may be placed near the patient's head, facing east towards Mecca; sacred ash may be applied to the forehead.
- A few drops of water from the sacred Ganges River may be placed in the dying person's mouth, while a mantra is softly chanted in the patient's right ear.
- Prayer and incense are part of the rituals of the dying process.

After death, family members should be the only ones to touch the body and ideally a family member of the same sex should clean the body. After the body is cleansed, a cloth is tied under the chin and over the top of the head, and the body is wrapped in red cloth. Embalming and organ donation are prohibited, and there is a preference is for cremation. Following the death, religious pictures at home are turned toward the wall and mirrors may be covered. It is believed that for 12 days the soul wanders in the home, trying to let go of life and the material world. During this time, the family prays and chants and on the 12th day, the soul is reincarnated (Bhungalia & Kemp, 2002).

Research Regarding Culture and End-of-Life Issues

Based on a study of 800 older individuals from four ethnic groups—specifically European Americans, African Americans, Korean Americans, and Mexican Americans—Blackhall, Murphy, Frank, Michel, and Azen (1995) examined the relationship between ethnicity and attitudes toward patient autonomy. The finding indicated that Korean Americans and Mexican Americans were significantly less likely than European Americans and African Americans to believe that patients should be told of their diagnosis of metastatic cancer and were less likely to believe that the patient should make decisions about the use of life-supporting technology. Korean and Mexican Americans believe that the family should make the decisions to use life support, holding a family-centered model of decision making rather than a patient-autonomy model favored by European Americans and African Americans.

With regard to attitudes toward life-sustaining treatments, Caralis, Davis, Wright, and Marcial (1993) found that non-Hispanic Whites were more likely to agree to withhold life-sustaining treatments in various clinical scenarios than were Hispanics and African Americans. Klessig (1992) found that European Americans were also less likely to start life support under hopeless and terminal conditions than African Americans, Chinese Americans, Filipino Americans, Korean Americans, and Mexican Americans were.

McGrath, Vun, and McLeod (2001) found similar end of life concerns across cultural groups of patients and caregivers, despite the differences in cultural backgrounds of Indian,

Filipino, Chinese, and Italian participants. These concerns included the importance of support from families; the pressures on family members to care for relatives at the end of life; lack of knowledge about hospice and palliative care services; lack of choice in how they wished to care for their family member; difficulty in talking about dying; and desire to care for a family member at home. Health professionals in hospice and palliative care need to be aware of these shared concerns and assist patients and families in recognizing the supports and resources that are being offered to enhance their quality of life (Kagawa-Singer & Blackhall, 2001).

QUALITY NURSING CARE: DEVELOPING CULTURAL COMPETENCE

A culturally competent health care system "acknowledges and incorporates at all levels the importance of culture, the assessment of cross-cultural relations, vigilance toward the dynamics that result from cultural differences, and the expansion of cultural knowledge, and adaptation of services to meet culturally unique needs" (Cort, 2004, p. 68). Achieving cultural competence is a dynamic state in which health professions gain knowledge of their own cultural and social backgrounds and become aware of the history, traditions, and values of other groups, including understanding the history, food, and lifestyles of people from other countries (Cort, 2004).

According to the Schim and Miller cultural competence model, there are four components of cultural competence:

1. Cultural diversity, which is reflected in every aspect of the health care system in the United States and recognizes diverse populations with unique values, beliefs, and customs

2. Cultural awareness, which implies knowledge and information exchange regarding health, beliefs, and practices specific to various communities, and cultural variations within groups

3. Cultural sensitivity, which requires the recognition of individual attitudes and beliefs and a refinement of communication skills related to active listening, use of silence and touch, conversational distance, language patterns, and the effective use of translators

4. Cultural competence, which is the ultimate goal and incorporates diversity (fact), awareness (knowledge), and sensitivity (attitude) into everyday practice and behaviors. (Doorenbos & Schim, 2004)

The National Organization of Nurse Practitioner Faculties (NONPF) (2000) reinforces the integration of cultural competency into nursing care by the following:

1. Showing respect for the dignity of every human being, whatever the age, gender, religion, sexual orientation, socioeconomic class, or ethnic or cultural group

2. Accepting the rights of individuals to choose their health care provider, participate in care, and refuse care

3. Acknowledging personal biases and preventing these from interfering with quality care

4. Recognizing cultural issues and interacting in culturally sensitive ways

5. Incorporating cultural preferences, health beliefs, and behaviors and traditional practices into patient's plan of care

6. Developing appropriate educational materials that reflect the language and belief of the patient

7. Accessing culturally appropriate resources

Nurses' Cultural Self-Awareness and Development of Cultural Competency

The key to accommodating cultural diversity is for nurses to understand their own values, beliefs, and customs related to the celebration of life, and coping with illness and death. Irish, Lundquist, and Nelsen (1993) suggest that health professionals assess the degree in which they are proactive in their attitudes and activities toward diversity by asking themselves the following questions:

- Have I actively sought information to enhance my own awareness and understanding of multicultural diversity?
- Have I consciously pondered my own attitudes and behaviors as they either enhance or hinder my relationships with others?
- Have I evaluated my use of terms or phrases that may be perceived by others as degrading or hurtful?
- Have I suggested or initiated workshops or discussions about multicultural diversity?
- Have I openly disagreed with racial, cultural, or religious jokes, comments, or slurs?
- Have I utilized in my work setting appropriate occasions to discuss the multicultural climate in the organizations with my colleagues and with institutional administration?
- Have I complained to the author when I see a broadcast, advertisement, or newspaper article that is racially, culturally, or religiously biased? (p. 45)

Furthermore, DeSpelder (1998) suggests that health care professionals develop end-of-life cultural competence, when they reflect on their own attitudes, beliefs, and practices toward dying and death. Nurses may explore for themselves

- their own beliefs about death and what influenced these attitudes;
- how significant religion is in their attitudes toward death;
- what kind of death they would prefer;
- if diagnosed with a terminal illness, whom they would want to tell;
- what efforts should be made to keep a seriously ill person alive;
- how they would want their bodies to be disposed; and
- what their experience is of participating in rituals to remember the dead.

By awareness of one's own feelings, attitudes, preferences, and biases, nurses can be more in touch with themselves, acknowledging their right to their own beliefs, but not allowing those values and beliefs to take precedence over those expressed by patients and families. In order for nurses to care effectively for patients from diverse cultural groups, they also must be willing to learn about the cultures of their patients and presuppositions. The first step is to find educational sources that provide information about the various cultures, while recognizing that there are individual differences even within the same culture because of differences in social stratum, personal experiences with illness and death, and individual preferences and values. By asking someone of a particular culture to help them understand the taboos and meanings of experiences and events, nurses can actively learn about other cultures. Nurses must also recognize that losses have different meanings from person to person and culture to culture and may be viewed as major or minor.

In providing culturally competent care, general principles include the need to

- listen with sympathy and understanding;
- be nonjudgmental;

- determine what is appropriate and polite caring behavior;
- recognize differences in communication styles related to such behaviors as handshaking, use of surnames, and eye contact;
- acknowledge and discuss differences and similarities between perceptions, recommending treatments while remembering the patient's cultural perspectives;
- negotiate and compromise when worldviews are in conflict. (American Medical Student Association [AMSA], 2001; Crawley et al., 2002)

Cultural Assessment and Interventions

Developing cultural competency also requires that nurses listen carefully and gather cultural information. The patient's background may provide clues about a person's beliefs; however, these are only assumptions unless validated by asking patients about their beliefs, needs, expectations, and wishes. Knowledge about a person's cultural group should serve only as a starting point or guideline in assessing individual beliefs and behaviors (Kagawa-Singer, 1998; Lipson, Dibble, & Minarik, 1996).

In conducting a cultural assessment, there are several areas to be addressed:

- Identify the birthplace of the patient.
- Ask a patient about their immigration experience.
- Determine their level of ethnic identity.
- Evaluate their degree of acculturation as evidenced by their use of the English language, the length of time in the United States, and their adaptation.
- Determine their family structure.
- Identify the use of informal networks and sources of support within the community.

- Identify who makes decisions, such as the individual patient, the family or another social unit.
- Assess their primary and secondary language.
- Determine the person's verbal and nonverbal communication patterns.
- Consider gender and power issues within relationships.
- Evaluate the patient's sense of self-esteem.
- Identify the influence of religion or spirituality on patients' and families' expectations and behaviors.
- Ascertain the patient's perceptions regarding discrimination or racism.
- Identify cooking and dining traditions and the meaning of food.
- Determine the patient's educational level and socioeconomic status.
- Assess attitudes, beliefs, and practices related to health, illness, suffering, and death.
- Determine patients' and families' preferences regarding location of death.
- Discuss expectations regarding health care.
- Determine the degree of fatalism or activism in accepting or controlling care and death.
- Evaluate the patient's knowledge and trust regarding the health care system.
- Assess the value and use of pharmacologic, nonpharmacologic, and complementary therapies.
- Discuss how hope is maintained. (AMSA, 2001; ELNEC, 2001; Ersek et al., 1998)

In providing culturally sensitive care, DeSpelder (1998) also suggests that health professionals listen for and mirror the language patterns based on an individual's culture. Small differences in language, such as saying "passed away" or "passed on" can in-dicate much about the speaker's experience. For example, "passed away" may describe the deceased from the survivor's perspective, whereas "passed on" may imply a belief in life after death. Nurses also can attend to the cultural needs of their patients by gathering information about distinctive rituals, practices, and beliefs, particularly an understanding of what is meaningful to the individual person. This assessment involves listening, observing, and asking about practices of patients and families that may be unfamiliar to the nurse. Furthermore, nurses can determine the strengths an individual draws on when encountering death, dying, or bereavement, such as internal resources provided by the individual's belief system or past experiences; and external resources, such as the comfort provided by cultural customs (DeSpelder & Strickland, 1999). As nurses interact with patients and families from diverse cultures, they have the experiential opportunity to learn about cultural values, expectations, and needs regarding illness, dying, and death. In caring for patients and families at the end of life, nurses can enhance the quality of life and quality of dying by promoting a respectful and peaceful death through the recognition of their spiritual and cultural needs.

Cultural mistrust is a dynamic that has implications not only for individual health care providers but also for administrators of health care systems (Cort, 2004). Measures carried out by hospices to overcome cultural mistrust may include (1) hiring competent African American staff and minority volunteers; (2) respecting differences in cultural preferences; (3) conducting public education campaigns, by television or community and local organizations, newsletters, and church presentations; (4) involving African American pastors in capacities that permit them to serve as bridges of trust between their communities and the health care system; and (5) avoiding perceptions of injustice and inequality by promising only the services that can be delivered (Cort, 2004).

NURSES' NEED FOR SELF-REFLECTION AND SELF-HEALING IN PALLIATIVE CARE

Doka and Morgan (1993) describe the caregivers' assumptions and principles of spiritual care. First, nurses represent diverse spiritual or cultural backgrounds and like patients have the right to expect respect for their belief systems. Second, nurses should be offered opportunities to explore their own values and attitudes about life and death and their meaning and purpose in life. Third, nurses should be aware that they have the potential for providing spiritual care, and should be encouraged to offer spiritual care to dying patients and their families, as needed. Fourth, just as all caregivers, nurses should be flexible and realistic in setting spiritual goals. Fifth, ongoing care of the dying and bereaved may cause a severe drain of energy and uncover old and new spiritual issues for the caregiver. Spiritual growth and renewal is, therefore, a necessary part of staff support and a personal priority for each caregiver.

Indeed, in caring for dying patients and bereaved families, nurses may have experiences that create a grief response of their own because they have lost someone in whom they have invested themselves emotionally. Nurses' grief response, like that of their patients, will be influenced by their spiritual and cultural values and beliefs. If accumulated grief is not worked through, the nurse is vulnerable to the same manifestations of unresolved grief as any other individual who has had a loss but failed to complete the grief work (Rando, 1984; Sherman, 2004b). Nurses, therefore, need to resolve their own feelings of loss, with their spiritual convictions supported, sense of failure alleviated,

and emotional strength replenished (Rando, 1984; Sherman, 2004b).

In coping with the stress of caring for the dying, Rando (1984) believes that nurses progress through five stages: (1) focusing on professional knowledge and factual information; (2) experiencing the trauma of the patient's illness, often accompanied by guilt and frustration as the nurse confronts the patient's impending death; (3) moving through the pain and coming to an acceptance of the reality of death; (4) identifying the pain and suffering with sensitivity, but freeing themselves from the incapacitating effects; and (5) relating compassionately with the dying person in full acceptance of impending death. In caring for patients in palliative care, nurses must develop an awareness of their own emotional, physical, or spiritual limits, and develop an awareness of their own energy levels. By realizing the need for self-care, acknowledging their own feelings about dying and death and the stresses in caring for the dying that are most troublesome to them individually, nurses can prevent caregiver burnout (Rando, 1984).

In developing awareness and supporting nurses' spiritual well-being, nurse educators may ask their students or nursing colleagues the following questions:

- What expectations do you have about yourself in caring for the dying and bereaved?
- What would define success in your work?
- What are the three most difficult aspects of your work in caring for patients with life-threatening illness?
- What are you doing to help yourself cope with stress and replenish yourself to avoid becoming overstressed?

"Nurses must recognize their stress reactions and symptoms and employ self-care strategies to replenish themselves in physical, emotional, mental, and spiritual ways to overcome the various sources of stress" (Sherman, 2004b, p. 53).

According to Sherman (2004b), *physical health* is promoted as nurses care for their bodies by eating well, engaging in restful and relaxing activities, and counterbalancing fatigue by making improvements in lifestyle. *Emotional health* is bolstered by developing a calm mind with peaceful thoughts through such activities as meditation or listening to quiet music, as well as consciously letting go of negative thoughts and emotions. *Mental health* is strengthened by making choices, setting priorities, letting go of conflict, and saying no, while keeping open to new opportunities and possibilities; and *intuitional health* is nurtured by listening to the soul's wisdom and recognizing the need for balance and wholeness.

In overcoming interpersonal stressors, particularly when relations with others are difficult, nurses may find it helpful to reflect on the rewards of their work and the moments in which they have made the greatest difference in the lives of their patients and families. To cope with feelings of grief and loss, nurses can take time to reflect on what happened at the time of the patient's death and lessons learned and speak to colleagues or journal about feelings, perceptions, and experiences (Sherman, 2004b).

Within the context of end-of-life care, and given that spirituality has emerged as a vital component of health, it becomes necessary for nurses to acknowledge their own spiritual beliefs and values and to deal with their own spiritual and cultural issues. Based on a sample of 155 Israeli oncology nurses, Musgrave and McFarlane (2004) reported that nurses' attitudes toward spiritual care are influenced by their spiritual well-being, intrinsic and extrinsic religiosity, and education. In caring for people with life-threatening and progressive illness, nurses must remain in tune with their own spiritual needs, healing themselves as well as others. To do so, Halifax (1999) suggests a contemplative exercise for nurses to remain centered, renewed, and whole as they care for others. Sitting in a relaxed position, with eyes closed and aware of the rhythm of the breath, the nurse focuses one at a time on each of the following five phrases, which are repeated slowly twice. The nurse then allows the phrase to pass into the background of her or his awareness, moving attention to the breath and to the next phrase. The phrases are as follows:

- May I offer my care and presence unconditionally, knowing that it may be met with gratitude, indifference, anger, or anguish.
- May I offer love knowing that I cannot control the course of life's suffering or death.
- May I remain in ease and let go of my expectations.
- May I view my own suffering with compassion just as I do the suffering of others.
- May I be aware that my suffering does not limit my good heart.
- May I forgive myself for things left undone.
- May I forgive all who have hurt me.
- May those whom I have hurt forgive me.
- May all beings and I live and die in peace.

Spiritually and culturally competent care, therefore, requires self-reflection and self-care of nurses. Replenishing one's own vessel in spiritually and culturally renewing ways is important in supporting nurses' caregiving potential. For it is only by doing so that nurses will come to the bedside with the strong healing presence and true compassion needed to alleviate the suffering of patients and their families.

CONCLUSION

Illness and dying are occurrences that take us to the very core of our being. Although they are intensely personal experiences, they occur within the context of our spiritual and cultural traditions. Spirituality and culture can therefore not be separated from who we are, as they are often the very source of our nourishment and physical, emotional, social, and spiritual well-being. Through sensitive and competent spiritual and cultural care, nurses can protect patients and families from the ultimate tragedy of depersonalization.

They will be able to sustain them in a personalized environment that recognizes their individual needs, reduces their fears, and offers them hope and dignity. Sulmasy (1997) believes that

> when patients collapse spiritually in the face of illness, a clinician with the right perspective will understand much more acutely how desperate their plight really is and will treat the wounds of such patients with even more liberal applications of the wine of fervent zeal and the oil of compassion. (p. 52)

To identify the knowledge, attitudes and skills of undergrade and graduate nurses' behavioral outcomes and teaching/learning strategies, please refer to the Education Plan (Table 1.1).

EDUCATION PLAN 1.1   Plan for Achieving Competencies: Spiritually and Culturally Competent Palliative Care

Knowledge Needed	Attitude	Skills	Undergraduate Behavioral Outcomes	Graduate Behavioral Outcomes	Teaching/Learning Strategies
Spirituality and culture as factors that structure responses to life-threatening illness.	★Affirm nurses' commitment to holistic practice. ★Emphasize the value of spirituality and culture in providing end of life care.	★Act in accordance with the patients' and families' spiritual and cultural values and wishes.	★Incorporate spiritual and cultural care in nursing practice.	★Role model and expect of others spiritually and culturally competent care for patients and families.	★Write a position paper about the role of spirituality and culture in providing nursing care.
The Spiritual Nature of the Person	★Value and support the spirituality of human beings. ★Appreciate the needs of the dying to make peace with life and death.		★Provide spiritually competent care to patients and families experiencing life threatening illness by considering spiritual well-being.	★Create an environment in which the spiritual nature of people is recognized, valued, and supported. ★Assist patients and families to find a source of spiritual energy or reaffirm students'/ nurses'/spiritual focus.	★Based on the spiritual assessment of a particular patient and family, develop a spiritual plan of care. Review the plan of care with clergy/chaplain.

(continued)

EDUCATION PLAN 1.1 *(continued)*

Knowledge Needed	Attitude	Skills	Undergraduate Behavioral Outcomes	Graduate Behavioral Outcomes	Teaching/Learning Strategies
Suffering as a Human Condition —Reciprocal suffering of patients and family; —Care of those who are suffering.	*Acknowledge suffering as a multidimensional experience. *Recognize that suffering may be personal or experienced as witness to another's suffering. *Appreciate that suffering and pain are not identical. *Consider the effect of suffering on health and quality of life of patients, families, and health care providers.	*Demonstrate therapeutic use of self in alleviating suffering.	*Assist patients and family to identify the meaning of suffering and refer to members of other disciplines as appropriate.	*Assess the impact of suffering on patient, family, health care providers, and community. *Implement the role of nurse as a coach in caring for those who are suffering. *Support patients and family in achieving some transcendent meaning to their suffering.	*Based on a case study, identify the dimensions of suffering and nursing strategies to alleviate suffering.

| Spiritual and religious perspectives of death: —Jewish —Roman Catholic —Protestant —Eastern —No conventional religious beliefs —Research regarding spirituality | *Appreciate varying spiritual and religious perspectives of death. *Value research in informing spiritual care. | *Demonstrate sensitivity to spiritual and religious beliefs and customs. | *Develop a plan of care with the patient and family that addresses their spiritual and religious perspectives on death and associated needs. *Critique and utilize research in guiding spiritual caregiving. | *Address conflicts that result from differences in spiritual and religious perspectives on death of patients, families, and health care providers. *Participate in conducting research regarding spirituality and health-related outcomes. | *Role play as a way of learning about different spiritual/religious beliefs and values in a nonjudgmental way. Self-critique attitudes and interaction followed by feedback from faculty and peers. *Critique five research articles related to spiritual or religious beliefs and health care issues. Synthesize the findings and discuss the implications for nursing practice. |

(continued)

EDUCATION PLAN 1.1   *(continued)*

Knowledge Needed	Attitude	Skills	Undergraduate Behavioral Outcomes	Graduate Behavioral Outcomes	Teaching/Learning Strategies
					*Distribute 3 × 5 cards and ask the students what happens at the time of death on side one and how that belief serves them on side two of the card. Ask the students to pass the card to another student. They are to take on the belief of the other student as their own. They are now asked how this new belief may benefit them.

Quality Nursing Care: Addressing Spiritual Needs of Patients and Families: —Spiritual caregiving —Spiritual assessment —Spiritual interventions and care —Educating nurses and physicians regarding spirituality.	*Recognize students'/nurses' own spiritual and religious beliefs and values. *Value nurses' presence, compassion, and hopefulness in providing quality spiritual care. *Appreciate the role of chaplains and clergy in offering spiritual care.	*Convey unconditional acceptance of patients and families of diverse spiritual and religious beliefs and backgrounds. *Demonstrate the completion of a spiritual history/assessment.	*Create an environment that nurtures the the patient's exploration of spiritual needs and concerns. *Address patients' and families' spiritual and religious needs through presencing, active listening, unconditional regard, and support of meaningful rituals.	*Identify patients and family who are at risk for spiritual distress. *Develop a comprehensive plan of care to alleviate spiritual suffering. *Education other health care in providing spiritually competent care.	*Write a position statement identifying students'/nurses' personal beliefs and assumptions as it relates to spirituality or religiosity. *Conduct a values clarification exercise for students/nurses to identify their own spiritual values. *Discuss the role of clergy as members of the interdisciplinary team in post-conference or seminar. *Discuss illustrative cases where patient's spirituality or religiosity negatively affected their health outcomes and potential spiritual interventions.

(continued)

EDUCATION PLAN 1.1 *(continued)*

Knowledge Needed	Attitude	Skills	Undergraduate Behavioral Outcomes	Graduate Behavioral Outcomes	Teaching/Learning Strategies
Cultural Perspectives Regarding Illness and Death: —Native American; —African and African American; —Hispanic; —Asian; —Cultural values underlying advanced directives and medical decision making; —Research regarding culture and end of life issues.	*Appreciate varying cultural perspectives of death. *Value research in informing cultural care.	*Demonstrate sensitivity to cultural beliefs and customs.	*Develop a plan of care with the patient and family that addresses their cultural perspectives on death and cultural needs. *Critique and utilize research in guiding culturally competent care.	*Address conflicts that result from differences in cultural perspectives on death of patients, families, and health care providers. *Participate in conducting research regarding culture and health-related outcomes.	*Have students interview two individuals of diverse cultural backgrounds and compare beliefs, values, expectations and traditions related to illness and death. Compare the information obtained from information written in textbooks or journal articles. Share findings in class. *Critique five research articles related to cultural beliefs and health care issues. Synthesize the findings and discuss the implications for nursing practice.

Quality Nursing Care: Addressing Cultural Needs of Patients and their Families —Nurses' Cultural Self-Awareness and Development of Cultural Competency —Cultural Assessment and Interventions.	*Recognize students'/nurses' own cultural beliefs and values.	*Convey unconditional acceptance of patients and families of various cultural backgrounds. *Demonstrate the completion of a cultural assessment.	*Create an environment which supports cultural beliefs, values, traditions, and rituals.	*Develop a comprehensive plan of care which takes into account cultural values, needs, and expectation. *Educate other health care providers in providing culturally competent care.	*In post-conference or seminar, encourage students to express feelings of appreciation regarding their own cultural heritage while introducing the topic of ethnocentrism in connection with the value of cultural diversity. *Have students identify who was significant in teaching or transmitting to them their cultural identity and discuss the impact of their identity on their present life. *Have students identify how members of their cultural group approach personal or emotional problems.

(continued)

EDUCATION PLAN 1.1   *(continued)*

Knowledge Needed	Attitude	Skills	Undergraduate Behavioral Outcomes	Graduate Behavioral Outcomes	Teaching/Learning Strategies
					*In the clinical setting, conduct a cultural assessment of a patient/family and report findings in post-conference or seminar. *In post-conference or seminar, create and discuss a list of behaviors or comments which may be viewed as culturally insensitive based on past, personal, or professional experiences. Role play compassionate and effective communication regarding cultural issues relevant to palliative care.

| Nurses' Needs for Self-Reflection and Self-Healing in Palliative Care. | ★Affirm nurses' right to be respected for their belief systems. ★Acknowledge students'/nurses' personal potential for providing spiritual and and cultural care. ★Appreciate the potential drain of energy and resurfacing of personal spiritual issues related to care giving. | ★Develop an awareness of students'/nurses' own spiritual, emotional, and physical limits. ★Establish a personal plan of care for maintaining health and promoting personal and professional growth. | ★Assess colleagues at risk for caregiving burnout. ★Advocate for systems that support students'/nurses' self-care and personal and professional growth. | ★Write a personal plan of care to address the students'/nurses' physical, emotional, social, and spiritual needs, and strategies to promote personal and professional growth within the next 6 months. ★Create a suggestion box and contribute one recommended change, which would support the nurses' caregiving potential within the educational setting. |

(continued)

EDUCATION PLAN 1.1 *(continued)*

Knowledge Needed	Attitude	Skills	Undergraduate Behavioral Outcomes	Graduate Behavioral Outcomes	Teaching/Learning Strategies
					*Discuss in the classroom, post-conference, or seminar ways in which students/nurses have been able to provide spiritual care and the responses of the individual and family. *Beginning with a 5 minute relaxation exercise, have students/nurses write a poem asking a transcendent life force for support. Have each student/nurse read their poem, twice slowly.

REFERENCES

Abrums, M. (2000). Death and meaning in a storefront church. *Public Health Nursing, 17*(2), 132–142.

Albuagh, J. (2003). Spirituality and life-threatening illness: A phenomenologic study. *Oncology Nursing Forum, 30,* 593–598.

American Medical Student Association. (2001). Cultural competency in medicine. Retrieved from http://www.amsa.org/programs/gpit/cultural

Arnold, E. (1989). Burnout as a spiritual issue: Rediscovering meaning in nursing practice. In V. Carson (Ed.), *Spiritual dimensions of nursing practice* (pp. 320–353). Philadelphia: Saunders.

Beeney, L., Butow, P., & Dunn, S. (1997). Normal adjustment to cancer: Characteristics and assessment. In R. K. Portenoy & E. Bruera (Eds.), *Topics in palliative care: Vol. 1* (pp. 213–244). New York: Oxford University Press.

Bhungalia, S., & Kemp, C. (2002). (Asian) Indian health beliefs and practices related to end of life. *Journal of Hospice and Palliative Nursing, 4*(1), 54–58.

Bird, L. (1986). Suffering, thanatology, and whole-person medicine. In R. DeBellis, E. Marcus, A. Kutscher, C. Smith Torres, V. Barrett, & M. Siegel (Eds.), *Suffering: Psychological and social aspects in loss, grief, and care* (pp. 31–39). New York: Haworth Press.

Blackhall, L., Murphy, S., Frank, G., Michel, V., & Azen, S. (1995). Ethnicity and attitudes toward patient autonomy. *Journal of the American Medical Association, 274,* 820–825.

Born, W., Greiner, A., Sylvia, E., Butler, J., & Ahuwalia, J. (2004). Knowledge, attitudes, and beliefs about end of life care among inner-city African Americans and Latinos. *Journal of Palliative Medicine, 7,* 247–256.

Brokenleg, M., & Middleton, D. (1993). Native Americans: Adapting, yet retaining. In D. Irish, K. Lundquist, & V. Nelsen (Eds.) *Ethnic variations in dying, death, and grief* (pp. 101–112). Philadelphia: Taylor & Francis.

Burkhardt, M. A. (1989). Spirituality: An analysis of the concept. *Holistic Nursing Practice, 3*(3), 69–75.

Caralis, P. V., Davis, B., Wright, K., & Marcial, E. (1993). The influence of ethnicity and race on attitudes towards advance directives, life-prolonging treatments, and euthanasia. *Journal of Clinical Ethics, 4,* 155–165.

Carson, V. B. (1989). *Spiritual dimensions of nursing practice.* Philadelphia: Saunders.

Cassell, E. (1982). The nature of suffering and the goals of medicine. *New England Journal of Medicine, 306,* 639–645.

Conrad, N. L. (1985). Spiritual support for the dying. *Nursing Clinics of North America, 20,* 415–425.

Corr, C., Nabe, C., & Corr, D. (2003). *Death and dying; life and living.* CA: Brooks/Cole.

Cort, M. (2004). Cultural mistrust and use of hospice care: Challenges and remedies. *Journal of Palliative Medicine, 7*(1), 63–71.

Cousins, N. (1979). *Anatomy of an illness.* New York: Norton.

Coyle, N. (1995). Suffering in the first person. In B. R. Ferrell (Ed.), *Suffering* (pp. Sudbury, MA: Jones and Bartlett.

Crawley, L., Marshall, P., Lo, B., & Koenig, B. (2002). Strategies for culturally effective end of life care. *Annals of Internal Medicine, 136,* 673–679.

Davies, B., Reimer, J., & Marten, N. (1994). Family functioning and its implications for palliative care. *Journal of Palliative Care, 10,* 35–36.

DeBellis, R., Marcus, E., Kutscher, A., Smith Torres, C., Barrett, V., & Siegel, M. (1986). *Suffering: Psychological and social aspects in loss, grief, and care.* New York: Haworth Press.

DeSpelder, L. (1998). Developing cultural competency. In K. Doka & J. Davidson (Eds.), *Living with grief* (pp. 97–106). Washington, DC: Hospice Foundation of America.

DeSpelder, L., & Strickland, A. (1999). *The last dance: Encountering death and dying.* Mountain View, CA: Mayfield.

Doka, K. (1993). The spiritual needs of the dying. In K. Doka & J. Morgan (Eds.), *Death and spirituality* (pp. 143–150). Amityville, NY: Baywood.

Doka, K., & Davidson, J. (1998). *Living with grief.* Philadelphia: Hospice Foundation of America.

Doka, K., & Morgan, J. (1993). *Death and spirituality.* Amityville, NY: Baywood.

Dombeck, M. B. (1995). Dream telling: A means of spiritual awareness. *Holistic Nursing Practice, 9*(2), 37–47.

Doorenbos, A., & Schim, S. (2004). Cultural competence in hospice. *American Journal of Hospice and Palliative Care, 21*(1), 28–32.

Doyle, D. (1994). *Caring for a dying relative: A guide for families.* New York: Oxford University Press.

Driscoll, J. (1999, March). *Chaplain-physician partnerships.* Paper presented at the Harvard University Spirituality and Healing Conference, Denver, CO.

Driscoll, J. (2001). Spirituality and religion in end of life care. *Journal of Palliative Medicine, 4,* 333–335.

Dunn, K., and Harzas, A. (2000). The prevalence of prayer as a spiritual self-care modality of elders. *Journal of Holistic Nursing, 18(4),* 337–351.

End of Life Nursing Education Consortium (ELNEC) (2001). *Module 5: Cultural considerations.* City of Hope Medical Center and American Association of Colleges of Nursing. Available from the American Association of Colleges of Nursing: www.aacn.nche.edu/elnec.

Ersek, M., Kagawa-Singer, M., Barnes, D., Blackhall, L., & Koenig, B. (1998). Multicultural considerations in the use of advance directives. *Oncology Nursing Forum, 25,* 1683–1689.

Ferris, F., & Cummings, I. (1995). *Palliative care: Towards a consensus in standardized principles of practice.* Ottawa, Ontario: Canadian Palliative Care Association.

Foley, K. (1995). Pain, physician-assisted suicide, and euthanasia. *Pain Forum, 4,* 163–176.

Fricchione, G. L. (1999, March). *Spirituality and healing at the bedside.* Paper presented at the Harvard University Spirituality and Healing Conference, Denver, CO.

Gallop, G. (1990). *Religion in America.* Princeton, NJ: Princeton Religion and Research Center.

Gallop, G. (1997). *Spiritual beliefs and the dying process. A national survey conducted for the Nathan Cummings Foundation and the Fetzer Institute.* New York: Nathan Cummings Foundation.

Grollman, E. (1993). Death in Jewish thought. In K. Doka & J. Morgan (Eds.), *Death and spirituality* (pp. 21–32). Amityville, NY: Baywood.

Halifax, J. (1999, October). *Being with dying: Contemplations on death and dying.* Presentation at the Art of Dying III Conference: Spiritual, Scientific and Practical Approaches to Living and Dying by the New York Open Center and Tibet House, New York, NY.

Hermann, C. (2000). A guide to the spiritual needs of elderly cancer patients. *Geriatric Nursing, 21,* 324–325.

Highfield, M. (2000). Providing spiritual care to patients with cancer. *Clinical Journal of Oncology Nursing. 4(3),* 115–120.

Higginson, I. J. (1998). Introduction: Defining the unit of care: Who are we supporting and how? In E. Bruera & R. K. Portenoy (Eds.), *Topics in palliative care: Vol. 2* (pp. 205–207). New York: Oxford University Press.

Irish, D., Lundquist, K., & Nelsen, V. (1993). *Ethnic variations in dying, death, and grief.* Philadelphia: Taylor & Francis.

Johnson, P. (2002). The use of humor and its influences on spirituality and coping in breast cancer survivors. *Oncology Nursing Forum, 29,* 691–695.

Kagawa-Singer, M. (1998). The cultural context of death rituals and mourning practices. *Oncology Nursing Forum, 25,* 1752–1756.

Kagawa-Singer, M., & Blackhall, L. (2001). Negotiating cross-cultural issues at the end of life. *Journal of the American Medical Association, 286,* 2993–3001.

Kahn, D. L., & Steeves, R. (1996). An understanding of suffering grounded in clinical practice and research. In B. R. Ferrell (Ed.), *Suffering* (pp. 3–27). Sudbury, MA: Jones and Bartlett.

Kaldjian, L. C. (1998). End of life decisions in HIV-positive patients: The role of spiritual beliefs. *AIDS, 12*(1), 103–107.

Kemp, C., & Chang, B. (2002). Culture and the end of life: Chinese. *Journal of Hospice and Palliative Nursing, 4,* 173–177.

Klass, D. (1993). Spirituality, Protestantism, and death. In K. Doka & J. Morgan (Eds.), *Death and spirituality* (pp. 51–73). Amityville, NY: Baywood.

Klass, D., & Goss, R. (1998). Asian ways of grief. In K. Doka & J. Davidson (Eds.), *Living with grief* (pp. 13–26). Philadelphia: Hospice Foundation of America.

Klein, S. J. (1998). *Heavenly hurts: Surviving AIDS-related deaths and losses.* New York: Baywood.

Klessig, J. (1992). The effects of values and culture on life support decisions. *Western Journal of Medicine, 163,* 316–322.

Koenig, H. G. (1998). Religious coping and health status in medically ill hospitalized older adults. *Journal of Nervous Mental Disease, 186,* 513–518.

Koenig, H. G. (1999, March). *The healing power of faith: When serious illness strikes.* Paper presented at the Harvard University Spirituality and Healing Conference, Denver, CO.

Koenig, H. G. (2002). An 83-year old woman with chronic illness and strong religious beliefs. *Journal of the American Medical Association, 288,* 487–493.

Koenig, H. G., Cohen, H. J., Blazer, D., Pieper, C., Meador, K., Shelp, G., et al. (1992). Religious coping and depression among hospitalized elderly medically ill men. *American Journal of Psychiatry, 149,* 1693–1700.

Lederberg, M. (1998). The family of the cancer patient. In J. Holland (Ed.), *Psychooncology* (pp. 981–993). New York: Oxford University Press.

Lipson, J., Dibble, S., & Minarik, P. A. (1996). *Culture and nursing care: A pocket guide.* St. Louis, MO: Mosby.

Lo, B., Uston, D., Kates, L., Arnold, R., Cohen, C., Faber-Langendoen, K. et al. (2002). Discussing religious and spiritual issues at the end of life: A practical guide for physicians. *Journal of the American Medical Association, 287,* 749–754.

Loscalzo, M., & Zabora, J. (1998). Care of the cancer patient: Response of family and staff. In E. Bruera & R. K. Portenoy (Eds.), *Topics in palliative care: Vol. 2* (pp. 209–246). New York: Oxford University Press.

Lowe, J., & Struthers, R. (2001). A conceptual framework of nursing in Native American culture. *Journal of Nursing Scholarship, 33,* 279–283.

Macrae, J. (1999, March). *Nursing with emphasis on Florence Nightingale.* Paper presented at the Harvard University Spirituality and Healing Conference, Denver, CO.

Martinez, R. (1995). *Close friends of God: An ethnography of health of older Hispanic people.* Unpublished doctoral dissertation, University of Colorado.

Matthews, D. (1999, March). *The faith factor: Is religion good for your health.* Paper presented at the Harvard University Spirituality and Healing Conference, Denver, CO.

McGann, J. (1997). *Comfort my people: Finding peace as life ends.* Rockville Center, New York: Long Island Catholic.

McGrath, P., Vun, M., and McLeod, L. (2001). Needs and experiences of non-English speaking hospice patients and families in an English speaking country. *American Journal of Hospice and Palliative Care, 18(5),* 305–312.

Meraviglia, M. (2004). The effects of spirituality on well-being of people with lung cancer. *Oncology Nursing Forum, 31(1),* 89–94.

Miller, E. (1993). A Roman Catholic view of death. In K. Doka & J. Morgan (Eds.), *Death and spirituality* (pp. 33–49). Amityville, NY: Baywood.

Moberg, D. O. (1984). Subjective measures for spiritual well-being. *Review of Religious Research, 25,* 351–364.

Moore, T. (1992). *Care of the soul: A guide for cultivating depth and sacredness in everyday life.* New York: Harper-Collins.

Munley, A. (1983). *The hospice alternative.* New York: Basic Books.

Musgrave, C., & McFarlane, E. (2004). Israeli oncology nurses' religiosity, spiritual well-being, and attitudes toward spiritual care: A path analysis. *Oncology Nursing Forum, 31,* 321–327.

Nathan Cummings Foundation. (1999 February 12). Spiritual beliefs and the dying process: Key findings. Retrieved from http://www.ncf.org/ncf/publications/reports/fetzer/fetzer_keyfindings.html

National Organization of Nurse Practitioner Faculties. (2000). *Cultural guidelines.* Washington, DC: Author.

O'Connor, P. (1993). A clinical paradigm for exploring spiritual concerns. In K. Doka & J. Morgan (Eds.), *Death and spirituality* (pp. 133–150). Amityville, NY: Baywood.

O'Neill, D., & Kenny, E. (1998). Spirituality and chronic illness. *Image: Journal of Nursing Scholarship, 30,* 275–279.

Orion, P. (1993). Spiritual issues in death and dying for those who do not have conventional religious beliefs. In K. Doka & J. Morgan (Eds.), *Death and spirituality* (pp. 93–112). Amityville, NY: Baywood.

Poloma, M. M., & Pendleton, B. F. (1989). Exploring types of prayer and quality of life. *Review of Religious Research, 31(1),* 46–53.

Puchalski, C. (1998a). Facing death with dignity. *The World and I, 3,* 34–39.

Puchalski, C. (1998b). FICA: A spiritual assessment. Unpublished manuscript.

Puchalski, C. (2001). Spirituality and health: The art of compassionate medicine. *Hospital Physician, 37(3),* 30–36.

Puchalski, C. (2002). Spirituality and end of life care: A time for listening and caring. *Journal of Palliative Medicine, 5,* 289–294.

Puchalski, C., & Larson, D. (1998). Developing curricula in spirituality and medicine. *Academic Medicine, 73,* 970–974.

Purdy, W. (2002). Spiritual discernment in palliative care. *Journal of Palliative Medicine, 5,* 139–141.

Rando, T. (1984). *Grief, dying, and death: Clinical interventions for caregivers.* Champaign, IL: Research Press.

Roberts, J. A. (1997). Coping with gynecologic cancer. *American Journal of Obstetrics and Gynecology, 176,* 166–172.

Rosenblatt, P. (1993). Cross-cultural variation in the experience, expression, and understanding of grief. In D. Irish, K. Lundquist, & V. Nelsen (Eds.), *Ethnic variations in dying, death and grief* (pp. 13–19). Philadelphia: Taylor & Francis.

Ryan, D. (1993). Death: Eastern perspectives. In K. Doka & J. Morgan (Eds.), *Death and spirituality* (pp. 75–92). Amityville, NY: Baywood.

Ryan, S. (1997). Chaplains are more than what chaplains do. *Visions, (3)7,* 8–9.

Schroeder-Sheker, T. (1999, October). *I die awake: The luminous wound.* Presentation at the Art of Dying III Conference: Spiritual,

Scientific and Practical Approaches to Living and Dying by the New York Open Center and Tibet House, New York, NY.

Sherman, D. W. (1998). Reciprocal suffering: The need to improve family caregiver's quality of life through palliative care. *Journal of Palliative Medicine, 1,* 357–366.

Sherman, D. W. (2004a). Cultural and spiritual backgrounds of older adults: Considerations for quality palliative care. In M. L. Matzo & D. W. Sherman (Eds.), *Gerontological palliative care nursing* (pp. 3–30). St. Louis, MO: Mosby.

Sherman, D. W. (2004b). Nurses' stress & burnout: How to care for yourself when caring for patients and their families experiencing life-threatening illness. *American Journal of Nursing, 104*(5), 48–57.

Showalter, S. (1998). Looking through different eyes: Beyond cultural diversity. In K. Doka & J. Davidson (Eds.), *Living with grief* (pp. 71–82). Washington, DC: Hospice Foundation of America.

Smith, R. (1996). Theological perspectives. In B. R. Ferrell (Ed.), *Suffering* (pp. 159–171). Sudbury, MA: Jones and Bartlett.

Spross, J. (1996). Coaching and suffering: The role of the nurse in helping people face illness. In B. R. Ferrell (Ed.), *Suffering* (pp. 173–208). Sudbury, MA: Jones and Bartlett.

Sulmasy, D. (1997). *The healer's calling: A spirituality for physicians and other health care professionals.* New York: Paulist Press.

Taylor, E. J. (2003). Nurses caring for the spirit: Patients with cancer and family caregiver expectations. *Oncology Nursing Forum, 30,* 585–590.

Taylor, E. J. (2003, July/August). Prayer's clinical issues and implications. *Holistic Nursing Practice,* 179–188.

Taylor, E., & Outlaw, F. (2002). Use of prayer among persons with cancer. *Holistic Nursing Practice, 16*(3), 46–60.

Thorson, J. A., & Powell, F. C. (1992). Meanings of death and intrinsic religiosity. *Journal of Clinical Psychology, 46,* 379–391.

Urdang, L. (1972). *Random House college dictionary.* New York: Random House.

Watson, J. (1986). Suffering and the quest for meaning. In R. DeBellis, E. Marcus, A. Kutscher, C. Smith Torres, V. Barrett, & M. Siegel (Eds.), *Suffering: Psychological and social aspects in loss, grief, and care* (pp. 175–187). New York: Haworth Press.

Weaver, J. Flannelly, L., & Flannelly, K. (2001). A review of research on religious and spiritual values in two primary gerontological journals. *Journal of Gerontological Nursing, 27*(9), 47–54.

Wink, P. (1999). Addressing end of life issues: Spirituality and inner life. *Generations, 23*(1), 75–80.

Winslow, G., & Winslow, B. (2003, July/August). Examining the ethics of praying with patients. *Holistic Nursing Practice,* 170–177.

2

Holistic Integrative Therapies in Palliative Care

Carla Mariano

AACN Competency

#9: Evaluate the impact of traditional, complementary, and technological therapies on patient-centered outcomes.

> *The greatest discovery of any generation is that human beings can alter their lives by altering the attitudes of their minds.*
> —Albert Schweitzer

This chapter introduces the reader to a variety of holistic modalities that are used in nursing practice today and that can be used in palliative care. The modalities are defined and shown where they are most useful. In addition, this chapter includes a section on exercises that can be used readily by nurses and incorporated into their practice. It also includes resources where more information on each of these modalities can be obtained. In the education of nurses, it is particularly important for nursing faculty to incorporate these healing modalities into the curriculum for both undergraduate and graduate-level students.

Holism focuses on unity, mutuality, meaning, and the interrelationship of all beings, events, and things. The words heal and health come from *haelan*, which means to be or become whole. Holism emphasizes the basic wholeness and integrity of the individual. It views the body, mind, emotion, and spirit as inseparable and interdependent. All behaviors, including health, illness, and dying are manifestations of the life process of the whole person (Quinn, 1995).

Holistic nursing care draws on nursing knowledge, theories, expertise, and intuition as nurses and clients become therapeutic partners in a shared evolving process toward healing. Holistic care

- believes that people can grow and learn from health, illness, and dying;
- promotes clients' active participation in their own health care, wellness, and healing;
- uses appropriate interventions in the context of the client's total needs;
- works to alleviate clients' physical signs and symptoms; and
- concentrates on the underlying meanings of symptoms and illness events, and changes in the clients' life patterns and perceptions. (Mariano, 1998)

Numerous modalities are used in the provision of holistic care. Some of these that are particularly useful in end-of-life care are discussed in a subsequent section of this chapter. Nurses can practice holistic care in any setting where healing occurs.

"Healing the dying sounds like an oxymoron. . . . But to heal is not necessarily to cure. . . . To heal is to bring various levels of oneself—cellular, physical, intrapersonal, interpersonal, societal, spiritual, perhaps even cosmic—into new relationship with each other" (Olson, 2001, p. 3). The nurse must assess the relationship of the individual who is dying with self, others, a higher power, and provide appropriate interventions to assist in the development or maintenance of new or right relationships.

"Dying healed means that a person has finished the business of life, said good goodbyes, and reached life's goals. An individual knows who he is, and has a sense of integration of self and life" (Olson, 2001, p. 3). She or he realizes that one's life was unique and one's death matters to someone. One looks inward and realizes that life's difficulties have created a certain wisdom. Significant others have had time to grieve and plan for changes, and comfort and peace are attained. Control of the dying process is maintained as long as possible by the individual and as much as possible as the person is willing. Dying is seen as a stage of life. It is part of a larger philosophy and perception in which both life and death have meaning.

As mentioned previously, healing the dying necessitates regard for relationships and connectedness. We speak of transcendence when implying a sense of connectedness between self and a greater reality. Transcendence "integrates self with past and future, giving meaning to life. It is a set of introspective activities that reflect concern for others or for meaning" (Olson, 1997, p. 128). Many of the integrative modalities described in this chapter facilitate self-transcendence. As noted by Olson (1997), positive outcomes for the self-transcendent person, even when nearing death, include less depression, neglect, and hopelessness; a greater sense of well-being and ability to cope with grief and death; and the ability to live and find meaning in the present and connect with a higher power.

This caring relationship emphasizes quality rather than length of life. Healing the dying includes palliative care, and focuses on relationships of all kinds. There is the provision for opportunities and choices where the dying person can live life to its fullest, and at some point comfortably forgive, let go, release, and experience a peaceful death.

The nurse is in a partnership with the dying client, sharing rather than denying the experience. The focus of nursing care is on providing sacred space and the milieu for a calm and peaceful death. The nurse works with the client to foster hope and cultivate an appreciation of the seemingly irrelevant things in life. Learning to appreciate simple occurrences such as a sunset or the joys of life can cultivate a more positive view of life and one's present experience. Enhancing avenues of support, whether professional, social (family and friends), or support groups, can often facilitate grieving and increase a sense of meaning in illness. Developing unrecognized inner strengths and resources is of great importance to the person who is dying or grieving.

The Chinese symbol for crisis indicates that crisis offers an opportunity for growth and a different perspective. Grief can serve as a building block for personal growth and healing. Asking the dying person about spiritual needs gives the client an occasion to verbalize unmet needs. All of this requires skill, knowledge, compassion, caring, anticipation and organization on the part of the nurse, as well as a willingness to face one's own impermanence and mortality. It also necessitates caring for oneself.

SPECIFIC HOLISTIC HEALING MODALITIES

Holism is the theoretical and philosophical foundation for alternative/complementary integrative healing modalities. Numerous kinds of these modalities are used in health care today. This chapter will cover only a few of those that are most useful in end-of-life care. Many of these modalities can be used effectively by the nurse as well as the client, for example, centering, relaxation, imagery, meditation, prayer, herbology, and homeopathy. Others are described in use with clients, such as sense therapies, reminiscence and life review, touch, and Reiki. In addition to their calming influence and physiological benefits, these techniques also may alter the perception of pain. Another valuable aspect of these modalities is that their use can empower clients and families. When clients learn to heal themselves, they are empowered. When they learn these techniques, they can do it themselves, which oftentimes gives them a sense of control (Mariano, 2004). And when families are taught to use these modalities, they feel as if they are contributing something to the care of their loved ones.

Centering

Centering is a process by which one quiets the mind and focuses one's thoughts. It calms the mind and allows the practitioner to access inmost resources that are powerful forces in healing. Krieger (1997) notes that

> Being on-center does not mean being still, immobile, rigid. . . . In centering, we are quiet and 'listen' to another language. Our attention goes to the heart region, where we find our own center of peace and know it as an attribute of our true self. We find that this sense of deep serenity is reminiscent to the truer

peace we find in untrammeled nature and, with a thrill of personal discovery, realize that it is through such profound natural experiences that we can be at-one with the universe. (p. 22)

Centering is a shift in consciousness, an integrated sense of being. Bodily movements become quieted, and yet one is in an actively conscious state. One feels a unique stillness and peace. There is a sense of inner equilibrium and well-being. Perception deepens and one is less aware of the chaos of the moment, the day, and the mind's chatter. Practice in the act of centering (closing eyes, quieting one's mind and activities, focusing on one's center or inner peace) leads to intuition and inner wisdom (Krieger, 1997, 2002).

By remaining "on-center," the nurse is able to convey to the client an awareness, a sensitivity, an empathy and deep sense of peace and regard that often creates a relaxation response in the client. One must give oneself permission to center, as the environment is always calling us to be present for it rather than for ourselves. But when one is centered and personally present, compassion becomes real and this state is needed for those who would facilitate healing. One important exercise that the nurse can practice is to center before entering into each client encounter—detaching from any prior encounter, to approach each client with awareness and with, as Carl Rogers says, "unconditional positive regard" (Laurant & Shlien, 1984).

Relaxation

Relaxation is a state where there is an absence of physical, mental, and emotional tension. A pleasant sensation and the lack of stressful or uncomfortable thoughts also accompany relaxation. It is often referred to as the opposite of the fight-or-flight response.

Relaxation makes it possible to quiet the body/mind and focus inward. One learns to retreat mentally from one's surroundings, still thoughts, relax muscles, and maintain the state of relaxation . . . to reap the benefits of decreased tension, anxiety, and pain. Regardless of the approach [use of meditation, yoga, muscle and breathing exercises, hypnosis, prayer, and other forms of stress management], the end result is a movement of the person toward balance and healing. (Kolkmeier, 1995, p. 575)

Relaxation techniques are the basis of many holistic modalities.

Relaxation has three aims (Payne, 2001): (1) as a prevention to protect body organs from unnecessary stress and wear; (2) as a treatment to alleviate stress in numerous conditions, for example, hypertension, tension headache, insomnia, asthma, immune deficiency, panic, pain; and (3) as a coping skill to calm the mind and to help thinking become more clear and effective. Positive information in memory also becomes more accessible when a person is relaxed.

There are numerous benefits to the relaxed state, including lowered blood pressure, decreased heat rate, increased body temperature, decreased anxiety associated with painful situations, easing of muscle tension pain such as in contractures, a general sense of intense calm, decreased symptoms of depression and stress, decreasing fatigue. Other benefits include helping the client to sleep, increasing the effects of medications, improvements in side effects of cancer therapy (decreased nausea, vomiting, and anxiety) and AIDS therapy, assisting in preparation for surgery or other treatments, and helping to dissociate from pain (Freeman, 2004; Payne, 2001). In addition to the therapeutic benefits, relaxation techniques also give clients a sense of control by enabling them to bring about certain psychological and mental responses by themselves.

Payne (2000), Anselmo (2005), and Lawson and Horneffer (2002) provide excellent guidelines for the nurse in preparing the client for relaxation and actual scripts to guide one through various relaxation exercises. Table 2.1 includes guidelines or key points for relaxation.

Imagery

Imagining is a powerful technique of focusing and directing the imagination. One uses all the senses—vision, sound, smell, taste, movement, position, and touch. Imagery influences an individual's attitudes, feelings, behaviors, and anxiety, which can either lead to a sense of hopelessness or promote a perception of well-being that assists in changing opinions about disease, treatment, and healing potential. "Imagery [is the] internal experience of memories, dreams, fantasies, and visions—sometimes involving one, several, or all the senses that serve as the bridge for connecting body, mind, and spirit" (Schaub & Dossey, 2005, p. 567). Imagery can affect people physically, emotionally, mentally, and biochemically, and the body and mind respond as if the event is actually occurring.

Guided imagery and interactive guided imagery (having the client directly interact with the image) are techniques to access the imagination through a guide. There are numerous types of imagery (Schaub & Dossey, 2005):

- Receptive imagery (inner knowing or "bubble-up" images)
- Active imagery (a focus on the conscious formation of an image)
- Correct biological imagery (recognizing the impact of negative images on physiology and creating positive correct biological images)
- Symbolic imagery (images emerging from both the unconscious and conscious that shape attitudes, belief sys-

TABLE 2.1   Guidelines for Relaxation

Be familiar with the relaxation exercise before introducing it to the client.

Encourage use of familiar relaxation techniques that the client knows.

Assess the client's level of tension, level of readiness to learn to relax, pain, anxiety, fear, and perception of reality or history of depersonalization.

Ask the client what it means for him/her to be relaxed.

Assess the client's ability to remain comfortably in one position for 10–20 minutes. Decrease as much environmental stimuli as possible.

Assist the client to develop a positive expectation of what is to occur. Describe the potential benefits of relaxation and enlist cooperation.

Reduce the opportunity for self-blame if the session does not go as expected.

Have the client close his or her eyes

Use a tone of voice that is quiet and calm, conversational at first, and decreasing in volume as the session goes on.

Use either tapes or a live voice. Music can provide background if desired.

Guide the client through a basic breathing exercise (see Exercises section).

Phrase all suggestions in a positive form, e.g., "*Let go* of your tension," "Feel the tightness *melting away*," "*Loosen and soften* your muscles," "Allow the tension to *drift* away."

Clients may experience a release of emotion as they relax such as tears, vomiting, or faster and more shallow breathing. Gently ask if the client can put words to those feelings. Allow time for expression before continuing.

At the completion of the session, bring the client gradually back to reality by having the client take deep breaths, move the hands and feet, and stretch if able.

Have the client evaluate the experience.

Engage the client's cooperation in continuing practice until the next session.

A basic breathing exercise and relaxation exercise that can be used with the client or by the nurse is found in the *Exercise* section of this chapter.

tems, and cultural experiences, often mythic symbols)

- Process imagery (a step-by-step rehearsal of any procedure, treatment, surgery, or other event prior to its occurrence)
- End-state imagery (rehearsal of an image of being in a final, healed state)
- General healing imagery (images that have a personal healing significance such as a wise person, an animal, the sun, etc.)
- Packaged imagery (another person's images such as commercial tapes)
- Customized imagery (images specific to an individual)

Guided imagery has many applications in end-of-life care, including relaxation, stress reduction, pain relief, symptom management, grief work, and assisting clients to comprehend meaning in their illness experience (Van Kuiken, 2004). It is useful not only in mobilizing latent, innate healing abilities of the client by intensifying the impact of healing messages that the autonomic nervous system sends to the immune system and other bodily functions, but also in the self-care of the nurse. It has been found helpful in relieving chronic pain and headaches, stimulating healing, tolerating medical procedures, exploring emotions that may have caused illness, solving difficult problems, envisioning and planning for the future, and listening to one's inner advisor.

It is usually helpful for the nurse to have training in the use of interactive guided imagery because of possibly overwhelming effects with this type of imagery (Rossman, 1999). Otherwise, as Schaub and Dossey (2005) note, imagery scripts are more effective when one learns the speaking skills of voice modulation, specific word emphasis, and the use of pauses. Guidelines for the nurse to use in teaching the client the imagery process are presented in Table 2.2.

Meditation

Meditation is a quiet turning inward. It is the practice of focusing one's attention internally to achieve clearer consciousness and inner stillness. There are numerous methods and schools of meditation, all having an individual interpretation of the practice. However, all methods believe in emptying the mind and letting go of the mind's chatter that preoccupies us.

Meditation originated in the Eastern tradition and is integral to Hinduism, Taoism, and Buddhism and is both a state of mind and a method. The state is one where the mind is quiet and listening to itself. The practitioner is relaxed but alert. The method involves the focusing of attention on something such as

---

TABLE 2.2   Guidelines to Imagery

Have the client relax. Help the client to identify the problem or goal of imagery.

Develop a basic understanding of the physiology involved in the healing process. Begin with a few minutes of relaxation, meditation, or paying attention to the breath exercise.

Assist the client to develop images of

—the problem

—inner healing resources (beliefs, coping strategies, etc.)

—external healing resources (medications, treatments, family, etc.)

End with images of the desired state of well-being.

Basic imagery exercises that nurses can use with clients are under the *Exercises* section of this chapter.

---

the breath, an image, a word, or action such as tai chi or qigong. There is a sustained concentration but it should be effortless.

The objective of meditation is to detach from external events as well as one's own mental activity. Rather than examining thoughts that may enter the mind, the person disregards them and allows them to drift away. There is no criticism or judgment, but an attitude of a beginner's mind: a mind that is open and receptive, clear of attachment to any thoughts. The body is relaxed and the mind is emptied of all thought except awareness of the image, word, or breath. "Passive concentration" keeps the meditator in a state of awareness and alertness rather than drowsiness, and intently focused on the present moment. There should be no blame, guilt, or recrimination if the meditator loses focus or if the mind wanders; one is instructed simply to return the mind to its original focus. Reentry into the normal waking state should be gentle and relaxed. Meditation requires practice on a regular schedule, usually once or twice daily to achieve maximal results.

There are various reasons for practicing meditation: to find peace, achieve awareness and enlightenment, find oneself, experience true reality, and enhance a sense of well-being. Research has demonstrated that relaxed forms of meditation decrease heart rate and blood pressure, increase breathing volume while decreasing the number of breaths per minute, increase peripheral blood flow, and improve immune function; decrease skeletal muscle tension, epinephrine level, gastric acidity, motility, anxiety, depression, traumatic stress, and alcohol and drug consumption (Anselmo, 2005; Bonadonna, 2003; Freeman, 2004; Gatchel & Maddrey, 1998; Gross et al., 2004). It is believed that meditation activates the right cerebral hemisphere and the parasympathetic nervous system, thereby quieting the nerves and allowing intuitive, wordless thinking to occur. In addition to physiological benefits, the advantages of meditation cited by Payne (2000) are listed in Table 2.3.

Sense Therapies

Sense therapies use the senses to treat physical and psychological problems and to adjust chemical or other imbalances within the body. These can include behavioral vision therapy, eye movement, desensitization, flower remedies, hydrotherapy, and light therapy. Two therapies will be explored under sense therapies: Music therapy and music thanatology, and aromatherapy.

Music Therapy and Music Thanatology

Guzzetta (2005) defines music therapy as the "behavioral science concerned with the systematic application of music to produce relaxation and desired changes in emotions, behavior, and physiology" (p. 617). The elements of music, sound, rhythm, hearing,

TABLE 2.3   Advantages of Meditation

A better understanding of the self and increased receptivity to insights arising from one's deeper being. Practicing meditation can bring the experience of self for the dying; where the individual may attain calm and often a sense of purpose.

A new sense of relaxation and inner peace.

A clearer mind and improved concentration.

More harmony with and within the self.

As a result of the detachment, an acceptance that many unpleasant emotional responses are short-lived sensations created by one's thoughts.

An emphasis on living in the present and valuing the here and now.

A simple meditation that can be practiced by the nurse or with a client is in the *Exercises* section of this chapter.

melody, harmony, and movement are part of people's primary experiences. Listening to, creating, or moving to music assists people in improving, changing, or better integrating aspects of themselves. Music has a power that cannot be expressed in verbal language.

There are references to the therapeutic powers of music in philosophy, art, and literature throughout the ages. Music is used in healing ceremonies throughout the world. Our own experiences demonstrates the psychological effect that music has on us. Despite varying musical tastes, certain types of music create specific moods, for example, a march, ominous music, lively music at sports events, quiet relaxing music in waiting rooms, or a mother's singing and rocking her baby in times of distress (a, Barrios-Chaplin, Atkinson, & Tomasino, 1998).

Music therapy can reduce biopsychological stress, pain, anxiety, and isolation. It assists clients in reaching a deep state of relaxation, developing self-awareness and creativity, improving learning, clarifying personal values, and coping with a variety of psychophysiological problems. It also provides clients with integrated body/mind episodes and encourages them to become active participants in their own healing. Appropriate music produces the relaxation response, often removing a client's inner restlessness and quieting ceaseless thinking. It is used as a healing technique to quiet the mind and bring about inner relaxation (Guzzetta, 2005). Research has demonstrated that music reduces acute and chronic pain (Freeman, 2004), is beneficial in treating or managing dementia symptoms (Koger & Brotons, 2000), reduces agitated behaviors in elderly individuals (Remington, 2002) and reduces pain and nausea (Sahlar, Hunter, & Liesveld, 2003).

Because music therapy focuses on process and not on outcome, one need not have any musical skills or talents to derive benefits. Frank-Schwebel (1999) recommends that clients be induced to a relaxed state through breathing, suggestive imagery, or a relaxation exercise. Music selected by the client or the nurse is played, and the client is invited to explore images, sensations, emotions, memories, and visions brought on by the music. No one type of music works well for all individuals in all situations. A variety of soothing selections (popular, New Age, classical, country, opera, folk, jazz, choral hymns, etc.) should be available because one cannot always predict a client's particular preference or response to the music. Often the client experiences an altered state of consciousness, which is usually very relaxing. After the listening, the client is brought back to reality to discuss the experience. In some instances, the client chooses the music and moves or paints to the music. The nurse should assess the factors described next in preparing to use music therapy (Guzzetta, 2005) as presented in Table 2.4.

Music has the greatest effect when the client is appropriately prepared. Find a quiet

TABLE 2.4   Assessment for Music Therapy

The client's music history and music preferences

The client's identification of music that make the client happy, excited, sad, or relaxed

The client's identification of music that is distasteful and that makes the client tense

Assessment of the importance of music in the client's life

The frequency of music playing in the client's life

Previous participation in relaxation/imagery techniques combined with music; the client's mood—this will determine the type of music to be played

environment and have the client assume a comfortable position. Suggest that the client maintain a passive attitude, neither forcing nor resisting the experience, and remind the client to focus all concentration on the music.

Music Thanatology

Music thanatology, developed by Therese Schroeder-Sheker (1994), is a relatively new field that addresses the needs of the dying by assisting the client in completing the transition between life and death. Specially trained therapists, using harp, voice, and chanting, assist the client in leave-taking during the last hours of life by reinforcing peace, acceptance, and a calm anticipation of death. Schroeder-Sheker (1994) describes music thanatology as a "palliative medical modality employing prescriptive music to tend the complex physical and spiritual needs of the dying . . . music thanatology is concerned with the possibility of a blessed death and the gift that conscious dying can bring to the fullness of life" (p. 83). This music is live (not taped), dynamic, and prescriptive. It is individual to each patient and each death, much like childbirth. According to Schroeder-Sheker, music-thanatology has been found to be most effective in deaths from cancer, AIDS, burns, and slowly degenerative diseases.

Schroeder-Sheker identifies six foundational assumptions of music thanatology:

1. A recognition of dying as a spiritual process and as an opportunity for growth.
2. The musical deathbed vigil, often called "musical-sacramental-midwifery," is a contemplative practice requiring serious inner work and integration of the physical, emotional, mental, and spiritual aspects of the caregiver.
3. Death is not an enemy and it is not a failure. It is a critical chapter of human biography.
4. The way in which each person dies is equally important as the way in which that person lived. Beauty, reverence, dignity, and intimacy are central to life and especially so for death. The infirmary music can bring things to the surface in a nonthreatening way or serve the role of meditation. Music is a flow, weaving body, soul, and spirit together.
5. This work is a vocation, not merely a career. It requires clear intention and attention at each deathbed vigil.
6. Death and dying should be returned to the human, personal realm rather than denying or ignoring loss and leavetaking and thus reducing them to legal or corporate medical matters.

Music thanatology focuses on music for the dying versus music for the living. The dying person should not spend energy, only receive energy.

The entire surface of the skin can become an extension of the ear, thus enabling the patient to absorb infirmary music, creating the possibility for even deeper emotional, mental, and spiritual reception. . . . The sole focus is to help the person move toward completion and to unbind from anything that prevents, impedes, or clouds a tranquil passage. (Schroeder-Sheker, 1994, pp. 93–94)

Aromatherapy

Aromatherapy is an offshoot of herbal medicine

in which aromatic plant extracts are inhaled or applied to the skin as a means of treating illness and promoting beneficial changes in mood and outlook. Though aromatherapy and herbal medicine use many of the same plants, in aromatherapy the plants are distilled into oils of exceptional potency. (Allison, 1999, p. 86)

The benefit of these oils comes from their influence on the limbic system, which coordinates mind and body activity. This system is very sensitive to odors and encodes them into associations and memories, which when awakened alter basic physical functions such as heart rate, blood pressure, breathing, and hormone level. When these oils are rubbed into the skin or inhaled, they set off a reaction leading to rapid and significant alterations in memory, heart rate, and other bodily mechanisms. Some boost energy, some promote relaxation, and others have pharmaceutical effects. However, no treatment should ever involve more than a few drops of oil.

There are hundreds of plants used for aromatherapy. Some of the more common ones that are useful in the care of the dying include chamomile, which is used to overcome anxiety, anger, tension, stress, and insomnia; lavender, for exhaustion, depression, and stress; marjoram, used for those who are physically debilitated; neroli, for countering depression, anxiety, nervous tension, and fearfulness; peppermint and rosewood for treating nausea; and chamomile, camphor, fennel, lavender, peppermint, and rose for relieving vomiting (Duke, 1997). Aromatherapy also is used in the relief of pain (lavender, capsicum, bergamot, chamomile, rose, ginger, rosemary, lemongrass, sage, and camphor) (Buckle, 2004; Duke, 1997; Huebscher & Schuler, 2004). It is most useful in the enhancement of mood, increasing vitality, and relaxation (Robins, 1999). These plants and oils can be found in natural or health food stores.

Reminiscence and Life Review

Life review or reminiscence therapy is the remembering of significant past events that enable one to reintegrate past issues and experiences in the present for the purpose of achieving a sense of meaning and ego integrity. The concept has been most frequently used with elderly individuals but is just as effective with those nearing the end of life. Reminiscence is a natural phenomenon. It is the process of recounting past events to someone else or it can be a more complex process of transpersonal focusing and inward reflection. The level of complexity depends on the wish of the client and the training of the nurse. Life review can be oral, including audio and video recordings, or written. Journal and letter writing can also be useful techniques in life review. Photographs and personal items often provide the opportunity for reminiscence and give information about the client that assists the nurse in providing personal and meaningful care.

Life review is a process of unfolding and emerging and therefore cannot be hurried. A life review can be one or many sessions. Olson (2001) provides a guide for a structured life review that usually includes six to eight sessions:

- Use open-ended questions. Ask about childhood and earliest memories and be sure to be supportive if the client recalls sad events.

- Again using open-ended questions, proceed through their life history by asking about adolescence, family and home, adulthood, and later life.
- Have a summary session inquiring about the following: "Generally, what kind of life do you think you have had? What would you do over again?"

To promote the process, the nurse should encourage the client to express himself or herself, involve significant others, assure confidentiality of the information, be sure the client has sufficient physical strength and a desire for sharing, listen carefully, use touch as appropriate, and allow the client periods of silence to reflect. Life review provides integration, a feeling that this life was individual and unique. The client may verbalize sadness as well as achievement, but the objective is to allow a person to see the meaning in their life.

Journal Writing

Keeping a log or journal is a very healing technique to use for individuals who are experiencing life-threatening illness and during the grieving process. It allows the person to express innermost feelings and thoughts without fear of criticism. It is often helpful for those who are uncomfortable or unable to articulate how they feel or what they are going through. The healing emanates from the actual writing and expression, and not from an analysis of the content of the journal. The writing may be totally private or shared with others. Many clients do not think of this technique and the nurse may suggest it. Roach and Nieto (1997) offer some suggested topics for journal writing:

- special thoughts of the dying person or about the deceased
- feelings that were never expressed
- saying good-bye

- ways that grief or dying has helped me grow
- positive aspects of the past, present, and future

There are numerous topics for journal writing or the client can just write thoughts and feelings as they occur. The individual may find comfort in writing when difficult times occur, for example, unanticipated news about diagnosis or prognosis, dealing with family members, or writing to God, a loved one, or one's disease. Often the journal becomes one's own record of grieving. It often serves as a chronicle of personal growth, insights, and wisdom gleaned from the experience of dying or loss.

Touch

In the later stages of life, individuals are often deprived of tender and nurturing physical contact such as being touched in a way that is healing, nourishing, relaxing, and pleasurable. Touch is essential to one's quality of existence. It provides comfort, warmth, and renewed vitality—a sense of security and assurance that we are not alone. Reasons for the lack of touch of the dying include fear, discomfort, stereotypes about dying people, and a sense of one's own vulnerability. However, the benefits of touch on individuals are many. There is an increase of circulation and mobility (e.g., range of motion or hand grasp); a decrease in pain, increase in vitality, increase in physical functioning (Cook, Guerrerio, & Slater, 2004), the experience of being nurtured and cared for; a boost in self-esteem; increased motivation to receive and give attention to self and others; energy and emotional release; a sense memory triggering relaxation response; relief from loneliness and isolation; decreased feelings of abandonment and deprivation; verbal interaction; and calming reassurance and support (Giasson & Bouchard, 1998). It often induces much-needed sleep. In this day of technological care, touch may be the one caring tool to help a client feel better.

There are many forms of touch considered to be holistic/integrative modalities (Allison, 1999; Aspen, 2003; Dossey, Keegan, & Guzzetta, 2005; Fontaine, 2000; Micozzi, 2001; Walker & Walker, 2003). These include but are not limited to the following:

Acupressure—the application of pressure, using fingers, thumbs, palms, or elbows to specific sites along the body's energy meridians to stimulate, disperse, and regulate the body's healing energy for the purpose of relieving tension and reestablishing the flow of energy along the meridian lines.

Body therapy—a general term used for approaches (e.g., Alexander technique, chiropractic, Rolfing, shiatsu, Feldenkrais, etc.) that use hands-on techniques to manipulate and balance the musculoskeletal system to facilitate healing, increase energy, relieve pain, and promote relaxation and well-being.

Reflexology—the application of pressure to specific reflex areas on the feet or hands that correspond to other parts of the body in order to locate and correct problems in the body.

Massage—the practice of kneading or otherwise manipulating a person's muscles and other soft tissue with the intent of inducing physical and psychological relaxation, improving circulation, relieving pain and sore muscles, and improving the individual's well-being. Procedural massage is done to diagnose, monitor, or treat the illness itself, focusing on the end result of curing the illness or preventing further complications. In the past, massage has been one of nurses' most important interventions for pain reduction, comfort, tension release, prevention of atrophy of muscles and stiffness of joints, and inducing sleep. A back massage has left many a patient refreshed and feeling cared for. It would behoove us in nursing to reintroduce massage into our practice armamentarium.

Therapeutic touch (TT)—developed by Dolores Krieger and Dora Kunz. This is a specific modality of centering intention while the practitioner moves the hands through the client's energy field for the purpose of assessment and treatment. It is based on the philosophy that universal life energy flows through and around us, and any interruption in this free flow of energy leads to illness. The goal is to balance and repattern the body's energy so that it flows most efficiently to promote health and prevent disease. The TT practitioner scans the client's energy flow, replenishing it where necessary, releasing congestion, removing obstructions, and restoring order and balance in the ill system. This approach is also an effective complementary care approach for facilitation of the body's natural restorative processes, thereby accelerating healing, promoting relaxation, reducing pain and anxiety, and treating chronic conditions (Denison, 2004; Krieger, 1997, 2002; Newshan, 2003).

According to Janet Macrae (1987), a well-known TT practitioner,

Since therapeutic touch is an interaction, it has the potential to heal the practitioner as well as the patient. . . . You can also use the principles of TT to assist in healing yourself . . . the use of mental imagery can facilitate both the energy transfer and the rebalancing of the [practitioner's] field. If you have pain or discomfort somewhere: (1) Sit quietly and center yourself; (2) Visualize the healing energy (as light, if you wish) coming down from above and flowing through you; (3) Visualize the energy clearing away the pain or discomfort (as light shines through a dark area). (pp. 79–80)

Compassionate touch, developed by Nelson (1994) specifically for hands-on care given to those who are elderly, ill, or dying, is described as

a gentle, sensitive, and non-intrusive program of massage, attentive touch, and supportive

comfort care for those individuals who are temporarily or permanently less active. . . . It also includes individuals of any age who are actively beginning the mysterious life transition that we call death. (p. 1)

Compassionate touch is a hands-on technique stemming not from the hands but from the heart. It combines massage and attentive touch with active listening, reflective communication, relaxation, imagery, and breathing awareness exercises. It focuses on not only the physical condition of the client, but also on the psychosocial, emotional, and spiritual needs as well.

According to Nelson (1994),

compassion for another implies a feeling of unconditional regard for that other; it also implies a genuine, sincere interest in that person's well-being. The compassionate heart shares in, and is affected by the suffering of another. . . . The compassionate individual is able to put aside his or her own concerns for a time in order to give attention to someone else. Some say compassion is love in action. (p. 1)

Compassionate touch is not something we give; it is a way of being. It is a way of providing contact, reassurance, relief, and comfort for those who may be frightened, depressed, out of control, abandoned, overwhelmed, confused, or in despair. It is a means of relating to others rather than a prescribed set of techniques to be practiced on others. It is a spontaneous event of relationship that unfolds moment to moment. Compassionate touch can be administered by anyone who feels inspired to reach out toward a fellow human being in need.

Reiki is based on Buddhist teachings, using hands-on touch to support and intensify energy in the physical, emotional, intellectual, and spiritual areas. "Universal and individual energy are aligned and balanced through the application of gentle hands-on touch to energy pathways of the body" (Abrahms, 1999, p. 133). Those who use Reiki attribute it with reducing stress and stress-related illnesses, including acute and chronic conditions; helping in debilitating disease because it bolsters the immune system by increasing energy; and contributing to an overall sense of well-being in the client.

The philosophy of Reiki contends that a person is vitalized by an essential energy that comes from the universal life force. Everyone has access to this life force, and one becomes ill when the energy flow is interrupted or stopped. Opening pathways for energy flow is the prime objective of Reiki. Learners of Reiki must themselves receive an attunement by an expert Reiki master in an initiation ceremony so that they are attuned to the energy transfer process.

Reiki bodywork is not massage. The touch is gentle and

> aims not to manipulate tissue, but rather to transmit universal life force to the client. The practitioner uses both hands, palms down, fingers held together, and proceeds in a pattern over the client's body. Each positioning of the hands is maintained for 3 to 5 minutes without any movement of the fingers or change in the initial gentle touch. During these hand placements, the universal life force flows through the practitioner to the client to balance the client's energy where necessary. (Micozzi, 2001; Miles & True, 2003)

Reiki bodywork is very individualized and the client's perception of the energy transfer is unique to each person. Most find it rejuvenating and relaxing. The effects may be felt immediately or several days later. Following attunement/initiation of the caregiver, Reiki can be used as a method of self-healing as well as caring for others.

As can be seen, numerous holistic healing modalities can be used during end-of-life care.

HERBOLOGY

Herbology is also known as *phytotherapy* or *phytomedicine*. Herbal remedies have been used in various cultures for centuries and are increasingly popular in the United States as health products and medicines. In fact, herbal use is the fastest growing category of alternative/complementary therapy in the U.S. McCaleb, Leigh, and Morien (2000) define herbs as plants or plant parts (bark, fruit, stem, root, or seed) that are used in fresh, dried, or extracted form for promoting, maintaining, or restoring health. Herbs are prepared in many forms: tinctures, extracts, capsules, tablets, lozenges, teas, juices, vapor treatments, poultices, compresses, salves, liniments, and bath products (Bascom, 2002; Springhouse, 2001).

Herbs are classified for their effects as follows (Springhouse, 2001):

- Adaptogenic herbs (which increase the body's resistance to illness)
- Anti-inflammatory herbs
- Antimicrobial herbs
- Antispasmodic herbs
- Astringent herbs (which are applied externally)
- Bitter herbs to increase the secretion of digestive juices, stimulate appetite, and promote liver detoxification
- Carminative herbs (aromatic oils) to soothe the lining of the GI tract and reduce gas, inflammation, and pain
- Demulcent herbs to soothe and protect inflamed and irritated tissue and mucous membranes
- Diuretic herbs
- Expectorant herbs
- Hepatic herbs to tone the liver and increase the production of hepatocytes
- Hypotensive herbs
- Laxative herbs

- Nervine herbs to (a) strengthen and restore, (b) ease anxiety and tension; and (c) stimulate nerve activity
- Stimulating herbs to stimulate physiologic and metabolic activities
- Tonic herbs, which enliven and invigorate by promoting the "vital force," the key to health and longevity
- Pain-relieving herbs

Although herbs are natural substances and overall risk seems to be low, they cannot be used indiscriminately. Herbs are medicinal and may have serious side effects and interactions with prescription drugs. Additionally, there is a lack of regulation of commercial herbal products in the United States and lack of standardized dosage ranges and preparations. Yet so many Americans choose to take herbal remedies because they are much less costly than prescription drugs, access is virtually unlimited and unrestricted, they are effective, and many people are becoming disenchanted with traditional health care. However, before taking any herbal remedy one must know what it does, how to use it, and the possible adverse effects.

Many clients may hesitate to inform their health care provider that they are using herbs. It is therefore important for the nurse to assess clients' use of herbs and advise them accordingly. Several researchers offer the following guidelines (Bascom, 2002; Skidmore-Roth, 2004; Springhouse, 2001):

1. In a nonjudgmental manner, encourage the client to disclose use of herbal treatments and obtain a history of herb use as complete as possible, including all products taken, amounts, and brand names. If the client is seeing an herbalist, report any prescription drugs.
2. Determine if the client is using herbal remedies instead of, or as an adjunct to, conventional treatment. Is the herb being used to treat a specific condition or for general health?
3. Inform the client of various benefits, risks, and side effects of the herbal remedy, and any potentially serious adverse reactions that may occur when herbs are used with other drugs or substances the client is using. Labels on the products should contain information about product ingredients and use. Recommend standardized herbs.
4. Warn elderly clients, pregnant women, children, and those with known adverse drug reactions, allergies, chronic skin rashes, or preexisting liver disease that they have an increased risk of adverse effects from herbal medicines.
5. Advise the client to notice any unusual symptoms and to report these to the health provider immediately.
6. Advise the client not to take herbal products for serious medical conditions unless they are used under the care of a well-trained health care provider. Urge clients to take only the recommended dosages of herbal remedies.
7. Advise the client to be informed of reputable herbal companies and careful about products sold through magazines, brochures, and the Internet.
8. Tell the client to see a health provider well-trained in herbology when using herbal remedies. Health food store clerks are salespersons, not trained practitioners.
9. Keep a referral list of knowledgeable herbologists.

The field of herbology is expanding at an enormous rate and many books are now available for the nurse to refer to in the care of clients. It is important that the nurse become informed about herbs because increasingly our clients will be coming to us while concurrently using herbal remedies.

HOMEOPATHY

"Homeopathy" comes from the Greek words *homeo*, which means similar, and *pathos*, which means disease or suffering. (Boiron, 2004). It is based on the law of similars, or like cures like, where stimulating the natural healing properties in the body cures a disease or alleviates a symptom (Freeman, 2004). In other words, when a substance identical to the symptoms of the disease is introduced into the body in very small or minute doses, it stimulates the person's healing energy. This is very different from what Hahnemann (the father of homeopathy) called allopathy, from the Greek words *allos*, meaning different, and *pathein* or *pathos*, meaning disease or suffering (Weiner, 1996).

The philosophy of homeopathy strongly contends that health and disease are a holistic phenomenon and the individual must be considered from a body, mind, and spirit perspective; that there is an inherent capacity in all living things to respond to illness in a self-curative way; that there is an "unknowability" about certain disease processes; and that rather than focusing on the disease, treatment may begin with the symptom but the client is treated as a whole and as an individual rather than as a diagnosis with common symptoms. Treatment is individualized and tailored to the uniqueness of each person.

Homeopathic remedies are prepared from natural substances—plant, animal, and mineral. The use of micro doses, that is, highly diluted doses, assures the minimization of toxicity and side effects. Homeopathic medicines are available in various dosage forms: pellets, tablets, liquids, suppositories, and ointments. The U.S. Food and Drug Administration (FDA) recognizes homeopathic remedies as official drugs and regulates the manufacturing, labeling, and dispensing of homeopathic remedies. Simple homeopathic medications of low potencies are available over the counter; however, dilutions for more complicated and chronic conditions are available only from a homeopathic practitioner. Homeopathic remedies are safe, economical, simple to administer, mild in action, and have very few serious or prolonged adverse effects (Micozzi, 2001).

Homeopathic remedies are valuable for a number of symptoms: arnica (marked muscle soreness and acute pain); hypericum (nerve pain, shooting pain); bryonia (trauma, pain on movement); bellis perennis (muscle injury from surgery); ipecacuanha (nausea and vomiting); aconite (fear and shock); calendula (bleeding, preventing infection, increasing granulation); chamomilla (irritability, sensitivity); belladonna (fever); nux vomica (insomnia).

PRAYER

Whatever holistic/complementary therapy we use may not be as important as how we use it. Our providing safe space where healing can occur is what is most important—and that means using ourselves as an instrument of healing. Clients with life-threatening illness often question "Why?" and may need support in their desire to connect with something larger and outside of themselves. Focusing on them as spiritual beings allows them to explore the meaning and purpose of their illness and can bring comfort, often alleviating pain.

As O'Brien (2003) notes, "Prayer is as unique as the individual who prays. Whether one's prayer is of petition, adoration, reparation, or thanksgiving, both the form and the content may vary greatly" (p. 105). Prayer is a simple act of turning our attention to the sacred. Depending on one's beliefs, this can be the God of whatever religion or culture, a higher power, or the ultimate reality. Prayer can be active or passive, involve words, or be wordless. It can involve asking something for oneself or another, expressing repentance for wrongdoing and asking for forgiveness, giving praise and honor, summoning the presence of the Almighty, or offering gratitude (Ameling, 2000). Many forms of prayer are meditative in nature e.g. centering prayer, mantra, prayer beads, and have the benefits of meditation previously discussed in the section on *Meditation*. Others are intercessory, an active form of prayer that seeks an outcome through intentionality where we ask for healing for another or ourselves. This also can be done at a distance which is referred to as non-local healing (Dossey, 1999). Clients also can benefit from prayerful listening to sacred music or sounds, writing or art, or expressing their intent toward the sacred through some body movement or posture (Taylor, 2003).

Prayer is often an important solace to clients who are ill; however, illness may create a barrier to prayer. In those instances, nurse's prayer for and with the client can be a meaningful spiritual intervention as long as permission is obtained when possible. The nurse should assess the client to ascertain if prayer is desired and then follow the client's expressed wish. Taylor (2003) suggests some assessment questions that the nurse can use:

- "How important or helpful is prayer to you?"
- "Would praying together now be comforting?"
- "What type of prayer would be helpful or comforting to you now?"
- "What helps or hinders you as you pray?"
- "How has your illness affected the way you pray or think about prayer?"
- "Have your prayers changed since you became sick?"
- "Do you find it harder to pray sometimes? How do you deal with that?"

- "Have your beliefs about prayer been challenged or changed by illness?" (p. 182)
- "At times like this, some start thinking about if and how their prayers 'get answered.' Have you thought about this?"
- A few minutes spent on assessing and possibly praying with a client can often lower a client's anxiety or assist the nurse's understanding of how prayer facilitates the client's coping.

THE HEALING JOURNEY AT THE END OF LIFE

Individuals become aware of their own deaths in phases, and this awareness can lead to consciousness in dying. Olson (1997) and Olson and Dossey (2005) identify some tasks for dying consciously, specifically:

1. *Live fully* until death comes. Direct or participate in treatment decisions, determinations about the kinds of care, and other decisions, until you are comfortable with accepting the assistance of others.
2. *Plan* to say good-bye to family and friends, finish things one wanted to do, make final decisions, regarding the last will and testament, the estate, organ donation, and so forth. Consider what an ideal death would be like. Who do you want with you, or do you want to be alone? Who are the important people in your life and have you told them? Are there certain rituals you want at your death, for example, a memorial service, cremation? What kind of ceremony do you want? Are there certain treasures that you want particular people to have? Are there particular prayers, poems, or music you want read or played?

3. *Participate* in emotional and spiritual tasks such as forgiving oneself and others, feeling that life mattered and the world is different because you were here, and knowing and accepting love as one changes. Forgiving oneself and others necessitates recognizing that we are responsible for what we are holding onto; confessing one's story to self and others, looking for the good points in ourselves and others; making amends where possible; looking to a higher power for help; and considering what we have learned (Borysenko, 1990). Forgiving others and ourselves helps one recognize unconditional love and connect more with the source of our joy instead of focusing on loss, sadness, and pain. Unconditional love helps release one from fear and anxiety.

4. *Rehearse* the dying process. Through an awareness of dying learn to diminish the fear of death and to "let go of this life" when it is time to do so. Imagery, relaxation, meditation, and prayer scripts on learning forgiveness in peace, letting go, opening the heart, forgiving self and others, releasing pain and grief, conscious dying, moving into the light, and closure can facilitate the detachment from pain and grief, the establishment of comfort and peace, and the achievement of closure. Olson and Dossey (2005) is an excellent source for some of these scripts. However, the nurse should have some practice experience prior to their use with clients.

SELF-CARE FOR THE HEALER

Working with the dying and their families can create much stress for the nurse. It is sometimes referred to as "death overload." Olson (1997) notes that caregivers of dying persons often reexamine their own belief systems and may suffer an existential crisis of faith. Health professionals grieve the loss of their clients, and when the losses come too quickly they may not complete the grieving process before the next death. This may lead to feelings of guilt, anger, irritability, frustration, helplessness, inadequacy, sleeplessness, and depression. Problems may arise in interaction with clients, family members, and other staff. Olson (1997) further notes consequences when staff are not dealing well with the deaths of clients (p. 207):

- avoiding patients
- poor clinical judgment
- unrealistic expectations
- staff absences
- outbursts of anger
- lack of anticipatory planning
- staff conflict
- scapegoating
- interdisciplinary power struggles
- staff fatigue
- ambivalence toward patients

These problems can affect an individual or an entire team. Therefore, it is imperative that health professionals learn self-care techniques. In discussing bereavement care and the role of nurse healers, Roach and Nieto (1997), identify five self-care areas and questions that need to be explored when working with the dying and their families:

1. Spiritual self-care—Is spirituality important in my life? What is my relationship with God or a higher power? Why am I here and what is my purpose? What is my relationship to the universe?

2. Emotional self-care—Can I identify my emotions? How do I deal with them? Am I usually in control? Can I discuss my emotions? Am I open to others and do I respect the feelings of others or do

I jump to conclusions? When do my emotions get out of control?

3. Physical self-care—What areas of my lifestyle are unhealthy or do I have a healthy lifestyle? What can I do to improve my lifestyle?

4. Mental self-care—Am I knowledgeable and do I continually increase my knowledge? Am I satisfied with the status quo or am I open to new ideas? What am I doing to stimulate my mind?

5. Relationships self-care—Am I open and honest with myself and others? Do I have satisfying relationships with others? Am I willing to accept the thoughts and feelings of others even though they are different from my own or am I judgmental? Must I have all the control or can I share it? Do I have a balance between work, home, and leisure? (pp. 171–175)

Worden (1982) identified four tasks of mourning that are equally applicable to staff. Accepting the reality of the loss, although painful, is necessary for healing to occur. It may sometimes feel as if the nurse in end-of-life care is in chronic grieving because of the number of dying clients. But denying the emotional pain, especially of a favored patient, only slows or inhibits the healing process from occurring.

Although more obvious in the significant others, experiencing the pain of the loss also occurs in the staff, including anger, depression, and guilt. Healing support of each other involves encouraging the expression of feelings and emotions such as sadness, anger, guilt, resentment, and pain. Validating the normalcy of the feelings and emotions is also important. One should identify coping strategies that might work or are not working; forgive oneself and others; and remember shared experiences with the deceased client.

Rediscovering meaning is a period of yearning, searching, and discovery. One yearns for the lost person(s) or assumed state of ordinariness, searches for some type of normalcy to reenter the everyday living or working situation, and then discovers the meaning of the loss or losses. Meaning to each of us is individual, unique, and personal. But if one can find meaning, one seems to adjust more easily. Some find meaning in religion, some in support or supportive groups, and some in going inward. Some may never find the answer to the questions "Why did they have to die?" or "Why am I surrounded by so much death?" However, even if these questions are not answered, one may find a new meaning to life—to the present and to the future.

Reinvesting in life or work is somewhat like hope (Roach & Nieto, 1997). One realizes that there is a purpose to this type of work, that the future can be full and good. There is a letting go of remorse and fear of the future, a sense of empowerment, and a sense of one's place in the world. With letting go, the nurse is free to remember the meaningful times with clients and the lessons learned. Although many techniques described above help in reinvesting in work, it also is useful for one to engage in an area of interest outside of work: enroll in a class, take a trip, do special things for oneself, or review one's job goals and setting. Reinvesting in work doesn't necessarily mean that everything is solved; however, it can be the motivation for growth. This growth can be expressed as feeling more intensely, empathizing more completely, caring more fully, and developing more sensitivity to and compassion for others.

As noted earlier, those who care for the terminally ill are at risk for stress associated with many losses. There is also opportunity for a career leading to joy, a sense of personal and professional proficiency, and a capability of living life to the fullest. Olson (1997) identifies three aspects of developing growth when working with the dying. Identifying one's motivation for practicing end-of-life care is important. Is it unresolved personal issues; a professional challenge beyond the physical that involves a search for meaning and peace; a desire to witness the growth of each individual as one comes to terms with mortality and the nature of life; a spiritual calling; a joy in physical care that involves a variety of techniques including complementary modalities such as breathing, TT, and relaxation? Whatever the motivation, exploring this question leads the nurse in end-of-life care to a certain insight and wisdom.

Coping techniques include those strategies used to change the negative effects of stress. It can be forgiving self and others, maintaining health through good nutrition, weight control, regular exercise, adequate sleep, and sufficient resources to maintain oneself in a healthy state. Other kinds of physical activities include massage, diaphragmatic breathing, and distraction. Time needs to be scheduled so that the staff can focus on themselves. An example of diaphragmatic breathing is found in the Exercises section of this chapter. Those who use this technique regularly can do so on cue, even at the bedside of a dying patient. Distraction includes humor, a massage break, having lunch out, a day off, or just a break. One needs these distractions to rest and refresh one's spirit. Scheduling things that are not reminders of patients, death, or dying are important aspects in addition to grieving and remembering.

Developing the spiritual self includes knowing that one's life has meaning and confronting one's mortality. These are key aspects in caring for the dying and their significant others. "*Healing the Dying* means healing oneself by forming connections with the Universe and all that it is. It means a path one can count on, a way one travels with confidence" (Olson, 2001, p. 252). Searching for meaning necessitates learning to listen, quiet-ing the mind's chatter, hearing the whisper of the inner self, and connecting to one's spirituality. A sense of connection with meaningfulness and purpose can be with an organized religion, with a group, or the path of an inner process. There are many ways to develop an ability to listen to the inner self: meditation, creating an environment that supports peace, for example, nature or sound; reading literature about the development of a spiritual path; setting a regular time to practice; keeping a journal; sharing one's spiritual journey with like-minded people; and enjoying life. Whatever the technique, there is a growing sense of unity and purpose in being. One belongs here, one has a mission and a purpose.

This chapter has presented some of the more common alternative/complementary/integrative healing modalities that are and can be used by nurses and by students of nursing. It should be noted that centering, relaxation, imagery, meditation, reminiscence and life review, and journal writing are basic and can be practiced by nurses and students with little or no experience. The sense therapies, touch therapies, and Reiki bodywork necessitate further study, which are offered through a few master's degree programs and workshops. Whenever one learns these therapies, it is imperative that nurses practicing end-of-life care be familiar with healing modalities and their beneficial effects for clients during the dying process.

EXERCISES

Passive Relaxation[1]

Procedure for participants who are lying down:

---

[1]R. Payne, 2000, *Relaxation Techniques: A Practical Handbook for the Health Care Professional.* Copyright 2000 by Churchill Livingston. Reprinted with permission.

- With your eyes closed, let your attention focus on your breathing . . . notice how gentle, slow, and regular it is becoming . . . imagine each breath out carrying your tensions away, leaving you more relaxed than you were before . . . if you want to, take one deep breath . . . then allow your breathing to settle into its own rhythm . . . easy, calm, and even . . . and forget about it.

- I'm going to ask you to take a trip around the body, checking that all the muscle groups are as relaxed as possible and letting go any tension that might still remain. If outside thoughts creep in, hold them in a bubble and let them flow away. I'll begin with the feet.

- Bring your attention to your toes . . . are they lying still? If they are curled or stretched out in some way not entirely comfortable, wiggle them gently. As they come to rest, feel all the tension leaving them . . . feel them sinking down, heavy and motionless.

- Let your feet roll out at the ankles. This is the most relaxed position for them. Let all the tension flow out of them . . . enjoy the sensation of just letting them go.

- Moving on to the lower legs: Feel the tension leaving the calf muscles and the shins. As the tension goes, so they feel heavier . . . so they feel warm and pleasantly tingling.

- The thighs next: to be fully relaxed they need to be slightly rolling outwards . . . feel the relaxing effect of this position . . . make sure you have released all tension, and feel your thighs resting heavily on the surface you are resting on.

- Focus for a moment on the sensation of sagging heaviness throughout your legs . . . let the muscles shed their last remaining hint of tension and settle into a deep relaxation.

- And now, think of your hips. Let them settle into the surface you are lying on . . . recognize any tension that lingers in the muscles . . . then relax it away . . . let it go on relaxing a bit further than you thought possible.

- Settle your spine into the rug or mattress . . . become aware of how it is resting on a surface. Let it sink down, making contact whenever it wants to . . . all tension draining out of it.

- Let your abdominal muscles lose their tension. Let them go soft and loose. Feel them spreading as they give their last vestige of tension . . . notice how your relaxed abdomen rises and falls with your breathing . . . rises as the air is drawn in and falls as the air is expelled . . . abdominal breathing is relaxed breathing.

- Move up to your chest and shoulders, to muscles that are prone to carry tension . . . feel them letting go . . . feel them spreading . . . feel them easing into the surface, limp and heavy . . . feel them drooping down towards your feet . . . imagine them shedding their burdens . . . and as the space between your shoulders and your neck opens out, imagine your neck a bit longer than it was before.

- Now, direct your thoughts to the muscles of your left arm. Check that it lies limply on a surface. Notice the feeling of relaxation and allow this feeling to sweep down to your wrist and hand. Think of the fingers, are they curved and still? . . . neither drawn up nor stretched out . . . neither opened nor closed, but gently resting . . . totally relaxed. As you breathe out, let the arm relax a little bit more . . . let it lie heavy and loose . . . so heavy and loose that if someone were to pick it up, then let it go, it would flop down again like the arm of a rag doll.

- Repeat the last paragraph with the muscles of the right arm.

- Your neck muscles have no need to work with your head supported, so let them go . . . enjoy the feeling of letting go in muscles that work so hard the rest of the time to keep your head upright. If you find any tension in the neck, release it and let this process of releasing continue, even below the surface . . . feel how pleasant it is when you let go the tension in these muscles.

- Bring your attention now to your face, to the many small muscles whose job it is to manage your expressions. At the moment there's no need to have any expression at all on your face, so allow your muscles to feel relaxed . . . imagine how your face is when you are asleep . . . calm and motionless.

- Now, think about the jaw . . . and as you do, allow it to drop slightly so that your teeth are separated . . . feel it relaxing with your lips gently touching. Check that your tongue is still, and lying in the middle of your mouth, soft and shapeless. Relax your throat so that all tension leaves it and the muscles feel smooth and resting.

- With no expression on your face, your cheeks are relaxed and soft. If you think of your nose, it is just to register the passage of cool air traveling up your nostrils while the warmer air passes down . . . breathe tension out with the warm air . . . breathe stillness in with cool air.

- Check that your forehead is smooth . . . not furrowed in any direction . . . and as you release its remaining tension, imagine it being a little higher and a little wider than it was before . . . continue this feeling into your scalp and behind your ears . . . feel a sense of calm as you do this.

- Let your thoughts focus on your eyes as they lie behind gently closed lids. Think of them resting in their sockets, floating rather than fixed . . . and as they come to rest, so do your thoughts.

- Spend a few minutes continuing to relax, deepening the effect of the above sequences . . .

- You now have relaxed all the major muscle groups in your body. Think about them now as a whole . . . a totally relaxed whole . . . soothed by your gentle breathing rhythm, feel the peacefulness of this idea . . .

- Images may drift in and out of your mind . . . see them as thoughts passing through. Feel yourself letting go of them. Say to yourself: "I am feeling calm, I am feeling peaceful." Let your mind conjure up a sense of contentment.

Imagery

The instructor picks one of the following: a sunny beach, a river bank, or a scented garden. If trainees suffer from hay fever, the first item is the best choice. Imagery is best used after a short relaxation exercise.

A Sunny Beach

- See yourself lying on the hot sand of a sunny beach within an enclosed bay. It is sheltered from storms and protected from ocean currents. It is safe. You watch the light dancing on the water; you smell the sea air as it fills your nostrils; you hear the gulls calling above the sound of waves; you feel the warm sun on your skin. The grains of dry sand run through your fingers, forming little bumps and hollows beneath your hand.

A River Bank

- Imagine you are lying in the soft, juicy long grass of early summer. You are in a green meadow that rolls down to the river. Scents rise up from the wildflowers, sweeping over you in waves. The sun is warm but a gentle breeze softens its intensity. Closing your eyes, you become aware of the sound of water flowing, of birds calling, and of leaves rustling.

A Scented Garden

- Picture yourself lying on a newly mown lawn with the sun beating down on the moist cuttings, drawing out their fragrance. Reach out and feel the coolness of the damp grass. Through your half-closed eyelids you can see the tops of the trees swaying against the sky. Light breezes carry the scent of honeysuckle.

Following one of these short passages of visualization, trainees can relax for a few minutes, before the session is brought to an end.

Relaxation[2]

I would like for you to be as comfortable as you possibly can. Take a couple of deep breaths. Inhale deeply. Exhale very slowly and very completely. Focus on your breathing. Again, inhale very deeply and exhale very slowly. Become aware of your ability to relax your muscles. Allow every muscle in your body to be as relaxed as possible, starting with the feet. Allow the feet to become very, very comfortable. Relax the feet completely. As the muscles relax you may notice a tingling sensation in the soles and toes of the feet. This simply indicates that the muscles are relaxing.

Be aware as this sensation of relaxation begins to move upward from the feet to the ankles. This sensation of relaxation flows from the ankles to the calves of the legs. The muscles of the calves release the tension and

relax. The calves become very comfortable as the tension is released.

This comfortable, relaxed sensation moves from the calves to the upper legs and thighs. These muscles also relax and become very comfortable. Feel the muscles on the sides of the legs, the outside of the legs, the inner legs, and on the top of the legs become very comfortable and relaxed.

The sensation of relaxation moves up towards the buttocks and toward the pelvic area. Occasionally you may feel a muscle twitch. This is just another sign that relaxation is occurring. The tension of the muscles of the buttocks, pelvic area, and the lower abdomen is released. The internal organs relax and the muscles that surround them feel completely tension free.

The sensation of relaxation moves up the body to the upper abdomen, to the chest, and from the lower back toward the upper back. The muscles are relaxing from the chest and the upper back to the shoulders.

This relaxation extends to the neck and the throat. Feel the tension draining from the back of the neck. Tension is draining away from the back of the neck and the back of the head. As tension drains away, a sense of relaxation settles in. These feelings are so comfortable and so pleasant. Feel the muscles of the throat, the jaw, and across the bridge of the nose relaxing.

The tension in the arms is released and these muscles feel relaxed. Relaxation spreads to the hands and the fingers as the tension is released.

From the feet, to the head, to the arms, to the fingertips, the whole body is completely and totally relaxed. Take a few moments to savor this comfortable state of total relaxation of body and mind.

Closure

Allow time for the client to appreciate this restful state of complete relaxation. After a

---

[2]S. Roach & B. Nieto, 1997, *Healing and the Grief Process.* Copyright 1997 by Delmar Publications.

few minutes instruct the client to bring his attention back to the present. At times, the nurse may want to count slowly from one to ten as the client progressively returns to a more wakeful state.

Meditation[3]

Using a Mantra

1. Select a word to focus on. It can be a neutral word, such as "one," or a Sanskrit mantra such as "Om Shanti," "Sri Ram," "So-Hum." It could also be a word or phrase that has some special significance within your personal belief system. In his recent book, *Beyond the Relaxation Response,* Benson (1985) describes how a word or phrase of special personal significance (such as "I am at peace" or "Let go, let God") deepens the effects of meditation.

2. Repeat this word or phrase, ideally on each exhalation.

3. As any thoughts come to mind, just let them pass over and through you and gently bring your attention back to the repetitive word or phrase.

Continuing Breaths

1. As you sit quietly, focus on the inflow and outflow of your breath. Each time you breathe out, count the breath. You can count up to 10 and start over again, or keep counting as high as you like, or you can use Benson's method of repeating "one" on each exhalation.

2. Each time your focus wanders, bring it back to your breathing and counting. If you get caught in an internal monologue or fantasy, don't worry about it or

judge yourself. Just relax and return to the count again.

3. If you lose track of the count, start over at 1 or at a round number like 50 or 100.

4. After practicing breath-counting meditation for a while, you may want to let go of the counting and just focus on the inflow and outflow of your breathing.

Whichever form of meditation you try, you might want to start out with short periods of 5 to 10 minutes and gradually lengthen them to 20 to 30 minutes over a period of 2 to 3 weeks. Most people find that it takes persistent and disciplined effort over a period of several months to become proficient at meditating. Even though meditation is the most demanding of relaxation techniques to learn, it is for many people the most rewarding. Research has found that among all relaxation techniques, meditation is the one that people are most likely to persist in doing regularly.

If you are truly interested in establishing a meditation practice, you may want to find a class, group, or teacher to study with. This will make it easier for you to continue your practice.

Script for Breathing for Relaxation and Health[4]

- Close your eyes . . . Focus your mind on your breath . . . Just follow the air as it goes in . . . and as it goes out.

---

[3]Edmund J. Bourne, 1995, *The Anxiety and Phobia Workbook* (2nd Ed.), Copyright 1995 by New Harbinger Publications, Inc. All rights reserved.

[4]Julie T. Lusk, *30 Scripts for Relaxation, Imagery and Inner Healing,* Vol. 1. Copyright 1992 by Julie T. Lusk, Vols. 1 and 2 are available from Whole Persons Associates, 210 W. Michigan, Duluth, Minnesota 55802, 800-247-6789. Julie T. Lusk is also the author of *Refreshing Journeys,* a relaxation audiotape available from Whole Persons Associates, and *Desktop Yoga*™, available from Perigee Books, 800-631-8751.

- Feel it as it comes in . . . and as it goes out . . . If your mind begins to wander, just bring it back to your breath.
- Feel your stomach rise . . . your ribs expand . . . and your collarbone rise . . . Breathe in naturally and slowly.
- On your next exhalation, release all the air from your lungs without straining . . . Let it all go . . . Let it all out . . . Prepare your lungs to receive fresh oxygen.
- Now take in a full, deep breath and let the air go to the bottom of your lungs . . . Feel your stomach rise . . . your chest expand, and the collarbone area fill.
- Now empty your lungs from top to bottom . . . Let all the air out . . . Compress your stomach to squeeze out all the stale air and carbon dioxide. Squeeze out every bit of air . . . Let it all go.
- Take in another deep breath . . . As you breathe in, your diaphragm expands and massages all the internal organs in the abdominal region . . . aiding your digestion.
- Breathe out . . . Relax . . . Feel the knots in your stomach untie . . . Let go.
- Breath in . . . Your diaphragm is stimulating your vagus nerve, slowing down the beating of your heart . . . relaxing you.
- Breath out . . . Let it all go . . . Relax . . . Relax more and more . . . Breathing heals you . . . calms you . . . soothes you.
- Breathe in again, fully and completely. Oxygen is entering your bloodstream, nourishing all your organs and cells . . . protecting you.
- Breath out . . . Release all the poisons and toxins with your breath . . . Your breathing is cleansing you . . . healing you.
- Breathe in.
- Now imagine exhaling confusion . . . and inhaling clarity.

- Imagine exhaling darkness . . . and inhaling light.
- Imagine exhaling hatred . . . and inhaling love.
- Exhaling anxiety . . . and inhaling peace.
- Exhaling selfishness . . . and inhaling generosity.
- Exhaling guilt . . . and inhaling forgiveness.
- Exhaling weakness . . . and inhaling courage.
- Breathe in through your nose and sigh out through your mouth. Let the air stay out of your lungs as long as it is comfortable, and then take another breath.
- Let your breath return to its normal and natural pace. Continue to breathe in slowly, smoothly, and deeply . . . Your breathing is steady, easy, silent.
- Each time you exhale . . . allow yourself to feel peaceful . . . calm . . . and completely relaxed . . . If your mind wanders, bring your attention back to your breath.
- Stretch and open your eyes, feeling refreshed and rejuvenated, alert, and fully alive.

Repeat the above instructions until everyone is alert.

White Light of Healing Energy Imagery[5]

Begin to imagine that there is a sphere of white light of healing energy about 4 inches above your head. The white light is now

---

[5]Barbara Montgomery Dossey, "Imagery," in *Holistic Nursing: A Handbook for Practice,* (2nd Ed.), edited by Barbara Montgomery Dossey, Lynn Keegan, Cathie E. Guzetta, and L. Kolkmeier. Copyright 1995 by Aspen Publishers.

touching the top of your head. Begin to feel this light as it flows from the top of your head and allow it to flow down through the entire inside of the body.

The healing light has filled the inside of your head ... and it now flows down your shoulders, back, down your arms, and into your fingertips. The white light is now flowing into your chest ... around your sides ... into your middle and lower back ... below your waist ... around your sides flowing into your abdomen ... into your buttocks ... and into your pelvis. The light now flows down your thighs ... to your lower legs ... and to your feet.

The white light has now completely filled the inside of your body. There is now a wonderful abundance of this healing light . . . and it begins to bubble up and flow back out through the top of your head ... down the outside of your body ... coating the entire outside of your body. The more you allow it to flow throughout your body ... the more abundant it is. Send the healing white light to specific areas that need extra attention, such as places of discomfort or disease.

Inner Guide Imagery[6]

As you begin to feel even more relaxed now ... going to a greater depth of inner being ... more relaxed ... more secure and safe ... let yourself become aware of the presence of not being alone. With you right now is a guide ... who is wise and concerned with your well-being. Let yourself begin to see this wise being with whom you can share your fears or your joys. You have trust in this wise guide.

If you do not see anyone, let yourself be aware of hearing or feeling this wise being, noticing the presence of care and concern. In whatever way seems best for you ... proceed to make contact with the wise inner guide. Let yourself establish contact with your guide now ... in any way that comes. Your guide may appear to you in any form, such as a person, an animal, or inner presence/peace ... or as an image of the very wisest part of you.

Notice the love and wisdom with which you are surrounded. This wisdom and love are present for you now ... Let yourself ask for advice ... about anything that is important for you just now. Be receptive to what emerges ... Let yourself receive some new information. This inner guide may have a special message to share with you ... Listen with openness and pure intention to receive.

Allow yourself to look at any issue in your life. It may be a symptom, a choice, or decision . . . Tell your wise guide anything that you wish . . . Listen to the answers that emerge. Imagine yourself acting on the answers and directions that you received . . . Imagine yourself calling upon the wisdom and love of this wise guide to help you in the days to come. Now in whatever way is best for you ... bring closure to the visit with this inner guide. You can come back here any time you wish. All you have to do is take the time.

Imagery Finding One's Special Place[7]

Begin by placing your body in a comfortable position, arms and legs uncrossed, your back well-supported. Now take three deep breaths, and during each breath relax even more. Let the exhalation be a letting-go kind of breath, letting go of tension. With each breath, take in what you need and with each exhalation, release anything you don't need. Bring your attention to the top of your head. Feel your

---

[6]Ibid. [Adapted]

[7]K. Shames, 1996. *Creative Imagery in Nursing.* Copyright 1996 by Delmar Publications.

scalp relax and let your brow soften and smooth out. Allow the muscles around your eyes to relax. And let any tension flow out through your cheeks as you exhale. Suggest that your jaw relax. Imagine a wave of relaxation flowing down your shoulders, into your arms, elbows, and forearms, all the way into your hands and fingers. Now focus on your chest, releasing any tension around your heart or lungs, relax the muscles around your ribs. Wrap that relaxation around your back and let a wave of relaxation travel down the spine. Allow the muscles along the spine to lengthen and release. Soften and relax the buttocks and pelvis. Let the belly be very soft so that the breath moves easily down into the abdomen. Invite the legs to join in the relaxation now, as it moves through the thighs, knees, calves, ankles, and feet. Let any last bit of tension or tightness drain out through your feet or toes. When you feel relaxed and comfortable, let me know with a nod of your head. As your body remains relaxed and comfortable, imagine yourself in a very special place, somewhere that is full of natural beauty, safety, and peace. It may be a place you have been to before or it may be a place you want to create in your imagination. Take some time and let yourself be drawn to one place that is just right for you today. Let me know when you are present there (wait for response). Describe what it is like there. What do you see? Are there any smells? Are there any sounds? What is the temperature like? Where are you in this special place? How do you feel here? Take some time to do whatever you would like to do here, to relax or do some activity. Feel free to do whatever you want. This is your place. (Pause 3 to 4 minutes).

In a few moments, it will be time to come back into a waking state. Know that you can return to this place again anytime you want. Now gently bring yourself back, letting the images fade but keeping with you this re-laxed and peaceful feeling. Remember what has been important about this experience. Become aware of the current time and place. Begin to move your body, take a deep breath, open your eyes, and feel relaxed and awake.

At this point, the guide can take a few minutes to allow the person to share his experience.

Imagery in Oncology[8]

Cancer might well be the most feared disease of our time. Many people live their lives in dread and fear of cancer. The traditional medical treatments are terrifying and excruciating. Many nurses find it beneficial to work with the client's negative images and beliefs.

Some nurses have reported making tapes (there are also some available commercially) in which the client is encouraged to imagine chemotherapy or radiation therapy as something positive. Some clients prefer to view it as beams of energy or light.

The practitioner might ask "How do you imagine the chemotherapy?" Despite the response, the nurse can be helpful in supporting the transformation of the images into something beneficial and positive. "Imagine the medicine going into exactly the cells that most need it. The side effects will be minimal." There are a great variety of techniques and applications that enhance the healing journey through the experience of cancer.

Quick Uses of Imagery in the Clinical Setting

IVs

When a patient is receiving intravenous fluids, he can envision fluid flowing to every

---

[8]Ibid.

part of his body, removing toxins and flushing them out. The patient can see nutrients providing nourishment to every cell.

Pain Medications

Similarly, the patient can enhance the benefits of pain medication by envisioning its soothing effects as it travels through the bloodstream, sedating any irritated areas and bringing a deep sense of relief throughout. It is suggested that relaxation be used at the first sign of discomfort; focus the patient on the breath. Imagine the body releasing its natural medicine to all areas that are tense or uncomfortable. If pain begins to interfere with activity or rest, ask for medication before becoming so uncomfortable that it would be difficult to work with relaxation and the following imagery:

Imagine the pain medication to be exactly the strength it needs to be. See, feel, or sense the muscles around the painful area softening and relaxing as you breathe into the discomfort. See or feel the pain medication moving to that area, numbing the pain as if it had deposited a layer of frost.

Imagining a dial registering a number from 1 to 10 that represents your pain now. See the number come down to your tolerance level. Allow an image to form of a special, quiet, restful place and allow yourself to be there as you rest.

Antibiotics

Some patients like to imagine their antibiotic medication in the bloodstream as hunters stalking their prey. They can envision that the medication stays where the most protection is needed, particularly around burns or incisions, ready to pounce. If more medication is needed, there is an endless supply in the imagination.

Anticoagulants

Likewise, clients using anticoagulant agents can envision their blood becoming thinner, flowing to exactly the right places to prevent clotting. They can see the medication as extraordinarily efficient and relish watching as it does its magic.

Oxygen

As you take a deep breath, send nourishing healing oxygen into every cell of your lungs, expanding each cell like a balloon. As you exhale, imagine letting the balloons completely deflate and blow any tension or toxins that remain in the body out into the air. Continue doing this slowly for a few minutes, watching the balloons expand and contract.

Healing Image

Imagine little workers repairing the muscles and bones while they are resting, allowing the healing process to begin. See the bone rich in calcium, and see little bone cells growing like coral, increasing in number and density.

Ideal Images

Many clients continue to envision their healing process long after the crises have passed. One way to do this is to imagine themselves in 3 or 6 months. They can imagine themselves exactly as they would wish to be. They can observe how they look, how they walk, their facial expressions. They might imagine themselves running or swimming, looking healthy and happy.

It is also a good practice for nurses to see themselves as they want to be. Focus on the image; how does it feel to be whole? Many nurses find that using imagery supports their patients totally and empowers them in their work. According to one nurse, after incorporating imagery frequently, "I finally felt as if I were making a difference, despite the disempowering aspect of the environment."

Diaphragmatic Breathing

Diaphragmatic breathing is a useful technique for relaxing and beginning the centering process. Consciously realizing the path each inhalation takes through the respiratory passages, and inhaling so that the abdomen and lungs expand, allowing each breath to move to the bottom of the respiratory tree by moving the diaphragm downward and outward moves the whole person toward feeling more relaxed. As the slow, long exhalation occurs, a person feels shoulders moving downward and tensions slowly leaving the body. To help with stress at work, a nurse should practice diaphragmatic breathing at home, in either a supine or sitting position. Putting one's hand on the abdomen is an easy way to know if the abdomen is involved in the breath, or if shallow, tense breaths are a pattern. Once a pattern of abdominal breathing is the norm, the nurse can think of phrases such as, "I can feel this way whenever I take a deep breath and cross my fingers." Connecting the relaxed feeling to the physical act of crossing fingers (or another physical cue) helps the body remember how it feels to relax. A nurse who regularly practices this technique will have the ability to break the cycle of stress and muscle tension in just a few seconds, even at the bedside of a dying patient. The pattern is as follows:

- Recognize the feeling of tension.
- Take an abdominal breath—on inhalation the stomach expands.
- On exhalation the stomach contracts—allow the shoulders to sag and relaxation to be experienced during the exhalation.
- Use a physical cue that has been practiced.

This technique, or pattern, is useful by itself to help relax for a few minutes or to lead to more profound states of relaxation.

KEY POINTS

1. Holism focuses on unity, mutuality, meaning, and the interrelationship of all beings, events and things.
2. People can grow and learn from illness and dying. Individuals can die healed.
3. Holism is the theoretical and philosophical foundation for all alternative/complementary integrative healing modalities.
4. Holistic integrative therapies can be used by the nurse, client, and family. They are therapies of healing and empowerment.
5. Relaxation is the basis for most holistic modalities.
6. Imagination can play a powerful role in healing.
7. Although there are many forms of meditation, all attempt to quiet the mind and focus one's attention inward.
8. Sense therapies such as music (sound), aromas (smell), and touch (kinesthetics) have very potent natural healing properties that can adjust chemical or other imbalances with the body.
9. Reminiscence and life review allow one to reintegrate past issues and experiences in the present to achieve a sense of meaning and ego integrity.
10. Journal writing often helps those who cannot express verbally how they feel or what they are experiencing.
11. Touch is essential to the quality of one's existence. It needs to be reintroduced as a significant modality in nursing practice.
12. Herbs have many healing qualities but should be used knowledgeably.

13. Homeopathy is a longstanding method of holistic medicine in which "like cures like" and remedies are tailored to the individual.
14. Prayer is unique to each individual both in form and in content.
15. There is a consciousness in dying where individuals become aware of their own deaths in phases.
16. Self-care for health professionals who care for dying persons is imperative. Self-care areas include spiritual, emotional, physical, mental, and relationships.

EDUCATION PLAN 2.1   Plan for Achieving Competencies: Holistic Integrative Therapies in Palliative Care

Knowledge Needed	Attitude	Skills	Undergraduate Behavioral Outcomes	Graduate Behavioral Outcomes	Teaching/Learning Strategies
Assumptions and philosophy of holistic care and healing within the context of dying.	*Accept the assumptions and philosophy of holistic therapies in end-of-life care. *Appreciate the ability to heal within the context of dying.		*Verbalize an appreciation for holistic, complementary care for patients and families.	*Evaluate the relationship between the use of holistic, complementary modalities and quality of life for patients and families.	*Document personal assumptions/philosophy regarding healing, holistic care, and the value of complementary therapies in a journal.
Discussion of specific holistic therapies and application to palliative care.	*Affirm the benefits of holistic, complementary therapies at the end of life.	*Demonstrate the steps of simple holistic, complementary therapies.	*Inform patient and family about the value and availability of holistic healing therapies. *Administer simple holistic integrative therapies in the care of patients and families at the end of life.	*Administer more complex holistic healing therapies.	*Develop a case study that reveals healing at the end of life. *Conduct a selected holistic, complementary therapy in class, seminar, or post-conference each week.

Healing journey: tasks for dying consciously.	*Personally consider the tasks for dying consciously.	*Engage in activities that promote emotional or spiritual tasks of dying consciously.	*Role model activities that promote emotional or spiritual tasks of dying consciously.	*Rehearse the dying process by creating a story of students'/nurses' own death and sharing this story and associated feelings with a fellow student, faculty, or colleague. *Document in a journal a written plan to complete unfinished business.
Self-care for the healer.	*Value self-care.	*Perform healing therapies with colleagues to reduce caregiver stress. *Engage in self-care activities daily.	*Role model comprehensive self-care behaviors. *Identify alternative self-care strategies.	*Create an inventory of self-care activities within the last month and evaluate their adequacy. *Perform one self-care activity each day with journal documentation.

RESOURCES

Academy for Guided Imagery
P.O. Box 2070
Mill Valley, CA 94942
(800)726-2070; fax (415)389-9342
www.healthy.net/agi/index_explorer.html

American Association for Music Therapy
    (AAMT)
P.O. Box 27177
Philadelphia, PA 19918
(215)265-4006

American Herbalist Guild
1931 Gaddis Road
Canton, GA 30115
(770)751-6021
www.americanherbalist.com

American Holistic Nurses Association
PO Box 2130
Flagstaff, AZ 86003-2130
(800)526-2462
www.ahna.org

American Massage Therapy Association
820 Davis Street, Suite 100
Evanston, IL 60201-4444
(847)864-0123
www.amtamassage.org

American Psychological Association
750 First Street NE
Washington, DC 20002-4242
(800)374-2721

Association for Applied Psychophysiology
    and Biofeedback
Biofeedback Certification Institute of
    America
10200 W. 44th Avenue, Suite 304
Wheat Ridge, CO 80003
(303)420-2902
www.bcia.org

Center for Mindfulness in Medicine, Health
    Care and Society
University of Massachusetts Medical
    Center
419 Belmond Avenue
Worcester, MA 01604
www.mindfulnesstapes.com

Compassionate Touch
20 Swan Court
Walnut Creek, CA 94596
(510)935-3906

Contemplative Outreach, Ltd.
    [centering prayer]
P.O. Box 737
10 Park Place, Suite 2B
Butler, NJ 07405
(973)838-3384; e-mail: office@coutreach.
    org
www.centeringprayer.com/cntrgpryr.htm

International Center for Reiki Training
29209 Northwestern Highway, #592
Southfield, MI 48034
(800)332-8112

Maharishi Vedic School
    [TM program]
636 Michigan Avenue
Chicago, IL 60605
(312)431-0110
www.maharishi.org

National Association for Holistic
    Aromatherapy
836 Hanley Industrial Court
St. Louis, MO 63144
(888)ASK-NAHA; (888)275-6242

National Association of Music Therapy
    (NAMT)
8455 Colesville Road, Suite 930
Silver Springs, MD 20910
(301) 589-3300

National Association of Nurse Massage
 Therapists
(800)262-4017
http://members.aol.com/naumtl

National Center for Complementary and
 Alternative Medicine (NCCAM)
P.O. Box 7923
Gaithersburg, MD 20898
(888)644-6226; e-mail: info@nccam.nih.gov/

National Center for Homeopathy
801 N. Fairfax Street, Suite 306
Alexandria, VA 22314
(703)548-7790
www.homeopathic.org

National Certification for Acupuncture and
 Oriental Medicine (NCCAOM)
11 Canal Center Plaza, Suite 300
Alexandria, VA 22314
(703)548-9004
www.nccaom.org

Nurse Healers - Professional Associates
 International [therapeutic touch]
3760 South Highland Drive, Suite 429
Salt Lake City, UT 84106
(801)942-5900 (801)273-3399; e-mail:
 rmgood@worldnet.att.net
www.therapeutictouch.org

Transcendental Meditation
(888)532-7686

Transcendental Meditation Program
(888)LEARN TM
www.tm.org

REFERENCES

Abrahms, E. (1999). Reiki. In N. Allison (Ed.), *The illustrated encyclopedia of body-mind disciplines* (pp. 133–136). New York: Rosen.

Allison, N. (1999). Guided imagery. In N. Allison (Ed.), *The illustrated encyclopedia of body-mind disciplines* (pp. 71–73). New York: Rosen.

Ameling, A. (2000). Prayer: An ancient healing practice becomes new age again. Holistic Nursing Practice, *14*(3), 40–48.

Anselmo, J. (2005). Relaxation: The first step to restore, renew, and self heal. In B. Dossey, L. Keegan, & C. Guzzetta (Eds.), *Holistic nursing a handbook for practice* (4th ed., pp. 523–564). Sudbury, MA: Jones and Bartlett.

Aspen Reference Group. (2003). *Holistic health promotion and complementary therapies: A resource for integrated practice.* Gaithersburg MD: Aspen.

Bascom, A. (2002). *Incorporating herbal medicine into clinical practice.* Philadelphia: Davis.

Benson, H. (1995). *Beyond the relaxation process.* New York: Berkley Books.

Boiron Group. (2004). *The smart guide to homeopathy.* Newtown Square, PA: Author.

Bonadonna, R. (2003). Meditation's impact on chronic illness. *Holistic Nursing Practice, 17,* 309–319.

Borysenko, J. (1990). *Guilt is the teacher, love is the lesson.* New York: Warner Books.

Bourne, E. (1995). The *anxiety & phobia workbook* (2nd ed.). Oakland, CA: New Harbinger.

Buckle, J. (2004). Aromatherapy. In L. Freeman (Ed.), *Mosby's complementary and alternative medicine: A research-based approach* (2nd ed.) St. Louis, MO: Mosby.

Cook, C., Guerrerio, J., & Slater, U. (2004). Healing touch and quality of life in women receiving radiation treatment for cancer. *Alternative Therapies in Health and Medicine, (10)*3, 34–41.

Denison, B. (2004). Touch the pain away: New research on therapeutic touch and persons with fibromyalgia syndrome. *Holistic Nursing Practice, 18,*142–150.

Dossey (1998). *Reinventing medicine: Beyond mind-body to a new era of healing.* San Francisco: Harper.

Dossey, B., Keegan, L., & Guzzetta, C. (2005). *Holistic nursing: A handbook for practice* (4th ed.). Sudbury, MA: Jones and Bartlett.

Duke, J. (1997). *The green pharmacy.* New York: St. Martin's Press.

Frank-Schwebel, A. (1999). Music therapy. In N. Allison (Ed.), *The illustrated encyclopedia of body-mind disciplines* (pp. 366–369). New York: Rosen.

Fontaine, K. (2000). *Healing practice: Alternative therapies for nursing.* Upper Saddle River, NJ: Prentice-Hall.

Freeman, L. (2004). *Complementary and alternative medicine: A research-based approach* (2nd ed.). St. Louis, MO: Mosby.

Gatchel, R., & Maddrey, A. (1998). Clinical outcome research in complementary and alternative medicine: An overview of experimental design and analysis. *Alternative Therapies, 4*(5), 36–43.

Giasson, M., & Bouchard, L. (1998). Effect of therapeutic touch on the well-being of persons with terminal cancer. *Journal of Holistic Nursing, 16,* 393–398.

Gross, C., Kritzer, M. J., Russas, V., Treesak, C., Frazier, P., & Hertz, M. (2004). Mindfulness meditation to reduce symptoms after organ transplant. *Alternative Therapies in Health and Medicine, (10)*3, 58–66.

Guzzetta, C. (2005). Music therapy: Healing the melody of the soul. In B. Dossey, L. Keegan, & C. Guzzetta (Eds.), *Holistic nursing a handbook for practice* (4th ed., pp. 617–640). Sudbury, MA: Jones and Bartlett.

Huebscher, R., & Schuler, P. (2004). *Natural, alternative and complementary health care practices.* St. Louis, MO: Mosby.

Koger, S. M., & Brotons, M. (2000). *Music therapy for dementia symptoms.* Cochrane Database Systematic Review. CD001121

Kolkmeier, L. (1995). Self-reflection: Consulting the truth within. In B. Dossey, L. Keegan, C. Guzzetta, & L. Kolkmeier (Eds.), *Holistic nursing a handbook for practice* (2nd ed.). Gaithersburg, MD: Aspen.

Krieger, D. (2002). *Therapeutic touch: A transpersonal healing.* New York: Lantern Books.

Krieger, D. (1997). *Therapeutic touch inner workbook.* Santa Fe, NM: Bear.

Laurant, R., & Shlien, J. (1984). *Client centered therapy and the person centered approach.* New York: Praeger.

Lawson, K., & Horneffer, K. (2002). Roots and viewing a pilot of a mind-body-spirit program. *Journal of Holistic Nursing, 20,* 250–263.

Lusk, J. (1992) *30 scripts for relaxation, imagery, and inner healing.* Duluth, MN: Whole Persons Associates.

Macrae, J. (1987). *Therapeutic touch: A practical guide.* New York: Knopf.

Mariano, C. (1998). Preparing nurses to deliver holistic care. *Spectrum, 10*(22), 14–15.

Mariano, C. (2004). Holistic nursing today. *Creative Nursing, 10*(1), 4–8.

McCaleb, R., Leigh, E., & Morien, K. (2000). *The encyclopedia of popular herbs.* Roseville, CA: Prima.

McCraty, R., Barrios-Chaplin, B., Atkinson, M., & Tomasino, D. (1998). The effects of different types of music on mood, tension and mental clarity. *Alternative Therapies, 4*(1), 75–84.

Micozzi, M. (2001). *Fundamentals of complementary and alternative medicine* (2nd ed.). New York: Churchill Livingston.

Miles, P., & True, G. (2003). Reiki—Review of a biofield therapy history, theory, practice, and research. *Alternative Therapies, 9*(2), 62–72.

Nelson, D. (1994). *Compassionate touch: Hands-on caregiving for the elderly, the ill and the dying.* Barrytown, NY: Station Hill Press.

Newshan, G. (2003). Large clinical study shows value of therapeutic touch program. *Holistic Nursing Practice, 17,* 189–192.

O'Brien, M. (2003). *Spirituality in nursing standing on holy ground.* Sudbury, MA: Jones and Bartlett.

Olson, M. (1997). Death and grief. In B. Dossey (Ed.), *Core curriculum for holistic nursing.* Gaithersburg, MD: Aspen.

Olson, M. (2001). *Healing the dying* (2nd ed.). New York: Delmar Thompson Learning.

Olson, M., & Dossey, B. (2005). Dying in peace. In B. Dossey, L. Keegan, & C. Guzzetta (Eds.), *Holistic nursing a handbook for practice* (3rd ed., pp. 429–454). Gaithersburg, MD: Aspen.

Payne, R. (2001). *Relaxation techniques: A practical handbook for the health care professional.* (2nd ed.). New York: Churchill Livingston.

Quinn, J. (1995). The Healing Arts in Modern Health Care. In D. Kunz (Ed.), *Spiritual aspects of the healing arts.* Wheaton, IL: Quest Books. pp. 176–192.

Remington, R. (2002). Calming music and hand massage with agitated elderly. *Nursing Research, 51,* 317.

Roach, S., & Nieto, B. (1997). *Healing and the grief process.* New York: Delmar.

Rossman, M. (1999). Interactive guided imagery. In N. Allison (Ed.), *The illustrated encyclopedia of body-mind disciplines* (pp. 77–78). New York: Rosen.

Sahler, J., Hunter, B., & Liesveld, J. (2003). The effects of using music therapy with relaxation imagery in the management of patients undergoing bone transplantation. *Alternative Therapies in Health and Medicine, 9*(6), 70–74.

Schaub, B., & Dossey, B. (2005). Imagery: Awakening the inner healer. In B. Dossey, L. Keegan, & C. Guzzetta (Eds.), *Holistic nursing: A handbook for practice* (4th ed., pp. 567–613). Sudbury, MA: Jones and Bartlett.

Schroeder-Sheker, T. (1994). Music for the dying. *Journal of Holistic Nursing, 12*(1), 83–99.

Shames, K. (1996). *Creative imagery in nursing.* New York: Delmar.

Skidmore-Roth, L. (2004). *Mosby's handbook of herbs and natural supplements* (2nd ed.). St. Louis, MO: Mosby.

Springhouse Corporation. (2001). *Nursing herbal medicine handbook.* Springhouse, PA; Springhouse.

Taylor, E. (2003). Prayer's clinical issues and implications. *Holistic Nursing Practice, 17,* 179–188.

Van Kuiken, D. (2004). A meta-analysis of the effect of guided imagery on practice outcomes. *Journal of Holistic Nursing, 22,* 164–179.

Walker, M., & Walker, J. (2003). *Healing massage.* Scarborough, Ontario: Thompson Delmar Learning.

Weiner, M. (1996). *The complete book of homeopathy.* Arden City Park, NY: Avery.

Worden, J. (1982). *Grief counseling and grief therapy: A handbook for the mental health practitioner.* New York: Springer.

Section II

Social and Professional Issues in Palliative Care

3

Death and Society

Marilyn Bookbinder, Margaret Kiss, and Marianne LaPorte Matzo

AACN Competencies

#1: Recognize dynamic changes in population demographics, health care economics, and service delivery that necessitate improved professional preparation for end-of-life care.

#13: Identify barriers and facilitators to patients' and caregivers' effective use of resources.

#15: Apply knowledge gained from palliative care research to end-of-life education and care.

> *In the end, the question comes down to one of control over how a particular life ends and who has the power to make that decision and implement it.*
>
> —Robinson

At the turn of the twentieth century, Americans died from diseases such as yellow fever, small pox, diphtheria, and cholera. Death was often rapid with little time to say good-bye to loved ones. In 1900, life expectancy was less than 50 years of age for both men and women, while in the year 2000, the median age of death was 77 years old. Currently, Americans are struggling to develop a health care system that is both cost-effective and can ensure a "good life" and a "good death." This chapter addresses the changes and issues surrounding death in society in the twentieth century, their impact on quality patient care,

and the role of educators in preparing nurses to care for patients and families experiencing life-threatening illness. Two landmark studies from the 1990s—specifically, the "Study to Understand Prognosis and Preferences for Outcomes and Risks of Treatments" (SUPPORT, 1995) and the Institute of Medicine's report "Approaching Death: Improving Care at the End of Life" (IOM, 1997)—provide evidence of the need to improve the care of the dying in America. This is the challenge of nurses and all health professionals in the twenty-first century.

CHANGES IN THE DEFINITION OF DEATH IN SOCIETY

Over the last few decades, the concept of death has raised many moral and ethical dilemmas for society. The *Encyclopedia Britannica* (2005) defines death as "the total cessation of life processes that eventually occurs in all living organisms." It goes on to say that "human death has always been obscured by mystery and superstition, and its precise definition remains controversial, differing according to culture and legal systems." Indeed, the experience of death has changed: death in the first half of the century usually occurred from an acute or unexpected event, while today many deaths occur following degenerative diseases that entail a long and declining course. In 1967, Kubler-Ross's seminal research and interviews with dying patients raised our awareness about the dual concept of death: death,the event, and dying, the process. Though questioned today, her psychological stages of dying, specifically denial, anger, bargaining, depression, and acceptance, revolutionized our thinking about death. Although no consensus currently exists about when dying or end of life begins, the American Geriatrics Society (AGS) (1997) offers clinicians guidelines for making this determination with the following statement: "people are considered to be dying when they have a progressive illness that is expected to end in death and for which there is no treatment that can substantially alter the outcome (p. 87)."

Although the precise determination of death is not a focus of this chapter, nurses may care for patients whose families' fear the patient's being declared dead prematurely, for example, when the determination of death is extended to assure viability of organs for transplantation. The ability to prolong life and sustain life with artificial means necessitates the need for additional definitions of death. For legal purposes, brain death is considered to be the irreversible cessation of circulatory and respiratory function or the irreversible cessation of all functions of the entire brain, including the brain stem. Bioethicists and sociologists recommend the notion of "social death," referring to individuals who have lost their personhood by losing function of their cortex (Brody, 1988). Botkin and Post (1992) proposed that death be viewed as a syndrome, requiring that a cluster of related attributes be present before a diagnosis of brain death can be made.

The different views of death reflect the multidimensional nature of the concept. Professionals need to be cognizant of varying definitions of death and the issues raised by each perspective, such as the following:

- When should we remove life support and how should we support families?
- What are the risks and benefits of feeding versus not feeding patients at the end of life?
- When and from whom should we remove organs for transplantation?
- What skills and training do nurses need to serve as advocates to dying patients and families?
- What evidence is available to help nurses provide best practices in caring for patients and families experiencing life-threatening and terminal illness?

In palliative care, death is also viewed as an outcome measure for improving end-of-life care. The Institute of Medicine's report (IOM, 1997) provides some conceptual benchmarks from which quality outcome indicators can be developed. A "good death" is defined as one free from avoidable stress and suffering for patients and families and caregivers; in general accord with patients' and families' wishes; and reasonably consistent with clinical, cultural, and ethical standards. In contrast, a "bad death" is one in which there is needless suffering, disregard for patients' or family's wishes or values, and a sense among participants or observers that the norms of decency have been offended.

The fear of experiencing a "bad death" seems warranted by the conclusions of a 5-year study of the end-of-life care received by 9,000 dying hospitalized patients. The *Study to Understand Prognosis and Preferences for Outcomes and Risks of Treatments* (SUPPORT, 1995) was designed both to increase understanding of hospitalized dying and to devise an intervention to promote more humane care of dying patients. The SUPPORT data confirmed the high reports of pain among dying patients (more than 50%), clinicians' lack of training in pain management, and institutional limitations on the delivery of pain-control interventions. In addition, the SUPPORT data confirmed that patients' end-of-life treatment preferences, whether written or verbally communicated to nurses or family members, were often ignored by physicians or were otherwise ineffective in furthering the autonomous choices made by patients (SUPPORT, 1995).

BEYOND TABOOS IN ACKNOWLEDGING DEATH

Death in the United States is a taboo topic for many. Taboo, a Polynesian word, refers to something sacred or unclean. The object of a taboo in Polynesia is believed to have a power, or *mana,* so strong that only priests approach it. It is believed in some cultures that breaking the taboo requires ritual purification, or even death of the offender, to cleanse the community (*Concise Columbia Electronic Encyclopedia,* 1994). Awareness of the objects, words, or acts associated with religious or cultural rituals are important in supporting and communicating with members of varying social and religious groups and planning end-of-life (EOL) care. For example, early American Indians shot arrows in the air to ward off evil spirits; military funerals often use this same ritual when guns are fired in the air as the last salute. Indeed, the traditional tombstone may have originated to keep the bad spirits deep in the ground.

As death approaches, some individuals are inspired to search for meaning, peace, or transcendence that can replace fear and despair with hope and serenity (Byock, 1997). For others, grief, shame, guilt, and anger become overwhelming emotions, which prolong the period of grief or surface later in other areas of the mourner's life. In many households, it is taboo to speak of death, especially in the presence of children. Parents often consider death as morbid, and too much for children to handle. Children may even be sent off to a relative and told a lie such as "Mommy has gone on a long trip" to avoid the topic. Unfortunately, when the child eventually learns the truth, problems can arise such as unresolved guilt, distrust for grown-ups, and poor coping skills. Discussions about death make most people uncomfortable, including health care providers, and can trigger people's feelings about their own demise. Clearly, the SUPPORT study (1995) findings validate the need for improved physician-patient communication regarding goals of care and end-of-life decision-making.

America is a country of many races and cultures, and with each passing year more health care providers are recognizing the challenge of caring for patients from diverse linguistic and cultural backgrounds. In addition to providing quality care to an aging and diverse population, clinicians need to integrate patients' and families' racial, ethnic, cultural, and religious and nonreligious rituals and beliefs into care planning. Nurses should assess patients' perceptions, preferences, and behaviors and individualize communication and care strategies so as to respect these differences in the context of their organizational systems. Consumers are becoming more educated and vocal about their needs and options, especially those having Internet access to sophisticated medical information. Although information empowers some patients, it can create confusion for others and place them in a quandary regarding decision making (Desbeins, Mueller-Rizner, Hamel, & Connors, 1998).

All cultures have developed ways to cope with death. Interfering with these practices may interfere with the necessary grieving processes. Understanding different cultural responses to death can help professionals recognize the grieving process in patients of other cultures. The National Cancer Institute (www.Cancer.gov) offers professional and patient information on grief, loss, and bereavement. Helping families cope with the death of a loved one includes showing respect for the family's cultural heritage and encouraging them to decide how to honor the death. Important questions that should be asked of people who are dealing with the loss of a loved one include the following:

1. What are the cultural rituals for coping with dying, the deceased person's body, the final arrangements for the body, and honoring the death?
2. What are the family's beliefs about what happens after death?
3. What does the family feel is a normal expression of grief and the acceptance of the loss?
4. What does the family consider to be the roles of each family member in handling the death?
5. Are certain types of death less acceptable (for example, suicide), or are certain types of death especially hard to handle for that culture (for example, the death of a child)?

In a cross-cultural patient/provider relationship, both parties (patient and professional) may be called upon to acknowledge and respect health concepts and practices different from their own. Although this is an opportunity for growth and enrichment, it can also cause discomfort. Tension arises when different health belief systems confront one another. Common responses to the unknown or unfamiliar are anxiety, wariness, and even anger or fear.

To address the need for culturally and linguistically appropriate services (CLAS) in health care, national standards were published in the Federal Register, (2000). All health care personnel should learn to regard the patient and his or her family as unique and aim to develop skills to assess the role of culture in any given situation. It is important that clinicians develop consensus about how they will evaluate patient and family education regarding end-of-life issues, and provide culturally relevant resources and other sources of support.

Morbidity and Mortality Statistics for the United States: Leading Causes of Death

Life expectancy in the United States was the highest ever in 2002, but infant mortality increased from a rate of 6.8 infant deaths per 1,000 live births in 2001 to a rate of 7.0 per 1,000 births in 2002. A new report prepared by the Centers for Disease Control and Prevention's (CDC) National Center for Health Statistics (NCHS), entitled "Deaths: Preliminary Data for 2002," finds that in 2002, life expectancy in the United States reached a new high of 77.4 years, up from 77.2 in 2001. Life expectancy increased for both men and women, and for African Americans and Whites. Statistics from 2001 show that Black women can expect to live to 75 years compared to 80 years for White women; Black men can expect to live 68.6 years compared to 75 years for White males. These data reflect an increase of nearly a quarter of a century in life expectancy in the United States that can be attributed in part to advances in sanitation, nutrition, and immunization, which have eradicated or greatly reduced diseases. The report attributes the rise in infant mortality to an increase in neonatal infant deaths (infants less than 28 days old), particularly infants who died within the first week of life. However, there was continued decrease in late-term fetal deaths, defined as 28 or more weeks of gestation.

Three causes of death accounted for most of the increase in infant mortality: congenital anomalies (birth defects), disorders related to short gestation and low birth weight, and maternal complications of pregnancy. Deaths from sudden infant death syndrome (SIDS) declined between 2001 and 2002, continuing a long-term downward trend.

Overall, death rates for the total U.S. population dropped in 2002. The national age-adjusted death rate decreased slightly from 855 deaths per 100,000 population in 2001 to 847 deaths per 100,000 in 2002. In 1996, the death rate reached an all-time low of 491.6 deaths per 100,000.

The four leading causes of death in the United States continue to be heart disease (33%), cancer (23%), cerebrovascular disease (7%), and chronic obstructive pulmonary disease (4.6%). Accidents account for another 4.0% and pneumonia another 3.7%. The 2002 report shows declines in mortality from heart disease (3%), stroke (nearly 3 %), accidents/unintentional injuries (nearly 2%), and cancer (1%). The biggest decline in mortality among the leading cause of deaths was for homicides—down 17%. That number had increased sharply in 2001 due to the September 11 terrorist attacks. Excluding the September 11 deaths, the decrease from 2001 to 2002 would have been 3%, which still reflects a continuing downward trend in homicides that began in 1991.

There has also been a continued decline in the preliminary age-adjusted death rate from HIV/AIDS, which dropped 2% between 2001 and 2002. HIV mortality has decreased approximately 70% since 1995, but remains the fifth leading cause of death for people ages 25 to 44. Mortality rates increased for some leading causes of death, including Alzheimer's disease (up 5.8%), influenza and pneumonia (up 3.2%), high blood pressure (up 2.9%), and septicemia or blood poisoning (up 2.6%).

WHERE PEOPLE DIE

Little is known about where dying patients spend their last few months of life; however, mortality statistics from 1992 indicate that 57% of deaths occurred in hospitals, 15% in nursing homes, 20% in residences, and 6% elsewhere, including those declared dead on arrival at the hospital (IOM, 1997). About 55% to 60% of persons older than age 65 die in the hospital (Kaufman, 1998). Recent findings from SUPPORT investigators (Pritchard et al., 1998) support the national polls that although most people prefer to die at home. the majority died in the hospital. The number of patients dying in-hospital varied between 29% and 66% in the five research sites across the United States, with 23% to 54% of these cases being Medicare beneficiaries. Investigators found that measures of hospital availability and use were the most powerful predictors of the place of death. The chance of dying in a hospital was increased for residents of regions with a greater availability of hospital beds. The risk was decreased in regions that had greater nursing home and hospice availability and use. Variations within groups were not explained by sociodemographic, clinical, or patient preferences.

In previous centuries the majority of people died at home. By the mid 1970s, more than 70% of deaths were occurring in hospitals and other institutional settings (National Hospice Organization [NHO], 1997a). The shift in the location of dying had a dramatic impact on the nature of dying. Patients dying at home were usually cared for by family members with little or no high-technology equipment. The institutionalization of death raised a new set of challenges and problems for caregivers. Challenges include increased decision making about the extent of aggressive treatments; how to support and provide proper care for the dying; how to deal with the isolation and depersonalization of institutions; and how best to meet the nonphysical but critically important sociological, spiritual, and emotional needs of patients and family members. Additional regulations placed on institutions from managed care organizations often resulted in earlier discharges, shortened lengths of stay, and follow-up home care needs far greater than previously experienced. This is validated in data from 1988 through 1994, in which program payments for Medicare-covered home care services grew more than 500%, from $1.7 billion to $12.7 billion, and the number of certified home-health agencies grew from approximately 5,700 to 7,800 (Health Care Financing Administration [HCFA], 1996; IOM, 1997).

The literature describes an often fragmented approach to the care of the dying in institutions that led to undermining the patient's identity, wishes, and sense of self-worth. Institutionalization often served to isolate the family and to rob them of the opportunity to confront their own impending loss and adapt to the new roles and responsibilities ahead. Given proper support, most experts agree that families are able to resolve issues and become a strong source of support and caregiving for the patient. Ira Byock's (1997) book *Dying Well* illustrates through stories the prospect for growth and ability to achieve death-with-dignity at the end of life for patients and families. The hospice movement grew in response to this fragmentation of health care; the two strongest proponents for change came from the community and health care professionals who recognized inadequacies in end-of-life care.

DEATH TRAJECTORIES

Americans are living longer with chronic or terminal illnesses, resulting in the need for increases in assistance, symptom management, and hospice care services. There are many paths leading toward death. Patients who understand that they have a progressive disease from which they will likely die may not see themselves, or be seen by their families and friends, as dying. This group is differentiated from those thought to be imminently dying (i.e., likely to die within minutes to days), and those who are terminally ill but not thought to be actively dying (i.e., having a life expectancy of days to months and sometimes years). The latter group may have a period of prolonged "chronic living-dying" between the diagnosis of incurable illness and imminent death (McCormick & Conley, 1995). Patients in this group may be able to carry out their daily activities while coping with the prospect of death. Pediatric patients, for example, can live years to decades with illness such as cystic fibrosis. In the case of chronically ill older adults, premature death may suddenly occur from a superimposed viral illness, such as pneumonia.

The National Institute on Aging's agenda (NIA, 2000) for the years 2001 to 2005 has targeted three areas for research: (1) preventing or reducing age-related diseases, disorders, and disability; (2) maintaining physical health and function; and (3) enhancing older adults' societal roles and interpersonal support and reducing social isolation. The aging population is at increased risk for developing multiple chronic or life-threatening diseases, including heart disease, cancer, stroke, respiratory diseases, and other terminal illnesses, such as Alzheimer's disease. Health care costs can increase and quality of life and independence may be compromised for older adults and the terminally ill by weakness, falls, delirium, urinary incontinence, sleep disturbances, and serious depression. Living months or years with disease presents patients, families, and clinicians with social, moral, ethical, and medical dilemmas.

Technologies that sustain life by artificial means have increased our ability to prolong life, yet they have raised many moral, ethical, and legal dilemmas for Americans. Some bioethicists contend that the real political struggles of the twentieth century have not been over legal rights, but over control in the "way" individuals live their lives. Supreme Court rulings regarding the right to abortion, to die or cause death, to make family decisions, to live, to control one's own body, to health care, to refuse hydration, and to self-determination are examples of health care issues brought forth in the last few decades (Annas, 1993).

Nurses are an essential voice in these discussions in their roles as patient and family advocates, clinicians, leaders, health care policy-makers, educators, and as researchers. Education in the legal, moral and ethical principles, and decision-making models are essential for nurses to have an impact in determining the quality of care offered to individuals at the end of life and empowering patients to take an active role in achieving this outcome.

PATIENT-REQUESTED EUTHANASIA AND ASSISTED SUICIDE

Assisted suicide is described as a practice by which health care providers supply, but do not directly administer, the means for a patient to voluntarily hasten his or her own death. This is usually done by prescribing lethal doses of medication that the patient then ingests (IOM, 1997). Patient-requested euthanasia refers to a practice in which the means of hastening death are administered directly by the health care provider (Matzo & Emmanuel, 1997), for example, by injecting the patient with a lethal dose of medication. Brody (1992), a nationally known physician/ethicist, originated the term "assistance in dying" and claimed that patients capable of decision making could request assistance to achieve a "good death."

Since the 1970s notable events have shaped a new conceptualization and legal system related to the end of life and causing or assisting death (Table 3.1). The activities of Dr. Jack Kevorkian, a nonlicensed pathologist who has admitted to assisting more than 130 people to commit suicide, fueled the media and heightened public awareness about euthanasia and assisted suicide. Although he was found guilty in 1999 of second-degree murder and sentenced to 10 to 25 years of imprisonment, many Americans still view assisted dying as a "responsible alternative" to their fear of dying a lonely, undignified, prolonged, painful, or institutionalized death (Annas, 1995).

Oregon became the first state to legalize assisted suicide (but not euthanasia) in 1997 via the Death with Dignity Act, which allows physicians to prescribe lethal dosages of medication to competent, terminally ill patients who request them. Two surveys since the new law have provided some evidence about actual practices. Ganzini et al. (2000) found that physicians granted approximately one in six requests for a prescription for a lethal dose of medication, and one in ten requests actually resulted in suicide. The authors reported that effective palliative care interventions led most patients to change their minds about committing suicide.

In a second study, to understand physicians' reactions to requests for assisted suicide, 35 Oregon physicians who had received requests from patients were interviewed (Dobscha, Heintz, Press, & Ganzini, 2000). Requests for assisted suicide had a powerful impact on physicians and their practices. Physicians reported feeling unprepared, and experienced

TABLE 3.1   Events Raising Public Awareness About Assisted Dying

- The first "right to die" case of Karen Ann Quinlan, NJ. Parents request permission to withdraw use of a respirator on their comatose young daughter.

- California "Natural Death Act" empowered patients to specify end-of-life wishes in a living will.

- Patient Self-Determination Act. Hospital patients are informed of their right to make treatment decisions.

- Opinion poll shows majority of Americans support assisted suicide.

- Study to Understand Prognosis and Preferences for Outcomes and Risks of Treatments (SUPPORT). Five-year study results include inadequate pain management at end of life.

- Dr. Kevorkian's activities criticized by physicians and ethicists for assisting more than 130 people to commit suicide.

- Americans continue to view assisted dying as a reasonable alternative to the fear of dying a lonely, undignified, prolonged, and painful, institutionalized death.

- Death with Dignity Act legalizes physician-assisted suicide in Oregon.

- Dr. Kevorkian found guilty of second-degree murder and sentenced to 10 to 25 years in prison.

apprehension and discomfort before and after receiving requests. Frequent sources of discomfort included concerns about adequately managing symptoms and suffering, not wanting to abandon patients, and incomplete understanding of patients' preferences, especially when physicians did not know the patients well. Participation in assisted suicide required a large investment of time and was emotionally intense. Physicians did not express major regrets about their decisions to assist or not. Many physicians felt that the process and discussions increased their confidence and assertiveness in discussing end-of-life issues with other patients. Physicians rarely sought support from their spouses about the emotional aspects of their experiences. The data also confirm other results that suggest patients who receive good symptom control at the end of life choose life over death (Coyle, 1992; Foley, 1995).

Although public debates about assisted dying have focused almost exclusively on physician practices (Bachman et al., 1996), nurses' reports of their experiences with as-sisted dying are increasing. Schwarz's (1999) integrated review of bioethics and nursing literature (from 1990 to 1999) reveals the dilemmas faced by many nurses in discriminating between "hastening" and "assisting" death when caring for patients with severe symptom distress at the end of life. When 80 nurses were interviewed about the circumstances under which they felt justified in performing patient-requested euthanasia, 21% of the nurses were ethically able to justify active euthanasia and 16% indicated that they viewed patient autonomy and the presence of severe suffering as justifications (Davis et al., 1995). In Asch's 1996 study of 1,139 critical care nurses' self-reported clinical experiences with assisted dying, 16% ($n = 129$) reported participating in assisted suicide or patient-requested euthanasia. Recurring themes in their comments included concerns about overuse of life-sustaining technology, a profound sense of responsibility for the patient's welfare, and a desire to relieve patient suffering to overcome the perceived unresponsiveness of physicians toward that suffering. Matzo and Emmanuel's (1997) survey of 441 oncology nurses (71% response rate) revealed that 131 nurses (30%) received up to 20 requests for lethal drugs in the previous year. Of this group, 1% ($n = 6$) acknowledged helping a patient to commit suicide and 4.5% ($n = 20$) reported performing patient-requested euthanasia.

Ferrell, Virani, Grant, Coyne, and Uman (2000) surveyed 2,333 nurses' perspectives on end-of-life care; their results support the need for closer examination of nurses' participation in assisted dying. Fewer than 1% of the nurses report participation but these findings are troubling and indicate the need to understand nurses' conduct better, despite the prohibition of such practices by the ANA Code for Nurses. There is much support for the argument that if good symptom management were provided to dying patients, requests for assisted dying could be virtually eliminated (Coyle, 1992; Hall, 1996; Kazanowski, 1997; Kowalski, 1997; Murphy, 1992). This is especially important because skilled palliative care and hospice clinicians report being capable of making the dying process tolerable, if not completely comfortable, for almost 95% of their patients (Coyle, 1992; Foley, 1996; Quill, 1993).

Understanding why a terminally ill patient wishes to die has become a focus for improving end-of-life care and a key component of the physician-assisted-suicide debate. In identifying the factors that contribute to a patient's desire for hastened death, the psychological factors of depression and hopelessness have been discovered to be as, if not more, important than physical pain in influencing a patient's wish to die (Brietbart et al., 2000).

Coyle and Sculco's (2004) qualitative study of 7 patients living with advanced cancer revealed the many meanings of the expression "desire for hastened death." These include (a) a manifestation of the will to live; (b) a dying process so difficult that an early death was preferred; c) an intolerable immediate situation; (d) to extract themselves from an unendurable situation; (e) a last control effort; (f) a way to draw attention to one's uniqueness; (g) a gesture of altruism; (h) an attempt to manipulate a family situation; and (i) a despairing cry depicting the misery of the situation. Coyle recommends that nurses assess the context of the patient's situation, life history, and experiences and use the expression "desire for hastened death" as a communication tool, not necessarily as a literal request.

Research regarding nurses' practices are needed. The statements to be answered involve the barriers that nurses encounter when trying to provide the best end-of-life care and access to palliative or hospice care for dying patients. Nurse educators, in particular, are challenged to help their students who are caring for highly symptomatic dying patients to distinguish between those acts presumed to be morally and professionally permissible and illegal acts of "assisted" dying (Schwarz, 1999).

Evidence of the Need to Improve End-of-Life Care

Two major studies within the last decade have identified priority areas for end-of-life care: the SUPPORT study (1995) and the Institute of Medicine Report (1997). Few clinical research projects have generated as much public interest or as many published articles as the SUPPORT study. This $29 million multiyear research project (funded by the Robert Wood Johnson Foundation) was the first to reveal the failure of the American health care system to provide effective and compassionate care to seriously ill and dying patients. The study began with a 2-year prospective observational study (Phase 1) of 4,301 patients, followed by a 2-year controlled clinical trial (Phase 2) in which 4,804 patients and their physicians were randomized by specialty group to an intervention group ($n = 2,652$) or control group ($n = 2,152$). The "intervention" took the form of a specially trained nurse who had multiple contacts with patient, family, physician, and hospital staff to elicit preferences, encourage attention to pain control, and facilitate advance care planning and physician/patient communication.

Results from Phase 1 documented the lack of communication between patients and physicians and provided characteristics about hospital deaths. Specifically, the results indicated that 46% of Do Not Resuscitate (DNR) orders were written within 2 days of death; 47% of physicians knew when their patient wanted to avoid CPR; 38% of patients who died spent at least 10 days in the ICU; 50% of patients who died in the hospital had moderate to severe pain (reported by families) at least half the time; and there was a high use of hospital resources. No improvements were found in the above outcomes following the Phase 2 nurse intervention. The findings from the SUPPORT study have provided the impetus for leaders in all health disciplines to develop and implement initiatives in research, education, and practice to improve end-of-life care for patients and their families.

The Institute of Medicine has produced the second series of landmark reports. The first report, "Approaching Death: Improving Care at the End of Life" (1997), is based on the collaborative efforts of a committee of 12 experts in medicine and nursing who cared for chronically ill and severely ill patients. The IOM report summarized issues that needed to be addressed regarding end-of-life care: (1) a review of the state of the knowledge in EOL care, including (2) evaluation methods for measuring outcomes; (3) factors impeding high-quality care; and (4) steps toward agreement on what constitutes "appropriate care" at end of life. The committee's four major findings, listed below, suggest starting points for quality improvement (QI) work in terms of patient care, organizations, education, and research:

1. Too many people suffer endlessly at the end of life both from errors of omission (when caregivers fail to provide palliative and supportive care known to be effective) and from errors of commission (when caregivers do what is known to be ineffective and even harmful).
2. Legal, organizational, and economic obstacles conspire to obstruct reliably excellent care at the end of life.
3. The education and training of physicians and other health care professionals fail to provide them with knowledge, skills, and attitudes required to care for the dying patient.
4. Current knowledge and understanding are inadequate to guide and support consistent practice of evidence-based medicine at the end of life. (IOM, 1997)

Two reports that followed—"Improving Palliative Care for Cancer" (2001) and "When Children Die: Improving Palliative and End-of-Life Care for Children and Their Families" (2002)—continued their arguments that medical and other support for people with fatal or potentially fatal conditions often fall short of what is reasonably if not simply attainable. The IOM reports highlight the inadequacy of current knowledge to guide the practice of clinicians in end-of-life care and the need for support from policy makers. Federal and private sources of funding to improve care at the end of life have increased. Examples include private foundations such as the Open Society Institute's Project on Death in America, the Commonwealth Fund, and the United Hospital Fund of New York. Requests for applications are available from federal and professional organizations in targeted areas such as reducing barriers to symptom management in palliative care and improving end-of-life care in the underserved elderly.

During the Clinton Administration (1992–2000), health care spending and allocation of resources resulted in the rapid expansion of managed care organizations in the United States. Managed care offers a broad menu of ways that health services are accessed and paid for. This system is designed to save money by controlling patient access to expensive secondary and tertiary services and technology, and by setting limits on reimbursement. Managed care systems utilize management trends such as product-line management, total quality management (TQM) or continuous quality improvement (CQI), and innovations that streamline delivery systems. Goals are aimed at reducing waste and cost, increasing customer satisfaction, and improving clinical outcomes (Johnsson, 1992). Health care providers are challenged with balancing the needs of their patients and the constraints of what insurers will provide. Reducing cost and providing quality care is the goal of hospital management; it is estimated that about 70% of nurse manager responsibilities will be allocated to quality improvement activities in the next decade.

The cost of end-of-life care in the United States is projected to escalate with the population's life expectancy. The National Medical Care Expenditure Survey (Cohen, Carlson, & Porter, 1995) found that for those persons 65 or older who died in 1987, spending during the last 6 months of their lives accounted for an estimated 5.5% of total spending or $32.6 billion. Other data sources (Scitovsky, 1996) suggest that expenditures may not increase so much by age alone, but rather by the cause of death. For example, cancer, chronic obstructive pulmonary disease (COPD), and renal disease cost more in Medicare payments than accidents and heart attacks.

End-of-life care is primarily funded through Medicare, Medicaid, the Veterans Administration and other public programs, with an estimated 60% of hospice patients being covered by Medicare (Vladeck, 1995). Although hospice coverage is now offered by nearly 80% of large- and medium-size employers (IOM, 1997), many patients and families miss the opportunity to access hospice services because of inadequate end-of-life discussions with their health care providers.

THE EVOLUTION OF HOSPICE AND PALLIATIVE CARE

The hospice concept originated in the Middle Ages when pilgrims traveling to the Holy Land found their minds and bodies restored when they stopped at way stations attended by religious orders. Hospices, originally opened by the Irish Sisters of Charity in Dublin, Ireland, in 1879, moved to London by 1905. Dame Cicely Saunders, a nurse who later became a social worker and physician, is credited with opening Saint Christopher's Hospice in London where she championed the need for a multidisciplinary approach and around-the-clock administration of opioids when caring for dying patients. Her approach to care focused on comfort, skilled nursing, family counseling, physical therapy, and addressing spiritual needs (Storey, 1996). These fundamental elements of care characterize quality palliative care.

Florence Wald, another nurse recognized for her pioneer work in the hospice movement in the United States, envisioned the need to maximize the quality of life for the terminally ill. Following a trip to Saint Christopher's in the 1960s, she returned home to conduct a feasibility study of the need for a hospice in Connecticut. The United States subsequently opened its first hospice in Branford, Connecticut, in 1974 (Friedrich, 1999). Inducted into the Women's Hall of Fame in 1998, Wald is known for her exemplary work in influencing hospices throughout the country, promoting holistic and humanistic care for the dying, and advocating for nurses' education regarding care at the end of life. The hospice model serves as the gold standard for offering the best end-of-life care to patients and their families.

Access to hospice traditionally has been limited to patients who have a life expectancy of less than 6 months and are no longer pursuing active treatment. Palliative care, however, can begin from the time a patient is diagnosed with a life-threatening illness. Due to a typically late referral to hospice, the median length of stay for hospice patients is relatively short and averages only about 22 days (National Hospice and Palliative Care Organization [NHPCO], 2003). Physicians are less reluctant to refer patients to the palliative care team because it does not carry the absolute association with death that hospice care does. Hospice programs typically require a Do Not Resuscitate order, insurers may not allow high-tech life-prolonging therapies, or they may limit access to medical specialists. Although palliative care programs also strive to relieve the pain and suffering associated with any life-threatening illness, they do not mandate foregoing life-prolonging therapies. The goal of treatment remains achieving the optimal quality of life for patients and families.

The Medicare hospice benefit is based on a probability prediction that an individual with a terminal or incurable illness will not survive for longer than 6 months. Palliative care experts, however, have long recognized the need to provide access to comprehensive services earlier in the disease trajectory.

Newer models of palliative care address both disease-specific therapies as well as supportive-comfort therapies that promote the optimal function and well-being of patients and their family caregivers. The Canadian Palliative Care Association's model (1995) documents how palliative care needs intensify at the end of life. The core issues of palliation, comfort, and function are salient throughout the course of the disease. A palliative care model recognizes the need to address symptom distress, physical impairments, and psychosocial disturbance even during the period of aggressive primary therapy with goals of cure or the prolongation of life (Portenoy, 1998).

National Hospice Foundation research on end-of-life care found that Americans are more willing to talk about safe sex and drugs with their children than to discuss end-of-life care with their terminally ill parents. Only 24% of Americans put into writing how they want to be cared for at the end of life. A substantial proportion, 19%, have not thought about end-of-life care at all, while 16% have thought about it, but have not told anyone their wishes.

In 2003, there were nearly 40 million seniors in the U.S. In the next 30 years, that number is expected to double, as baby boomers successively reach age 65. Considering the discussions taking place in the media, online, and in other arenas, these boomers will place importance on dying well, just as they have emphasized living well. Hospice provides the quality care that allows people to live well at the end of life (NHPCO, 2003).

Palliative care found its roots in the hospice movement. The World Health Organization (WHO, 2002) defines palliative care as

an approach that improves the quality of life of patients and families who face life-threatening illness, by providing pain and symptom relief, spiritual and psychosocial support to from diagnosis to the end of life and bereavement.

Palliative care

- provides relief from pain and other distressing symptoms;
- affirms life and regards dying as a normal process;
- intends neither to hasten nor postpone death;
- integrates the psychological and spiritual aspects of patient care;
- offers a support system to help patients live as actively as possible until death;
- offers a support system to help the family cope during the patient's illness and in their own bereavement;
- uses a team approach to address the needs of patients and their families, including bereavement counselling, if indicated;
- will enhance quality of life, and may also positively influence the course of illness;
- is applicable early in the course of illness, in conjunction with other therapies that are intended to prolong life, such as chemotherapy or radiation therapy, and includes those investigations needed to better understand and manage distressing clinical complications.

Definitions of palliative care have evolved based on the work of the National Consensus Project (NCP) for palliative care (2004). Palliative care and hospice programs have grown in the United States in response to a population living with chronic, debilitating, and life-threatening illness and to clinician interest in effective approaches to providing care. Most recently, five major palliative care organizations led a National Consensus Project for Quality Palliative Care to improve the quality of palliative care in the U.S. Efforts resulted in "Clinical Practice Guidelines for Quality Palliative Care" (2004). The guidelines are organized into eight domains of care (see Table 3.2) and aim to promote quality and reduce variation in new and existing programs, develop

TABLE 3.2 Domains of Quality Palliative Care

- Structure and Processes of Care
- Physical Aspects of Care
- Psychological and Psychiatric Aspects of Care
- Social Aspects of Care
- Spiritual, Religious, and Existential Aspects of Care
- Cultural Aspects of Care
- Care of the Imminently Dying Patient
- Ethical and Legal Aspects of Care

and encourage continuity of care across settings, and facilitate collaborative partnerships among palliative care programs, community hospices, and other health care settings. Fundamental processes that cross all domains include assessment, information sharing, decision making, care planning, and care delivery. Developers incorporated established standards of care from Australia, New Zealand, Canadian, Children's Hospital International, and the National Hospice and Palliative Care organizations. Studies will be needed to evaluate the usefulness of the guidelines to foster access to care; continuity across settings, such as home, residential, hospital, and hospice; development of national benchmarks for care; uniform definitions that assure reliable quality care and encourage performance measurement and quality improvement initiatives for palliative care services.

Factors that have contributed to the palliative care movement in the United States include the growing aging population, the assisted suicide debate, reduced patient autonomy, and inappropriate end-of-life care (i.e., overtreatment of medical conditions and undertreatment of pain and depression). Quality outcomes of good palliative care ensure that patients' values and decisions are respected; comfort is a priority; psychosocial, spiritual, and practical needs will be addressed; and opportunities will be encouraged for growth and completion of unfinished business (NCP, 2004).

GENERALIST AND SPECIALIST PALLIATIVE CARE

Palliative care specialists (advance practice nurses and physicians) address diverse quality-of-life concerns and promote interdisciplinary care emphasizing distinction of life and of dying, promotion of comfort and relief of suffering, and respect for autonomy and family involvement. As specialists they serve as role models and educators in clinical practice. They work to develop the theoretical and empirical body of knowledge in palliative care through research, develop and implement institution-based models of palliative care, and institute quality improvement programs. Palliative care specialists focus on complex patients, such as those with multiple or difficult symptom-control problems who require comprehensive care for multiple needs (e.g., needing family support or nursing-home-based management for monitoring and titration of medication), and comprehensive care of the imminently dying. Although palliative care is now recognized as a specialty, palliative care as a model of care is a therapeutic approach ideally integrated into the care of all patients with life-threatening disease across the illness/dying trajectory (NCP, 2004).

Improving Education of Professionals

The SUPPORT (1995) study documented nurses' opinions that improved communication, time, and repeated information about end-of-life issues were necessary for families to make decisions regarding interventions for life-threatening illnesses (Hiltunen et al., 1995). These findings highlight the role of the nurse as companion and confidant to patients and families and support a shared decision-making model in end-of-life treatment discussions. This is especially relevant given that only 15% of patients nationally have an advance directive. National efforts are increasing to educate professionals in the United States. The American Medical Association's Education for Physicians on End-of-Life Care (EPEC) (Emanuel, von Gunten, & Ferris, 1999) curriculum, supported by a grant from the Robert Wood Johnson Foundation, is designed to educate physicians across the United States on essential clinical competencies in end-of-life care. The American Society of Clinical Oncology, in collaboration with the National Cancer Institute and the EPEC Project, offer workshops to help optimize care for patients throughout the course of their illness. A complementary program entitled the End of Life Nursing Education Consortium (ELNEC), also funded by the Robert Wood Johnson Foundation, is a partnership of the American Association of Colleges of Nursing (AACN) and the City of Hope National Medical Center (COH). As of 2003, courses have been tailored to oncology and pediatrics.

CHANGES IN HEALTH CARE ECONOMICS

Treatment Decision-Making: Estimating Prognosis

Physicians and nurses struggle with decisions about appropriate care for patients who are near death. Predicting how long someone will live with an incurable illness is a difficult and complex task. Lynn, Teno, and

Harrell (1995) describe the construction of a model for more accurate prognostications of death. It includes a risk of death estimate plus 14 patient characteristics: diagnosis, serum sodium level, temperature, respiratory rate, heart rate, oxygenation, creatinine level, mean blood pressure, bilirubin and albumin levels, Glasgow coma score, age, days in hospital, and having cancer as a comorbidity. These authors assert that their statistical model coupled with the physician's estimates is better than either one alone.

Weeks and colleagues (1998) examined data from 917 adults with stage III or IV non–small-cell lung and metastatic colon cancer in phases 1 and 2 of the SUPPORT study across five U.S. teaching sites. Results indicated that patients were substantially more optimistic about their prognosis than their physicians were. In 82% of the physician-patient pairs, the patients' estimate of their chance of living 6 months was higher than the physicians; in 59% of the pairs, the patient estimate exceeded the physician estimate by two prognostic categories. Patients who were more optimistic about their prognosis lived longer than patients who were less optimistic. Patients who believed that they would survive at least 6 months favored life-extending therapy over comfort care at more than double the rate of those who believed they had less than 6 months to live. Patients greatly overestimated their chances of surviving 6 months while physicians' prognostic estimates were more precise: physicians (estimating 90% survival) accurately predicted 71% of the deaths.

These studies indicate two important findings. First is the need for better communication between physicians and their patients about prognosis. This discussion could help patients make more informed treatment decisions consistent with their values and could facilitate earlier access to palliative or hospice care. The second relates to the need to understand better the source of patients' beliefs, preferences, and the ways in which they arrive at decisions about their care. This may be critical in designing interventions that are effective in changing end-of-life patterns of communication and care.

PROMOTING QUALITY PALLIATIVE CARE

Research results indicate that there is an overwhelming need for improved symptom management at the end of life for both adults and children. Patients at the end-of-life experience many of the same symptoms and syndromes regardless of their underlying condition. To decrease patient and family suffering at the end of life and improve symptom control, in-hospital programs are adopting a palliative care model that offers comprehensive care for seriously ill patients and their families. Nine case studies of pioneer palliative care programs are described in a Milbank Memorial Fund Report (2000) sponsored by the Robert Wood Johnson Foundation. More nurses with specialized palliative and hospice care expertise are being trained to provide patient care, serve as role models for staff, assure that standards are evidence-based, and develop monitoring and evaluation programs to meet benchmarks set by professional organizations for quality care at the end of life. This work is especially important because nearly 35 years after the start of the hospice movement in the United States, only half of adults who die of cancer receive hospice care. Nurses have an important role in identifying patients eligible for hospice and palliative care and facilitating access to specialty services for patients and families.

Palliative care services are lacking for children as well. In a Boston study of 165 children with cancer, 49% died in the hospital, and half of these were in the ICU. According to parents, 89% of the children suffered "a lot" or a "great deal" from at least one symptom in the last month of life, mostly pain, fatigue, and dyspnea (Wolfe et al., 2000). Currently only a handful of organized palliative care services for children exist in the United States. Palliative care programs designed for adults are inappropriate and ineffective for children (Stevens, Dalla Poza, Caelletto, Cooper, & Kilham, 1994; Whitman, 1993). One reason cited was the unwillingness of providers and parents to relinquish curative, invasive therapies even when there was little or no realistic hope for favorable outcomes. Often aggressive therapy is not abandoned until shortly before death so families and providers have little or no time to address their emotions or begin to grieve.

Removing Barriers to Providing Excellent End-of-Life Care

Several structures, processes, and outcome measures are needed in organizations to identify and remove barriers to providing effective end-of-life care. A "top-down, bottom-up" approach is necessary. This means a mandate is needed from top administration that includes support and resources, coupled with a multidisciplinary team of experts, masterful in using a systematic process for creating change (Bookbinder et al., 2005). Structures geared toward reducing variation in practice and optimizing the achievement of best practices and outcomes can serve as a benchmark against which we can measure and constantly improve. In addition to hospital-required policies and procedures, structures include standards of care, guidelines, and tools that direct patient care management such as protocols, algorithms, care paths, flow charts, and standardized orders.

Quality structures can be internally initiated or externally imposed. By 2001, the Joint Commission on Accreditation of Healthcare Organizations (JCAHO, 2004) required hospitals to implement new pain-management standards, including routine assessment and reassessment of pain and care at the end of life. This national initiative requiring relief of pain and suffering occurred within 15 years of the American Pain Society's quality-assurance pain standards for acute and cancer pain guidelines (Max et al., 1995; WHO, 2002). This dramatic change in society's culture regarding the need for pain relief offers hope to palliative care initiatives aimed at good end-of-life care.

Protocols and algorithms have become popular clinical tools in a managed care era of "doing more with less time and resources." These tools aim to streamline processes of care, deliver consistent and timely interventions, and improve quality of life, particularly at the end of life. Tools such as the *Palliative Care Clinical Practice Protocol for Dyspnea* (Hospice Nurse Association, 1996), *Symptom Management Algorithms for Palliative Care* (Wrede-Seaman, 1999), and the *Pocket Guide to Hospice/Palliative Medicine* (American Association of Hospice and Palliative Medicine [AAHPM], 2003) offer clinicians a methodology for assessing symptoms, etiology, directions for treatment options, and guidelines for pharmacological and nonpharmacological interventions.

Family perception of end-of-life care is increasingly being used to measure outcomes of care. Teno et al. (2004) conducted a mortality follow-back survey of family members or other knowledgeable informants representing 1,578 decedents. They found that family perceptions of patients who were involved in end-of-life decision making have reported positive end-of-life outcomes, for example, peaceful death, patient preferences were met, and goals of care were agreed upon, grief resolution.

Pathways (care paths), flow sheets, and standardized orders are products of a managed care era that intend to "reduce variation" in services and practices, and thereby reduce costs (Association of Community Cancer Centers, 1999; Blancett & Flarey, 1998; Gordon, 1996; Haward, 1998; Janken, Grubbs, & Haldeman, 1999; Wakefield, Johnson, Kron-Chalupa, & Paulsen, 1998; Zander, 1991). Although the many needs of dying patients have been identified (SUPPORT, 1995), few end-of-life clinical pathways have been developed and tested (Bookbinder, 2000; NHO, 1997b;). Goals for these pathways include (1) respecting patient autonomy, values, decisions; (2) continually clarifying goals of care; (3) minimizing symptom distress at the end of life; (4) optimizing appropriate supportive interventions and consultations; (5) reducing unnecessary interventions; (6) supporting families by coordinating services; (7) eliminating unnecessary regulations; (8) providing bereavement services for families and staff; and (9) facilitating the transition to alternate care settings, such as hospice, when appropriate (Bookbinder, 2000).

Palliative and hospice care experts are working to produce and implement the materials needed to build "safe and competent" infrastructures that will improve patients' and families' quality of living and dying. As members of multidisciplinary teams, nurses can lead efforts to implement structures that can improve the care of dying patients. This includes selecting and evaluating tools for practice and determining the strength of the evidence to reliably predict positive patient outcomes. Evaluation and testing of palliative care structures and their appropriateness, effectiveness, and cost of care are greatly needed (Higginson, 1993; Kristjanson, 1986).

Kirchhoff and Beckstrand's (2000) survey of 199 critical care nurses (69% response rate) documented perceptions of obstacles and helpful behaviors regarding the provision of end-of-life care. Six of the top ten obstacles that made patient care at the end of life more difficult were related to issues involving the patient's families. Examples cited included the family's not fully understanding the meaning of life support, not accepting the patient's poor prognosis, requesting more technical treatment than the patient wished, and being angry. Additional barriers related to problems with physicians. The "most helpful" behaviors were those that made dying easier for patients and their families, such as, agreement among physicians about care, dying with dignity, and the family's acceptance of the prognosis.

Building Evidence-Based Practice

Although few end-of-life care practices are currently based upon strong scientific evidence (IOM, 1997), research is available to help nurses shape their role in providing state-of-the-art care to patients and their families at the end of life. Research results indicate the need for health care settings to (a) systematically identify and remove obstacles to excellent care at the end of life; (b) identify end-of-life issues in vulnerable populations such as children, older adults, and those who are chemically dependent; (d) test models and tools (algorithms and care paths) aimed to improve symptom control and end-of-life outcomes such as comfort and distress; (e) develop programs to educate professionals in end-of-life care and evaluate the various formats for education; and (f) develop professional competencies which demonstrate "best practices" at the bedside. Also important is the need for professionals to: a) improve communication and understanding about treatment goals and outcomes among physicians, nurses, patients, and families; b) understand the contributing factors to nurses' reported behaviors in assisted suicide; and c) determine patient prognosis and earlier preparation for end-of-life care planning, especially in the "chronic-living-dying" population.

CONCLUSIONS

Views toward death and dying in American culture continue to change at a relatively consistent pace as evidence is compiled documenting the need to improve the care of the dying and their families. This challenge to nurses and nurse educators is a formidable one in the decade ahead. Nurses leading the field need advanced education and training in palliative care. All nurses need to know when the services of an interdisciplinary specialist-level palliative care team is indicated and how to access them. They need to be aware of evidence-based clinical practice guidelines in palliative care and how to implement and evaluate them to achieve desirable patient and family outcomes.

EDUCATION PLAN 3.1 Plan for Achieving Competencies: Death and Society

Knowledge Needed	Attitudes	Skills	Undergraduate Behavioral Outcomes	Graduate Behavioral Outcomes	Teaching/Learning Strategies
Changes related to death in American society and the taboo in acknowledging death.	*Consider changes related to death in society of the 21st century as compared to the previous century. *Appreciate death as a normal part of the life cycle. *Validate the need for improved health care provider-patient/family communication regarding dying and death.		*Discuss dying and death with patients and families as a normal part of the life cycle rather than something that should be feared.	*Raise public awareness of the negative consequences of avoiding the discussion of dying and death.	*Explore the students'/nurses' first experience with death and their related perceptions. *Discuss taboos about death from students'/nurses' own cultural/religious perspectives. *Have students report on societal perspectives of dying and death as presented by mass media, i.e., television, newspapers.

(continued)

EDUCATION PLAN 3.1   *(continued)*

Knowledge Needed	Attitudes	Skills	Undergraduate Behavioral Outcomes	Graduate Behavioral Outcomes	Teaching/Learning Strategies
Changing Demographics Related to Death: —Morbidity and mortality statistics; —Leading causes of death; —Where people die; —Different dying trajectories.	*Value patients' and families' desires to die at home with necessary support. *Support patients and families who are experiencing varying dying trajectories.		*Describe the changes in morbidity and mortality rates, leading causes of death, patient/family preferences of where to die, and different dying trajectories as they relate to nursing practice and health care delivery.	*Collaborate in research studies that provide epidemiological data related to dying and death.	*In small groups, have students/nurses discuss feelings and attitudes regarding different dying situations. Elicit their perceptions regarding nursings' roles and responsibilities in caring for patients and families experiencing varying dying trajectories.

Desire for Hastened Death: —Euthanasia; —Physician-assisted suicide.	*Appreciate the need for quality palliative care so that the need for hastened death will not be perceived as necessary by patients with terminal illness. *Affirm the ANA Code of Ethics which states that nurses' participation in assisted suicide or euthanasia is unethical.	*Communicate to patients that palliative care will be provided to alleviate end of life suffering.	*Collaborate with other health professionals for greater access to palliative care for all patient populations.	*Discuss the Oregon Death with Dignity Act, the reasons individuals requested physician-assisted suicide, and implications for nursing practice.

(continued)

EDUCATION PLAN 3.1 (*continued*)

Knowledge Needed	Attitudes	Skills	Undergraduate Behavioral Outcomes	Graduate Behavioral Outcomes	Teaching/Learning Strategies
Changes in health care economics: —Cost containment in practice settings. —Treatment decisions based on estimate of prognoses.	*Appreciate the impact of managed care on quality care offered at the end of life. *Acknowledge the difficulties in determining prognoses and estimating life expectancy.		*Balance the needs of patients and families at the end of life within the constraints of managed care systems. *Discuss with patients and families their role and responsibilities as members of an HMO. *Encourage patients and families to advocate for their end of life needs to their insurance companies. *Assist patients/families in selecting an HMO through discussion of relevant criteria.	*Address economic barriers to palliative care for all populations across all health care settings by proactive strategies at the administrative, institutional, and community levels. *Advocate for the needs of patients and families enrolled in HMOs who are experiencing life-threatening illness. *Evaluate models that prognosticate death for varying disease states in diverse patient populations.	*Invite an administrator of an HMO to class or conduct a telephone interview to discuss the care available to patients and families experiencing life-threatening illnesses. *Analyze newspaper and media reports regarding access to palliative care across populations and health care settings.

| Changes in service delivery to improve end of life care: —Improving patient suffering; —Removing barriers to end of life care; —Improving education of health professionals; —Building evidence based practice. | *Express commitment to changes in service delivery that will improve end of life care. | *Participate in nursing initiatives which will improve patient suffering, remove barriers to end of life care, improve nursing knowledge regarding palliative care, and build evidence-based practice. | *Provide expert palliative care. *Serve as role models for staff. *Insure that standards are evidence based. *Set up monitoring and evaluation programs to meet benchmarks set by professional organizations for quality care at the end of life. | *Assist students/ nurses to identify leadership opportunities related to palliative care. *Have students/ nurses develop continuous quality improvement with their clinical setting to evaluate an aspect of palliative care. |

(continued)

REFERENCES

American Academy of Hospice and Palliative Medicine. (2003). *Pocket Guide to Hospice/ Palliative Medicine.* Glenview, IL: Author.

American Association of Colleges of Nursing. (2002). *Peaceful death. Recommended competencies and curricula guidelines for end-of-life nursing care* [Electronic version]. Retrieved 12/28/04 from http:/www.aacn.niche.edu./ Publications/deathfin.htm

American Geriatrics Society. (1997). *Measuring quality of care at end-of-life: A statement of principles* [Electronic version]. Retrieved 12/28/04 from http://www.americangeriatrics.org

Annas, G. J. (1993). *Standard of care: The law of American bioethics.* New York: Oxford University Press.

Annas, G. J. (1995). How we die. *Hastings Center Report, 25,* 512–514.

Asch, D. A. (1996). The role of critical care nurses in euthanasia and assisted suicide. *New England Journal of Medicine, 334,* 1374–1401.

Association of Community Cancer Centers. (1998). *Oncology Critical Pathways.* Rockville, MD: Author.

Avellanet, C. (2000). *1999 Annual report of Jacob Perlow Hospice.* New York: Beth Israel Medical Center.

Bachman, J., Alcser, K., Doukis, D., Lichtenstein, R., Corning, A., & Brody, H. (1996). Attitudes of Michigan physicians and the public towards legalizing physician-assisted suicide and voluntary euthanasia. *New England Journal of Medicine, 334,* 303–309.

Blancett, S. S., & Flarey, D. L. (1998). *Health care outcomes: Collaborative, path-based approaches.* Gaithersburg, MD: Aspen.

Bookbinder, M. (2000). Quality care at end-of-life. In. B. R. Ferrell & N. Coyle (Eds.), *Palliative care nursing* (pp. 503–530). New York: Oxford University Press.

Bookbinder, M., Blank, A. E., Arney, E., Wollner, D., Lesage, P., McHugh, M., Indelicato, R. A., Harding, S., Barenboim, A., Mirozvev, T., Portenoy, R. K. Improving end-of-life care: development and pilot-test of a clinical pathway. *Journal of Pain & Symptom Management.* 29(6):529–43, 2005 Jun.

Bookbinder, M., Kiss, M., Coyle, N., Brown, M., Gianella, A., & Thaler, H. (1995). Improving pain management practices. In D. McGuire, C. Yarbro, & B. Ferrell (Eds.), *Cancer pain management* (2nd ed., pp. 321–361). Boston: Jones and Bartlett.

Botkin, J. R., & Post, S. G. (1992, Autumn). Confusion in the determination of death. *Perspective in Biology and Medicine, 36*(1), 129–138.

Breitbart, William MD; Rosenfeld, Barry PhD; Kaim, Monique PhD; Funesti-Esch, Julie RNA. Randomized, double-blind, placebo-controlled trial of psychostimulants for the treatment of fatigue in ambulatory patients with human immunodeficiency virus disease. *Archives of Internal Medicine.* 161(3):411–420, February 12, 2001.

Breitbart, W., Rosenfeld, B., Pessin, H., et al. (2000). Depression, hopelessness, and desire for hastened death in terminally ill patients with cancer. *Journal of the American Medical Association, 284,* 2907.

Brody, H. (1988). Brain death and personal existence: A reply to Green and Wikler. *Journal of Medicine and Philosophy, 4,* 8.

Brody, H. (1992). Assisted dying—A compassionate response to a medical failure. *New England Journal of Medicine, 327,* 1384–1388.

Byock, I. R. (1997). *Dying well.* New York: Riverhead Books.

Canadian Palliative Care Association. (1995). Palliative care: Towards a consensus in standardized principles of practice.

Cohen, S. B., Carlson, B. L., & Porter, D. E. B. (1995). Health care expenditures in the last six months of life. *American Statistical Association, Health Policy Review, 1*(2), 1–13.

Concise Columbia Electronic Encyclopedia. (2001, 2005). New York: Columbia University Press.

Coyle, N. (1992). The euthanasia and physician suicide debate: Issues for nursing. *Oncology Nursing Forum, 19*(Suppl. 7), 41–46.

Coyle, N., & Sculco, L. (2004). Expressed desire for hastened death in seven patients living with advanced cancer: A phenomenolgic inquiry. *Oncology Nursing Forum, 31*(4), 1–8.

Davis, A. J., Phillips, L., Drought, T. S., Sellin, S., Ronsman, K., & Hershberger, A. K. (1995). Nurses' attitudes toward active euthanasia. *Nursing Outlook, 43,* 174–179.

Desbeins, N. A., Mueller-Rizner, N., Hamel, M. B., & Connors, A. F. (1998). Preference for comfort care does not affect the pain experience of seriously ill patients. *Journal of Pain and Symptom Management, 16,* 281–289.

Dobscha, S. K., Heintz, R. T., Press, N., & Ganzini, L. (2004). Oregon physicians' responses to requests for assisted suicide: A qualitative study. *Journal of Palliative Medicine, 7,* 469–471.

Emanuel, L. L., von Gunten, C. F., & Ferris, F. D. (1999). *The education for physicians on Encyclopedia Britannica,* V 32, Encyclodia Britannica, Inc. *end-of-life care (EPEC) curriculum.* From the EPEC Project, Feinberg School of Medicine, Northwestern University, Chicago.

Encyclopedia Britannica, V. 32, Encyclopedia Britannica, Inc.

Ferrell, B., Virani, R., Grant, M., Coyne, P., & Uman, G. (2000). Beyond the Supreme Court decision: Nursing perspectives on end-of-life care. *Oncology Nursing Forum, 27,* 445–455.

Foley, K. M. (1995). Pain, physician-assisted suicide, and euthanasia. *Pain Forum, 4,* 163–178.

Foley, K. M. (1996). Controlling the pain of cancer. *Scientific American,* 164–165.

Friedrich, M. J. (1999). Hospice care in the U.S.: A conversation with Florence S. Wald. *Journal of the American Medical Association, 281,* 1683–1685.

Ganzini, L., Nelson, H. D., Schmidt, T. A., Kraemer, D. F., Delorit, M. A., & Lee, M. A. (2000). Physicians' experiences with the Oregon Death with Dignity Act. *New England Journal of Medicine, 342,* 557–563.

Gordon, D. B. (1996). Critical pathways: A road to institutionalizing pain management. *Journal of Pain and Symptom Management, 11,* 252–259.

Hainsworth, D. S. (1996). The effect of death education on attitudes of hospital nurses toward care of the dying. *Oncology Nursing Forum, 23,* 963–967.

Hall, J. (1996). Assisted suicide: Nurse practitioners as providers? *Nurse Practitioner, 21,* 63–71.

Haward, R. A. (1998). Review of evidence-based cancer medline. *Annals of Oncology, 9,* 1073–1078.

Health Care Financing Administration. (1996). Trends in Medicare home health agency utilization and payment: CYs 1974–1994. *Health Care Financing Review 1996* (Statistical Suppl.), 76–77, 1996b.

Higginson, I. (Ed.). (1993). *Clinical audit in palliative care.* Oxford, UK: Radcliffe Medical Press.

Hiltunen, E. F., Puopolo, A. L., Marks, G. K., Marsden, C., Kennard, M. J., Follen, M. A., et al. (1995). The nurse's role in end-of-life treatment discussions: Preliminary report from the SUPPORT project. *Journal of Cardiovascular Nursing, 9*(3), 68–77.

Hospice Nurses' Association. (1996). *Hospice and palliative care clinical practice protocol: Dyspnea.* Pittsburgh, PA: Author.

Institute of Medicine. (1997). In M. J. Field & C. K. Cassel (Eds.), *Approaching death: Improving care at the end of life* (pp.). Washington, DC: National Academies Press.

Institute of Medicine. (1999). In M. Hewitt & J. V. Simone (Eds.), *Ensuring quality cancer care* (pp.). Washington, DC: National Academies Press.

Institute of Medicine. (2002a). In K. M. Foley & H. Gelband (Eds.). *Improving palliative care for cancer.* Washington, DC: National Academies Press.

Institute of Medicine. (2002 b). In M. J. Field & R. E. Behrman (Eds.). *When children die: Improving palliative and end-of-life care for children and their families.* Washington, DC: National Academies Press.

Janken, J. K., Grubbs, J. H., & Haldeman, K. (1999). Toward a research-based critical pathway: A case study. *Online Journal of Knowledge Synthesis.* Clinical Column. Document Number 1C.

Johnsson, J. (1992). TQM approach may help solve physician practice problems. *Trustee, 45*(4), 11.

Joint Commission on Accreditation of Hospitals Organization. (2004). Retrieved 12/28/04 from http:// www.jcaho.org

Kaufman, S. (1998). Intensive care, old age, and the problem in America. *Gerontologist, 38,* 715–725.

Kazanowski, M. (1997). A commitment to palliative care: Could it impact assisted suicide? *Journal of Gerontological Nursing, 23*(3), 36–42.

Kirchhoff, K. T., & Beckstrand, R. L. (2000). Critical care nurses perceptions of obstacles and helpful behaviors in providing end-of-life care to dying patients. *American Journal of Critical Care, 9*(2), 96–105.

Kowalski, S. (1997). Assisted suicide: Where do nurses draw the line? *Nursing and Health Care, 14,* 70–76.

Kristjanson, L. J. (1986). Indicators of quality of palliative care from a family perspective. *Journal of Palliative Care, 2,* 7–19.

Kubler-Ross, E. (1967). *On death and dying.* New York: Touchstone.

Lynn, J., Teno, J. M., & Harrell, F. E. (1995). Accurate prognostications of death: Opportunities and challenges from clinicians. *Western Journal of Medicine, 163,* 250–257.

Matzo, L. M., & Emanual, E. J. (1997). Oncology nurses practices of assisted suicide and patient-requested euthanasia. *Oncology Nursing Forum, 24,* 1725–1732.

Max, M. B., Donovan, M., Miaskowski, C. A., Ward, S. E., Gordon, D., Bookbinder, M., et al. (1995). American Pain Society quality improvement guidelines for the treatment of acute pain and chronic pain. *Journal of the American Medical Association, 274,* 1874–1880.

McCormick, T. R., & Conley, B. J. (1995). Patients' perspectives on dying and on the care of dying patients. *Western Journal of Medicine, 163,* 236–243.

Milbank Memorial Fund Report. (2000). *Pioneer programs in palliative care: Nine case studies.*

Murphy, P. A. (1992). Perspective: Nursing—the real issue. *Trends in Health Care, Law, and Ethics, 10,* 124–127.

National Consensus Project for Quality Palliative Care. (2004). *Clinical practice guidelines for quality palliative care.* Brooklyn, NY: Author.

National Hospice and Palliative Care Organization. (2003). *Hospice facts and figures.* Retrieved 12/28/04 from http://www.nhpco.org/files/public/Hospice_Facts_110104.pdf

National Hospice Organization. (1997a). *Changing gears: Guidelines for managing care in the last days of life in adults.* Arlington, VA: National Hospice Organization, Working Party on Clinical Guidelines in End-of-Life Care.

National Hospice Organization (1997b). *A pathway for patients and families facing terminal illness.* Arlington, VA: Author.

National Institute on Aging. (2000). Research agenda for 2001–2005 [Electronic version].

Retrieved February 3, 2000, from http://www.nih.gov/nia/strat-plan *New Encyclopedia Britannica.* (1999). Chicago: Encyclopedia Britannica.

Portenoy, R. K. (1998). *Defining palliative care.* Retrieved from http://www.stoppain.org

Pritchard, R. S., Fisher, E. S., Teno, J. M., Sharp, S. M., Reding, D. J., Knaus, W. A., et al. (1998). Influence of patient preferences and local health system characteristics on place of death. *Journal of the American Geriatric Society, 46,* 1242–1250.

Quill, T. E. (1993). Doctor, I want to die. Will you help me? *Journal of the American Medical Association, 270,* 870–873.

Schwarz, J. K. (1999). Assisted dying and nursing practice. *Image: Journal of Nursing Scholarship, 31,* 367–373.

Scitovsky, A. (1996, October). *Age and the high cost of health care.* Paper presented at the First International Conference on Priorities in Health Care, Stockholm, Sweden.

Stevens, M. M., Dalla Pozza, L., Caelletto, B., Cooper, M. G., & Kilham, H. A. (1994). Pain and symptom control in pediatric palliative care. *Cancer Survey, 21,* 211–231.

Storey, P. (1996). *Primer of palliative care* (2nd ed.). IA: Kendall/Hunt, Dubuque, Iowa.

SUPPORT Principal Investigators. (1995). A controlled trial to improve care for seriously ill hospitalized patients: The Study to Understand Prognoses and Preferences for Outcomes and Risks of Treatments (SUPPORT). *Journal of the American Medical Association, 274,* 1591–1598.

Teno J. M., Clarridge, B. R., Casey V., Welch L. C., Wetle T., Shield, R., et al. (2004). Family perspectives on end-of-life care at the last place of care. *Journal of the American Medical Association, 291*(1), 88–93.

Vladeck, B. (1995). Medicare and managed care: Working together for the future. *Medical Interface, 8*(1), 50–52.

Wakefield, B., Johnson, J. A., Kron-Chalupa, J., & Paulsen, L. (1998). A research-based guideline for appropriate use of transdermal fentanyl to treat chronic pain. *Oncology Nursing Forum, 25,* 1505–1512.

Weeks, J., Cook, F., O'Day, S. J., Peterson, L., Wenger, N., Reding, D., et al. (1998). Relationship between cancer patients' predictions of prognosis and their treatment preferences. *Journal of the American Medical Association, 278,* 1709–1714.

Whitman, E. H. (1993). Terminal care of the dying child: Psychosocial implications of care. *Cancer, 71,* 3450–3462.

Wolfe, J., Holcombe, G. E., Klar, N., Levin, S., Ellenbogen, J. M., Salen-Schatz, S., et al. (2000). Symptoms and suffering at the end of life in children with cancer. *New England Journal of Medicine, 342,* 326–333.

World Health Organization. (2002). *Palliative care.* Retrieved 12/28/04 from http://www.who.int/cancer/palliative/en/

Wrede-Seaman, L. (1999). *Symptom management algorithms: A handbook for palliative care.* Yakima, WA: Intellicard.

Zander, K. (1991). CareMaps. The core of cost/quality care. *New Definition, 6*(3), 1–3.

4

Professional Organizations and Certifications in Hospice and Palliative Care

Judy Lentz and Deborah Sherman

The scope of hospice and palliative care nursing continues to evolve as the science and art of palliative care develop. Hospice and palliative care nursing reflects a holistic philosophy of care implemented across the life span and across diverse health settings. Within a matrix of affiliation, including the patient and family and other members of the interdisciplinary team, hospice and palliative care nurses provide evidence-based physical, emotional, psychosocial, and spiritual and existential care to individuals and families experiencing life-limiting, progressive illness. The goal of hospice and palliative care nursing is to promote the quality of life through the relief of suffering along the illness trajectory, through the death of a patient, and into the bereavement period of the family. Relief of suffering and quality of life for individuals and families are enhanced by

- providing effective pain and symptom management;
- addressing psychosocial and spiritual needs of patient and family;
- incorporating cultural values and attitudes in developing a plan of care;
- creating a healing environment to promote a peaceful death;
- supporting those who are experiencing loss, grief, and bereavement;

- promoting ethical and legal decision-making;
- advocating for personal wishes and preferences;
- utilizing therapeutic communication skills in all interactions;
- facilitating collaborative practice;
- insuring access to care and community resources through influencing and developing health and social policy;
- contributing to improved quality and cost-effective services;
- creating opportunities and implementing initiatives for palliative care education for patients, families, colleagues, and community; and
- participating in the generation, testing, and evaluation of palliative care knowledge and practice.

Hospice and palliative nursing is provided for patients and their families in a variety of care settings including but not limited to settings such as acute care hospital units; long-term-care facilities; assisted living facilities; inpatient, home, or residential hospices; palliative care clinics or ambulatory settings; private practices; and prisons. Practice settings for palliative and hospice care nursing are changing in response to the dynamic nature of today's health care environment.

Hospice and palliative nurses are licensed registered nurses who are educationally prepared and licensed in nursing and are qualified for specialty practice at two levels—generalist and advanced. These levels are differentiated by educational preparation, complexity of practice, and performance of certain nursing functions.

Hospice- and palliative-licensed practical/vocational nurses are also educationally prepared and licensed but at a different level of complexity in their practice. Hospice and palliative nursing assistants are educationally prepared through local- and state-mandated processes to meet the requirements of the specific setting in which they function. These requirements differ significantly across the United States, although hours of educational requirements are specifically defined in the home care, hospice, and long-term-care settings on a national basis. There are no licensure requirements for the nursing-assistant level of hospice and palliative caregiver.

According to the article entitled "History of the Hospice Nurses Association, 1986–1996" (Amenta, 2001), the founding of the Hospice Nurses Association occurred as follows:

> . . . in spring 1986 a group of nurses attending the Third Western Hospice Nursing Conference sponsored by the Hospice Organization of Southern California in San Diego, frustrated by the failure of national groups to develop adequate standards and networking structures for hospice nurse, put out the call to start a national hospice nursing organization. (p. 13)

Membership in the organization grew rapidly. In 1998, the word palliative was added to the organization's name, now known as the Hospice and Palliative Nurses Association (HPNA). By 2000, 2,800 nurses had joined this growing organization with more than 1,000 new members added each year thereafter to the current date. With a pattern of continued growth, membership varies between 7,000 and 7,500. The mission of HPNA relates to providing leadership in the specialty by

- promoting the highest professional standards of hospice and palliative nursing;
- studying, researching, and exchanging information, experiences, and ideas leading to improved nursing practice;
- encouraging nurses to specialize in the practices of hospice and palliative nursing;
- fostering the professional development of nurses, individually and collectively;
- responding to the changing needs of HPNA members and the population they represent; and
- promoting the recognition of hospice and palliative care as essential components within the health care system.

Within this mission are educational products and services designed for all levels of nursing caregivers. Many of these educational services offer continuing education credits as well.

EVOLUTIONARY PERSPECTIVE OF HOSPICE AND PALLIATIVE CARE NURSING

Nationally, there has been a growing interest in palliative and hospice care and an emphasis on the education of health professionals in this area. Billings and Block (1997) have identified the following forces that have increased national attention regarding palliative care:

- a growing interest in death and dying
- the development of hospice programs
- increasing integration of pain and symptom management into conventional care

- concern about the high cost of dying
- increasing national focus on pain management
- greater attention to the role of medicine in caring rather than curing
- national debates on physician-assisted suicide and euthanasia

These factors combine to create a dramatically increased demand for health care providers, including nurses, who are educated at all levels to provide expert, comprehensive palliative and hospice care.

The landmark Study to Understand Prognoses and Preferences for Outcomes and Risks of Treatment (SUPPORT) by (Support Study Investigators, 1995) (1995) highlights an urgent need for health care professionals who are prepared and committed to improving the quality of life for seriously ill and dying patients and their families. Knaus et al. (1995) conducted a 2-year prospective observational study with 4,301 patients from teaching hospitals in the United States, followed by a 2-year controlled clinical trial with 4,804 patients and their physicians who were randomized either to a control group or to an intervention group that received educational information related to end of life. The findings indicated that despite the SUPPORT intervention, there was a continued lack of communication between patients and their providers, particularly related to end-of-life preferences, aggressiveness of medical treatments, and a high level of reported pain by seriously ill and dying patients. The Support Study Investigators (1995) believe that improving the experience of seriously ill and dying patients requires an individual and collective commitment of health care providers, as well as proactive efforts at shaping the caregiving process.

In 1997, the Institute of Medicine (IOM) released a significant report entitled "Approaching Death: Improving Care at the End of Life" (Field & Cassel, 1997). This re-

port identified gaps of knowledge in many areas about caring for those at end of life. Based on this report, Field and Cassel reiterated that "the need for consensus and action to improve care for those approaching death is growing more urgent" (p. 17). On average, Americans live longer than they did in the nineteenth century, with more than 70% of the population dying after the age of 65 and with an average life expectancy in the United States of nearly 77 years (Field & Cassel, 1997). Over the last 100 years, the leading causes of death have changed from primarily infectious processes to chronic illnesses experienced by an aging population. Although some people die suddenly and unexpectedly, the dying process for many has been extended, with some individuals—such as those with cancer—facing a steady and fairly predictable decline, while others have long periods of chronic illness punctuated by crises that are often fatal (Field & Cassel, 1997). The result is a national increase in the number of individuals who require palliative care. Although hospice and palliative care has been delivered mainly to patients with cancer, other patients with incurable diseases are candidates for these services, including the growing number of elderly, those suffering from chronic diseases such as cardiovascular, pulmonary, neurological, and renal disease, as well as patients with AIDS Doyle, Hanks, (Cherney & Colman, 2001). More recently, the Institute of Medicine collaborated with the National Cancer Policy Board and the National Research Council to release a follow-up report called "Improving Palliative Care for (Cancer" Foley & Gelband, 2001), which further supports the need for changes in caring for the dying. The report details the undertreatment of distressing symptoms resulting from the continued deficiencies in the training of health care professionals. In the IOM report (Foley & Gelband, 2001) titled "Crossing the Quality Chasm: A New Health System for the 21st Century," the IOM argued that professional associations should commit to professional development and competency enhancement by developing curriculums, disseminating information, and promoting practice guidelines and standards.

The field of palliative care is one response to the changing profile of death in the twentieth century as it focuses on the prevention and relief of suffering through the management of pain and other symptoms and attention to the emotional, spiritual, and practical needs of patients and family from the early through the final stages of an illness (Field & Cassel, 1997). Palliative care builds upon the template of hospice care, with hospice care now recognized as a type of palliative care that is offered toward the end of life. Palliative care is the combination of active and compassionate therapies intended to comfort and support individuals who are living with and dying from life-threatening illness. During periods of illness and bereavement, palliative care strives to meet the physical, emotional, social, and spiritual needs of patients and their families. Palliative care may be combined with therapies aimed at reducing or curing illness or it may be the total focus of care (Ferris & Cumming, 1995). Indeed, specialty organizations of hospice medicine and nursing have now incorporated palliative care in their titles (Sherman, 2001). The rise in hospice programs in the United States from one program in 1979 to more than 3,200 programs in 2003, and a rise in the number of patients and families served from 128,000 in 1985 to 885,000 in 2003 support the projection of future needs for hospice/palliative care services. (National Hospice and Palliative Care Organization [NHPCO], 2003).

It has been recognized that educational preparation for end-of-life care is inconsistent at best, and neglected for the most part, in both undergraduate and graduate cur-

ricula (American Association of Colleges of Nursing [AACN], 1997). In accord with the International Council of Nurses' mandate that nurses have a unique and primary responsibility for ensuring the peaceful death of patients, the AACN, supported by the Robert Wood Johnson Foundation, convened a roundtable of expert nurses to discuss and initiate educational change related to palliative care. It was concluded that precepts underlying hospice care are essential principles for all end-of-life care. Such precepts include the assumptions that persons are living until the moment of death; that coordinated care should be offered by a variety of professionals with attention to the physical, psychological, social, and spiritual needs of patients and their families; and that care be sensitive to patient and family diversity. It was proposed that these precepts be foundational to the educational preparation of nurses. Based on these precepts, the document entitled "Peaceful Death" was developed, which outlined baccalaureate competencies for palliative and hospice care and content areas where competencies can be taught (AACN, 1997).

Emphasizing the role of nursing in end-of-life care, the American Nurses Association formulated a position statement regarding the promotion of comfort and relief of pain of dying patients, reinforcing nurses' obligation to promote comfort and insure aggressive efforts to relieve pain and suffering. Specialized palliative care educational initiatives have also begun in medicine and nursing, such as Education for Physicians on End of Life Care, known as EPEC; and the nursing initiative End of Life Nursing Education Consortium, known as ELNEC. The goal of ELNEC is to train 1,000 nurse educators from associate and baccalaureate programs in end-of-life care, supported by a grant from the Robert Wood Johnson Foundation to the AACN and the City of Hope Medical Center.

ELNEC has been adapted since for other nursing specialists in geriatrics, pediatrics, and oncology. In November 2004 a proposal was written for a grant from the National Institutes of Health to provide ELNEC to nursing educators in hospice and palliative care in hopes of reaching those in long-term-care settings. There was a paucity of educational resources such as textbooks for hospice and palliative nursing practice prior to the beginning of this century. A study conducted by Ferrell, Virani, and Grant (2000), revealed that only 2% of the text in nursing textbooks and teaching resources reflected content on end-of-life care. Initiatives are also underway in both medicine and nursing to revise medical and nursing textbooks to include palliative care content and to include palliative care content in licensing examinations. Most nursing curricula has been limited in terms of content or clinical experiences in end-of-life care, despite consensus reports, standards, and position statements from leading nursing specialty organizations indicating this need (Ferrell, Grant, & Virani, 2001).

Within the past 5 years, numerous palliative and hospice nursing-care resources have been published. Among the many are the following:

- *Textbook of Palliative Nursing* by Betty Ferrell and Nessa Coyle
- *Palliative Care Nursing: Quality Care to the End of Life* by Marianne LaPorte Matzo and Deborah Witt Sherman
- *Gerontological Palliative Care Nursing* by Marianne LaPorte Matzo and Deborah Witt Sherman
- *Palliative Practices from A–Z for the Bedside Clinician* by Kim Kuebler and Peg Esper
- *Hospice Concepts: A Guide to Palliative Care in Terminal Illness* by Shirley Ann Smith

- *Hospice Care for Children* by Ann Armstrong-Dailey and Sarah Zarbock
- *Terminal Illness: A Guide to Nursing Care* by Charles Kemp
- Numerous clinical resources from the Hospice and Palliative Nurses Association available through Kendall Hunt Publishers (www.hpna.org); and from the Oncology Nursing Society available through the Oncology Education Services (www.ons.org)

In April 2004, the standards and guidelines of palliative care were defined by the National Consensus Project Steering Committee in its Clinical Practice Guidelines for Quality Palliative Care. This document was the culmination of 2 years of collaboration by 20 representatives from five leading national hospice and palliative care organizations, specifically the American Academy of Hospice and Palliative Medicine, Center to Advance Palliative Care, Hospice and Palliative Nurses Association, National Hospice and Palliative Care Organization, and the former Last Acts organization. A need for consensus had been defined by practitioners to provide credible, broad-based guidelines for practice in an effort to standardize and improve the quality of palliative care in the United States. That need was affirmed when in the first 2 weeks following publication, 90,000 copies of the guidelines were downloaded from the National Consensus Web site (www.nationalconsensusproject.org). One of the baseline assumptions of these guidelines is that the qualifications of caregivers are determined by the organizations that grant professional credentials and programmatic accreditation. As a specialty organization, the Hospice and Palliative Care Nurses Association has identified the scope and standards of hospice and palliative care nursing and the competencies at all levels of nursing practice, specifically nursing assistants, licensed vocational nurses, professional registered nurses, and advance practice nurses.

DEVELOPING THE SCOPE, STANDARDS, AND COMPETENCIES OF PALLIATIVE AND HOSPICE NURSING PRACTICE

By developing and articulating the scope and standards of professional nursing practice, the specialty defines its boundaries, informs society about the parameters of nursing practice, and guides the development of rules and regulations for the specialty. As in all nursing specialties, palliative care nurses must accept professional practice accountability and ensure that their practice remains within the scope of their state's nurse-practice act, their professional code of ethics, and professional practice standards. The first standards of hospice nursing generalist practice were developed in 1987 by HPNA for the American Nurses Association and were revised in 1995. The publication was revised again in 2002 to include the advanced practice level of practice (HPNA, 2002a).

The scope of hospice and palliative care nursing continues to evolve as the science and art of palliative care develop. Palliative care nursing reflects a holistic philosophy of care implemented across the life span and across diverse health settings. Within a matrix of affiliation, including the patient and family and other members of the interdisciplinary team, hospice and palliative care nurses provide evidence-based physical, emotional, psychological, and spiritual and existential care to individuals and families experiencing life-limiting progressive illness. The goal of hospice and palliative care nursing is to promote the quality of life through the relief of suffering along the illness trajectory, through

the death of the patient, and into the bereavement period of the family.

In order to provide quality hospice and palliative nursing care, standards have been defined by a credible body of peers who were charged with this responsibility. The standards of hospice care were defined by the National Hospice and Palliative Care Organization in 1986. The standards of hospice and palliative nursing practice were first defined by the Hospice Nurses Association in 1995 with subsequent revisions to the name of the organization to include palliative care. Scope and standards of hospice and palliative nursing care define the body of knowledge needed in terms of the standards of care and the standards of performance. Standards of care refer to the basic level of care that should be provided to all hospice and palliative care patients and families. Standards of performance for palliative and hospice care nurses describe the standards for activities related to quality of care, performance appraisal, education, collegiality, ethics, collaboration, participation in research, and resource utilization. Documents such as agency standards, guidelines, policies, procedures, and protocols may further direct the individual's performance. Standards are defined in broad terms to define the scope of the specialty of palliative and hospice care nursing

The standards of palliative and hospice care nursing practice are authoritative statements described by the Hospice and Palliative Nurses Association for the nursing profession, which identifies the responsibilities for which palliative and hospice care nurses are accountable. Standards reflect the values and priorities of palliative care nursing and provide a framework for the evaluation of practice. The standards are written in measurable terms and define the palliative and hospice care nurses' accountability to the public and the individual and family outcomes for which they are responsible.

The standards are divided into two sections: The Standards of Care and the Standards of Professional Performance. Each section has identified criteria that allow the standards to be measured. Criteria include key indicators of competent practice. Standards remain stable over time as they reflect the philosophical values of the profession; however, the criteria should be revised to incorporate advancements in scientific knowledge, technology, and clinical practice. Criteria must be consistent with current nursing practice, and reflect evidence-based practice.

Standards of Care

Standards of care describe a competent level of basic and advanced-practice registered nursing care as demonstrated by the nursing process, involving assessment, diagnosis, outcomes identification, planning, implementation, and evaluation. The development of the relationship between the therapeutic nurse and patient and family is essential throughout the nursing process. The nursing process encompasses all significant actions taken by palliative care nurses in providing care to individuals and families, and forms the foundation of clinical decision-making. Several themes of nursing practice provide additional dimensions for attention and include the following:

- providing age-appropriate and culturally, ethnically, and spiritually sensitive care and support
- maintaining a safe environment
- educating patients and families about setting
- assuring continuity of care
- coordinating the care across all settings and among caregivers
- managing information
- communicating effectively

Registered nurses at the generalist level have completed a nursing program and passed the state licensure examination for registered nurses. Registered nurses who practice in palliative care settings may provide direct patient and family care, and may function as educators, case managers, administrators, and in other nursing roles. Advance practice nurses develop and implement advanced plans of care based on the synthesis of complex health-assessment data. Advanced practice nurses are expert clinicians, leaders, educator, consultants, and researchers. Differences in the level of practice are reflected in the scope and standards of palliative care nursing of the generalist nurse and advanced practice nurse as delineated below.

Standard I: Assessment

Palliative and hospice care nurses educated at the generalist level collect individual and family data. At the advanced level, palliative and hospice care nurses conduct an in-depth and comprehensive assessment based on a synthesis of individual and family health data.

Standard II: Diagnosis

Palliative and hospice care nurses educated at the generalist level analyze the assessment data in determining diagnoses. At the advanced level, palliative and hospice care nurses utilize an accepted framework that supports palliative and hospice care nursing knowledge and judgment used in critically analyzing the data.

Standard III: Outcome Identification

Palliative and hospice care nurses educated at the generalist level identify expected outcomes relevant to the individual and family and with the interdisciplinary or health care team, when appropriate. At the advanced level, palliative and hospice care nurses identify expected outcomes based on a critical analysis of both complex assessment data and diagnoses that are relevant to the individual and family and the interdisciplinary or health care team, when appropriate.

Standard IV: Planning

Palliative and hospice care nurses educated at the generalist level develop a plan of care that is negotiated among the individual, family, and interdisciplinary or health care team that includes interventions and treatments to attain expected outcomes. At the advanced level, palliative and hospice care nurses develop a comprehensive plan of care that prescribes evidence-based interventions to attain expected outcomes, and review with individuals and families the relative risks, benefits, burdens, and costs of interventions.

Standard V: Implementation

Palliative and hospice care nurses educated at the generalist level implement the interventions identified in the plan of care. At the advanced level, palliative and hospice care nurses prescribe, order, or implement interventions and treatments identified in the plan of care.

Standard VI: Evaluation

Palliative and hospice care nurses educated at the generalist level evaluate the individuals' and families' progress in attaining expected outcomes. At the advanced level, the palliative and hospice care nurses critically appraise and comprehensively evaluate all relevant and available data related to the attainment of expected outcomes.

Standards of Professional Performance

Standards of professional performance describe competent professional role behaviors, including activities related to quality of care, performance appraisal, education, collegiality, ethics, collaboration, research, and resource utilization. It is expected that all palliative and hospice care nurses engage in professional role activities that are appropriate to their education, position, and practice setting. Therefore, some standards or measurement criteria identify these activities. Palliative and hospice care nurses should be self-directed and purposeful in seeking necessary knowledge and skills to develop and maintain their competency. Their professionalism may be enhanced through membership in their professional organizations, certification in their specialty, and professional development through academic and continuing education.

Standard I: Quality of Care

Palliative and hospice care nurses educated at the generalist level evaluate the quality and effectiveness of nursing practice. At the advanced level, palliative and hospice care nurses develop criteria for evaluating the quality of care and effectiveness.

Standard II: Performance Appraisal

Palliative and hospice care nurses educated at the generalist level evaluate their own nursing practices in relation to professional practice standards and relevant standards and regulations. At the advanced level, palliative and hospice care nurses continuously evaluate their own nursing practice and the practice of subordinates in relation to professional standards and relevant statues and regulations, and are accountable to the public and to the profession for providing competent clinical care.

Standard III: Education

Palliative and hospice care nurses educated at the generalist level acquire and maintain current knowledge and competency in palliative and hospice care nursing. At the advanced level, palliative and hospice care nurses maintain knowledge related to current research, scientific findings, and advanced clinical practice in the areas of palliative and hospice care nursing and related disciplines.

Standard IV: Collegiality

Palliative and hospice care nurses educated at the generalist level interact and contribute to the professional development of peers and other health care providers as colleagues. At the advanced level, palliative and hospice care nurses serve as leaders and role models for the professional development of peers, colleagues, and others.

Standard V: Ethics

Palliative and hospice care nurses educated at the generalist level make decisions and act on behalf of the patient and family in an ethical manner. At the advanced level, palliative and hospice care nurses demonstrate moral discernment, critical reasoning, and discriminating judgment in integrating ethics during all interactions with the patient, family, organization, and community.

Standard VI: Collaboration

Palliative and hospice care nurses educated at the generalist level collaborate with patient and family, members of the interdisciplinary health-care team and other health care providers in providing patient and family care. At the advanced level, palliative and hospice care nurses promote an interdisciplinary or health care team approach to providing advanced palliative and hospice nursing care to the patient, family, community, and environment related to potential or actual disease process and treatments.

Standard VII: Research

Palliative and hospice care nurses educated at the generalist level use research findings in practice. At the advanced level, palliative and hospice care nurses utilize research to identify, examine, validate, and evaluate knowledge, theories, and creative approaches to health care providers related to advanced practice with the goal of improving outcomes for the patient, family, community, and environment.

Standard VIII: Resource Utilization

In planning and delivering patient and family care, palliative and hospice care nurses educated at the generalist level consider factors related to safety, effectiveness, and cost. At the advanced level, palliative and hospice care nurses provide cost-effective, quality care by using the most appropriate resources and delegating care to the most appropriate, qualified health care clinician.

Standards of Care and Standards of Professional Performance are also written for the palliative- and hospice-licensed practical/vocational nurses and for the palliative and hospice nursing assistants. Variations to each standard are made to adapt to scopes of practice and statutory regulations.

COMPETENCIES

According to HPNA (2002b) competencies represent the "quantifiable knowledge, attitudes, and skills that practitioners demonstrate in the performance of safe, consistent, compassionate, state-of-the-art, evidence-based end-of-life care which conforms to the patients' and their families' wishes." This definition applies to all levels of nursing practice although the specific clinical judgments and core competencies vary with each level. The competencies for the palliative and hospice generalist and advanced practice nurse were initiated in 2001. Subsequently, competencies for the palliative- and hospice-licensed practical/vocational nurse and nursing assistant were also written.

Competencies must reflect the breadth of the standards, but are written in general domain statements with clinical judgments and core statements to demonstrate accomplishments of the particular domain of competence.

Why are competencies needed? The reason for competencies are discussed in the publication "Professional Competencies for Generalist Hospice and Palliative Nurses" (HPNA, 2001):

The use of standards, competencies and the process of accreditation are necessary and important strategies to meet stated goals. Identifying the intellectual, interpersonal, technical and moral competencies needed to practice quality end-of-life care will help to ensure these standards are met. These competencies need to be outcome specific and therefore are more measurable than the objectives or goals of the past. Identified national competencies will be the benchmark to make explicit the areas of knowledge and skills a nurse needs in order to provide quality hospice and palliative care. (p. 2)

The basic competencies of palliative care nursing represent the knowledge, skills, and attitudes demonstrated when providing evidence-based physical, emotional, psychosocial, and spiritual care. The care is provided in a collaborative manner across the life span in diverse settings, to individuals and families experiencing, progressive illness. The generalist-level competencies and the related general statements are as follows:

Clinical judgment. At the generalist level, the palliative and hospice nurse demonstrates critical thinking, analysis and clinical judgment in all aspects of palliative and hospice care of patients and families experiencing life-limiting illness through the use of the nursing process to address the physical, psychosocial, and spiritual/existential needs of patients and families. At the advanced practice level, the palliative and hospice nurse must be able to respond to all disease processes with advanced clinical skills.

Advocacy and ethics. The palliative and hospice nurse incorporates ethical principles and professional standards in the care of patients and families who are experiencing life-limiting illnesses or progressive illness, as well as identifying and advocating for their wishes and preferences. Promoting ethical and legal decision-making, advocating for personal wishes and preferences, and ensuring access to care and community resources through influencing or developing health and social policy are ways for the nurse to incorporate ethical principles and professional standards in the care of patients and their families.

Professionalism. The palliative and hospice nurse demonstrates knowledge, attitude, behavior, and skills that are consistent with the professional standards, code of ethics, and scope of practice for palliative and hospice nursing.

Collaboration. The palliative and hospice nurse actively promotes dialogue with patients and families, the health care team, and the community to address and plan for issues related to living with and dying from chronic, life-limiting progressive illness.

Systems thinking. The palliative and hospice nurse utilizes resources necessary to enhance quality of life for patients and families experiencing life-limiting progressive illness through knowledge and negotiation within the health care system.

Cultural competence. The palliative and hospice nurse demonstrates cultural competence by respecting and honoring the unique diversity and characteristics of patients, families, and colleagues in palliative and hospice care.

Facilitation of learning. The palliative and hospice nurse facilitates learning of patient, family, self, members of the health care team, and the community through the development, implementation, and evaluation of formal and informal education related to living with and dying from life-limiting progressive illnesses.

Communication. The palliative and hospice nurse demonstrates the use of effective verbal, nonverbal, and written communication with patients and families, members of the health care team, and the community in order to address therapeutically and accurately convey the palliative and hospice care needs of patients and families.

Advanced practice hospice and palliative nurses are held to the same competencies but at an advanced level because they exercise a high degree of critical thinking, analysis, and independent judgment, within the framework of autonomous and collaborative interdisciplinary practice. The advanced practice nurses are distinguished by their ability to synthesize complex data, implement advanced plans of care, and provide leadership in palliative and hospice care. The roles of the advanced practice hospice and palliative nurse include, but are not limited to expert clinician, leader or facilitator of interdisciplinary teams, educator, researcher, consultant, collaborator, advocate, and administrator. Advanced practice palliative and hospice nurses who have fulfilled the requirements established by their state's nurse-practice acts may be authorized to assume autonomous responsibility for clinical role functions, which may include prescription of controlled substances, medications, or therapies. To practice as an advanced practice palliative and hospice nurse, national certification in advanced practice palliative and hospice nursing is recommended, although it is recognized that the advanced practice palliative and hospice nurse may have concurrent advanced practice certification in another specialty.

Competencies for the licensed practical nurse focus on decision making instead of clinical judgment. For the nursing assistant, clinical judgment is rooted in observation and reporting. Although the core competencies are very similar in all four levels of nursing, the criteria are specific to the various scopes of practice.

CERTIFICATION IN HOSPICE AND PALLIATIVE CARE NURSING

Incorporated in 1987, the Hospice Nurses Association (HNA) became the first professional nursing organization dedicated to promoting excellence in the practice of hospice nursing. Consistent with that goal, the HNA Board of Directors appointed the National Board for the Certification of Hospice Nurses (NBCHN) in 1992. A sister organization of HPNA is the National Board for Certification of Hospice and Palliative Nurses (NBCHPN). The mission of this organization is to promote a certification process that advances quality in the provision of hospice and palliative care.

In March of 1994, the NBCHN offered the first certification examination and the credential of Certified Registered Nurse Hospice (CRNH). A decade later, HNA recognized the similarity in the nursing practice of the hospice and palliative nurse, and expanded its name to embrace palliative nursing practice, becoming the Hospice and Palliative Nurses Association (HPNA). Hospice and palliative nurses were providing patient and family care in more diverse settings, and the fundamental nursing concepts developed in hospices were applied to other practice environments such as in acute care hospitals, prisons, long-term care, and home care.

The results of the 1998 generalist hospice and palliative nurse Role Delineation Study, commissioned by NBCHN, scientifically demonstrated that only minor differences in practice activity existed between hospice and palliative nurses working in nonhospice settings. These differences correlated with requirements of the role or practice setting.

In 1999, the NBCHN became the National Board for Certification of Hospice and Palliative Nurses (NBCHPN), offering a new designation to recognize base competence in hospice and palliative nursing—Certified Hospice and Palliative Nurse (CHPN). The generalist must be licensed and it is recommended to have a minimum of 2 years of clinical experience in palliative and hospice care. By 2004, nearly 8,000 were certified.

Recognizing the need to offer an examination for advanced practice hospice and palliative nurses, in 2000 the NBCHPN began discussions with New York University and the American Nursing Credentialing Center (ANCC) to collaborate for this purpose. Following the role delineation study, development of the scope, standards, and competencies, a certification exam was initiated in May 2002. Eligibility for the exam includes holding a currently active registered nurse license, having graduated from a program offered by an accredited institution that includes both didactic and clinical components, and holding a master's degree or higher in nursing from an advanced-practice palliative-care program or a post-master's certificate with a minimum of 500 hours of clinical practice. The individual must also have 500 hours of palliative and hospice care practice in the year prior to applying for the examination. As of 2004, there were more than 200 certified advanced-practice hospice and palliative nurses with the credential of APRN, BC-PCM. In an effort to expand the portfolio of examinations, NBCHPN successfully negotiated a buy-out of the partnership with ANCC effective December 2004.

Through a commitment to a strategic plan to provide certification for all levels of caregivers, NBCHPN was fully funded by the Fan Fox and Leslie R. Samuels Foundation in October 2000 to certify nursing assistants in hospice and palliative care. Following development of the scope, standards, and competencies for the hospice and palliative nursing assistant, a role delineation study was completed and the first hospice and palliative nursing-assistant examination was offered in September 2001 and the credential of Certified Hospice and Palliative Nursing Assistant (CHPNA) was offered. To be eligible for the examination, the nursing assistant must have a minimum of 2,000 hours in palliative and hospice care as validated by the nursing supervisor. By 2004, more than 2,000 nursing assistants were certified as CHPNAs.

Continuing with the strategy of providing certification for all levels of caregivers, NBCHPN in 2002 began the process of developing the scope, standards, and competencies for the licensed practical/vocational hospice and palliative nurse. Upon completion, using additional funds from the Fan Fox and Leslie R. Samuels Foundation, a Role Delineation Study for the hospice and palliative LP/VN was completed and the first examination offered in September 2004, conferring the credential of CHPLN. To be eligible for the examination the palliative and hospice practical/vocational nurse must be licensed and it is recommended to have 2,000 clinical hours in the prior 2 years. In 2004, nearly 250 CHPLNs had successfully completed the certification requirements.

Certification, as defined by the American Board of Nursing Specialties, is "the formal recognition of the specialized knowledge, skills, and experience demonstrated by the achievement of standards identified by a nursing specialty to promote optimal patient care," and the standards were approved by the American Board of Nursing Specialties (ABNS) board of directors in June 2003. The ABNS further defines standards for accrediting nursing examinations to assure they are of the highest standard. NBCHPN's generalist nursing examination achieved accreditation by ABNS in February 2002.

In 2004, HPNA wrote a position statement supporting the certification of nurses and other qualified members of the nursing team in hospice and palliative care and encourages employers to support actively those individuals pursuing certification.

Certification is valued for the following reasons:

- The individual nurse has a tested and proven competency across the spectrum of hospice and palliative nursing care.
- The individual nurse increases his or her knowledge of hospice and palliative care by studying for the examination.
- The individual nurse has access to a national network of experienced and knowledgeable hospice and palliative nurses.
- The individual nurse has demonstrated a commitment to his or her specialty practice by pursuing certification.
- The individual nurse has demonstrated dedication to professional development in his or her nursing career by attaining the credential.
- The individual nurse is an asset to his or her employer in an atmosphere of increasing awareness regarding quality in health care.

Certification is valued by the employer and consumer because it offers a measure of knowledge translating to a professional who performs at a higher level of competence and therefore assures a higher quality of safe care for the patient and family.

As of 2005, NBCHPN can proudly proclaim to be the *only* nursing specialty certification organization offering certifications for all levels of hospice and palliative care nursing providers. As hospice and palliative care needs increase, NBCHPN seeks to provide assurance of competency within those nursing agents who administer nursing care.

FUTURE VISIONS FOR HOSPICE AND PALLIATIVE CARE NURSING

With the current nursing shortage and dire projections for the years ahead, the hospice and palliative specialty nursing organizations believe that all representatives of the nursing team must be competent. Therefore, four core curriculums have been written, four scope/standards of practice have been written, four competencies have been written, and four examinations have been developed to cover the four major areas of nursing—advanced practice, generalist, licensed practical/vocational nursing, and nursing assistants. Hospice and palliative care is unique in this regard.

The National Consensus Project's Clinical Practice Guidelines for Quality Palliative Care (which can be viewed at www.nationalconsensusproject.org) recommend that all palliative and hospice nursing care providers be educated and certified. Great progress has been made, with membership in the Hospice and Palliative Nurses Association nearly tripling over the past 5 years to more than 7,500 and nearly 10,000 nursing care providers certified. However, this recommendation has not yet been actualized. When estimating the numbers of registered nurses, licensed practical/vocational nurses, and nursing assistants employed in hospices, palliative care programs, long-term-care facilities, assisted living facilities, and prisons, our projected palliative and hospice nursing universe is far beyond our current successes. Much work is yet to be accomplished.

The vision for the future of advanced practice hospice and palliative care nursing, has been articulated in a monograph entitled "Promoting Excellence: A Position Statement From American Nursing Leaders in Palliative Care." This initiative was possible through the support of Dr. Ira Byock's Promoting Excellence in End of Life Care Program.

In the monograph, leaders in advanced-practice palliative-care nursing emphasize the role of advanced practice nurses in the national efforts to improve care and quality of life for Americans and their families living with advanced, life-limiting illness. Leaders in the clinical professions, nursing educators, health service providers, health care payers, and public policy advocates are asked to take the following actions:

1. Professional organizations in nursing, medicine, hospice, and palliative are called to engage in dialogue about the APN and opportunities and strategies to advance the role.
2. Nursing educators must become knowledgeable about palliative care and develop continuing education programs that support hospice and palliative care nursing competencies.
3. Payers of health care services are called on to recognize the specialty of palliative care and provide APNs with adequate and consistent compensation that is commensurate with APNs' scope of practice, authority, and responsibility, regardless of practice setting.
4. The National Council of State Boards of Nursing and individual state boards of nursing are called on to work collaboratively and consistently to recognize the scope and standards of advanced-practice palliative-care nursing.
5. Health care systems or health service providers are asked to develop or expand practice opportunities for APNs in all settings that care for patients who may experience life-threatening illness.
6. Advanced practice nurses who practice in hospice and palliative care are called on to document and disseminate the outcomes of their practice experience and roles, engage in interdisciplinary research, and translate research findings into practice.

These recommendations will not be enacted and our vision for hospice and palliative care nursing will not be actualized only at the advanced practice level. Indeed, it will require the collective expression of passion and commitment to quality care across all levels of hospice and palliative care nursing and related constituencies to actualize our nursing potential and create the envisioned reality.

Hospice and palliative nursing has a bright future. Although the specialty and nursing organization is still young, HPNA has established visibility, credibility, and recognition for hospice and palliative care nursing. With the graying of America, demands for our specialty will grow. The work of the National Consensus Project under the leadership of the Hospice and Palliative Care Coalition (consisting of AAHPM, HPNA, and NHPCO) will continue to challenge the delivery of palliative and hospice care in America. Quality indicators must be defined, earlier referrals to palliative and hospice care must be achieved, access to care must be addressed, and recognition of certification for advanced practice nurses leading to practice licensure and reimbursement must be assured Hospice and palliative nurses are being prepared and positioned to meet the challenges ahead.

EDUCATION PLAN 4.1   Plan for Achieving Competencies: Professional Organizations and Standards for Hospice and Palliative Nurses

Knowledge Needed	Attitude	Skills	Undergraduate Behavioral Outcomes	Graduate Behavioral Outcomes	Teaching/Learning Strategies
History of hospice and palliative care nursing	*Recognize the value of joining a specialty organization.		*Discuss the history of HPNA.	*Support HPNA through membership and leadership roles.	*Trace the evolution of HPNA and its role in the development of the specialty.
Components of the Scope and Standards of Hospice and Palliative Care Nursing	*Appreciate the application of the Scope and Standards in nursing practice.		*Articulate the Scope and Standards of Hospice and Palliative Care Nursing.	*Evaluate changes in the Scope and Standards as the specialty develops over time.	*Participate in a discussion of how the Scope and Standards influences nursing practice for generalist and advanced practice nurses.
Competencies of the generalist and advanced practice nurse in hospice and palliative care	*Identify the value of palliative care nursing competencies in guiding nursing practice.		*Describe the competencies for generalist and advanced practice nurses in hospice and palliative care nursing.	*Achieve the competencies in generalist and advance practice hospice and palliative care nursing.	*Present a hospice or palliative care case and discuss the application of nursing competencies in the role of the generalist and advanced practice hospice and palliative care nurse.

REFERENCES

Amenta, M. O. (2001). History of the Hospice Nurses Association. *Journal of Hospice and Palliative Nursing, 3,* 128–136.

American Association of Colleges of Nursing. (1997). *Peaceful death document.* Round table Discussion on Palliative Care, Washington, DC.

Billings, J. A., & Block, S. (1997) Palliative care in undergraduate medical education. *Journal of the American Medical Association, 278,* 733–736.

Doyle, D., Hanks, G., Cherney, N., & Calman, K. (2001). *Oxford textbook of palliative medicine.* New York: Oxford Medical Publications.

Ferrell, B. R., Virani, R., & Grant, M. (2000). Analysis of end-of-life content in nursing textbooks. *Oncology Nursing Forum, 26,* 869–876.

Ferrell, B. R., Grant, M., & Virani, R. (2001). Nurses urged to address improved end-of-life care in textbooks. *Oncology Nursing Forum, 28,* 1349.

Ferris, F., & Cummings, I. (1995). *Palliative care: Towards a consensus in standardized principles of practice.* Ottawa, Canada: Canadian Palliative Care Association.

Field M. J., & Cassel, C. K. (Eds.). (1997). *Approaching death: Improving care at the end of life.* Washington, DC: National Academies Press.

Foley, K.M., & Gelband, H. (Eds.). (2001). *Improving palliative care for cancer.* Washington, DC: National Academies Press.

Hospice and Palliative Care Association. (2001). *Professional competencies for generalist hospice and palliative nurses.* Pittsburgh, PA: HPNA.

Hospice and Palliative Care Association. (2002a). *Scope and standards of hospice and palliative care nursing practice.* Pittsburgh, PA: HPNA.

Hospice and Palliative Care Association. (2002b). *Competencies for advanced practice hospice and palliative care nurses.* Pittsburgh, PA: HPNA.

Support Study Investigators (1995). A controlled trial to improve care for seriously ill hospitalized patients: The Study to Understand Progress and Preference for Outcomes and Risks for Treatments (SUPPORT). *Journal of the American Medical Association, 274,* 1591–1598.

National Hospice and Palliative Care Organization. (2003). NHPCO national data set summary Report. Retrieved 5/5/03 from http://www.nhpco.org/files/members/2003nationaldataset.pdf

Sherman, D. W. (2001). Access to hospice care. *Journal of Palliative Medicine, 3,* 407–411.

5

The Nurse's Role as a Member of the Interdisciplinary Palliative Care Team

*Lisa M. Krammer, Jeanne Martinez, Eileen A. Ring,
Mary Beth Williams, and Mary Jo Jacobs*

AACN Competencies

#6: Collaborate with interdisciplinary team members while implementing the nursing role in end-of-life care.

#14: Demonstrate skill at implementing a plan for improved end-of-life care within a dynamic and complex health care delivery system.

> *Why are you afraid? I am the one who is dying! But please believe me, if you care, you can't go wrong. Death may get to be routine to you, but it is new to me.*
> —Anonymous

This chapter will describe the significance of the interdisciplinary team process and the fundamental elements of effective interdisciplinary team process. In conclusion, the complex dimensions within nursing roles involved in successful family care at the end of life are presented.

PALLIATIVE CARE FRAMEWORKS

Conceptual Model of Care

In order to relieve suffering, palliative care nursing utilizes a conceptual framework for end-of-life care practice. An effective model of care for the delivery of palliative nursing, adapted from hospice nursing, is Dame Cicely Saunder's conceptual model of "whole person" suffering. Saunders espouses that whole-person suffering has four dimensions: physical, psychological, spiritual, and social (Krammer, Muir, Gooding-Kellar, Williams, & von Gunten, 1999). Under this concept, suffering affects each domain of the biopsychosocial-spiritual aspects of care. This conceptual model forms the basis for the description of palliative care nursing practice in this chapter.

DELIVERY MODEL OF CARE

Within the traditional, medical model of care lies a perceived dichotomy between curative/death-defying care and palliative care. It is almost as though the goal of care is *first* and *only* cure, then only if unable to cure, to relieve suffering. Often, this perceived dichotomy prevents or delays the introduction of palliative care measures for patients and their families. In order to provide quality, comprehensive, whole-person care, should not the goals of curative and palliative care be woven together concurrently? It would seem to be generally appropriate to relieve suffering *at the same time* as pursuing curative life-prolonging therapies (von Gunten & Muir, 2000).

An effective framework for the delivery of palliative care throughout the disease continuum can be most readily visualized as an "umbrella of care." Debate exists as to the beginning and end of the umbrella's arch. For some health care clinicians, palliative care starts with the initial diagnosis of an illness, at which time the management of symptoms and the psychosocial stressors of the disease upon the patient and family are vigorously addressed with active, curative-focused therapy. Although this scope may be considered ideal, the majority of palliative care providers emphasize the maximization of function and quality of life in those with far-advanced disease. For all providers, palliative care culminates in the management of complex physical, psychological, social, and spiritual issues that patients and members of their families will experience during the final phase of life and will include bereavement care for the family (Krammer et al., 1999).

With the emergence of palliative care as a distinct medical specialty (Cairms & Yates, 2003; LeGrand, Walsh, Nelson, & Zhukovsky, 2000; Leslie, Adams, 2002; von Gunten & Muir, 2000), an ever growing number of hospitals have begun to develop comprehensive, academic palliative care programs (El Sayem et al., 2004; Walsh, 2001; Zhukovsky, 2000), consisting of one or all of the following program elements: acute palliative care inpatient units (Santa-Emma, Roach, Gill, Spayde & Dylon, 2002); palliative consultation teams (Virik & Glare, 2002; Weissman, 1997); outpatient palliative care clinics, and home hospice programs. This programmatic approach allows for patients with advanced progressive disease and their families to have access to palliative care expertise in all settings, including the acute care hospital, outpatient clinic, home, or nursing home. With a comprehensive palliative care program, the interdisciplinary team will utilize the same philosophy and model of care as they work throughout the continuum with the patient and family in a coordinated and collaborative manner to achieve mutually established goals.

PRINCIPLES OF PALLIATIVE CARE

A core principle of palliative care across the entire disease spectrum and in all settings is the concept that the patient and family constitute the unit of care. The patient and family rather than the disease are the primary focus of care. The constructs of family-centered care form the foundation of the palliative care philosophy. Palliative care addresses the meaning of disease, suffering, life, and death within the context of each family unit (National Consensus Project, 2004). Palliative care recognizes that each family member will experience the disease process and all of its implications within the context of his or her particular worldview, and individual care plans are developed to reflect these worldviews.

Another core palliative-care principle is the commitment to collaborate through an interdisciplinary team process (Cairms & Yates, 2003; Leslie et al., 2002; National Consensus Project, 2004). In order to facilitate a family in crisis to establish and then achieve mutually agreed upon goals, the palliative care team integrates and coordinates the assessment and interventions of each team member and creates a comprehensive plan of care. Good palliative care is significant in the manner in which it embraces cultural, ethnic, and faith differences and preferences, while interweaving the principles of ethics, humanities, and human values into every patient- and family-care experience (Loscalzo & Zabora, 1998; Rosen, 1998).

Further, clinical ethics is an essential footprint for the provision of end-of-life care. Whereas clinicians often learn the *theoreti-*

cal principles behind ethics (Beauchamp & Childress, 1994), palliative care necessitates that these principles be incorporated into the practice or "put into motion" 24 hours a day, 7 days a week (Roy & MacDonald, 1998). Palliative care embodies this concept of "ethics in motion" (C. Muir, personal communication, June 30, 2004) as each interdisciplinary team member, including patient and families, contemplate the ethical questions in advanced disease and in end-of-life decision making.

Ethical challenges present themselves to the palliative care interdisciplinary team on an hourly basis. The following vignettes are a sampling of the ethical issues faced by the interdisciplinary team in routine daily practice.

Professional Boundaries:

Ms. D. is a 35-year-old patient, admitted to the palliative care unit for the third time in the past 2 months. Ms. D. was diagnosed with breast cancer 3 years ago. She is now admitted for terminal delirium. She is expected to die this admission. One staff nurse who has cared for her on the three previous admissions has become very close to the patient and family. She tells the staff that she will be visiting the patient on her day off, and she is to be called at any time if the patient's status changes. She has given her home phone number to the family, promising to be there at the time of the patient's death. Are the nurse's actions appropriate? How should other members of the palliative care team respond to the nurse's request to be called? Should the patient's and family's desires about the nurse's presence be considered in deciding the appropriate boundaries of professional staff?

Physician-Assisted Suicide:

Mr. S., diagnosed with head and neck cancer, was admitted to the palliative care unit 3 weeks ago. Upon admission, he was found to have increased somnolence, dyspnea, fever, tachycardia, and low blood pressure. The tumor on his right neck recurred about 2 months go. At that time, the patient received radiation for palliation. However, since then the tumor has continued to grow through the skin and is now visible, about 12 cm in diameter, with a strong odor. The patient's wife of 47 years has been managing her husband's care at home, but now finds it difficult to move him, and distressing to do his dressing changes. Upon admission, the staff prepared the family that the patient may be imminently dying. However, Mr. S.'s condition became relatively stable after completing a short course of IV antibiotics. He remains somnolent and bedridden, but is arousable when spoken to. The nurses have begun to have difficulty caring for him; for example, the odor has increased and pieces of the patient's neck flesh and ear have been coming off with each dressing change. The nurses have begun to express feelings of helplessness, wondering why this patient "is taking so long to die". They feel particularly bad for his elderly wife who takes two buses to the hospital to see her husband every day. One nurse expressed that "if there is any patient who needed physician-assisted suicide, it is Mr. S." In retrospect, should Mr. S. have been treated with antibiotics? What is the best way for the nurses to manage their feelings about caring for Mr. S.? And who is suffering the most in this situation—Mr. S., his wife, or the nursing staff?

Autonomy in Decision Making:

Mr. L. is a 60-year-old widower diagnosed with recurrent colon cancer. He is in the final stages of dying and unable to communicate. Mr. L. has been in hospice care, and was admitted to a hospice bed in the hospital 2 days ago. A few months after his diagnosis, Mr. L. had previously completed a living will indicating that he did not want any heroic measures at the end of life. He also completed and signed documents appointing a close friend to be his power of attorney for health affairs. At that time, Mr. L. informed this friend that he and his attending physician had agreed to a DNR status when his disease no longer responded to treatment. Mr. L.'s 31-year-old son has now arrived from out of state to visit his father in the hospital. He is very upset that his father is in a hospice bed and is a DNR status. He is requesting that the DNR order be rescinded, and his father transferred to another unit in the hospital where he will be "actively treated." What rights does the patient's son have in making decisions for his father? Is the health care team obligated to follow the patient's living will when the patient can no longer make his own decisions? What is the role of this power of attorney?

Each member of the interdisciplinary team has a unique relationship with, and view of, the patient and family. These varied perspectives reveal vital information that is invaluable when identifying and clarifying potential conflicts and facilitating resolution. It is through the use of an interdisciplinary team process that each ethical issue in palliative care is collaboratively and interdependently addressed and evaluated.

THE INTERDISCIPLINARY TEAM

Palliative care's reliance upon the interdisciplinary team as a key factor for successful outcomes requires an understanding of the distinction between interdisciplinary and multidisciplinary practice. In the traditional multidisciplinary team, the physician primarily directs care of the patient, and the family needs may or may not be considered (see Figure 5.1). Multiple disciplines of the health care team may be involved in the individual assessments and in the delivery of care, although efforts by these team members are often uncoordinated and independent. The primary mode of communication between

disciplines is the medical chart. The result is often incomplete communication between professions, lack of accountability, and a tendency for each discipline to develop its own patient care goals. Family needs are often unidentified and most often are not incorporated into the overall plan of care.

In contrast, in an interdisciplinary model, communication and decision making between team members is collaborative, with leadership shared and based upon primary patient and family needs and goals. The identity of the interdisciplinary team supersedes personal identities and agendas (Cummings, 1998), and the concept of the "sum of the whole is greater than its parts" is valued and respected. The interdisciplinary model facilitates team members to (a) directly interact with the patient and family, (b) share information among team members, (c) provide consultation to one another, and (d) work interdependently together in order to achieve the goals identified by the patient and family.

Table 5.1 lists the most common members of the palliative care interdisciplinary team, explains their function within the team, and discusses their interrelationship with the palliative care nurse. As a coordinator of care and a core member of the interdisciplinary team, the nurse has the responsibility to spearhead the development of therapeutic relationships, not just between herself and the patient and family, but also with all pertinent members of the team, which in turn ensures effective and goal-driven supportive communication and patient outcomes. The goals of the patient and family, their treatment preferences, and support needs are continually reassessed by the palliative care nurse. A hallmark of quality palliative care is the collaborative role that the nurse develops with the physician and other interdisciplinary team members. Often, the physician has had a long-term relationship with the patient and family, and as the needs for traditional medi-

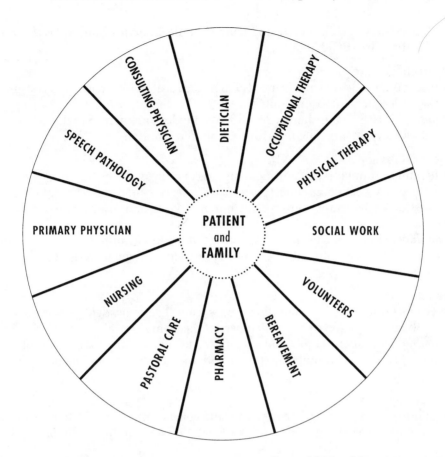

FIGURE 5.1   The multidisciplinary team. Various members of the health care team contribute as individuals to the care plan for each patient. However, the communication between each discipline is often lacking and/or fragmented as represented by the individual pie pieces separated by heavy dark lines. Additionally, there is no mechanism to facilitate communication between the disciplines.

cal-model "curative" care lessen and palliative care measures increase, this may represent a "loss" for the physician. As the nurse develops a relationship with the patient and family, the collaborative relationship with the physician may also be a source of support for the physician personally as well as professionally for decision making. The nurse is a primary conduit for information, critical assessments, and evaluation of the patient and family goals within the interdisciplinary team. A critical aspect of palliative care involves the identification and subsequent resolution of often divergent goals of the patient, family, or the

health care team. The palliative care nurse is often in the ideal position to be instrumental in coordinating and affecting a comprehensive family-focused plan of care.

CHARACTERISTICS OF AN EFFECTIVE INTERDISCIPLINARY TEAM

A dynamic and outcomes-oriented interdisciplinary team requires collaboration, leadership, coordinated decision making, and

TABLE 5.1   The Interdisciplinary Team Member's Role, Function, and Interrelationship with the Palliative Care (PC) Nurse

Advanced Practice Nurse
Function: Incorporates the role of advanced clinician, educator, researcher, and consultant to families, staff, colleagues, and communities.
Interrelationship: Acts as a consultant, educator, role model, and mentor to the PC nurse to synergistically achieve quality outcomes for patients and families.

Bereavement Counselor
Function: Identifies through IDT assessment high risk family members for bereavement and provides anticipatory grief counseling. Coordinates bereavement services for families including counseling sessions, grief support groups, memorial services, and community outreach programs.
Interrelationship: Relies on the PC nurse assessment of the family upon a patient's death in order to begin bereavement care. Values the PC nurse's role in identifying high risk family members for grief and bereavement.

Patient/Family
Function: The focus of care of the interdisciplinary team. The goals identified by the patient/family direct the participation of other members of the team.
Interrelationship: The patient/family understands the PC nurse is the coordinator of interdisciplinary care and continuously confers with the PC nurse regarding patient/family needs.

Palliative Care Physician
Function: Consults with primary care physician and collaborates with IDT to provide expertise in pain management, communication, and treatment decisions at the end of life for patients and families.
Interrelationship: Understands the PC nurse has the greatest prolonged contact with the patient and family and relies upon the holistic assessment and interventions of the nurse in order to develop a comprehensive medical care plan in collaboration with the interdisciplinary team.

Pastoral Care Counselor
Function: Provides in-depth assessment of spiritual needs of patient/family including search for meaning and purpose of life. Acts as a liaison with community clergy and a resource for the interdisciplinary team regarding ethical questions, faith traditions, and world religions.
Interrelationship: Respects the spiritual assessment of the PC nurse and is consulted when family issues require advanced assessment and intervention. Acts as a resource for PC nurse when needing to debrief after a difficult death or experience.

TABLE 5.1   *(continued)*

Primary Care Physician
Function: Initiates a relationship with the palliative care team with referral of a new patient/family. Provides a medical history of the patient's illness and any other pertinent medical and psychosocial information; continues to be the primary physician or transfers the role to the PC physician.
Interrelationship: Assessments and interventions of the PC nurse and those of the interdisciplinary team are coordinated with the primary physician to establish a comprehensive plan of care for the patient and family.

Social Worker
Function: Provides history (via genogram) regarding the strengths, resources, and realities of patient/family system. Interventions include emotional support through individual, family, high risk, and bereavement counseling. Provides referrals for families to the community as needed for social services.
Interrelationship: Delivery of care involves ongoing collaboration with PC nurse who is continuously identifying psychosocial needs and outcomes of the patient and family.

Therapies (Pharmacy, Occupational, Physical, Dietary, Speech, Art, Music, Touch, Massage)
Function: Provide education and/or "hands-on" therapy of specialized discipline to maximize independence and quality of life of patient and family.
Interrelationship: Participates in plan of care when consulted by PC nurse and reports outcomes of interventions through collaboration with the PC nurse.

Volunteer
Function: Gives of time freely to contribute to patient and family needs by direct service, administrative support of the palliative care program, public relations, and community education.
Interrelationship: Reports observed family dynamics to PC nurse in order to revise plan of care if needed.

Volunteer Coordinator
Function: Recruits, screens, educates, supervises, and retains volunteer staff to provide supportive services to patients and families.
Interrelationship: Plans assignments of volunteers based upon identified needs of family by PC nurse; Involves PC nurse in volunteer training.

conflict resolution. Collaboration is defined as the ability to work with others, especially on intellectual endeavors (Merriam-Webster, 1993). It is the process of collaboration that empowers team members to act as decision makers within the group. For example, if a question on nausea and vomiting arises, various members of the team may provide observations and opinions in an effort to maximize the relief of all components of nausea and vomiting. Using a true collaborative process, the ultimate decision maker regarding this aspect of care would not come to a conclusion solely benefiting one member or one member's own perspective, but rather would make a decision reflecting the team's total input. Through collaboration, effective patient- and family-driven quality outcomes are achieved.

Palliative care differs from the traditional medical model in which the physician is the sole leader of the multidisciplinary team. In the palliative care model, leadership is filled by the member of the interdisciplinary team who is best educated and qualified to address and focus upon specific patient or family goals. In addition to achieving patient and family outcomes, leadership is essential to facilitate and optimize the professional potential of each team member's contribution (National Consensus Project, 2004).

Also, in the traditional multidisciplinary team, the physician, as team leader, is the primary decision maker for the care team. In contrast, in a true interdisciplinary team process, coordinated decision making among team members is necessary to achieve quality patient and family outcomes. In order to sort out which member or members of the team would be the most appropriate in contributing to the decision-making process, the following questions, developed by Ina Cummings (1998), should be considered: "Who has the information necessary to make the decision?" "Who needs to be consulted before the decision is made?" "Who needs to be informed of a decision after it is made?" Certain levels of decision making may be made by individual members of the team (e.g., titrating a pain medication based on patient needs), whereas other levels will require the input from the entire team as a whole (e.g., developing a care plan). Poor, fragmented decision making results from failure to include appropriate team members in the decision-making process (Cummings, 1998;).

Due to the interdependency among interdisciplinary team members, professional conflict will inevitably arise, which may be beneficial and stimulating to an interdisciplinary team. Respect and trust in each team member's skills, knowledge, expertise, and motivation are imperative. Lack of respectful conflict will result in group uniformity, which may stifle the creativity and the professional advancement and development of team members. Diverse ideas and opinions are often the impetus for innovative solutions for patient care problems, and in the process may deepen the professional dialogue within the team. However, conflict becomes destructive when it is personalized or viewed as a threat to a member's role. Thus, the art in managing conflict is not to avoid it, but to manage it effectively so that team members, patients, and families can receive its full benefits.

THE DEVELOPING ROLE OF NURSING IN PRACTICING PALLIATIVE CARE

In the book *Intimate Death*, the author writes

When death comes so close, and sadness and suffering rule, there is still room for life, and joy, and surges of feeling deeper and more intense than anything known before ... to witness the preciousness of these last moments of life and to the extraordinary privilege of being able to share them has some value ... to deepen our respect for the value of life itself. (deHennezel, 1997)

In order to identify the essence of palliative care nursing, the values and beliefs of the role of the palliative care nurse and the qualities and themes inherent to the person that provides end-of-life care are to be delineated. As deHennezel describes it, working with patients at the end of their lives and with the families who are adjusting to illness and eventual loss enables those who work with these families not only to learn about the value of life but also to transform themselves continuously in the process.

The palliative care nurse combines the science of nursing with ethics, philosophy, the humanities, diverse worldviews, and individual and family life experiences in order to provide holistic care to families who are coping with a life-limiting illness.

THE NURSE'S ROLE IN INTERDISCIPLINARY CARE

The following case example is that of an advanced practice nurse (APN) bringing a specific and well-defined set of qualities, knowledge, and judgments to caring for individuals and families at the end of life. This includes advanced scientific and biophysical knowledge, analytical skills, and mastery of a broad repertoire of communication and interpersonal skills. Specialized knowledge and proficiency in the ability to incorporate ethics, humanities, cultural diversity, family, spiritual, and psychological issues into care is also demanded (Coyne, 2003; Kuebler, 2003).

The J. D. Calkin model of advanced nursing practice (Spross & Baggerly, 1989) serves as an excellent model on which to base palliative care advanced practice nursing. Calkin defines the clinical judgment abilities of three nursing practice levels as novice, expert by experience, and the master's-prepared nurse.

The following case study illustrates Saunder's four dimensions of human suffering within the context of Calkin's model. The case study also will demonstrate the APN sub-roles of expert clinician, educator, consultant, researcher, and collaborator (Spross & Baggerly, 1989).

Clinical Case Study: A Woman with Neuropathic Pain Secondary to Metastatic Breast Cancer

Mrs. S. is a 52-year-old female who is suffering from the sequelae of stage 4 metastatic breast cancer for the past 3 years. All curative interventions including surgical resection, chemotherapy, radiotherapy, hormone therapy and experimental therapy have failed to halt the progression of her disease, which now affects her lung, liver, and bones, most notably her spine. Mrs. S.'s major distressing physical symptom is severe neuropathic pain, which radiates around her back to her abdomen. This pain has limited her ability to bathe, cook, eat, get dressed, and walk. Essentially all activities of daily living have been stripped from her and she is now confined to bed under the care of her husband. Prior to her cancer, she prided herself in being extremely independent. Currently, her neuropathic pain is being managed by steroids, tricyclic antidepressants, neuroleptics, and methadone.

Mrs. S. is married, has two teenage children, and has been on disability from her job as a television personality for the past several months. She is Baptist and is an active member in her church.

Assessment of the Patient and Family

Through daily interactions with Mrs. S. and her family, the APN on the palliative care unit built a therapeutic relationship that focused on all dimensions of human suffering: physical, psychological, spiritual, and psychosocial. Despite the aggressive titration of pharmacotherapy being used to treat Mrs. S.'s pain, she continued to suffer from intense neuropathic discomfort. Her pain rating consistently was 8/10 or above on a visual analog scale and over time her sense of despair about dying in such agony was increasing. In consultation with other interdisciplinary team members, the APN was analyzing current research and consulting with other pain experts for novel approaches in treating neuropathic pain. The use of intravenous lidocaine has successfully worked in similar scenarios and after critical analysis by the APN, the interdisciplinary team decided to trial this therapy. The APN presented all the literature regarding the use of intravenous lidocaine in refractory neuropathic pain to the hospital's quality committee. The committee granted permission for immediate use as long as the APN would commit to developing and implementing an institutional policy in the near future. The APN quickly developed an evidence-based guideline, as the neuropathic pain was escalating daily. The next step was to educate all team members, specifically the nursing and pharmacy staff, and the patient and family about the etiology, sequelae, and rationale for choosing this intervention. Mrs. S. received a test dose of the lidocaine and her pain decreased about 10% within 1 hour. Thus, the intravenous lidocaine was deemed appropriate to continue use. Over the next days, her pain level decreased to 2/10.

Respecting the value of nonpharmacological measures in relieving pain, the APN assisted in having Mrs. S. be offered massage and music therapy. She declined guided imagery.

While Mrs. S. was experiencing her pain crisis, the APN spent a lot of time with her being present, thus allowing an opportunity for Mrs. S. to express her feelings and fears. She revealed that she felt close to death and was struggling with guilt about one of her desires upon dying—that of spending her last minutes alone, if possible. She was fearful that this request would offend her very protective and involved family. But she had lived a very independent life and wanted to die that way. The APN listened, reflected, and assessed the situation and reported her findings to the interdisciplinary team. Based on the APN's observations and recommendations, the interdisciplinary team members set forth a plan to help Mrs. S. and her family deal with these very important issues. Social work and chaplaincy intensified their involvement.

Through interventions by the interdisciplinary team, Mrs. S.'s family was learning to become more comfortable with respecting their mother's request and were working through their feelings of "abandoning" their wife and mother in time of need. This would continue to be a process.

With in-depth knowledge of family systems theory, the APN identified the need for the interdisciplinary team to address the already actualized loss of Mrs. S.'s role within the family, including mother and wife. The APN consulted the bereavement counselor as an early intervention for high-risk grief status, as Mrs. S.'s family was still dealing with their loved one's request of dying alone.

Progressively, Mrs. S. showed signs and symptoms of nearing death. As her pain increased, the APN adjusted Mrs. S.'s pain regimen so that she would remain comfortable. The APN and the interdisciplinary team increased support to Mrs. S.'s family to help them honor her wish at the time of death.

Outcome

Mrs. S.'s death occurred without pain and she was able to spend the last minutes of her life by herself, as requested. Through the coordinated efforts of the interdisciplinary team, Mrs. S.'s family was able to begin to work through their feelings of having abandoned their loved one in the last moments of life and giving her a final gift: death by her terms with dignity, respect, comfort, and adoration. Mrs. S.'s family has agreed to participate actively in bereavement counseling to continue to work on the issues surrounding the death and how it impacts their grieving process.

Discussion of the APN Role

Clinician.

The APN utilized sophisticated and appropriate assessment strategies to evaluate pain and symptoms. The APN interfaced with other interdisciplinary team members to develop and implement a comprehensive plan of care. The APN identified novel approaches to the treatment of neuropathic pain and developed hospital-based standards of care to reflect and support this treatment strategy, and executed interventions. Advanced clinical knowledge of complex pain syndromes and comfort measures to address symptoms was demonstrated through utilization of innovated, ethically sound, scientifically based practice.

Educator.

The APN facilitated complex philosophical, ethical, and clinical management discussions, assisting the patient and family and all interdisciplinary team members to achieve a positive outcome. The APN assessed the learning needs of Mrs. S. and her family and the entire staff. The APN presented scientifically based education on the following issues: (a) the management of neuropathic pain, (b) po-

tential for role conflict, (c) actual loss/anticipatory grief, and (d) potential for high-risk bereavement. The APN educated other disciplines also, for example, the quality committee and pharmacy staff through in-services and guidelines on the philosophy of palliative care and individualized treatment strategies, and most notably, the use of intravenous lidocaine for intractable neuropathic pain.

Researcher.

The APN generated new knowledge through identifying research questions and by instituting novel approaches that address these questions. The APN investigated and integrated palliative care research strategies, for example, the use of intravenous lidocaine, to formulate an individualized plan of care for Mrs. S.

Collaborator.

The APN mentored staff in biopsychosocial and spiritual assessments and interventions. The APN built and preserved collaborative relationships, and identified resources and opportunities to work with palliative care colleagues. The APN facilitated the development and implementation of staff forums, in-services, physician/nurse collaboration, and quality committee consultation. The APN demonstrated the value of collaboration with the patient and family, the interdisciplinary team, and other health care professionals in order to facilitate the best possible outcome.

Consultant.

The APN consulted with the palliative care physician, palliative care colleagues, and quality committee representatives to determine the appropriate treatment strategies for meeting the needs of the patient and family. Also, the bereavement counselor was consulted after the APN identified the actualized loss experienced by Mrs. S.'s family. As a consultant, the APN was consistently available to the patient and family, interdisciplinary team members, and other health care professionals to discuss and explain issues surrounding the palliative care philosophy.

By maintaining a consistent presence with the patient and family and among interdisciplinary team members, the APN helped to minimize decision-making conflicts. With advanced knowledge in the humanities, the APN through language and image gave expression to the experience of illness, death, grief, and human suffering.

CONTINUING PROFESSIONAL EDUCATION

Knowledge, public opinion, and changes in health care are generating rapid changes and developments in the area of how we understand and treat patients and families who face life-threatening illnesses. In order to fulfill the constantly expanding responsibilities of a palliative care nurse, the nurse is challenged to keep well informed of new developments in bioethics, symptom management, family care, and public policy. Various forums and educational resources are available to support the palliative care nurse in keeping abreast of evolving issues in palliative care. Participation in professional societies (e.g., Hospice and Palliative Care Nurses Association) and continuing education strategies (journals, national conferences, etc.) along with attainment of specialty certification (for instance, National Board for Certification of Hospice and Palliative Nurses) collectively enhances the palliative care nurse's ability to deliver quality bio-psychosocial and spiritual care for patients and families.

CONCLUSION AND FUTURE DIRECTION

Palliative care is an emerging specialty within health care, especially nursing. The philosophy and delivery of palliative care transcends all areas of nursing where suffering accompanies illness. The palliative care nurse is a true leader within the interdisciplinary team and hence is in an ideal position to establish standards for consistent practice, foster education, and promote research. It is a professional privilege to be in the field of palliative care nursing, as it brings hopefulness to areas of end-of-life care that traditionally have been avoided, for example, ethics, pain, and human suffering. Equally applicable to the art of palliative care nursing practice is Henry David Thoreau's (1943) prose in which he states:

> It is something to be able to paint a picture, or to carve a statue, and to make a few objects beautiful. But it is far more glorious to carve and paint the atmosphere in which we work, to effect the quality of the day—this is the highest of the arts. (p. 90)

EDUCATION PLAN 5.1   Plan for Achieving Competencies: Interdisciplinary Palliative Care

Knowledge Needed	Attitudes	Skills	Undergraduate Behavioral Outcomes	Graduate Behavioral Outcomes	Teaching/Learning Strategies
Palliative Care Movement	*Affirm the need for improved care of the dying and their family.	*Participate in activities supportive of palliative care nursing.	*Demonstrate commitment to offering quality care at the end of life.	*Assume leadership roles in organizing, implementing, and evaluating palliative care nursing initiatives.	*Report on information and resources available at three web sites related to palliative care. *Identify local initiatives targeting change in end of life care. *Participate in an advisory or board of directors meeting related to hospice/palliative care to identify the needs and planned initiatives/responses.

(continued)

EDUCATION PLAN 5.1 *(continued)*

Knowledge Needed	Attitudes	Skills	Undergraduate Behavioral Outcomes	Graduate Behavioral Outcomes	Teaching/Learning Strategies
Ethical issues related to palliative care.	*Consider nursing's position regarding ethical issues associated with palliative care.	*Act in accordance with published nursing position statements related to end of life care.	*Communicate nursing's position regarding ethical issues to the patient, families, and other health care providers.	*Analyze the implications of published nursing position statements related to end of life care. *Participate in the development of nursing position statements, policies, and standards related to ethical issues associated with palliative care.	*Debate ethical issues and nursing's position related to care at the end of life. Write a personal position statement regarding an ethical issue related to end of life care.

Role development as a palliative care nurse.	*Affirm students' or nurses' own personal and professional growth as a palliative care nurse.	*Demonstrate the integration of palliative care knowledge, attitudes, and skills in nursing practice.	*Provide competent, holistic, and compassionate end of life care for patients and families.	*Provide competent, holistic, and compassionate end of life care for patients and families in complex caregiving situations.	*Document through journaling an introspective narrative of students'/nurses' own personal and professional growth as a palliative care nurse. *Analyze a case study that documents the responses and practices of the nurse from novice to expert.

(continued)

EDUCATION PLAN 5.1   *(continued)*

Knowledge Needed	Attitudes	Skills	Undergraduate Behavioral Outcomes	Graduate Behavioral Outcomes	Teaching/Learning Strategies
Development, characteristics, and roles of an interdisciplinary palliative care team.	*Appreciate the unique contribution of each member of the interdisciplinary palliative care team. *Affirm the value of nursing's role on the interdisciplinary care team.	*Effectively communicate with all members of the interdisciplinary team.	*Collaborate with members of the interdisciplinary palliative care team in determining goals and plans of care for patients and families experiencing life-threatening illness.	*Assume a leadership position as a member of the interdisciplinary palliative care team.	*Interview individual members of the palliative care team and discuss their unique contributions in post-conference or seminar. *Invite members of the interdisciplinary palliative care team to attend class to discuss their unique contributions, and barriers and facilitators to effective team functioning. *Attend an interdisciplinary team meeting and evaluate effective and ineffective methods of communication. Share findings in class or seminar.

REFERENCES

Beauchamp, T. L., & Childress, J. F. (1994). *The principles of biomedical ethics* (4th ed.). Oxford, UK: Oxford University Press.

Cairms, W., & Yates, P. M. (2003). Education and training in palliative care. *Medical Journal of Australia, 179*(1), 26–28.

Coyne, P. (2003). The evolution of the advanced practice nurse within palliative care. *Journal of Palliative Medicine, 6,* 769–770.

Cummings, I. (1998). The interdisciplinary team. In D. Doyle, G. Hanks, & N. Mac-Donald (Eds.), *Oxford textbook of palliative medicine* (2nd ed., pp. 3–8). Oxford, UK: Oxford University Press.

deHennezel, M. (1997). *Intimate death.* New York: Vintage Books.

El Sayem, A., Swint, K., Fisch, M. J., Palmer, J. L., Reddy, S., Walker, P., et al. (2004). Palliative care inpatient service in a comprehensive cancer center: Clinical and financial outcomes. *Journal of Clinical Oncology, 22,* 2008–2014.

Krammer, L. M., Muir, J. C., Gooding-Kellar, N., Williams, M. B., & von Gunten, C. F. (1999). Palliative care and oncology: Opportunities for oncology nursing. *Oncology Nursing Updates, 6*(3), 1–12.

Kuebler, K. (2003). The palliative care advanced practice nurse. *Journal of Palliative Medicine, 6,* 707–714.

LeGrand, S. B., Walsh, D., Nelson, K., & Zhukovsky, D. S. (2000). Development of a clinical fellowship program in palliative medicine. *Journal of Pain and Symptom Management, 20,* 345–352.

Leslie, B., Adams, L., & Canter, J. S. (2002). Integrating an end of life curriculum into the internal medicine clerkship. *Journal of Palliative Medicine, 5,* 752–753.

Loscalzo, M. J., & Zabora, J. R. (1998). Care of the cancer patient: Response of family and staff. In R. K. Portenoy & E. Bruera, (Eds.), *Topics in palliative care* (Vol. 2 , pp. 209–245). Oxford, UK: Oxford University Press.

Merriam-Webster. (1993). *Merriam-Webster's collegiate dictionary* (10th ed.). Springfield, MA: Merriam-Webster.

National Consensus Project. (2004). *Guidelines.* Retrieved 6/20/05 from http://www.nationalconsensusproject.org

Rosen, E. J. (1998) *Families facing death: A guide for healthcare professionals and volunteers* (Rev. ed.). San Francisco: Jossey-Bass.

Roy, D. J., & MacDonald, N. (1998). Ethical issues in palliative care. In D. Doyle, G. Hanks, & N. MacDonald (Eds.), *Oxford textbook of palliative medicine* (2nd ed., pp. 97–138). Oxford, UK: Oxford University Press.

Santa-Emma, P., Roach, R., Gill, M. A., Spayde, P., & Taylor, R. (2002). Development and implementation of an inpatient acute palliative care service. *Journal of Palliative Medicine, 5,* 93–100.

Spross, J. A., & Baggerly, J. (1989) Models of advanced nursing practice. In A. B. Hamric & J. A. Spross (Eds.), *The clinical nurse specialist in theory and practice* (2nd ed., pp. 19–40). Philadelphia: Saunders.

Thoreau, H. D. (1971). Where I lived, and what I lived for. In J. Lyndon (Ed.), *Walden.* Princeton, NJ: Princeton University Press.

Virik, K., & Glare, P. (2002). Profile and evaluation of a palliative medicine consultation service within a tertiary teaching hospital in Sydney, Australia. *Journal of Pain and Symptom Management, 23,*(3), 17–25.

von Gunten, C. F., & Muir, J. C. (2000). Palliative medicine—An emerging field of specialization. *Cancer Investigation, 18,* 761–767.

Walsh, D. (2001). The Harry R. Horvitz Center for Palliative Medicine 1987–1999: Development of a novel comprehensive integrated program. *American Journal of Hospice and Palliative Care, 18,* 239–250.

Weissman, D. (1997). Consultation in palliative medicine. *Archives of Internal Medicine, 157,* 733–737.

Zhukovsky, D. S. (2000). A model of palliative care: The palliative medicine program of the Cleveland Clinic Foundation. A WHO Demonstration Project. *Supportive Care Cancer, 8,* 268–277.

6

Ethical Aspects of Palliative Care

Judith Kennedy Schwarz

AACN Competencies

#12: Apply legal and ethical principles in the analysis of complex issues in end-of-life care, recognizing the influence of personal values, professional codes, and patient preferences.

#13: Identify barriers and facilitators to patients' and caregivers' effective use of resources.

> *Should we inquire into the truth of the matter, or merely accept it on our own authority and that of others?*
> —Socrates, in Plato's *Euthypro* (c. 400 BC)

Some decisions nurses make when providing end-of-life care seem particularly difficult; even experienced nurses may feel uncertain about whether they made the "right" decision. When the issue is what, all things considered, is the *right* thing to do, a moral or ethical question is asked. It is often exquisitely difficult to determine what the right response is when, for example, a terminally ill and suffering patient pleads with you to help speed her dying; you feel unable to help without causing her harm. An ethically hard case is one in which the good that you want to bring about can only be realized if the harm you seek to avoid is also brought about, that is, when benefiting the patient cannot be disentangled from harming (Cavanaugh, 1996).

Advances in scientific knowledge and developments in medical technology far exceed any social consensus about the circumstances for their appropriate use. The process of dying can now be prolonged almost indefinitely; this technological imperative (*can* do implies *ought to*) has given rise to an unprecedented array of professional, moral, and legal questions within health care. Many Americans fear the possibility of dying a painful, protracted, or undignified death, in an institutional setting, absent personal control or meaning (Schwarz, 2004a). Studies indicate that nurses also have concerns about how best to provide care for dying patients. In one study, more than half of the sample of 759 nurses reported acting against their consciences when providing end-of-life care and were concerned that they were providing overly burdensome interventions to their dying patients (Solomon et al., 1993). More recently, Tilden, Tolle, Nelson, and Fields (2001) noted that approximately 70% of hospital deaths follow decisions to limit aggressive end-of-life treatments; thus, most hospital deaths follow a period of discussion among family members, clinicians, and patients (if they are able to participate) in deciding how long to pursue, and when to forgo, life-sustaining treatments.

Ethical aspects of end-of-life decision-making pose compelling challenges for nurses because they frequently involve conflicts among values, principles, and priorities of care; such conflicts require reasoned deliberation for their resolution. This chapter provides practicing nurses with the tools needed to identify and address the ethical issues in end-of-life care. In order to identify ethically relevant aspects of complex cases, nurses are encouraged to engage in values clarification and personal reflection. To address the ethical issues in end-of-life care effectively, nurses should use a decision-making framework that incorporates ethical theories, clearly defined moral concepts, and an understanding of the Code for Nurses (American Nurses Association [ANA], 2001).

Ethical and legal issues often seem intertwined in many end-of-life decisions. For example, the selection of who is permitted to speak for a person who is decisionally incapable is a legally determined question, but which treatment the decision maker chooses is often a moral issue. Often the most difficult clinical conflicts occur at the junction of law and ethics, where an act that is illegal may seem morally required, or one that is legally required may seem morally inappropriate. Many of these cases resist satisfactory solutions. Although ethics and law function similarly in society in that they both sanction and guide behavior, they also differ in important ways. This chapter will focus on ethical issues in nursing care for those at the end of their lives.

ETHICS AND ETHICAL THEORY

Ethics is a branch of philosophy that considers and examines the moral life. The word ethics comes from the Greek *ethos*, and origi-nally meant character or conduct; the word moral comes from the Latin *mores*, which means customs or habit (Davis, Aroskar, Liaschenko, & Drought, 1997). *Ethics* and *morals* are frequently used interchangeably in nursing ethics to refer to conduct, character, and motivations involved in moral acts, although there are distinctions that are sometimes made between these terms.

The concept of morality is often used to refer to personally embraced concepts of duty, obligation, and principles of conduct. *Morals* is frequently used interchangeably with *values*, and refers in particular to values or principles of conduct to which one is personally and actually committed (Jameton, 1984). Use of the word ethics is distinguished by reflective thinking and practical reasoning, and often includes overarching, publicly stated sets of rules or principles, such as those found in professional ethics codes. Stanley and Zoloth-Dorfman (2001) note that ethics seeks to logically justify choices for right behavior and rules—particularly in situations that challenge established norms of behavior, or in those that require a new paradigm for judging behavior. These authors add that ethical inquiry—which seeks to interpret acts and to answer such questions as "What is the right thing to do?"—traditionally include an evaluation of (1) the moral agent and his or her character, (2) the motive for the act itself, and (3) the effect of the action on others. *Normative* ethics seeks ways to answer questions about right and wrong or good or bad in situations that call for a moral decision. Nursing ethics is both normative and practical, in that it makes use of ethical theory and analysis to examine and resolve what *ought to be done* in situations involving moral conflict in nursing practice. *Bioethics* refers to the application of ethics and ethical analysis to moral and practical problems in biological sciences, medicine, and health care.

Values and Values Clarification

Values have been called the cornerstone of nursing's moral art (Uustal, 1987). Few aspects of our personal or professional lives are value free. Values are ubiquitous, although often unspoken and frequently unexamined; they determine the nature of our moral choices. Values are foundational to our notions of good and bad, and inform our understanding of what constitutes benefit and harm; thus they are instrumental to the ethical decisions we make. Because our values influence the choices we make, they may also bias our judgments about the worth of our own view and negatively influence our judgments about the merits of others' choices; hence the need for values clarification. In the absence of reflection we may simply assume that others believe and would (should) do as we do. Uustal (1987) states that the price paid for unexamined values often included "confusion, indecision, and inconsistency" (p. 149).

Values clarification is a process of self-reflection that helps individuals identify, consider, and articulate the belief, purposes, and attitudes they prize and that drive their actions. Beliefs about death and what makes life worth living, our conclusions about the nature and significance of truth, or the meaning of paths not chosen are all moral values. Fowler (1987) states that the purpose of values clarification is to assist individuals to identify those personal and professional values that influence behavior and their moral decision making. It is recognized that the essence of ethical conflict is the clash of values, principles, legal rules, and personal perspectives (Dubler, 1994). The need for values clarification is an essential first step in moral decision-making.

Every nursing act that intervenes in the life of a patient has at least the possibility of enhancing or transgressing some value cherished by that patient. In situations of moral uncertainty or ethical dilemmas, questions of value will always be foundational. *Moral uncertainty* occurs when nurses are uncertain *if* a moral problem exists, are unsure about its nature, and are unclear which values conflict and which principles might facilitate clarification. These situations often occur in nursing practice. Moral uncertainty may occur when a patient seems to be suffering unnecessarily, is refusing pain medication, but is unwilling or unable to explain their reason for refusing your efforts to help.

Moral dilemmas occur less frequently and are understood as a situation in which two or more clear moral or ethical principles apply that support mutually inconsistent courses of action. Each alternative course of action can be justified by a moral rule or principle, but one can choose or satisfy only one course of action at the expense of *not* satisfying the other. The nurse who believes he or she is duty-bound both to preserve life and reduce suffering may experience a dilemma when preserving life causes intense suffering or when suffering can only be reduced by interventions that may shorten life. There is no satisfying right answer to an ethical dilemma, but one should utilize reasoned (principled) thinking in order to be able to provide a rationale for the decision reached.

The third type of moral problem is the experience of *moral distress,* an emotion that occurs when nurses have identified and know what right response is called for, but institutional or other constraints make it almost impossible to pursue the right course of action (Jameton, 1984). The repeated experience of moral distress can lead nurses to experience moral passivity, burnout, or to leave the profession (Cameron, 1997). Nurses who experience moral distress from institutional constraints on their ability to practice as morally autonomous clinicians must seek

support from colleagues and from other institutional and professional resources such as
institutional and nursing ethics committees
and state nursing associations. The experience of organizational constraints on professional autonomy causes some nurse scholars
to rhetorically ask whether nurses who face
ethical dilemmas are able to be ethical (Davis,
1994).

Resources to assist the nurse to manage
moral problems effectively will be included
in subsequent sections of this chapter. However, whatever the conflict, knowing one's
own values and being sensitive to the values
of others is an essential first step in ethical
nursing practice.

ETHICAL THEORIES

Moral theories are methods of determining
what counts when a decision must be made,
and offer a method for weighing or ranking
considerations identified as morally relevant
to that decision. More succinctly, an ethical
theory provides a framework of principles
within which an agent can determine morally
appropriate actions (Beauchamp & Childress,
2001).

It should be noted that nurses regularly
explore and resolve ethical questions in their
practices without recourse to ethical theories
and without a formal consideration of the
nature of their foundational moral values.
Yet, people hold different foundational views,
which sometimes can heighten moral conflict
and diminish the options for resolution. The
following scenario by Benjamin and Curtis
(1992) illustrates the role that ethical theories
can play in facilitating or hampering decision making. The case involves the question
of whether everything should be done to prolong the life of an elder gentleman in a nursing home who is decisionally incapable. The
staff must make the decision because there

are no friends or family and no prior indication of his wishes. Person A argues that he
should be treated because not to do so would
violate the duty to protect and preserve life.
Person B agrees that the man should be
treated, but for a different reason. B argues
that he should be treated because he is not
in any pain, and although he is significantly
cognitively impaired, he seems fairly content.
In B's view, what one ought to do above all
is to maximize happiness, and therefore the
man's life should be prolonged. As presented,
the question about whether to continue treatment can be answered without agreement
about the nature of basic ethical values and
with dissimilar ethical theories.

Suppose the facts are changed a little, so
that the gentleman is experiencing intractable pain and distress. In this case, with her
foundational commitment to maximizing
happiness, B would revise her judgment and
conclude that they should no longer strenu-
ously attempt to extend the man's life. But
this change in facts would be irrelevant to
A, and her judgment that the patient's life
should be prolonged would remain the same.
This conflict is not likely to be resolved without further questions about the nature and
justification of ethical principles that are the
foundation to approaches of making ethical
decisions.

Within bioethics, there are two major approaches to theoretical considerations—deontological and teleological systems of ethics. The deontological (from *deon*, Greek for
duty), or Kantian, approach to ethics focuses
on duties and obligations. Teleological theories (from *telos*, Greek for end) base the determination of whether an action is right or
wrong on the action's consequences. These
two ethical theories are increasingly subject to
criticism for their overreliance on unrelated
and often conflicting principles in dealing
with moral problems in health care (Clouser
& Gert, 1990), and by feminist moral theo-

rists for their oppressiveness and indifference to the particularity of relationships (Gadow, 1996). These theories continue to dominate the ethical arguments used to resolve moral problems in health care, and nurses must recognize them and be familiar with their use in decision making. These two theories will be described and contrasted to a decisional theory based on caring.

Deontological Moral Theory

A deontological, or Kantian, approach to decision making focuses on duty and obligations. Kantian deontology is attributed to the eighteenth-century moral philosopher Immanuel Kant. Deontologists maintain that whether an act is right or wrong depends upon the nature of the act itself when considered in terms of its inherent moral worth. Kant argued further that consequences can never make an action right or wrong. Duty-based theories hold particular duties to be fundamental and make use of principles or their derivative rules in order to guide decision making. An example of duty-based theories include natural law, which identifies a duty to obey God's will and requires that one not kill; and the rules of traditional medical morality derived from the Hippocratic tradition, which maintain that above all we should do no harm.

A deontological position requires commitment to the principle of universalizability, which means that once a moral decision is made, that same decision must be made in all similar situations. The essence of this position is that morality requires that we cannot make exceptions for ourselves. Thus, if the proposed action is one that would be wrong if done generally, then the particular action is also wrong—even when the specific action has no harmful consequences. Such rules as "it is always wrong to directly take innocent human life" are considered valid when they

meet certain conditions, identified by Kant as categorical imperatives. Proposed by Kant as a means to resolve conflicts between rules and principles, this imperative means that for a rule to be valid it must be applicable to everyone universally. This principle can be illustrated as follows: If it is morally acceptable for me to act as I do for my patient (e.g., not charging for services, stealing medications for her use, skipping home visits, etc.), so must it also be acceptable for every other nurse to act similarly for their patients.

Another form of this categorical imperative requires that persons should always be treated (and valued) as ends in themselves, and never solely as means. Thus nurses are required to respect individuals and their beliefs regardless of consequences and they are similarly obliged to respect persons' autonomous choices. Kant identified these categorical imperatives as unconditional commands that are morally required and obligatory in any circumstance (Davis et al., 1997). Within this theoretical perspective, it is simply one's duty to obey categorical imperatives without any exceptions, without reference to the consequences of the act, and in the absence of external or guiding authority. The moral standard includes keeping promises, avoiding or preventing harm, and respecting persons; these are principles that are morally required and are consistent with the rules provided in our professional code of ethics.

Teleological Moral Theories

Teleological theories determine an action to be right or wrong based on the consequences of the action. The most important teleological theory for contemporary health care is utilitarian ethics (Aaras & Steinbock, 1995). Utilitarianism is best understood as a moral theory that asserts there is only one basic principle in ethics, the principle of utility, which declares that we ought always to produce the greatest possible balance of value over disvalue for the greatest number of persons (Beauchamp & Childress, 2001). This position assumes that one can weigh and measure harms and benefits and arrive at the greatest possible balance of good over evil for the most people (Davis et al., 1997).

Utilitarians are disinterested in considerations of the agent's intentions, feelings, or convictions; all are viewed as irrelevant to the question of "What is the right thing to do?" In the same fashion, utilitarians regard the question of whether a proposed action conforms to established social norms or ethical codes as relevant only to the extent that conforming (or not) has a bearing on the production of happiness or value over unhappiness (Aaras & Steinbock, 1995). At least in principle, utilitarians are able to provide definite answers to specific questions about how one ought to act. The question of whether it is ever morally permissible to be untruthful depends upon context and circumstances: in those situations where telling a lie would produce, overall, more happiness or value than unhappiness, then telling a lie would be morally justified.

As with deontological theories, there are two versions of this theory: an act-utilitarian is primarily concerned with the consequences of particular acts, while a rule-utilitarian is more concerned about the consequences of general policies. To illustrate the difference between these versions. imagine that a nurse is trying to decide if it would be morally right to help a terminally ill patient die. An act-utilitarian would try to determine which alternative in this particular situation would maximize happiness or minimize suffering, or both. The considerations included in making that determination would be the nature of the disease and the certainty of prognosis, the presence of a treatable depression, whether the patient really wanted to die or needed better palliative care, the impact in the patient's family, and the professional repercussions for the nurse.

By contrast, a rule-utilitarian uses the principle of utility to formulate and justify moral rules, and the correct moral rules are those that promote the greatest happiness for the greatest number (Aaras & Steinbock, 1995). In this particular case, the nurse would ask whether a general rule permitting assisted suicide would maximize happiness. Important considerations of this approach include questions about whether such a practice would put us on a slippery slope and threaten the lives of other terminally ill patients who do not really want to die but might feel obliged or are susceptible to being coerced. Thus a rule-utilitarian might agree that although helping this particular patient to die might maximize happiness (or minimize suffering) for the individual, it would still be wrong because of the larger negative consequences of a general policy permitting assisted suicide (Aaras & Steinbock, 1995).

How would a Kantian resolve this nurse's problem? Aaras and Steinbock (1995) suggest that the categorical imperative gives less guidance—it functions only to tell us what *cannot* be done, and not what *should* be done. The principle of universalizability is just one value in Kantian ethics; the other mandate is respect for persons. The question would then be reframed: Does a policy of assisted suicide promote respect for persons or would such a policy lead to the devaluing of human life and to nonvoluntary killing of the weak, the vulnerable, and the poor?

Each of these theories has strengths and limitations, but neither ethical theories nor principles alone will provide a formula for resolving ethical questions. What they do provide is a framework for trying to reach workable solutions to complex and difficult questions (Aaras & Steinbock, 1995).

Focus on Caring

An ethic of caring that focuses on relationships and responsibility is one aspect of the broader field of feminist ethics. This ethic stems in part from a criticism of traditional ethical theories as being biased in their representation of the experiences of men rather than women. Another dimension of feminist ethics is the analysis of oppression and dominance within relationships and social institutions. It is certain that power differentials between nurses (who are primarily women), physicians, patients, administrators, and payers illustrate just some of the relational inequalities that exist in most health care organizations (Davis et al., 1997). *Caring,* within the context of an *ethics of care,* refers to "care for, emotional commitment to, and willingness to act on behalf of persons with whom one has a significant relationship. Noticeably downplayed are Kantian universal rules, impartial utilitarian calculations, and individual rights" (Beauchamp & Childress, 2001, p. 369).

The idea of an ethic of caring is particularly appealing to nurses because caring is considered to be the very foundation of their practice. Sara Fry, a contemporary nurse philosopher, proposes caring as a fundamental value for the development of a theory of nursing ethics (Fry, 1989). Care for others is a core notion in an ethic of care, and is evident in the ANA Code for Nurses (2001), which mandates respectful care of the individual as its core tenet.

In an ethic of care, the decision maker focuses on identifying actions that promote and maintain relationships and views the patient as a unique individual within networks of relationships (Davis et al., 1997). Fry, Killen, and Robinson (1996) maintain that

> the actions and judgments made using care-based reasoning must be measured against what it means to be 'caring' within the context of the responsibilities the decision maker has to others . . . care-based reasoning does not involve the application of abstract ethical principles to the situation or impartiality on the part of the decision maker. (p. 42)

Other scholars criticize the rejection of ethical principles as "an invitation to capriciousness" (Held, 1994, p. 75). An ethic of care is not yet adequately developed to function as a conceptual theory for identifying "right" actions in morally troubling situations (Davis et al., 1997; Fry et al., 1996).

ETHICAL PRINCIPLES AND CONCEPTS

The major ethical principles of significance to nurses are respect for persons and autonomy, beneficence, nonmaleficence, and justice. The duties of veracity, fidelity, and confidentiality are moral rules derived from these principles that further guide and direct nursing actions. These moral rules are embedded in the provisions of the Code of Ethics for Nurses (ANA, 2001). One particular rule that resonates for nurses who care for patients at the end of life is the proscription that "nurses may not act with the sole intent of ending a patient's life even though such action may be motivated by compassion, respect for patient autonomy, and quality of life considerations" (p. 8).

There may be occasions when moral agents feel obliged to question these rules and their appropriateness in particular circumstances, and they may wish to "appeal" to a higher level of moral authority (Veatch & Fry, 1995). Perhaps a nurse may question whether it is *always* wrong to "act with the sole intent of ending a patient's life" and to ask whether other duties such as mercy and compassion might sometimes prevail. This higher level of authority within a moral framework consists of ethical principles.

Respect for Persons and the Principle of Autonomy

The most fundamental ethical principle within nursing practice is the principle of respect for persons. The first provision in the Code for Nurses (ANA, 2001) calls for nurses to "Practice with compassion and respect for the inherent dignity, worth and uniqueness of every individual, unrestricted by considerations of social, or economic status, personal attributes, or the nature of health problems" (p. 7).

The principle of respect for persons is broader and more abstract than the principle that addresses individual autonomy and self-determination. Respect for persons requires that each individual be treated as unique and entitled to treatment that is respectful of their human dignity. It is this principle of respect for persons that requires particular justification before we are permitted to interfere with the plans, privacy, or behavior of autonomous adult persons, and specifically constrains *paternalistic* decisions made by health professionals for patients with decision-making capacity.

The concept of autonomy is multidimensional and in its broadest sense incorporates the following: having a minimum of relevant information; self-determined choice; freedom to act on the basis of one's choices; and self-governance (Yeo, Moorhouse, & Dalzeil, 1996). Autonomous (or decisionally capable) persons determine their own course of action in accordance with a plan chosen by themselves. An autonomous action is understood as one done intentionally, made with understanding and without controlling influences that determine the action (Beauchamp & Childress, 2001).

How are nurses to understand and apply this principle? This principle guides nursing actions in that nurses are duty-bound to respect patients' autonomous choices in all situations unless this principle is overridden by another moral principle of greater weight or standing (Fry, 1987). Such would be the case when questions are raised about whether the choice is truly autonomous, whether the choice is perceived as harmful to the individual or others, and in other situations where autonomous choice is not possible. In these situations, the nurse's obligation to prevent harm to others or to benefit the patient may be determined to have greater moral weight.

It is the principle of respect for persons and autonomy that is the foundation of informed consent. According to this rule, persons must be given sufficient, accurate, and complete information necessary to make informed decisions about treatment choices. This includes decisions to accept, refuse, or to terminate treatments, whether or not these treatments are necessary for sustaining or prolonging life.

Limiting Autonomy

Nurses who care for patients at the end of life may sometime wonder whether they ought to intervene to prevent harm that they fear may result from a patient's decision. Put another way, are clinicians ever justified in limiting or interfering with a person's autonomy? The two most frequently occurring ways that health care professionals infringe upon patient autonomy are through control of information (e.g., withholding, deceiving, or equivocating), or through preventing a patient from acting upon his or her choice (e.g., refusing to comply or assist, constraining, or forcing treatment) (Yeo, Moorhouse, & Daziel, 1996). This type of interference, known as paternalism or parentalism, occurs often in health care and is done with the best of intentions; indeed, by definition it is understood as an intervention that is imposed for the patient's good or benefit.

In fact, paternalistic actions such as deception, breaking promises, or interfering with adult choices are violations of moral rules that morally are never permitted unless a morally adequate reason is provided. To justify such violations, philosophers Culver and Gert (1982) argue that we must determine whether we would publicly advocate this kind of violation in all similar situations. "If all rational persons would agree that the evil prevented by universally allowing this violation would be greater than the evil caused by universally allowing it, the violation is strongly justified" (p. 149). This would be a difficult standard to meet for those who presume justification exists for telling lies that we think benefit another.

In considering circumstances when limitations on autonomy may be justified, "weak" paternalism is sometimes accepted to prevent persons from causing themselves serious harm. In this view, one would be justified in interfering only to prevent a significant harm from occurring, but only when the person's conduct is substantially nonvoluntary or nonautonomous (Yeo, Moorhouse, & Daziel, 1996). To justify this type of interference, one would have to demonstrate that the presumption of autonomy or self-determination is no longer held, and that the person's choices were in fact no longer autonomous or freely chosen. Under this rule, we would be clearly justified in intervening if we discovered a patient attempting to jump out of a hospital window.

"Strong" paternalism, by contrast, involves limiting or interfering with the self-determination of someone whose autonomy is not in question (i.e., an adult capable of rational decision-making) and is very rarely justified. For example, a decisionally capable person who at the end of her life makes a thoughtful and considered decision to stop eating and drinking would be seriously wronged or harmed if a clinician were to override her decision and insert a feeding tube or intravenous line to prolong her life. Paternalistic behavior, regardless of how good the motives or the size of the benefit gained or the harm avoided, violates the right of an adult to be treated as a person. To disregard a person's life plans and values in such a fashion is to show contempt for them as persons, or in Kant's terms, it is to treat them as mere means to an end, rather than as an end in themselves.

Before an act of paternalism can be considered justified, each of the following conditions must be present:

1. The patient's capacity for rational reflection must be significantly impaired. This (*autonomy* condition) must be clinically determined and substantiated.
2. The patient is likely to be significantly harmed unless interfered with (the *harm* condition).
3. It is reasonable to assume that the patient will, at a later time, with recovery of capacity for rational reflection, ratify or agree to the decision made to interfere (the *ratification* condition). (Benjamin & Curtis, 1992)

Questions About Capacity for Autonomous Choice

Patients should be assumed to have the capacity to make decisions for themselves unless there is clear evidence to the contrary (Beauchamp & Childress, 2001). Clinical judgments about a person's decisional capacity serve as a gatekeeping role in health care by distinguishing those whose decisions should be solicited and honored from persons whose

decisions need not or should not be solicited or accepted (Beauchamp & Childress,
2001). Patient capacity is often neither completely present nor totally absent, as is particularly the case in some elderly persons who
may evidence a level of capacity that waxes
and wanes. When capacity waxes and wanes,
caregivers should take advantage of opportunities to engage the patient in decision making and advance-care planning when their
capacities are at their best (Lynn et al., 1999).
Capacity is best understood as task-specific,
in that a higher level of capacity is required
for decisions associated with serious consequences (i.e., agreeing to a proposed surgical
intervention) compared to decisions about
choosing meals or where to eat them (Mezey,
Mitty, & Ramsey, 1997). A capacity determination is a clinical judgment made by caregivers who know the patient best. When the
consequences of the capacity determinations
are particularly grave or the determination
is contentious, clinicians may wish to seek a
psychiatric consultation.

There are occasions when nurses may
question whether a decision reflects what
patients really want or whether their choice
was really made autonomously. They want to
know whether the patient is capable of making an autonomous choice and whether they
should comply with a decision that seems inconsistent with previously stated values or is
detached from contextual reality.

Assessing Decision-making Capacity

A decisionally capable person is able to understand a proposed intervention (or its termination), deliberate regarding major risks
and benefits, make a decision in light of that
deliberation, and communicate the choice
to others (Mezey et al., 1997). The following
is information that decisionally capable patients should understand:

- His or her condition for which the intervention is recommended
- The nature of the recommended intervention
- The risks and benefits of the recommended intervention, of alternative interventions, including no intervention
  or treatment

Caregivers should determine the following:

- The patient acknowledges that treatment is recommended.
- The patient understands how the proposed treatment or lack of treatment
  can affect their quality of life.
- The patient's decision is not substantially based on a delusional belief (Yeo,
  Moorhouse, & Daziel, 1996, pp. 99–
  100).

These criteria are intended to establish
whether the patient is capable of making a
rational choice, and not whether the choice
being made is rational.

Deciding for Others

If a patient lacks the capacity to make informed choices, other means must be identified for surrogate decision-making. There are
three standards for surrogate decision-making: written advance directives, substituted
judgment, or best interest. These three standards are ordered so that advance directives
have priority over the other two, and substituted judgment has priority over the best interest standard (Lynn et al., 1999). The best
of all situations is a thoughtfully drafted advance directive applied by a surrogate decision-maker who knows the patient's values
and wishes well.

The substituted judgment is a subjective
standard that is ideally based on knowledge

of the patient's wishes, values, views about particular interventions, and quality-of-life determinations. This standard allows the surrogate to decide as though the patient were speaking. Realistically, a surrogate's knowledge about the patient's goals and values is typically not entirely clear and decisive regarding a particular choice of treatment (Lynn et al., 1999). These authors state that "in practice, surrogate decision making for incompetent patients often has to draw on all three standards for decisions about an incompetent patient's care" (p. 273). The "best interests" standard is used when the patient's treatment wishes, or values, are unknown. Under these circumstances, the decision maker must objectively weigh the expected benefits and burdens associated with the treatment recommended by the health care team and determine what would be best for this patient.

Nurses have an important role to play in surrogate decision-making; the surrogate must be encouraged to focus on what the now incompetent patient would want if he or she were able to speak. It is often very difficult for grieving family members to put aside their own distress about the implications of honoring patient preference, especially when the decision involves withholding or withdrawing life-sustaining treatments. While the patient retains capacity, he or she should be encouraged and guided by nurses to discuss end-of-life choices with family members or other potential surrogate decision-makers. Nurses are well positioned to describe to patients and their loved ones the actual risks and benefits that are known to be associated with the use of interventions such as cardiopulmonary resuscitation, tube feedings, and mechanical ventilation. As Perrin (1997) notes, "advance directives are unlikely to have an effect on care if a health care provider, proxy or family member does not support and advo-

cate for following the person's wishes" (p. 25). Yet, even when patients complete advance directives (ADs), clinicians observe that the ADs often are unavailable or not applicable in many of the clinical situations faced by seriously ill adults (Tonelli, 1996).

Use of advance directives.

Researchers are beginning to investigate how advance directives actually function in various clinical settings, and are exploring whether the presence of an AD ensures compliance with patients' end-of-life wishes. For example, in a study by Tierney and colleagues (2001), investigators found that although discussions about ADs improved the "care satisfaction" of elderly patients with chronic illnesses, having completed a written living will did not increase the likelihood that family decision-makers would make treatment decisions that accurately reflected the patient's choice as stipulated in the AD.

A number of commentators agree that there are persistent difficulties associated with use of *written* directives that include incomplete information, the inability to anticipate future medical conditions, and uncertainty regarding the meaning and intent of written instructions. These problems of interpretation require clinicians to seek information from others in their attempt to determine what the patient "really meant" (Tonelli, 1996). Tonelli and others conclude that because of the limitations associated with use of written instructive directives, proxy or appointment directives are the preferred form of advance directive (Dexter, Wolinsky, Gramelspacher, Eckert, & Tierney, 2003; Perkins, 2000; Tonelli, 1996). Clearly, there is a need for further research to explore whether ADs facilitate good end-of-life care, and nurses are ideally situated to direct and participate in furthering understanding of these documents.

In the absence of a thoughtful discussion that includes general end-of-life values and specific preferences about use of interventions such as artificial nutrition and hydration, the legally appointed surrogate may be poorly prepared to identify or implement treatment decisions that conform with the patient's actual end-of-life preferences. In addition, family stress associated with decisions to withdraw life-sustaining treatments from decisionally incapacitated patients was highest in the absence of a completed advance directive (Tilden et al., 2001).

Beneficence and Nonmaleficence

Beneficence, known generically as doing good, is often hard to separate from nonmaleficence, or the duty not to inflict harm. Some philosophers argue that the principle of beneficence includes four rules:

1. One ought not to inflict evil or harm (what is bad).
2. One ought to prevent evil or harm.
3. One ought to remove evil.
4. One ought to do good or promote good. (Frankena, 1973)

These rules are prioritized in that the first takes precedence over the second, which is in turn more compelling than the third, which takes moral precedence over the fourth, all things being equal (Frankena, 1973). Although it can seem difficult in clinical practice to distinguish preventing harm from providing benefit, Benjamin and Curtis (1992) believe it is easier to get agreement on what constitutes a harm than on what constitutes a benefit. When the duty not to inflict harm conflicts with the duty to provide benefit, there is agreement that, all things being equal, there is a greater obligation not to injure others than to benefit them (Beauchamp & Childress, 2001).

In health care, the principle of maleficence is understood as requiring clinicians to avoid intentionally causing patients unnecessary harm or pain, whether psychological or physical. The principle of nonmaleficence and none of its derived moral rules are absolute. We often do harm to patients in order to benefit them or to prevent a greater harm from occurring—administering chemotherapy treatments is an obvious example. What is morally relevant is whether causing the harm is morally justified. Under most circumstances, death is considered a major harm; the question of whether causing death is ever justified is an issue of significance to nurses who provide care at the end of life.

Patients at the end of their lives may be particularly vulnerable to harm. They are harmed when they receive unwanted or unnecessary interventions, are overtreated with burdensome technological interventions that serve only to prolong dying, and also when treatments are withdrawn without their consent or agreement. Most certainly they are harmed when their pain is not managed adequately due to the nurse's fear that the patient's death might be hastened as a result of pain management with high-dose opiates. The Code of Ethics (ANA, 2001) stipulates that not only should they "not act with the sole intent of ending a patient's life," but also identifies an additional nursing duty: "the nurse should provide interventions to relieve pain and other symptoms in the dying client even when those interventions entail risks of hastening death" (p. 8).

Balancing Good and Evil—
The Principle of Double Effect

Any discussion that includes attempts to distinguish between harming and benefiting patients must consider the principle of double effect. Developed by Roman Catholic moral theologians in the Middle Ages, this principle is applied to situations in which it is impossible to avoid all harmful action and a decision must be made about whether one potentially harmful action is preferable to another (Quill, Dresser, & Brock, 1997). This principle is used to justify claims that the results of an act that would be morally wrong if caused intentionally are permissible if foreseen but unintended. The principle is often cited to explain why certain forms of care at the end of life that result in death are morally permissible and others are not (Coyle, 1992; Latimer, 1991; Quill, Lo, & Brock, 1997; Schwarz, 2004b).

The traditional formulation of this principle stipulates that the following four conditions be met before an act with both good and bad consequences may be morally justified (Schwarz, 2004b).

1. The action itself must be good or at least morally indifferent;
2. the individual must sincerely intend only the good effect and not the evil;
3. the evil effect cannot be the means to the good effect; and
4. there must be a proportionately grave reason for permitting the evil effect, that is, there must be a favorable balance between the good and the evil effects of the action.

The first condition determines whether the potential action is ever permissible, while the second and third conditions are used to determine whether the potential harm is intentional or unintentional, either as a means or as an end in itself. The fourth condition requires the agent to compare the net good and bad effects of the potential act to determine which course produces an effect of proportionally greater good (Quill, Dresser, et al., 1997).

Nurses may appeal to this principle in morally difficult situations where it is not possible

to benefit a patient by an action without at the same time causing harm. The classic example is that of the terminally ill pulmonary patient who is experiencing both great pain and a low respiratory rate. The treatment of choice, injecting morphine sulfate, will quell the pain but might also "quell" the respiratory rate. The nurse has a moral duty to prevent and remove evil (pain) that appears to conflict with the duty to benefit patients (protect and preserve life), a dilemma indeed. The answer to the question of whether the nurse may administer the morphine is clearly yes. Applying the criteria of double effect illustrates why this is so:

1. The action of giving an injection of morphine is itself morally indifferent.
2. The intended effect is to relieve the pain not to depress the respirations.
3. Respiratory depression is not the means by which the pain relief is obtained.
4. The relief of pain and the related reduction of suffering combine to provide a sufficiently important reason, or proportionately greater good than the harm that is incurred—respiratory depression and likely death. (Schwarz, 2004b)

Although this moral analysis is consistent with the position found within the Code for of Ethics (ANA, 2001), there are some who question the clinical usefulness of this principle as a guide to ethical decision making (Beauchamp & Childress, 2001). In particular, some clinical experts in palliative care challenge the purported "double effect" of opiate use in terminally ill patients and describe the likelihood of a secondarily associated hastened death as an "over blown myth" (Manfredi, Morrison, & Meier, 1998, p. 139). Others caution that "using the principle of double effect to justify using opioids to treat pain in dying patients contributes to the belief of pain medication, which in turn leads to fear of hastening death and the undertreatment of pain" (Fohr, 1998, p. 316).

Justice

The last principle that may facilitate nurses' decisions about end-of-life care is justice, which is understood broadly as fairness. Justice involves the determination of what someone or some group is owed, merits, deserves, or otherwise it entitled to (Yeo, Moorhouse, & Donner, 1996). At the societal (macro) level of resource allocation, the concept of justice includes questions of how scarce resources ought to be distributed and what should "count" as morally relevant differences between individuals in order to justify differences in treatment. Micro-allocation issues involve determining which particular person will receive a specific and limited resource. A number of criteria for making such selections include likelihood of medical benefit, random selection criteria, and present and future quality of life criteria (Yeo, Moorhouse, & Donner, 1996). It is generally agreed that if a treatment will not medically benefit a patient, it is considered futile, and as such its use is morally and professionally unwarranted. Medically futile interventions should not be proposed or offered to patients or families. As an illustration of how questions of futility have been clinically addressed, Choi and Billings (2002) describe a new Texas law cited by Fine and Mayo that attempts to remedy a situation that can occur when clinicians feel forced to provide medically inappropriate or futile care to terminally ill patients whose families insist that "everything be done" to avoid death. Under this Texas law, a detailed process of negotiation includes consultation with an ethics or medical committee; the option of family participation in the committee deliberations; and if the committee concludes that treatment is medically inappropriate, giving the family 10 days to transfer the patient, appeal to the courts, or accept that life support will be withdrawn.

At the individual level of end-of-life care, clinicians cite justice in support of claims for dying patients to receive access to a level of palliative care equal to that of curative care (Coyle, 1992). In the current era of cost containment and social injustice, some fear that those who are already marginalized and disadvantaged by poverty, chronic or terminal illness, old age, or by cultural and racial status may feel a duty to die in order to spare families financial or emotional strain (Robinson, 1990). Individual nurses at the bedside will not resolve these complex issues. Solution requires interdisciplinary understanding and cooperative effort among all affected parties within society (Aroskar, 1987). Meanwhile, the Code for Nurses (ANA, 2001) stresses that the nurse's commitment is to particular patients, "unrestricted by considerations of social or economic status, personal attributes, or the nature of their health problem" (p.7) and regardless of the cost of their care to society. The challenge for caregivers is to reach ethically supportable decisions that are fair to individual patients while using available resources responsibly.

ELEMENTS OF A DECISION-MAKING FRAMEWORK

When nurses must choose between alternative courses of action that seem equally unattractive, they experience an ethical dilemma. The decision will have significant implications for the well-being of the patient, involved family members, and for others affected by the choice. The nurse's ability to provide an ethically defensible rationale for decisions is recognized as a foundation to professional practice and the integrity of individual nurses (Davis et al., 1997). Rushton and Reigle (1993) argue in support of a shared decision-making model that promotes patient well-being and self-determination. According to this model, the health care team offers expert knowledge, treatment recommendations, and advice about medically available and appropriate options to the patient (patient/family unit). The patient decides which option will best promote his or her life goals and values. The nurse is particularly well positioned to understand the values that inform patients' choices and to appreciate the context of the patient's whole life, including the patient/family unit; their cultural, religious, and spiritual affiliations; and other unique preferences. The nurse is a vitally important member of this decision-making team.

When a clinical problem is identified as ethical and conflicts in moral values or ethical principles are present, the following steps will assist the nurse to discuss, analyze, and develop successfully an ethically supportable decision.

1. Review the overall situation—identify what is going on in this case.
2. Gather all relevant facts about the patient and her or his contextual situation, including
   - significant medical and social history,
   - decision-making capacity, and
   - existence of any advance treatment directives—written, appointed, or verbal, and any pertinent institutional policies.
3. Identify the parties or stakeholders involved in the situation, including those who will be affected by the decision(s) made.
4. Identify relevant legal data, including both state and federal laws.
5. Identify specific conflicts of ethical principles or values. Identify and consider nursing guidelines and the profession's code and position statements.
6. Identify possible choices, their purpose, and their probable consequences to the welfare of the patient, who is the focus of primary concern. Identify and make use of interdisciplinary and institutional resources such as institutional and nursing ethics committees, ethicists, chaplains, social workers, and other experienced colleagues.
7. Identify practical constraints to decision making, for example, institutional, legal, organizational, political, and economic.
8. Take action if you are the decision maker and implementer of the decision(s).
9. Review and evaluate the situation after action is taken in order to determine what was learned that will help in the resolution of similar situations in patient care and policy development. (Cassells & Gaul, 1998; Davis et al., 1997)

CONCEPTUAL CONFUSION AND DIFFICULT DECISIONS IN END-OF-LIFE CARE

The final segment of this chapter will explore issues of patient autonomy and decisions about end-of-life interventions that range from instances of allowing or permitting death, to hastening or intentionally causing death and how these decisions are understood by nurses.

Autonomy and the Refusal of Life-Sustaining Treatment

If the concept of autonomy means anything at all, it means the right to accept or refuse medical treatments. Decisions about the use or withdrawal of life-sustaining treatments (LST) are often complex and value-laden, in part because such decisions may forestall or hasten the time of death. Decisions regarding use of LST may also influence the patient's experience of the final stage of life by determining where death occurs, who is present, and whether the patient is able to communicate with loved ones (e.g., whether the patient is connected to a ventilator).

The concept of life-sustaining treatments includes any medical or nursing intervention, procedure, or medication, no matter how simple or complex, that is necessary for continued life. In the past, some treatments were considered ordinary and morally required, while others were called extraordinary and considered optional. This distinction between ordinary and extraordinary treatments has a prominent history within the Roman Catholic tradition and was used to determine whether a patient's refusal of treatment should be classified as suicide. Within that faith tradition, refusal of ordinary means was considered suicide (Beauchamp & Childress, 2001).

The terms *optional* or *nonburdensome treatments* include all medications, treatments, and operations that offer a reasonable hope of benefit and can be obtained and used without excessive expense, pain, or other inconvenience from the patient's perspective. *Extraordinary* (or *burdensome*) treatments are those that are very costly, unusual, difficult or dangerous, or do not offer a reasonable hope of benefit to the patient (Davis et al., 1997). What should be of moral concern for nurses is not what the intervention is, but whether the benefits of its continued use outweigh its associated burdens, as determined by the patient or surrogate decision-maker.

Withholding and Withdrawing Life-Prolonging Treatments

Many health care professionals and family members are more comfortable not initiating

life-sustaining treatments and then stopping them once begun. However, the question to be answered is whether this psychological fact has any moral significance (Beauchamp & Childress, 2001). Some clinicians regard withdrawing LST as "letting die," an act sometimes referred to as *passive euthanasia*, while others view withdrawing LST as an *act* that feels more like causing death, or killing. Withdrawing LST may be experienced as morally problematic for some nurses, particularly those who emphasize the "sanctity of life" and believe that continued life is an intrinsic good, regardless of burdens imposed by illness. However, nurses should be familiar with the legal and moral consensus that recognizes no moral distinction between withholding and withdrawing LST.

This consensus began to emerge in the early 1980s when a presidential commission was created to explore significant ethical issues in health care (President's Commission, 1983). One of their reports, entitled "Deciding to Forego Life-Sustaining Treatment," maintains that "neither criminal nor civil law—if properly interpreted and applied ... forces patients to undergo procedures that will increase their suffering when they wish to avoid this by foregoing life-sustaining treatments" (p. 89). The commission further held that "the distinction between failing to initiate and stopping therapy—that is, withholding versus withdrawing treatment—is not in itself of moral (or legal) importance. A justification that is adequate for not commencing a treatment is also sufficient for ceasing it" (p. 61).

There is a clear ethical consensus that LST may be withheld or withdrawn under certain circumstances; in particular, when its use is against the patient's wishes (provided the patient is fully informed and freely consenting), when it will or has begun to harm the patient, or when it does not or will not benefit the patient in the future (Beauchamp & Childress, 2001). The ANA (1994b) position statement on assisted suicide similarly encourages nurses to honor the refusal of treatments that an informed patient does not want, either because they are deemed overly burdensome or because they will not benefit the patient. This position statement specifically notes that when nurses participate in decisions to forgo life-sustaining treatments or provide other interventions aimed at relieving suffering that have an associated risk of hastening death, these acts are ethically acceptable and do not constitute assisted suicide.

Withdrawing Artificial Nutrition and Hydration

Often the most difficult decisions about withholding treatments are those that involve simple noninvasive therapies, such as the use of antibiotics, and those that are symbolically linked to caring and nurturing interventions, such as providing food and fluids. "Artificial" or technologically provided nutrition and hydration must be distinguished from the oral provision of food and water. Although dying patients typically experience a decline in appetite as death nears, nurses should continue to offer fluids and food so long as patients indicate any interest or derive pleasure in eating or in drinking fluids. The administration of artificial nutrition and hydration is viewed differently. A moral and legal consensus concludes that artificial nutrition and hydration is a medical treatment that may be refused or withdrawn on the same grounds as any other medical intervention, that is, on an estimation of its expected benefit or burden to the patient (Beauchamp & Childress, 2001). Ethical difficulties arise when it is unclear whether continued provision of nutrition is more beneficial or harmful to the patient.

A growing body of evidence suggests that routine use of artificial nutrition and hydration (ANH) in the care of terminally ill persons is unwarranted, and that providing ANH is unlikely to achieve the clinical outcomes for which it is most often employed, for example, to enhance comfort, prolong survival, and improve quality of life (Choi & Billings, 2002; Ersek, 2003).

In those cases where a patient is unable to make her or his wishes known, or is unable to evaluate the benefits or harms of refusing artificial nutrition and hydration, a surrogate decision-maker should be relied upon to determine what is in the patient's best interests. Nurses should know whether their state's legislative policy restricts or limits surrogates' rights to decide about the administrations of artificial nutrition and hydration. Twenty states have one or more explicit statutory provisions that require meeting a separate and more stringent standard before surrogates are permitted to refuse ANH (Seiger, Arnold, & Ahronheim, 2002).

FROM LETTING DIE TO ASSISTED DYING: BACKGROUND ISSUES

Nurses who regularly care for dying patients may experience requests for assistance in dying (AID) from patients or family members. Interest in clinician-provided assisted dying is thought, in part, to reflect an American public increasingly fearful of the process of dying, particularly the possibility of dying a painful, protracted, and undignified death that is absent personal control or meaning (Schwarz, 2004a). The most recently completed national survey reported that more than 60% of Americans supported legalization of assisted suicide (Reuters Health, 2002).

Since 1997, physician-assisted suicide (PAS) has been a legally available end-of-life option in Oregon for terminally ill, decision-ally capable citizens who make repeated, documented, voluntary requests for such assistance from those who are physically able to self-administer the lethal medication. In 2003, 67 prescriptions for lethal amounts of barbiturates were written and 42 patients died after ingesting the medication (Oregon Department of Human Resources, 2004). The majority of patients who used the Oregon Death with Dignity Act offered the following reason for their choice: concerns about loss of personal autonomy, inability to participate in activities that made life enjoyable, and desire to control the circumstances of dying (Hedberg, Hopkins, & Kohn, 2003; Oregon Department of Human Resources, 2004). The experience of unmanaged pain was not cited as a significant factor. Although only physicians are authorized to write the prescription for lethal medication, some warn that nurse practitioners with prescriptive authority will increasingly be asked by their patients as well as by physician colleagues to participate in assisted suicide (Hall, 1996). Oregon nurses must now decide whether and how they will participate in caring for dying patients who choose to ingest a lethal dose of medication, and how to respond in the event that the suicide attempt fails.

Definitions and the Need for Conceptual Clarity

Nurses experience uncertainty about the location of the moral, legal, and professional boundaries in end-of-life nursing care (Solomon et al., 1993). They may also find it difficult to distinguish professionally sanctioned end-of-life nursing interventions from those that are not (Schwarz, 1999a). This difficulty may be caused in part by imprecisely defined or understood terminology used in end-of-life interventions; thus for purposes

of clarification, use of the following definitions is recommended.

Assistance in dying is an act that directly and intentionally brings about the death of a decisionally capable adult who voluntarily requests such assistance as a means to end suffering that cannot be relieved otherwise in a manner acceptable to that person. This concept includes assisted suicide and voluntary active euthanasia (Brody, 1992).

Suicide is traditionally understood as the act of taking one's own life, and the act of doing so was decriminalized in 1961. Although the concept of "rational suicide" is increasingly acknowledged, most of those who commit suicide are irrational and suffer from clinically recognized psychiatric disorders, and clinicians are obliged to prevent them from harming themselves (Davis et al., 1997).

Assisted suicide is the provision of the means to end life (e.g., a prescription for a lethal amount of drug, the lethal drug itself, or other measures) to an adult who is capable of ending life, with knowledge of that person's intentions (ANA, 1994b; Brody, 1992; Quill, Lo, & Brock, 1997).

Voluntary active euthanasia is a deliberate and intentional act that causes the death (often by the administration of a lethal injection) at the voluntary request of an adult who is incapable of causing his or her own death (Brock, 1992; Brody, 1992; Quill, Lo, & Brock, 1997).

Nonvoluntary euthanasia is a deliberate and intentional act that causes the death of a person who is incapable of expressing his or her wishes about dying, and *involuntary euthanasia* would be direct and intentional killing of a competent person who explicitly refuses receiving euthanasia (Brock, 1992).

Each of these interventions is morally distinct from honoring a patient or authorized surrogate's refusal of treatment, withholding or withdrawing overly burdensome LST, and risking a hastening of death through treatments aimed at relieving suffering or controlling pain.

Nurse Participation in Assisted Dying—What Do We Know?

Until recently, little was known about how often nurses were asked by patients for help in dying or how they responded. Five empirical studies report American nurses' experiences and responses to patient or family members who requested their assistance in dying (Asch, 1996; Ferrell, Virani, Grant, Coyne, & Uman, 2000; Leiser, Mitchell, Hahn, Slome, & Abrams, 1998; Matzo & Emanuel, 1997; Volker, 2001). Findings from these studies confirm that nurses often get asked by patients or family members for assistance in dying and a small but persistent proportion of nurses acknowledge helping patients to die (Schwarz, 2004a).

A physician was the first to explore the clinical experiences of nurses and requests for AID. Asch (1996) received 1,139 completed questionnaires from critical care nurses (71% response) and reported that 16% of respondents indicated participation in assisted suicide or euthanasia on at least one occasion. Although this was a landmark study, the validity of these findings was challenged by concerns about the survey instrument and use of confusing and imprecise definitions (Scanlon, 1996). Leiser and colleagues (1998) surveyed 428 nurses who worked in facilities that served patients with HIV/AIDS in San Francisco. Of their 215 respondents, 15% reported assisting in the suicide of a patient with AIDS; 37% reported receiving a direct request to end the life of a person with HIV/AIDS. In another study, 440 New England oncology nurses returned completed questionnaires (response rate 74%) that explored their end-of-life experiences that included patient requests for AID (Matzo & Emanuel

1997). This study replicated a previously completed study of New England oncology physicians' responses to patient requests for AID, and facilitated the following comparison: more physicians than nurses assisted patient suicides (11% to 1%) and more nurses than physicians performed patient-requested euthanasia (4.5% to 1%). Eleven nurses (2%) acknowledged injecting a lethal drug into a patient more than once in the previous year (Matzo & Emanuel, 1997). Nurses reported that they did not discuss these experiences with their nurse colleagues. Of the 440 responding nurses, 110 wrote comments on their questionnaires They indicated among other things that they very much wanted to discuss this issue, and it was difficult to respond to questions about this topic with yes or no answers (Matzo & Schwarz, 2001).

In the largest American study to date, Ferrell and colleagues (2000) reported results of a survey completed by 2,333 oncology nurses. Respondents indicated their support for legalization of assisted suicide (30%) and active euthanasia (23%), and reported the frequency of patient requests for assisted suicide (23%) and for a lethal injection (22%). Of those respondents, 3% reported having helped a patient obtain a lethal prescription, and 3% reported administering a lethal injection. Ferrell and colleagues speculated that some of the respondents who acknowledged providing a lethal injection instead might have provided appropriate palliative analgesia that was incorrectly perceived to have hastened death.

Volker (2001) used naturalistic descriptive analysis of 48 stories that were anonymously submitted by 40 nurses who were identified as direct care providers or clinical nurses specialist members of the Oncology Nursing Society. She defined AID and asked respondents to provide stories that described their experience of being asked for AID by a terminally ill cancer patient.

In a study that used phenomenological analysis of stories told by 10 American nurses about their experiences of being asked by patients for AID, Schwarz (2004a) described how these nurses understood the meaning of their patients' requests, and given that understanding, how they determined what their response should be. The participants worked in a variety of clinical environments and provided care to seriously ill and dying patients in critical care, home hospice, and HIV/AIDS settings. Patients often withdrew their request for AID once they received good palliative care; thus persistent requests for AID were relatively uncommon, but when requests persisted, nurses provided a range of responses: refusing assistance, administering palliative drugs that might hasten dying, tacitly permitting and not interfering with patient or family plans to hasten death, and intentionally providing direct assistance in dying. Few participants unequivocally agreed or refused to help patients die; most struggled alone and in silence to find morally or legally acceptable ways to help their patients die well (Schwarz, 2003, 2004a).

In a national survey of physician practices regarding AID, Meier and colleagues (1998) report that more than half (57%) of the 38 physicians who described a recent experience with active euthanasia asked a nurse to inject the lethal drug. As this research was designed and implemented by physicians to explore physicians' experiences, the question of how these nurses responded to the physician's requests was not asked or answered (Schwarz, 1999b).

Professional Views About Assisted Dying

Nurses should know that it is not uncommon for incurably ill or dying patients to look forward to death, have occasional thoughts about suicide (Foley, 1995; Quill, 1995), or long for an end to the dying process (Coyle,

1992). Nurses and physicians are encouraged to recognize requests for assistance in dying. Requests for assisted suicide or active euthanasia can be viewed as pleas for help (Coyle, 1992; Foley, 1995), and the nurse should explore what the patients are actually telling them. Often there is a need for better pain management (Ersek, Scanlon, Glass, Ferrell, & Steeves, 1995), emotional support (Quill, 1993; Scanlon & Rushton, 1996), or active listening (Dixon, 1997).

Expert palliative care clinicians know that the experience of uncontrolled and persistent pain often results in patients with advanced disease feeling hopeless, becoming depressed, and likely to have thoughts about suicide (Coyle, 1992; Foley, 1995). When symptoms of pain and suffering are adequately managed most patients do not request AID. The dying process can be made tolerable, if not ideally comfortable, with good palliative or hospice care for 90% to 95% of dying patients (Coyle, 1992; Foley, 1996; Quill, 1993). Coyle (1992) cautions that "wanting to die is not the same as wanting to be killed" (p. 45) and maintains that nurses should not participate in assisted dying. She argues for greater access to comprehensive palliative care for symptom management in dying patients and acknowledges that a "small minority" of patients probably will continue to request AID despite adequate symptom control. "Intensive and ongoing supportive care is required for these patients and their families" (Coyle, 1992, p. 45).

Nurses hold varied views about nurse participation in assisted dying and often justify their position by referring to their own clinical experience (Schwarz, 1999a). Crucial to most who argue in support of assisting in dying are duties of beneficence, compassion for irremediable suffering, and the obligation to respect the autonomy of competent persons (Daly, Berry, Fitzpatrick, Drew, & Montgomery, 1997). Some experienced hospice nurses argue for those "very occasional" patients who, despite receiving skilled palliative care, prefer death to the life they are left with (Stephany, 1994). Most participants in the study by Schwarz (2003, 2004a) maintained that if patients were decisionally capable, had received good end-of-life palliative care, and made a voluntary and informed decision to end their own lives, they had the right to do that, but patients did not have the right to a nurse's assistance in dying (Schwarz, 2004a)

ANA Position Statements on Nurse Participation in Assisted Dying

The professional nursing organization opposes nurse involvement in both active euthanasia and assisted suicide; participation in either action is considered a breach of the Code for Nurses (ANA, 2001) and the ethical traditions of the profession. The justification for opposing nurse participation in active euthanasia is based on the principle of respect for persons, and nursing's historical commitment "to promote, preserve, and protect human life" (ANA, 1994a, p. 2).

Opposition to assisted suicide is based on the nurse's "obligation to provide comprehensive and compassionate end-of-life care which includes the promotion of comfort and the relief of pain, and at times, foregoing life-sustaining treatments" (ANA, 1994b, p. 1). The rationale for opposing nurse participation in assisted dying refers to the profession's central moral axiom—respect for persons—as well as the duty to "do no harm." The ethic of care and the profession's covenant with society that historically has been to promote, preserve, and protect human life (ANA, 1994b) are also factors.

Assisted Dying Distinguished From Hastening Death

Experienced palliative care nurses recognize that death sometimes occurs secondarily as an unintended though foreseen side effect of high-dose opiates used to manage refractory symptoms in dying patients. Despite the clear legal and moral consensus supporting the appropriateness of such interventions, when a patient dies immediately after a nurse provides additional analgesia, it can be a very disquieting experience. The fear of hastening death is well documented as one of the primary reasons nurses may be reluctant to provide adequate pain relief to suffering patients (Solomon et al., 1993).

In addition to reviewing the earlier discussion of the application of the principle of double effect to this issue, nurses are encouraged to also consult the ANA (1991) position statement on the promotion of comfort and relief of pain in dying patients. Nurses are supported in their obligation to provide "increasing titration of medication to achieve adequate symptom control, *even at the expense of life, thus hastening death secondarily*" (ANA, 1991, p. 1).

Barriers in the Practice Environment to Sound Ethical Practice

Nurses need to find ways to talk to each other and validate their experiences, tell their stories of despair or triumph, and share their experiences of moral uncertainty. Nurses may experience conflict between their own moral values and the values of the profession and they have the right to remain true to their conscientious moral and religious beliefs. Although prohibited from compromising legitimate patient choices or imposing their values on others, nurses who are ethically opposed to certain patient interventions will find support for their position in the Code for Nurses (ANA, 2001). They have the right to withdraw from providing care, assuming that arrangements can be made for the patient's safe transfer to the care of another.

It is undoubtedly true that some of the barriers that constrain nurses from participating in ethical decision-making are situations over which the nurse has no control. For example, most nurses practice as employees in health care organizations whose goals are business-oriented and whose focus is utilitarian (institutional values providing the greatest good for the greatest number). Nurses, by virtue of their education, experience, and moral commitment to caring, are focused on doing good for individual patients. Conflict inevitably arises between the nurses' role as caregivers and patient advocates, institutional employees, and as clinicians expected to implement physicians' orders. The experience of being the nurse in the middle combined with the moral distress of being unable to do the right thing may result in nurse' perceiving that they are unable to act as morally autonomous agents.

Preventing Burnout

Nurses who care for dying patients often may find themselves in situations of ethical conflict; burnout is one potential consequence. To avoid the experience of burnout, nurses should seek support from peers, share experiences of uncertainty, and seek ethics advice and support for the development of skills in identifying and resolving ethical problems in clinical practice. It is most important for nurses to acknowledge their own suffering and sense of frustration in caring for patients at the end of life. For example, it can be very upsetting and discouraging to identify a treatment approach that appears to be in a patient's best interest but then be unable to implement it (perhaps due to disagreements among team members or family members about what's in the patient's best interests). Sometimes, with reflection, a morally acceptable compromise can be identified, one that preserves the underlying values of the con-

cerned parties. Agreement to a trial therapy and to reassess within a specified time can help resolve some of the uncertainty.

Hospitals and health care organizations that provide support systems for nurses that encourage and facilitate moral growth and understanding will employ nurses who are less likely to succumb to moral passivity. Nurses should be encouraged to create their own opportunities for support regarding end-of-life issues and may consider the following interventions:

- Use of an ethics consultant can be a source of guidance and help nurses acquire the necessary skills for future application.
- Multidisciplinary and nursing ethics committees should be available to nurses for case consultation regarding ethical conflicts. Nurses should be members and work in concert with professional colleagues. Multidisciplinary institutional ethics committees also develop institutional policies and guidelines and plan programs for the ethics education of staff members.
- Interdisciplinary ethics rounds present an ideal opportunity for individuals working in different patient-care disciplines to discuss regularly troubling cases that may not require an immediate decision. Such meetings provide an opportunity for analysis, exploration, and sharing of different points of view. Thus, when ethical problems do occur, a foundation exists to provide guidance about the most effective way to respond.

CONCLUSION

In conclusion, nurses should be encouraged to continue to provide compassionate care and a caring presence as they struggle together with patients, family members, and professional colleagues, in the attempt to identify what, all things considered, ought to be done in situations of moral conflict. In doing so, we are reminded that "to the extent that care of the dying draws us into their lives, we experience the gifts and deprivations of their own deaths and painfully anticipate the death of our loved ones and even ourselves" (Dixon, 1997, p. 297).

EDUCATION PLAN 6.1   Plan for Achieving Competencies: Ethical Aspects of Palliative Care

Knowledge Needed	Attitudes	Skills	Undergraduate Behavioral Outcomes	Graduate Behavioral Outcomes	Teaching/Learning Strategies
Ethical decisions at the end-of-life: —Difficulties of right and wrong; —Influence of medical technology; —Conflicts between values, principles and priorities of care.	*Appreciate the difficulties regarding end-of-life decision making. *Recognize the utility and limitations of nurses' code of ethics. *Acknowledge how personal values influence behaviors and moral decision making.		*Address the ethical issues in end-of-life care. *Use a decision-making framework that incorporates ethical theories and moral concepts in end-of-life decision making.	*Assist nursing and other colleagues when faced with moral dilemmas or moral distress.	*Present cases that pose moral dilemmas and create moral distress related to end-of-life care. Discuss the conflicts, values, principles, and priorities inherent to the case.

Ethics and Ethical Theory: —Terms and definitions; —Normative ethics; —Values and values clarification; —Deontological and teleological theories; -Ethic of caring	*Be sensitive to the values of others.	*Engage in value clarification and personal reflection related to end-of-life care and decision making.	*Articulate the relationship of ethics and ethical theory to nursing practice and palliative care.	*Apply ethics and ethical theory and analysis to moral and practical problems in health care.	*Explore and debate ethical questions related to end-of-life care, i.e., physician-assisted suicide, euthanasia, withholding or withdrawing treatments, DNR. Ask students/nurses to defend a position other than their own. *Debate an ethical issue from a deontological, teleological, and feminist perspective.

(continued)

EDUCATION PLAN 9.1   *(continued)*

Knowledge Needed	Attitudes	Skills	Undergraduate Behavioral Outcomes	Graduate Behavioral Outcomes	Teaching/Learning Strategies
					★View films such as "Dax's Case: Who Should Decide," or "Is This Life Worth Living." ★Discuss the values presented, the ethical issues, and possible resolution of the ethical/moral problem using ethical theory to assist with decision making. ★Encourage students/nurses to relate an ethical issue from their personal history and explore how it has determined their present stand.

Ethical Principles and Concepts: —Respect for persons and the Principle of Autonomy; —Limiting autonomy as a result of paternalism.	*Respect human dignity and the uniqueness of all people. *Affirm patients' right to determine their course of actions in accordance with their values, beliefs, and preferences.	*Apply ethical principles and the nursing code of ethics in nursing practice. *Provide the patient/family with accurate and complete information necessary to make informed decisions about treatment choices.	*Participate on ethics committee to determine ethical decisions for patients in palliative care.	*Present cases in which patient autonomy has been undermined or not respected. Discuss appropriate nursing responses and actions to support autonomy.

(continued)

EDUCATION PLAN 6.1   *(continued)*

Knowledge Needed	Attitudes	Skills	Undergraduate Behavioral Outcomes	Graduate Behavioral Outcomes	Teaching/Learning Strategies
Assessing decision-making capacity	*Acknowledge that decision making capacity is often neither completely present nor completely absent.		*Collaborate with advanced practice nurses and other health professionals in determining the decision-making capacity of a patient. *Encourage patients who are competent to discuss their end of life wishes with family or other surrogate decision makers. *Discuss with patients and family the benefits and burdens of life-prolonging interventions.	*Assess decision-making capacity of the patient in conjunction with other members of the interdisciplinary team.	*Round with the interdisciplinary team to determine the decisional making capacity of selected patients. Discuss the process in class or post-conference.

Beneficence and Nonmaleficence and the Principle of Double Effect	*Affirm the principles of doing good and avoiding harm to the patient. *Acknowledge the Principle of Double Effect and its relationship to pain management. *Affirm nurses' moral duty to prevent/and or remove evil, such as pain.	*Avoid causing unnecessary harm or pain to the patient. *Refer the Principle of Double Effect in morally difficult situations regarding the provision of quality end-of-life care.	*Explain the Principle of Double Effect to health care providers, particularly in relationship to providing adequate pain management.	*Discuss cases of pain management with regard to the Principle of Double Effect.
The Principle of Justice	*Adhere to the principle of justice in the allocation of resources for all populations.	*Support access to resources for all patients.	*Collaborate with other health professionals to insure that access to health care and available resources are fairly distributed across all patient populations.	*Discuss an issue related to the allocation of health care resources, such as organs availability or access to opioids. Determine as a group the barriers to fair allocation, and strategies to overcome barriers.

(continued)

EDUCATION PLAN 6.1   *(continued)*

Knowledge Needed	Attitudes	Skills	Undergraduate Behavioral Outcomes	Graduate Behavioral Outcomes	Teaching/Learning Strategies
Elements of a Decision-Making Framework	*Appreciate the values that inform patient's choices.		*Utilize the steps of the decision-making process to discuss, analyze, and develop an ethically supportable decision regarding end-of-life conflicts.	*Educate other health professionals regarding the elements of the decision-making process regarding end-of-life conflicts.	*Identify an ethical conflict or problem. As a group utilize the steps of the decision-making process to arrive at a decision.

Controversies, complexities, and difficult decisions in end-of-life care: —Autonomy and life sustaining treatments; —Withholding and withdrawing life prolonging treatments; —From "Letting Die" to "Assisted Dying."	*Judge the benefits to burdens of life-sustaining treatments. *Consider life withholding and withdrawing of life-prolonging therapies as non-distinct and morally and legally appropriate options in end-of-life care. *Appreciate that nutrition and hydration are medical interventions that may be refused or withdrawn, whereas the provision of food and water is appropriate to offer so long as there is interest expressed by the patient.	*Refer difficult ethical situations to the institutional ethics committee.	*Participate on ethics committee to determine ethical decisions for patients in palliative care.	*Based on a case study, debate the issues of withholding or withdrawing life-sustaining therapies. Have students role play the family, physician, nurse, ethicist, and clergy presenting each perspective and determining a solution to the dilemma. *Have students/nurses attend an ethics committee meeting. Based on this meeting, have them present a case in question, the varying viewpoints, and the decision to the class.

(continued)

EDUCATION PLAN 6.1 *(continued)*

Knowledge Needed	Attitudes	Skills	Undergraduate Behavioral Outcomes	Graduate Behavioral Outcomes	Teaching/Learning Strategies
Nurse Participation in Assisted Dying: —The Profession's Position; —ANA Position Statements	*Affirm the ANA position regarding physician-assisted suicide and euthanasia.		*Respond to requests for physician-assisted suicide as patient's pleas for help for better pain management, emotional support, or the need for active listening or presence.	*Explore with patients their requests for assisted suicide. *Coordinate interdisciplinary team efforts to provide effective palliative care to decrease the requests for assisted suicide.	*Discuss professional experiences of students/nurses in which they were asked to participate in assisted suicide. Discuss the students/nurses' feelings and responses. *Review the ANA Position Statements related to End of Life Care. Identify the ethical/legal principles that support the position statements, and discuss the implication for palliative care.

REFERENCES

Aaras, J. D., & Steinbock, B. (1995). *Ethical issues in modern medicine* (4th ed.). Mountain View, CA: Mayfield.

American Nurses Association. (1991). *Position statement on the promotion of comfort and relief of pain in dying patients.* Washington, DC: American Nurses Association.

American Nurses Association. (1994a). *Position statement on active euthanasia.* Washington, DC: American Nurses Association.

American Nurses Association. (1994b). *Position statement on assisted suicide.* Washington, DC: American Nurses Association.

American Nurses Association. (2001). Code of ethics for nurses with interpretive statements. Washington, DC: American Nurses Association.

Aroskar, M. A. (1987). The interface of ethics and politics in nursing. *Nursing Outlook, 35,* 269.

Asch, D. A. (1996). The role of critical care nurses in euthanasia and assisted suicide. *New England Journal of Medicine, 334,* 1374–1401.

Beauchamp, T., & Childress, J. (2001). *Principles of biomedical ethics* (5th ed.). New York: Oxford University Press.

Benjamin, M., & Curtis, J. (1992). *Ethics in nursing* (3rd ed.). New York: Oxford University Press.

Brock, D. W. (1992). Voluntary active euthanasia. *The Hastings Center report, 22,* 10–23.

Brody, H. (1992). Assisted dying—A compassionate response to a medical failure. *New England Journal of Medicine, 327,* 1384–1388.

Cameron, M. E. (1997). Legal and ethical issues: Ethical distress in nursing. *Journal of Professional Nursing, 13,* 280.

Cassells, J., & Gaul, A. (1998, January). An ethical assessment framework for nursing practice. *Maryland Nurse, 6*(1), 9–12.

Cavanaugh, T. A. (1996). The ethics of death-hastening or death-causing palliative analgesic administration to the terminally ill. *Journal of Pain and Symptom Management, 12,* 248–254.

Choi, Y. S., & Billings, J. A. (2002). Changing perspective on palliative care. *Oncology, 16,* 515–527.

Clouser, K. D., & Gert, B. (1990). A critique of principlism. *Journal of Medical Philosophy, 15,* 219–236.

Coyle, N. (1992). The euthanasia and physician-assisted suicide debate: Issues for nursing. *Oncology Nursing Forum, 19,* 41–46.

Culver, C., & Gert, B. (1982). *Philosophy in medicine: Conceptual and ethical issues in medicine and psychiatry.* New York: Oxford University Press.

Daly, B. J., Berry, D., Fitzpatrick, J. L., Drew, B., & Montgomery, K. (1997). Assisted suicide: Implications for nurses and nursing. *Nursing Outlook, 45,* 209–214.

Davis, A. J. (1994). Selected issues in nursing ethics: Clinical, philosophical, political. *Bioethics Forum, 10,* 10–14.

Davis, A. J., Aroskar, M. A., Liaschenko, J., & Drought, T. S. (1997). *Ethical dilemmas and nursing practice* (4th ed.). Stamford, CT: Appleton & Lange.

Dexter, P. R., Wolinsky, F. D., Gramelspacher, G. J., Eckert, G. J., & Tierney, W. M. (2003). Opportunities for advance directives to influence acute medical care. *Journal of Clinical Ethics, 14,* 173–182.

Dixon, M. D. (1997). The quality of mercy: Reflections on provider-assisted suicide. *Journal of Clinical Ethics, 8,* 290–302.

Dubler, N. (1994, April). Introduction: Bioethics and alternative dispute resolution. In N. Dubler & L. Marcus (Eds.), *Mediating bioethical disputes* (p. 2). New York: United Hospital Fund of New York.

Ersek, M. (2003). Artificial nutrition and hydration: Clinical issues. *Journal of Hospice and Palliative Nursing, 5,* 221–230.

Ersek, M., Scanlon, C., Glass, E., Ferrell, B., & Steeves, R. (1995). Priority ethical issues in oncology nursing: Current and future directions. *Oncology Nursing Forum, 22,* 803–807.

Ferrell, B., Virani, R., Grant, M., Coyne, P., & Uman, G. (2000). Beyond the Supreme Court decision: Nursing perspectives on end-of-life care. *Oncology Nursing Forum 27,* 445–455.

Fohr, S. A. (1998). The double effect of pain medication: Separating myth from reality. *Journal of Palliative Medicine, 1,* 315–328.

Foley, K. M. (1995). The relationship of pain and symptom management to patient requests for physician-assisted suicide. *Journal of Pain and Symptom Management, 6,* 287–289.

Foley, K. M. (1996, September). Controlling the pain of cancer. *Scientific American,* 164–165.

Fowler, M. D. (1987). Introduction to ethics and ethical theory. In M. D. Fowler & J. Levine-Ariff (Eds.), *Ethics at the bedside: A source book for the critical care nurse* (pp. 24–38). Philadelphia: Lippincott.

Frankena, W. K. (1973). *Ethics* (2nd ed.). Englewood Cliffs, NJ: Prentice-Hall.

Fry, S. T. (1987). Autonomy, advocacy, and accountability: Ethics at the bedside. In M. D. Fowler & J. Levine-Ariff (Eds.), *Ethics at the bedside: A source book for the critical care nurse* (pp. 39–49). Philadelphia: Lippincott.

Fry, S. T. (1989). Towards a theory of nursing ethics. *Advances in Nursing Science, 11*(4), 9–22.

Fry, S. T., Killen, A. R., & Robinson, E. M. (1996). Care-based reasoning, caring and the ethic of care: A need for clarity. *Journal of Clinical Ethics, 7*(1), 41–47.

Gadow, S. (1996). Aging as death rehearsal: The oppressiveness of reason. *Journal of Clinical Ethics, 7*(1), 35–40.

Hall, J. (1996). Assisted suicide: Nurse practitioners as providers? *Nurse Practitioner, 21*(2), 63–71.

Hedberg, K., Hopkins, D., & Kohn, M. (2003). Five years of legal physician-assisted suicide in Oregon. *New England Journal of Medicine, 348,* 961–964.

Held, V. (1994). Feminism and moral theory. In J. E. White (Ed.), *Contemporary moral problems* (4th ed., pp.208–216). St. Paul, MN: West.

Jameton, A. (1984). *Nursing practice: The ethical issues.* Englewood Cliffs, NJ: Prentice-Hall.

Latimer, E. J. (1991). Ethical decision-making in the care of the dying and its application to clinical practice. *Journal of Pain and Symptom Management, 6,* 329–336.

Leiser, R. J., Mitchell, T. F., Hahn, J., Slome, L., & Abrams, D. I. (1998). Nurses' attitudes and beliefs toward assisted suicide in AIDS. *Journal Association of Nurses in AIDS Care 9*(6), 26–33.

Lynn, J., Teno, J., Dresser, R., Brock, D., Lindemann Nelson, H., Kielstein, R., et al. (1999). Dementia and advance-care planning: Perspective from three countries on ethics and epidemiology. *Journal of Clinical Ethics, 10,* 271–285.

Manfredi, P. L., Morrison, R. S., & Meier, D. E. (1998). The rule of double effect. [Letter to the editor]. *Journal of the American Medical Association, 338,* 1390.

Matzo, M. L., & Emanuel, E. J. (1997). Oncology nurses' practices of assisted suicide and patient-requested euthanasia. *Oncology Nursing Forum, 24,* 1725–1732.

Matzo, L. M., & Schwarz, J. K. (2001) In their own words: Oncology nurses respond to patient requests for assisted suicide and euthanasia. *Applied Nursing Research 14* (2), 64–71.

Meier, D. E., Emmons, C., Wallenstein, S., Quill, T., Morrison, R. S., & Cassel, C. K.

(1998). A national survey of physician-assisted suicide and euthanasia in the United States. *New England Journal of Medicine, 338,* 1193–1201.

Mezey, M., Mitty, E., & Ramsey, G. (1997). Assessment of decision-making capacity: Nursing's role. *Journal of Gerontological Nursing, 23*(3), 28–35.

Oregon Department of Human Resources. (2004). Oregon Death with Dignity: Sixth year report. Retrieved March 10, 2004, from www.dhs.or.us/news/2004–0309a.html

Perkins, H. S. (2000). Time to move advance care planning beyond advance directives. *Chest, 117,* 1228–1231.

Perrin, K. O. (1997). Giving voice to the wishes of elders for end-of-life care. *Journal of Gerontological Nursing, 23*(3), 18–27.

President's Commission for the Study of Ethical Problems in Medicine and Biomedical and Behavioral Research. (1983). *Deciding to forego life-sustaining treatment.* Washington, DC: U.S. Government Printing Office.

Quill, T. E. (1993). Doctor, I want to die. Will you help me? *Journal of the American Medical Association, 270,* 870–873.

Quill, T. E. (1995). When all else fails. *Pain Forum, 4,* 189–191.

Quill, T. E., Dresser, R., & Brock, D. W. (1997). The rule of double effect: A critique of its role in end-of-life decision making. *New England Journal of Medicine, 337,* 1763–1771.

Quill, T. E., Lo, B., & Brock, D. W. (1997). Palliative options of last resort: A comparison of voluntarily stopping eating and drinking, terminal sedation, physician-assisted suicide, and voluntary active euthanasia. *Journal of the American Medical Association, 278,* 2099–2104.

Reuters Health. (2002). New survey claims majority support assisted suicide. Retrieved October 22, 2003, from www.medscape.com/reuters/prof/2002/01/01.14/20020111ethc001.html

Robinson, B. (1990, Winter). Question of life and death: No easy answers. *Ageing International,* 27–35.

Rushton, C., & Reigle, J. (1993). Ethical issues in critical nursing. In M. Kinney, D. Packa, & S. Dunbar (Eds.), *AACN's clinical reference for critical care* (pp. 8–27). St. Louis, MO: Mosby.

Scanlon, C. (1996). Euthanasia and nursing practice-right question, wrong answer. *New England Journal of Medicine, 334,* 1401.

Scanlon, C., & Rushton, C. H. (1996). Assisted suicide: Clinical realities and ethical challenges. *American Journal of Critical Care, 5,* 397–405.

Schwarz, J. K. (1999a). Assisted dying and nursing practice. *Image, 31,* 367–373.

Schwarz, J. K. (1999b). The delegated providers' of assisted dying. *Viewpoint: American Journal of Nursing, 99*(6), 9.

Schwarz, J. K. (2003). Understanding and responding to patients' requests for assistance in dying. *Journal of Nursing Scholarship, 35,* 377–384.

Schwarz, J. K. (2004a). Responding to persistent requests for assistance in dying: A phenomenological inquiry. *International Journal of Palliative Nursing, 10,* 225–235.

Schwarz, J. K. (2004b). The rule of double effect and its role in facilitating good end-of-life care: A help or a hindrance? *Journal of Hospice and Palliative Nursing, 6,* 125–133.

Seiger, C. E., Arnold, J. F., & Ahronheim, J. C. (2002). Refusing artificial nutrition and hydration: Does statutory law send the wrong message? *Journal of the American Geriatrics Society, 50,* 544–550.

Solomon, M., O'Donnell, L., Jennings, B., Guilfoy, J., Wolf, S., Nolan, K., et al. (1993). Decisions near the end of life: Professional views on life-sustaining treatments.

American Journal of Public Health, 83(4), 14–22.

Stanley, J. K., & Zoloth-Dorfman, L. (2001). Ethical considerations. In B. R. Ferrell & N. Coyle (Eds.), *Textbook of palliative nursing* (pp. 663–681). New York: Oxford University Press.

Stephany, T. M. (1994). Assisted suicide: How hospice fails. *American Journal of Hospice and Palliative Care, 10*(6), 1–5.

Tierney, W. M., Dexter, P. R., Gramelspacher, G. P., Perkins, A. J., Zhou, X. H., & Wolinksy F. D. (2001). The effect of discussions about advance directives on patients' satisfaction with primary care. *Journal of General Internal Medicine,16*(1), 32–40.

Tilden, V. P., Tolle, S. W., Nelson, C. A., & Fields, J. (2001). Family decision-making to withdraw life-sustaining treatments from hospitalized patients. *Nursing Research, 50,* 105–115.

Tonelli, R. R. (1996). Pulling the plug on living wills: A critical analysis of advance directive. *Chest, 110,* 816–822.

Uustal, D. B. (1987). Values: The cornerstone of nursing's moral act. In M. D. Fowler & J. Levine-Ariff (Eds.), *Ethics at the bedside: A source book for the critical care nurse.* (pp. 136–170). Philadelphia: Lippincott.

Veatch, R. M., & Fry, S. T. (1995). *Case studies in nursing ethics.* Boston: Jones and Bartlett.

Volker, D. L. (2001) Perspectives on assisted dying: Oncology nurses' experiences with requests for assisted dying from terminally ill patients with cancer. *Oncology Nursing Forum, 28*(1), 39–49.

Yeo, M., Moorhouse, A., & Dalzeil, J. (1996). Autonomy. In M. Yeo & A. Moorhouse (Eds.), *Concepts and cases in nursing ethics* (2nd ed., pp. 91–138). Peterbourough, Ontario, Canada: Broadview Press.

Yeo, M., Moorhouse, A., & Donner, G. (1996). Justice. In M. Yeo & A. Moorhouse (Eds.), *Concepts and cases in nursing ethics* (2nd ed., pp. 211–266). Peterbourough, Ontario, Canada: Broadview Press.

7

Legal Aspects of End-of-Life Care

Marianne LaPorte Matzo and Gloria C. Ramsey

AACN Competencies

#12: Apply legal and ethical principles in the analysis of complex issues in end-of-life care, recognizing the influence of personal values, professional codes, and patient preferences.

#13: Identify barriers and facilitators to patients' and caregivers' effective use of resources.

> *Every Human being of adult years and of sound mind has a right to determine what shall be done with his own body.*
> —Justice Benjamin Cardozo[1]

Lay and professional communities throughout the world are struggling with bioethical and legal dilemmas brought about by the diffusion of medical technology. A heightened sense of self-determination and the decision making associated with: termination of life-sustaining treatment; care of the dying; patient-requested euthanasia and assisted suicide; organ transplantation; genetic testing and engineering; resource allocation; and confidentiality engender bioethical and legal dilemmas in health care. These dilemmas have different practice ramifications for different health care professionals. Patient's well-being, not only in hospitals, nursing homes, and home care but also in rapidly di-

versifying health care locations, will best be served only if health care professionals are able to collaborate with each other and the patient and family in examining and resolving bioethical issues.

For nurses, in particular, advance care planning is a moral as well as legal issue. The moral question of what is "right" or "best" for the patient, what ought to be done, and who is the best person suited to do the "right" or "best" thing evokes strong personal sentiments when discussing end-of-life care. These questions have the potential to provoke conflict among those involved in patient care—physicians, nurses, social workers, and others—and the questions for each are clouded by the individual's personal and professional ethics.

Moral questions pose a different dilemma for the family. Many times, families are faced with discussions regarding whether to stop treatment and "let" the patient die. A long drawn-out death can have a debilitating and at times devastating effect on family members. Whether expected or sudden, few people are truly prepared for death. Dealing with one's mortality evokes a level of discomfort that most people would rather avoid. However, if the family has accepted the patient's diagnosis, prognosis, and impending death, then the confusion, misunderstanding, and guilt they can experience may be mitigated.

---

[1]Schloendorff v. Society of New York Hospital (1914)

Decisions about advance care planning, and especially about forgoing treatment, call for careful thinking and communication. Decisions about care at the end of life ought to be made in accordance with an individual's wishes, preferences, beliefs, and values. No one should be subject to medical care against his or her wishes. Autonomy and self-determination are the foundation for such decisions.

Nursing faculty, nursing students, and practicing nurses address ethical and legal issues including advance care planning with patients and family members daily in clinical practice. With increased medical technology and competing interests of dying patients, their families, and significant others, the wish of many to die with dignity is a concern for health care professionals. Nurses are in a key position to address the escalation of bioethical dilemmas that result in wrenching situations for patients, families, providers, and the courts. Since the landmark cases of Karen Ann Quinlan (*In re Quinlan,* 1976) and Nancy Beth Cruzan (*Cruzan v. Director, Missouri Department of Health,* 1990), nurses, physicians, other health care professionals have shaped public policy regarding patient and surrogate participation in end-of-life decision-making even when the patient is incapacitated and unable to make decisions.

LAW AND ETHICS: SAME OR DIFFERENT?

Law and *ethics* are similar in that they have developed in the same historical, social, cultural and philosophical soil (Davis, Aroskar, Liaschenko, & Drought, 1997). Black's Law Dictionary defines law as "that which is laid down, ordained, or established; a body of rules of action or conduct prescribed by controlling authority and having binding legal forces; and that which must be obeyed and

followed by citizens subject to sanctions or legal consequences" (Garner, 2004, pp. 884–885). The law may be defined better as the sum total of rules and regulations by which a society is governed. Ethics, on the other hand, are informal or formal rules of behavior that guide individuals or groups of people.

Law and ethics are different in that actions may be (a) ethical and legal, (b) unethical and illegal, (c) ethical and illegal, or (d) unethical and legal. For the nurse, the latter two possibilities present the most difficult situations and are the most challenging. Legal rights are grounded in the law and ethical rights are grounded in ethical principles and values. The law establishes rules that define a person's rights, obligations, and the appropriate penalty for those who violate it. Moreover, the law describes how government will enforce the rules and penalties. There are many laws that affect the practice of nursing and nurses must be able to differentiate ethical issues from those that are strictly legal or clinical.

NURSING AND THE LAW

Legal and moral obligations are not new to nurses. The Nurse Practice Act, a legal statute regulating nursing, and the professional code of ethics are the foundations of nursing practice. Similarly, nurses are confronted with complex moral and legal questions on a regular basis when caring for dying patients, questions such as when does death occur? Does an individual have a right to choose death? Is there a difference between letting a person die and taking measures to hasten death? Do you disclose a terminal diagnosis to a patient? These are just a few of the ethical and legal issues in contemporary nursing.

Decision making at the end of life has been at the heart of many ethical-dilemma discussions and legal cases in bioethics in the past 25 years. Because nurses are legally responsible and accountable for the health care that patients and their families receive, nurses can no longer afford to view the questions of ethics and law as solely an academic exercise, nor should ethical and legal considerations of today's health care issues remain solely in the purview of the organization's ethics committee or risk management departments. Nurses must understand the basic concepts of ethical decision making and know the relevant laws that address the current controversies to ensure that individual and societal rights and values are protected.

THE RIGHT TO DIE

The term *right to die* is used in the legal context to mean that an individual has a right to refuse medical treatment and the refusal of such treatment will cause death. Meisel & Cerminara (2001) remind us that the term *right to die* has some unfortunate connotations. To the lawyer, the word *right* is almost sacred. However, to the health care professional, the word is often seen as antithetical to the interests (rights) of health care professionals. The language denotes an adversarial relationship between patients and health care professionals. Moreover, he argues that many health care providers and laypersons confuse the word *right* with *duty*. When *right* is used with *die,* the phrase connotes to some that death is preferable to life or that patients have a right to die, and health care professionals have a duty to let them die, to abandon them, or even to kill them (Miesel & Cerminara, 2001). Taking the lead from the Cruzan decision where the court used the term "right to refuse life-sustaining treatment" in preference to "right to die," the focus here is primarily on how laws may affect the right to refuse life-sustaining treatment and quality of care at the end of life.

PURPOSE AND TYPES OF ADVANCE DIRECTIVES

Before exploring the purpose and types of advance directives, nurses must know that each state has it own law regarding the use of advance directives. Nurses should know the formalities for executing an advance directive, which type is recognized in their state, and what the limitations are, if any, for honoring an advance directive.

Advance directives have three major purposes (Meisel & Cerminara, 2001). The first and perhaps most important is that they are a mechanism by which individuals can exercise control over their bodies. This document will allow them to direct the kind of medical care they want or do not want in the event they lack decision-making capacity at the time a medical decision needs to be made. They are directions to others about the kind of medical care one would like to receive in advance of the need for that care. Advance directives generally are discussed in the context of the right to forgo life-sustaining treatments. However, they also may be used to direct the administration of treatment. Advance directives pertain to decision making about any kind of health care and they may be executed by an adult who is in good or poor health as long as he or she possesses the requisite decision-making capacity to exercise the right to self-determination. Advance directives are intended to affect a person's own choice and self-determination even when the individual no longer possesses this capacity (Meisel & Cerminara, 2001).

The second purpose of advance directives is to provide guidance, especially to health care professionals, regarding how to proceed with decision making about life-sustaining treatment in the face of diminished capacity. When patients lack decision making capacity, a great deal of confusion can arise in the clinical setting as to how health care decisions are to be made, who has the authority to make them, and what the treatment decisions should be. Advance directives contribute significantly to the willingness of health care professionals to proceed with a clinical approach to decision making rather than requesting judicial intervention when patients lack decision-making capacity.

The third purpose of advance directives, and the one that might be identified as most important by health care professionals, is that they provide immunity from civil and criminal liability when certain stated conditions are met. All advance directive statutes contain provisions that grant immunity to health care professionals when they act in good faith and in accordance with state statutes respecting advance directives (Meisel & Cerminara, 2001). Most litigated right-to-die cases end up in court because of the fear of liability, and statutory immunity provisions provide an impetus for decision making by protecting health care professionals in the clinical setting.

There are two types of advance directives, the living will and the durable power of attorney for health care. Advance directives generally give instructions and guidance regarding end-of-life wishes and preferences and may also appoint a proxy to serve as a surrogate in decision making. This section will discuss each of these, as well as other relevant issues pertaining to advance directives.

THE SUPPORT STUDY

Even with the increased attention to end-of-life issues in lay and medical publications, physicians are often unaware of their patients' preferences concerning end-of-life care. The Study to Understand Prognoses and Preferences for Outcomes and Risks of Treatment (SUPPORT) and its companion study, the Hospitalized Elderly Longitudinal Project (HELP), both studies of seriously ill hospitalized patients, documented the lack of communication between physicians and their very ill patients about end-of-life issues (Haidet et al., 1998; Knaus et al., 1995). This landmark study, which produced significant data and 67 manuscripts published in the literature as of year-end 1999 (Phillips, Hamel, Covinsky, & Lynn, 2000), further documented the ineffectiveness of advance directives (Teno et al., 1994; Teno, Licks, et al, 1997; Teno, Lynn, et al., 1997), the effect of serious illness on patients and their families (Covinsky et al., 1994, 1996), the cost-effectiveness of life-extending interventions at the end of life (Hamel et al., 1997), and the influence of patient age and race on decision-making (Hamel et al., 1996, 1999; Phillips et al., 1996).

Although the SUPPORT study's intervention on five specific outcomes—physician understanding of patient preferences; incidence and time of documentation of Do Not Resuscitate (DNR) orders; pain; time spent in an intensive care unit (ICU); comatose or receiving mechanical ventilation before death; and hospital resource use—failed to make a difference, some of the SUPPORT/HELP findings did not influence clinical practice. For example, ineffectiveness of advance directives in SUPPORT has not dampened the importance for them in policy and clinical practice (Fins, Miller, Acres, Bacchetta, Huzzard, et al., 1999; Phillips et al., 2000). In fact, subsequent studies indicate that a durable power of attorney for health care was significantly associated with both DNR orders and comfort care plans (Fins et al., 1999). These findings support patients, nurses, and physicians to engage in conversation addressing end-of-life care. Advance directives are no substitute for careful and sensitive communication and thinking between patients, surrogates, and health care professionals. However, when physicians understood patient preferences and there was clear communication about patient preferences, patient's choices were respected (Wenger et al., 2000). Nurses play a seminal role in facilitating this important and much needed communication (Murphy et al., 2000).

Living Wills

A living will documents specific instructions to health care providers about particular kinds of health care treatment an individual would or would not want to prolong life. Living wills generally are used to declare wishes to refuse, limit, or withhold life-sustaining treatment under certain circumstances should the individual become incapacitated and unable to communicate. An individual may execute a living will to instruct health care professionals not to administer any "extraordinary treatment," "heroic treatment," "artificial treatment," or "life support" in the event of terminal illness. Furthermore, living wills also can be used to give instructions about what kind of treatment an individual wants to have administered, although there are no reported cases in which an individual has requested the administration of a particular treatment through a living will (Meisel & Cerminara, 2001). However, in light of the health care debate about "futile" treatment, such use may become more prevalent.

Although most states have detailed living-will statutes, living wills are not recognized by statute in New York, Massachusetts, and Michigan (Meisel & Cerminara, 2001). In New York, however, the court approved the use of living wills by stating that the "ideal situation is ... [where] patient's wishes [are] expressed in some form of writing" (*In re Westchester County Medical Center (O'Connor,* 1988). The "writing" provides a "clear and convincing" standard of proof (a very high standard of proof) to allow an individual's stated wishes to be respected.

Durable Power of Attorney for Health Care

Durable power of attorney for health care (DPAHC) is a document that permits individuals to designate another person to make health care decisions for them should they lose decision-making capacity. In order to be considered to have capacity (and therefore to be able to engage in the informed consent process), patients must have the requisite ability to comprehend information, to contemplate options, to evaluate risks and consequences, and to communicate decisions. Every adult is presumed to have capacity and decisional authority unless proven otherwise. Although *capacity* and *competence* are frequently used interchangeably, competence (a legal term) is determined by a court. Decisional capacity within health care is determined via clinical assessment (Cooney, Kennedy, Hawkins, Hurme, & Balch, 2004).

The person who is appointed by the patient to make decisions is called a health care proxy, health care agent, attorney-in-fact, or surrogate. The term "durable power of attorney" should be used to refer to the document used to appoint this person. The language used varies from state to state and nurses should become familiar with their own state's language.

One major distinction between a DPAHC and a living will is that the DPAHC may be used for all health care decisions, and is not limited to withholding or withdrawing life-sustaining treatment. Further, a DPAHC does not require that an individual know in advance all the decisions that may arise. In fact, a health care proxy can interpret the patient's wishes as medical circumstances change and can make treatment decisions as the need arises.

A DPAHC vests broad decision-making authority to one person. In states with family consent laws, it is not clear how health care providers are expected to resolve conflict between family members who bear the same relationship to the patient in the absence of an advance directive. Generally, in states with family consent statutes, the laws provide some mechanism whereby one may resort to the courts to resolve disputes among family members. There are times when health care professionals receive conflicting instructions from various members of the same family. Appointing a health care proxy is extremely important when an individual chooses not to appoint a family member. For example, it may be quite common for a patient who is HIV positive or a patient with AIDS to appoint a friend rather than a family member as a health care proxy under the DPAHC statute.

Advance directives should become effective only when it is determined that the individual is incompetent or lacks decision-making capacity. As long as the patient retains decision-making capacity, his or her decisions govern. When the patient is deemed to lack decision-making capacity, the health care proxy is authorized to make all treatment decisions on behalf of the patient and in accordance with the patients stated wishes, whether reduced to writing or verbally. The proxy is bound to make the kinds of decisions the patient would have made had he or she the capacity to do so.

Such decision-making employs the standard of "substituted judgement." In situations where the patient has never been competent, or there is no clear and convincing evidence of what the person would have wanted, the proxy will be called on to make decisions on the basis of what he or she believes to be in the best interest of the patient. Under this approach, it is impossible to analyze truly the proxy's decision based on the patient's right to self-determination. Rather, the effort is made to protect the interest of the patient and to carry out society's interest in providing appropriate health care for all.

The advocacy group Aging with Dignity has promoted the Five Wishes public information campaign so that individuals have a format to discuss their wishes related to end-of-life care. The five wishes are as follows:

My Wish For:
The person I want to make care decisions
   for me when I can't
The kind of medical treatment I want
   or don't want
How comfortable I want to be
How I want people to treat me
What I want my loved ones to know

Combination Directives

A number of states have a single advance directive statute that combines elements of a living will and a DPAHC into a single document. A combination document arguably avoids many of the pitfalls of each document alone. If the instructions are too general, the health care proxy has the authority to determine whether instructions should be applied under the specific circumstances. If the instructions are too specific and do not address the particular situation at hand, the health care proxy has the discretion to apply them or not. Nevertheless, a discussion between the patient and the health care proxy should occur regardless of whether there is a DPAHC or a combination directive. Communication is the most effective way to ensure that the patient's wishes are known and that the health care proxy is aware of their appointment.

Oral Advance Directives

Although a written advance directive is preferable, especially in the case of an emergency, courts view oral advance directives favorably, especially living wills. The courts either have enforced them per se or have heavily relied upon them in deciding whether to forgo life-sustaining treatment. Even when state statutes recognize written advance directives, oral directives have been found to be legally operative in a number of jurisdictions. The more specific the oral advance directive, the more likely it is to be enforced and have clinical and legal significance.

When made by individuals with full decision-making capacity, courts have considered patients' statements when making a decision to terminate life-prolonging treatments. Criteria for weighing these statements include the following (Furrow, Greaney, Johnson, Jost, & Schwartz, 2001):

- If the statements were made on serious occasions or were solemn pronouncements (were brought up when the parties were together)
- If they were consistently repeated
- If they were made by a mature person who understood the underlying issues
- If they were consistent with values demonstrated in other aspects of the patient's life (including the patient's religion)
- If they were made shortly before the need for the treatment decision
- If they addressed with some specificity the actual condition of the patient
- Accordingly, such statements should be considered and documented by the health care providers when discussing advance directives with patients. Figure 7.1 summarizes the clinical and legal distinctions between advance directives and DNR orders.

Family Consent Laws

Many people are under the impression that their family members will be allowed to make the proper decisions for them should the need arise and therefore see no need to execute an advance directive formally (Furrow et al., 2001). Traditionally, health care professionals and the courts have also relied on families to make health care decisions for family members throughout the years, without any legal authority. In 1982, the President's Commission concluded that given this practice, family decision-making had gained and should be accorded legal acceptance. The commission pointed out five reasons why deference to family members is appropriate when done in consultation with the physician and other health care professionals:

1. The family is generally most concerned about the good of the patient.
2. The family usually is the most knowledgeable about the patient's goals, preferences, and values.
3. The family deserves recognition as an important social unit that, within limits, ought to be treated as a responsible decision-maker in matters that intimately affect its members.
4. Especially in a society in which many other traditional forms of community have eroded, participation in a family often is an important dimension of personal fulfillment.
5. Because a protected sphere of privacy and autonomy is required for the flourishing of this interpersonal union, institutions and the state should be reluctant to intrude, particularly regarding matters that are personal and on which there is a wide range of opinion in society.

FIGURE 7.1   Summary of Clinical and Legal Distinctions between ADs and DNR Orders

	Advance Directives (e.g., Living Will)	Institutional-Based DNR Orderss	Community-Based DNR Orders
How does a person obtain one?	Can obtain from many sources including the web, hospital, MD, clinic, etc.	Physician writes as an order in the medical record.	Forms can be obtained *only* from a health care provider.
Who signs the documentation?	Only the person to whom it applies.	The physician.	The physician and the patient or their legal surrogate.
When does the document "take effect" or apply?	Only after the patient has been declared terminal or is in a state covered under state law (e.g., PVS or coma).	Immediately.	Immediately.
If the person should suffer a cardiopulmonary arrest, what should occur based on the document?	Start CPR and evaluate situation when stabilized and communication is possible with the patient or their legal surrogate.	Do not begin CPR.	Do not begin CPR.
Does the documentation represent informed consent?	No. Document is a written statement of person's wishes and does not require disclosure of specific information by a health care provider. Hence it does not represent an informed decision.	Yes. Order results from a discussion between MD (or team) and the patient or legal surrogate. Like any other order for treatment, informed consent should have occurred.	Yes. Form is signed by both the MD and the patient or the patient's legal surrogate. Form is written evidence that informed consent has occurred.

Motivated by concern over the formal legal status of family decision-making in the 1980s, state legislatures recognized and began to regulate it by statute. In 1995, with the exception of New York and Missouri, the courts authorized family members and others close to the patient to make decisions (New York State Task Force on Life and the Law, 1995). In fact, the District of Columbia and 24 other states have statutes that explicitly grant family members and others close to the patient the right to make decisions for patients who lack capacity. Family consent statutes vary from state to state. Some have been added to state living-will statutes to provide an alternative mechanism for making life-sustaining treatment decisions for individuals who do not have an advance directive, while others are freestanding statutes that apply either to life-sustaining treatment or health care decisions generally.

Who should complete an advance directive?

An advance directive can be likened to flood or fire insurance; one hopes never to have to use it but it is important to have the coverage should the need arise. Therefore, all persons should be encouraged to complete an advance directive, a DPAHC if someone is available to serve as a health care proxy, and, in the event that no such person exists or based on personal preference, a living will. A DPAHC is preferable to a living will because no one can accurately foretell the future, and interpretations of a living will may be difficult because of the lack of specificity and ambiguity in the terms used.

Even in states with family consent laws, people should be encouraged to complete an advance directive. This is especially important for persons who are concerned that their families would be unable or unwilling to comply with their wishes, or if the preferred health-care proxy is at variance with the hierarchy of family members stipulated in the state's family consent statute.

THE PATIENT SELF-DETERMINATION ACT

The Patient Self-Determination Act (PSDA), which became effective December 1, 1991, is the first federal law to focus on advance directives and the right of adults to refuse life-sustaining treatment. The act was motivated by concerns that in the absence of clear directives regarding their views on life-sustaining treatment, patients' views would not be re-

spected when they became incapacitated. The PSDA requires that facilities participating in the Medicare and Medicaid program must provide written information to individuals about their right to participate in medical decision-making and formulate advance directives. The key provisions of the legislation are as follows:

With regard to the Patient Self-Determination Act, facilities must provide the following:

1. *Written information* to each adult individual concerning "an individual's rights under State law (whether statutory or as recognized by the courts of the State) to make decisions concerning such medical care, including the right to accept or refuse medical or surgical treatment and the right to formulate advance directives."

2. *Written policies* of the provider or organization respecting the implementation of such advance directives.

3. *Inquiry* as to whether a person has an advance directive.

4. *Documentation* in the patient's medical records whether the individual has executed an advance directive.

5. *Nondiscrimination,* that is, not to condition the provision of care or otherwise discriminate against an individual based on whether the individual has executed an advance directive.

6. *Compliance* with requirements of state laws respecting advance directives at facilities of the provider or organization.

7. *Education* for staff on issues concerning advance directives and provision for community education regarding advance directives.

Procedural guidelines for implementation are provided within the PSDA. However, the legislation does not delineate roles for health care professionals in meeting the legislative mandate. This allows for flexibility and innovation in the law's implementation and the creation of appropriate mechanisms to facilitate its purpose. Who assumes responsibility for dissemination of the information, assists in executing advance directives, and places documentation in the health care record varies according to state and health care setting. Similarly, the PSDA does not provide guidance to resolve conflicts among family members and the patient nor does it address the difficult clinical and ethical questions related to decisionally incapacitated patients who have never executed an advanced directive. The PSDA neither creates nor effects requirements with respect to informed consent to medical care or determination of mental capacity. In sum, the PSDA's focus is narrow, that is, the handling of written directives for medical care made by persons who later become incapacitated.

DO NOT RESUSCITATE DIRECTIVES

Cardiopulmonary resuscitation (CPR) is an area in which nurses assume an active role in initiating or withholding treatment. Whether to initiate CPR calls for careful attention to ethical, legal, professional, and institutional policies. The ethical principles used to justify decisions regarding resuscitation are rooted in principles of autonomy, self-determination, respect for others, best interest, beneficence and nonmaleficence.

Cardiopulmonary resuscitation was established to be used with witnessed arrests, sudden death in the young, drowning, and predictable arrests, such as in anesthesia and cardioversion (Hall, 1996). Hall reminds us that all patients who have cardiopulmonary arrest—for any reason, of any age, or with any condition—will have CPR performed in almost all hospitals or nursing homes in the

United States unless there is a specific order written to the contrary (the DNR decision). "Slow codes" or "partial codes," or any actions that lead the patient's family to believe a full intensive code is being done when it is not, are unethical and could give rise to legal implications (Meisel & Cerminara, 2001). If such actions deceive or injure the family, those actions might be deemed illegal under a civil or criminal action for fraud (Hall, 1996).

Because CPR is automatic for every patient, physicians and nurses fear that if they do not start CPR on all patients they are at risk of being sued; this is not true. Health care professionals never are required legally to perform procedures that are clearly futile. In fact, nurses and other health care professionals might be sued for performing CPR without consent if the current medical literature indicates that such procedures are futile or the treatment will not be effective.

Similarly, with a policy of automatic resuscitation, obtaining a DNR order is critical if the patient wishes to avoid this type of treatment. In 1988, New York became the first state to enact DNR legislation and it required that consent to CPR be presumed; if physicians do not want to resuscitate patients, they must obtain patient's consent before writing such an order (Swidler, 1989). Many other states have enacted DNR legislation since New York did. The American Medical Association (1991) mandates that patients and families be consulted before a DNR order is written.

What nurses need to know about DNR directives is that patients have a right to refuse CPR and may request DNR orders after they have been informed of the risks and benefits involved. Open communication is important to ensure that the decision is acceptable to all parties involved. If the physician is unable to write a DNR directive or comply with the patient's request, the physician has a duty to notify the patient or family and assist the patient in obtaining another physician. Not all statutes address the duty of the physician to transfer the patient if the physician is unwilling to implement the directive. Thus, nurses ought to be aware when such dilemmas are present and act to advocate on behalf of the patient. Moreover, nurses need to know which patients have a DNR directive, the institutional policy and law governing the use of directives, the patient's wishes regarding interventions to be withheld, and their own values toward the decision to withhold treatment. The medical record should clearly indicate the terms of the directive and whether the terms accurately reflect the patients' current stated preferences.

In the mid 1990s, a task force of ethicists and clinicians at the Oregon Health Sciences University developed a new Do Not Resuscitate order form called POLST (Physician Orders for Life-Sustaining Treatment). The POLST is a comprehensive two-page order form that documents a patient's preference for life-sustaining treatments and is designed to record a patient's wishes clearly and simply (Ghusn, Teasdale, & Jordan, (1997). A complete POLST form and materials can be obtained from the Oregon Health Sciences University's Center for Ethics in Health Care (http://www.ohsu.edu/ethics/polst.htm).

Lee, Brummel-Smith, Meyer, Drew, and London (2000) studied the effectiveness of POLST in a Program of All-Inclusive Care for the Elderly (PACE) in Portland, Oregon. They retrospectively reviewed POLST instructions for each of the 58 participants and whether each of the treatments addressed by the POLST was administered in the final 2 weeks of life. The POLST specified DNR for 50 participants (93%); CPR use was consistent with these instructions for 49 participants (91%). The older adults in this study were also asked to designate the level of care they preferred (comfort care, limited, advanced, or full intervention). Interventions administered were consistent with patient preferences in only 25 cases (46%), with less frequent deviations in antibiotic administration, administration of IV fluids, and placement of feeding tubes. The investigators concluded that the POLST effectively limits the use of some life-sustaining interventions, but that further investigation is needed into the factors that lead physicians to deviate from patients' stated preferences about other treatment.

Surveys demonstrate strong support for advance directives among the public (Larson & Tobin, 2000). However, the low numbers of patients who complete advance directives is alarming. The literature suggests that more patients would complete advance directives if they had more information and assistance in completing them (Emanuel, Barry, & Stoeckle, 1991; Mezey, Ramsey, Mitty & Rapport, 1997). To that end, a number of educational interventions have been implemented to address these issues. Notwithstanding, few interventions increased advance directive completion by more than 18% (Hare & Nelson, 1991; Rubin, Strull, Fialkow, Weiss, & Lo, 1994; Sachs, Stocking, & Miles, 1992) and many did not increase completion at all (Robinson, DeHaven, & Koch, 1993; Stiller et al., 2001). Even patients at higher risk of becoming decisionally incapable and who were more likely to understand the need for advance directives were not more likely to complete advance directives. Completion, however, is more concentrated among White patients with higher education and income levels.

There is evidence to suggest that despite the seemingly low effectiveness rates of educational interventions, heath care providers can make a tremendous difference in whether patients discuss end-of-life care with their families or friends or complete advance directives. One outpatient home-care program elicited a 71% increase in advance directive completions among its 34 participants (Luptak & Bould, 1994). This intervention differed significantly from others by including multiple conversations with a regular health care provider during outpatient visits over a concentrated (2- to 4-month) period. Such conversations can have a positive effect on advance care planning discussions and advance directive completion.

According to Morrison (1998) physicians might avoid end-of-life conversations because they (1) fear causing pain and bearing bad news; (2) lack knowledge of advance directive laws and training in delivering bad news; (3) view death as an enemy to be defeated; (4) anticipate disagreement with the patient or family; (5) have medical and legal concerns; and (6) feel threatened by such discussions.

Patients and providers may fail to discuss advance directives because patients expect providers to initiate a discussion, while providers wait for patients to raise the issue. For that reason, nurses have a very important role in end-of-life care and their relationships with patients and families bear on the decision-making process. As advocates and educators, nurses must educate patients and families to communicate their treatment preferences to their physicians whether they choose to put it to writing or not. Nurses should facilitate dialogue to empower patients and families to communicate their values, goals, and treatment preferences. Patients want their physicians with whom they have a relationship to initiate and discuss end-of-life care and living wills (Emanuel et al., 1991; Kristjanson, 2001).

Although many patients discuss advance care planning with their families, other patients find it difficult to initiate such discussions (Elpern, Yellen, & Burton, 1993; Norton & Talerico, 2000). Health care professionals can open up discussions between families and patients by providing a format for such discussions or use advance directives to minimize conflicts between patients and their families. Patients indicate that they complete advance directives to ease the financial and emotional burden on their families and to support decision making (Elder, Schneider, Zweig, Peters, & Ely, 1992; Mezey, Mitty, Ramsey, 1997, 1996; Norton & Talerico, 2000). Patients may decide that an advance directive is unnecessary because they believe that family members would know what to do when the time came. Studies show that patients who feel that others will make appropriate decisions were more likely to have adult children than those who did not (Elder et al., 1992). Health care providers should be aware of these sentiments and, where appropriate, involve family members in these discussions.

Patients who lack critical information about health care interventions or who hold erroneous beliefs about treatments may be unwilling to execute a directive (Kayser-Jones, 1990). In such cases, education may change people's treatment preferences. For example, patients who received written information about CPR both appreciated the information and changed their treatment preferences regarding it (Schonwetter, Walker, Kramer, & Robinson, 1993).

The extent to which a patient's age influences his or her willingness to execute an advance directive is unclear (Ajaj, Singh, & Abdulla, 2001; Luptak & Bould, 1994); there is some evidence that older people are more likely to execute advance directives (U.S. Department of Health and Human Services [DHHS], 1993). Providers need to consider that older people's values about the importance of health may be different from younger individuals. Not uncommonly, an older person might refuse to formulate an advance directive out of concern for the family and the conflicts that such a document might generate (Stetler, Elliott, & Bruno, 1992); they would rather defer decisions to the family (Danis, Garrett, Harris, & Patrick, 1994; High, 1993).

Another issue that influences patients' or families' comfort or discomfort in discussing advance directives concerns how one defines autonomy. Most people who complete an advance directive do so to assure that their individual wishes are followed; however, the Western notion of autonomy is not applicable to cultures where the family rather than the individual is the locus of decision making. For such individuals, an advance directive may conflict directly with accepted norms of behavior and the decision-making process identified by that culture. Health care providers need to approach advanced directives with cultural sensitivity and cultural competence.

Fears that an advance directive permits providers to withhold care or will lead to substandard care may be at the root of the rejection of advance directives for some patients. People may be concerned that once an advance directive is completed and it contains a statement to withhold treatment, providers will devote less attention to their care and may withhold more treatment than was desired (Caralis, Davis, Wright, & Marcial, 1993; Patel, Sinuff, & Cook, 2004). In a study by Elder and colleagues (1992), some individuals feared that an advance directive might allow care to be withheld too soon and could result in a shirking of societal duties. One person commented that he would not want to hear, "Sorry, we don't have the time or money to treat you." This fear is not present among patients alone; nurses and other health care providers hold similar beliefs (Anderson, Walker, Pierce, & Mills, 1986; Davidson, Hackler, Caradine, & McCord, 1989; Louw, 2004).

Socioeconomic and cultural factors substantially influence decisions to complete an advance directive. Studies are confirming that people with less education, lower income, or who are African American or Hispanic are less likely to formulate advance directives (High, 1993; Mezey et al., 2000; Phipps et al., 2003; Robinson et al., 1993). Several explanations are plausible. Individuals with these sociodemographic characteristics are less likely to have regular access to care. For them, limiting any medical care would seem unnecessary because they already have too little, not too much. They are also less likely to have exposure to the concept of advance directives (Mezey et al., 1997). Furthermore, most physicians are White; people who have experienced discrimination throughout their lives may particularly distrust the intent of health care providers with respect to advance directives. Non-White patients are less likely than White patients to discuss end-of-life decisions with a White physician. Moreover, certain cultural factors in non-White communities may prohibit discussions of death and dying. For example, fears among the African American community that AIDS was developed to wipe out the community (Haas, Weissman, Cleary, Goldberg, Gatsonis, et al., 1993; Phipps et al., 2003).

The location and timing of when a patient receives information about advance directives is also important. It is well recognized that an acute episode or emergency admission is an inappropriate time to receive this information, yet this is the point at which most hospitals are fulfilling their responsibilities under the PSDA. Information may be better utilized during the preadmission period where patients can discuss advance directives in the comfort of their own homes. Alternatively, information can be presented as part of the discharge process when the impact of hospitalization is still new, but without the distraction of acute symptoms.

In long-term care, discussing advance directives poses particular issues. In some cases, nursing home residents may not have any family or friends with whom to discuss such issues; or a relative may live at some distance and rarely visit. Health care providers can sensitize residents to the need for advance directives under such circumstances. Should the resident decide to execute a DPAHC, providers need to be vigilant that the health care proxy will be available, willing, and able to act in the resident's best interest. Residents with fluctuating decision-making capacity may vary in their ability to participate fully or even partially in decisions about their care. If that is the case, providers need to work carefully and critically at not abrogating residents' rights while shielding those who are decisionally incapable from inappropriately making decisions

Although end-of-life decisions are made by some with little difficulty or conflict, the vast majority of people are reluctant to confront their own mortality and are unwilling to execute an advance directive. A similar phenomenon exists with organ donation; even though most people support donation, few actually fill out organ donor cards (Mackie, Sheridan, Alvaro, & Garlick, 2004). Some may feel that an advance directive will not be necessary in their individual case. Some may argue that no amount of education will be able to counteract the discomfort associated with discussing death and dying. However, nurses need to learn techniques to discuss death realistically and sensitively with patients and their families.

Health care providers, both professional and nonprofessional, raise a number of issues when they express their negative feelings about advance directives. Some may mistrust the validity of the information contained in the advance directive because they feel or fear that the patient did not fully understand the advance directives' content or purpose (Jacobson et al., 1994; Valente, 2004). The ability to predict specific treatment choices based upon generally stated values and beliefs is not uniformly congruent for patients and their proxies (Emanuel & Weinberg, 1993; Schneiderman, Pearlman,

Kaplan, Anderson, & Rosenberg, 1992. Overall, however, studies show that even if flawed, patients' wishes and decisions expressed by health care proxies more closely approximate the patient's own treatment preferences than do decisions of physicians or others. In general, patients' decisions seem to be fairly stable over time, especially among patients who have completed advance directives (Emanuel, Emanuel, Stoeckle, Hummel, & Barry, 1994; Danis et al., 1994). There is also some evidence that patients expect physicians to exercise some latitude in overriding their living will instructions if the physician thinks it would be best for the patient (Jacobson et al., 1994).

Providers are particularly hesitant to approach patients about directives when the issue of stopping or withdrawing treatment is imminent (Prendergast & Puntillo, 2004; Solomon, O'Donnell, Jennings, Guilfoy, Wolf, et al., 1993). Many providers erroneously perceive that there is a legal difference between forgoing treatment and discontinuing treatment. Under such circumstances, providers need to be concerned about the extent to which patients (and health care proxies) are informed correctly about treatment alternatives and consequences and know the relevant laws.

INFORMED CONSENT

Informed consent is not only a legal requirement, but also a moral imperative. The legal requirement of informed consent is based on the value of patient autonomy and self-determination. Every human being of adult years and sound mind has a right to determine what shall be done with his or her own body (*Schloendorff v. Society of New York Hospital*, 1914). Accordingly, the fundamental goals of informed consent are patient autonomy and self-determination (*In re Farrell*, 1987). This goal is effectuated by allowing patients to make their own decisions about their health care based on their own values for as long as they are able.

A second goal of informed consent is to empower patients to exercise their right to autonomy rationally and intelligently (Meisel & Cerminara, 2001). There is no guarantee that providing patients relevant information about treatment will result in patients' making intelligent decisions, nor does it guarantee that they will use the information provided; however, without such a requirement the likelihood of rational decision-making diminishes (Meisel & Cerminara, 2001). The patient's right to consent presumes that the patient has sufficient information to make a reasonable decision.

Consent to treatment is only valid when the patient has the capacity to consent (Meisel & Cerminara, 2001). "Competence" and "incompetence" are not the same yet they are frequently considered to be synonymous. Competency to make health care decisions is a legal term that is determined only by a court. The law presumes that all adults are competent and have the decision-making capacity (Applebaum & Grisso, 1988) to make health decisions and the assumption is ordinarily correct (Meisel & Cerminara, 2001). To be considered competent an individual must be able to comprehend the nature of the particular action in question and be able to understand its significance. One need not be adjudicated incompetent to lack the capacity to consent to medical treatment and one who is adjudicated incompetent does not necessarily lack the capacity to consent (Meisel & Cerminara, 2001).

Capacity, on the other hand, is determined not by the courts, but rather by clinicians who assess functional capabilities to determine whether capacity is lacking. Incapacity is not determined solely by a medical or psychiatric diagnosis; rather it rests on the judgments that an informed layperson might make (Mezey, Mitty, et al., 1997).

The basic elements of a valid consent—the determination that a patient has sufficient decisional capacity to consent or refuse treatment—are based on the observation of a specific set of abilities: (1) the patient appreciates/understands that he or she has the right to make a choice; (2) the patient understands the medical situation, prognosis, risks, benefits, and consequences of treatment (or not); (3) the patient can communicate the decision; and (4) the patient's decision is stable and consistent over a period of time (Roth, Meisel, & Lidz, 1977).

Not all health decisions require the same level of decision-making capacity in order to make a decision. Decision making capacity is not an "on-off switch" (Mezey, Mitty, et al., 1997); you do not either have it or not. Rather, during the past 20 years during the right-to-die movement, bioethicists and lawyers suggested that capacity be viewed as task-specific rather than in general terms (Mezey, et al., 1997). An individual may be able to perform some tasks adequately and may have the ability to make some decisions, but is unable to perform all tasks or make all decisions. The notion of "decision-specific capacity" assumes that an individual has or lacks capacity for a particular decision at a particular time and under a particular set of circumstances (Mezey, Mitty, et al., 1997; Mitty & Mezey, 2004). Most people have sufficient cognitive capability to make some but not all decisions (Mitty & Mezey, 2004; Miller, 1995).

Nurses can make a valuable contribution in ensuring that the informed consent process is accurately met (Davis, 1989; Virani, & Sofer, 2003). Yet, nurses have little training in assessing decision-making capacity (Mezey, Mitty, et al., 1997). Nurses must become proficient in assessing decisional capacity and in being active participants in discussions with other members of the health care team when determining decisional capacity. Those with the most knowledge of the patient should be asked to contribute meaningful and relevant information about the person. When nurses and other health care professionals learn how to assess capacity objectively, two types of mistakes will be avoided. First, mistakenly preventing persons who ought to be considered capacitated from directing the course of their treatment, and second, failing to protect incapacitated persons from the harmful effects of their decisions (President's Commission, 1982). Nurses at all educational levels should make efforts to meet their legal and ethical obligations so that patients will retain their rights to make decisions for as long as they are able.

INTRACTABLE PAIN LEGISLATION

All patients who suffer from pain, not just those who are dying, should be treated. The debate about patient-requested euthanasia and assisted suicide has drawn national and international attention to the fact that appropriate interventions can eliminate or drastically reduce the pain and suffering that many people experience. The need for appropriate types and amounts of pain medications was made clear in the U.S. Supreme Court ruling in *Vacco v. Quill* (1997). There is a relationship between pain and symptom management and the requests for assisted suicide (Foley, 1991).

Through the Federal Intractable Pain Regulation, the federal government in 1974 clarified the federal law that prohibits physicians from prescribing opioids to detoxify or maintain an opioid addiction. The regulation stated, in part, that the prohibitive regulations are "not intended to impose any limitation on a physician ... to administer or dispense narcotic drugs to persons with intractable pain in which no relief or cure is possible or none has been found after reasonable effort" (Institute of Medicine [IOM], 1997). Simi-

larly, some courts explicitly recognize that a patient's "right to be free from pain ... is inseparable from their right to refuse medical treatment" (Meisel & Cerminara, 2001), and have granted immunity to health care providers who treat pain with strong doses of analgesic medications that inadvertently end the patient's life (*McKay v. Bergstedt*, 1990). Moreover, several states have enacted intractable pain statutes to encourage those who treat patients who are terminally ill and have intractable pain to manage the pain without threat of legal liability if the treatment results in the patient's death. Nurses should also be aware of the legislation involving the treatment of pain and should advocate to treat patient's pain and to assist in the development of institutional policies that embrace the spirit of these laws.

The IOM report "Approaching Death: Improving Care at End of Life, (1997), coupled with other palliative care literature, asserts that change must occur at many levels if we are to improve care for the dying. The development of intractable pain statutes is a good first step to the undertreatment of pain. However, they are imperfect and there are problems associated with intractable pain statutes that include the following:

1. They do not, in all cases, mark a clear area of medical practice in which physicians feel free to manage their patients' pain. The more specific laws, for example, those that set out detailed prescription practices, may actually afford physicians less leeway in the practice of medicine. Additionally, by carving out an area of pain treatment that is immune from medical board discipline, there may be an implication that other forms of pain treatment should be subject to disciplinary review.
2. Even the strongest intractable-pain law is still limited by the term *intractable*. Many cases are ambiguous, and physi-

cians may believe they must delay opioid treatment until pain is far enough along to be called intractable.

3. An additional problem arises when state laws define addiction without regard to pain management. As noted earlier, California defines addicts as "habitual users," which might include patients taking opioids for chronic pain. Such confusing definitions . . . expose physicians to the threat of medical board discipline.

4. Finally, legal affirmations in these laws of the importance of pain control do not, in themselves, correct practice patterns or improve physician training. Laws could, however, encourage patients to expect diligence in pain relief, including use of generally effective medications. Medical boards could consider disciplining physicians who fail to apply proven methods of pain control. (IOM, 1997)

Thus, health care system changes are needed to improve access to care and to eliminate barriers to effective treatment. Nurses need to educate patients and families about their right to adequate palliative care. In states where there are intractable pain statutes, the PSDA requires all covered facilities to inform patients of their state law rights to adequate palliative care (Meisel & Cerminara, 2001). Health care providers need to "add the assessment of pain as the fifth vital sign" (Meisel & Cerminara, 2001), and national pain management standards ought to be followed (Joint Committee on Accreditation of Healthcare Organizations [JCAHO], 2000).

ETHICS COMMITTEES

Ethical issues in clinical practice often involve life-or-death decisions and such decisions give rise to a host of emotions. Just as physicians and patients turn to medical specialists and subspecialists for advice and consultations on questions of medicine, physicians and patients may need to consult ethics committees or ethics consultants to discuss today's perplexing ethical issues. Ethics consultations are more timely, less adversarial, and more flexible than court proceedings as a way to resolve disputes. According to one study in 1997 by Bernard Lo, 21 years after the New Jersey Supreme Court decision in the matter of Karen Ann Quinlan, between two thirds and three fourths of large hospitals have ethics committees (L. Rothenberg, Vasco, 1996). The JCAHO now requires institutions to have a mechanism to consider "ethical issues [that] arise in the care of patients," such as an ethics committee or consultation service. Moreover, some suggest that individuals with special training in clinical ethics may be an alternative to ethics committees. Institutions such as long-term-care facilities, which are not subject to the JCAHO requirements, also are establishing ethics committees or regional ethics networks in an effort to embrace the spirit of recent regulations and the need of health care providers to be knowledgeable and informed about ethical questions concerning life-sustaining treatments.

The goal of case consultations by ethics committees or consultants is to help resolve disagreements over ethical issues. One important question is who should serve on the committee. The committee should look like members of the health care team. In other words, an interdisciplinary ethics committee is needed. The committee members should include physicians, nurses, house officers, social workers, clergy, laypersons (community representatives), and members who have formal training in medical ethics, philosophy, religion, and law. The question about the relevance of having lawyers on the committee is mixed. However, if the hospital lawyer or risk manager is a committee member, it is essential that the potential legal risk to the institution does not dominate discussions and trump discussions that are ethically challenging and relevant to health care providers.

The Role of Ethics Committees

The overall role of an ethics committee is threefold. First, the committee may educate itself, the hospital administration, and the hospital staff about medical-ethical issues occurring in our current health care environment. For example, providers fear legal intervention when life-support systems are removed from a patient who is terminally ill (or even brain-dead) and the ethics committee can be alleviated of this fear arguably through education. Second, the committee may participate in policy development. For example, an institution may draft a DNR policy, a determination of brain death statute, or advance directive policy. Third, the committee has a role to participate in ethics consultation and to assist in the resolution of bioethical dilemmas. For example, a physician or family who are uncertain or unclear about whether it would be appropriate to discontinue therapy on a patient might consult with an ethics committee; the committee would assist by considering the issues, provide information to the physician and family, and revisit the physician's or family's previous decision, or it may move forward and decide the case itself.

Bernard Lo (1996) identifies five goals of ethics case consultations. First, the ethics committees can help the health care team identify and understand the specific ethical issues the case raises. For example, cases that involve questions about advance directives, surrogate decision-making, or disputes over life-sustaining treatments. Health care providers need to think carefully and critically through the ethical issues themselves before they try to resolve disagreements with the patient or family. Second, the ethics committee can suggest how health care providers

might improve communications with the patient and family. Some committees will hold a meeting with the family and the heath care team and not include the patient, even if he or she is available. Poor communications and lack of communication among the health care providers and members of the team may be a problem that the ethics committee can identify and help resolve. Third, the committee may provide emotional support to the physician, the nurses, and other health team members in a case. Some members of the team fear being sued and additional support is helpful and needed. Fourth, another role of the committee is to offer specific recommendations. Some committees or consultants help the health care team analyze the ethical issues and facilitate discussions with patients and families; however, they may stop short of giving recommendations. Most committees or consultants do offer specific recommendations for resolving ethics dilemmas and this should be the role of all committees. Finally, the committees or consultants have a role to improve patient care. They can prevent patient care decisions that contradict ethical guidelines. Patient care decisions do not necessarily need to change after consultations, nor is there a mandate that they must change. However, by participating in consultation, health care providers, patients, and families may feel that their concerns have been addressed and better understand the rationale for the treatment decision that is being proposed.

Committee members should be respected by colleagues and peers for their clinical judgment and their interpersonal skills. They should be receptive to different ideas and points of view, and most important, be able to deal with emotionally charged issues and interpersonal disagreements/conflicts, and be able to tolerate ambiguity and complexity (Lo, 1995). Ethics committees, generally, have found that they serve institutions best in their role as educator. Oftentimes, through education, policies are developed and people are willing to seek committees for consultation. Committees also are more likely to be accepted on pending substantive bioethics questions if they are an advisory group and not a formal and binding court of appeal.

Ethics committee should be voluntary, educational, and advisory in purpose so as not to interfere with the primary responsibility and relationship between physicians and patients. Some view ethics committees as intrusive, undermining the physician and resulting in loss of control and abdication of their responsibility as physicians. Medical staff bylaws and institutional policy and procedures should delineate the functions of the committee and the parameters of the committee's activities. Again, the function of the ethics committee is to consider and assist in resolving unusual, complicated ethical problems involving issues that affect the care and treatment of patients within the institution and to show concern for those who are responsible for their care and treatment. Typically, issues that involve quality of life, terminal illness, or life-sustaining treatments can give rise to disagreements and they are often complex and emotionally charged. Values and beliefs stemming from cultural, ethnic, and religious beliefs play a pivotal role in these discussions.

Emotional and psychological reactions to the decision-making process and treatment termination can also cause disagreement. Although the distinction between withdrawing and withholding treatment has no legal or ethical significance, it nevertheless can have a profound emotional effect on the health care team. Similarly, as set forth in *Cruzan,* despite widespread agreement that artificial nutrition and hydration are simply another form of life-sustaining medical treatment, many people feel strongly that these forms of treatment are fundamental and owed to all people.

Thus, patients and families are extremely resistant to suggestions to terminate them and the ethics committee may be the best forum to mediate such disputes.

In addition, disagreements that stem from uncertainty or miscommunications between patient and family may mandate that physicians consult with ethics committees. Uncertainty may arise because of the difficulty in determining the patient's medical condition or the effect of various treatment alternatives. Likewise, the patient's failure to state his or her treatment preferences explicitly can create uncertainty. A dilemma may result from miscommunication when the physician leader fails to convey clear and relevant information; when interested individuals do not have an accurate picture of the patient's treatment wishes, preferences, diagnosis, prognosis, and treatment options; or from the concerns, hopes, and fears of other interested individuals. Accordingly, regardless of the source of the disagreement, health care providers should be sensitive to warning signs of a brewing disagreement. When a seemingly irresolvable treatment termination disagreement arises, an ethics committee must be consulted and physicians must not view it as intrusive, but as clarifying and strengthening the relationship between the parties.

There are times when disagreements concerning life-sustaining treatments give rise to litigation. Then, the institution's lawyer is well suited to advise and educate the health care team about litigation and should be available to answer questions abut the legal process that the staff may encounter during litigation or to avoid litigation. Discussions with the lawyer may ease some of the fears and dispel some of the misconceptions that health care providers have about the law and litigation in this area. In addition, discussion with the lawyer may address the potential liability for members of the committee and available immunities.

EDUCATION OF NURSES AND OTHER HEALTH CARE PROFESSIONALS REGARDING ADVANCE DIRECTIVES

Education can change nurses' comfort with and willingness to approach patients about advance directives. When they are well informed and comfortable with their own feelings, they are more likely to initiate discussion about advance directives. Physicians who are educated about directives are more comfortable with such discussions, have more discussions with their patients, and their patients complete more advance directives than do patients of noneducated physicians (Emanuel, von Gunten, & Ferris, 1999; Greenberg, Doblin, Shapiro, Linn, & Wenger, 1993; Robinson et al., 1993).

Education of health care providers about advance directives must be multifaceted. For example, fewer than 50% of nursing homes in New York City provide ongoing education about advance directives for nurses and less than one third provide education for physicians (Mezey, Ramsey, et al., 1998). Much of the PSDA information available to institutions comes from legal departments, state departments of health, or from professional organizations (U.S. DHHS, 1993). The extent to which this information is sensitive to the needs of the institution, its subspecialty areas, or the cultural and socioeconomic differences of patients and families is unknown. Education requires more than a description of the law and the steps to be taken in formulating directives. Nurses and other health care providers need to learn how to discuss advance care planning with patients and families; assess decisional capacity to execute a directive; identify methods to help patients analyze the benefits and burdens of decisions; and resolve conflicts among staff with different values and beliefs about end-of-life treatment. Education should also include the dissemination and discussion of treatment guidelines,

attention to the psychology of decision making, and a dialogue between those who develop ethical recommendations and those who must carry them out at the bedside (Shapiro & Bowles, 2002; Solomon et al., 1993).

Finally, it is important that providers review with patients how and with whom they should communicate that a directive has been formulated. People need to be encouraged to discuss their values and health care preferences with their health care proxy (if one is appointed), their family, and a personal physician if they have one. A study of recently discharged hospital patients with advance directives documented that fewer than 15% were asked about an existing advance directive during their hospitalization, 60% of patients did not disclose to the hospital staff that they had a directive, and only 35% informed their physician about their advance directives (Mezey, Ramsey, et al., 1996). Though failure to communicate this information might be attributed to the patient's presumption that the directive would not be relevant for the hospital stay, selective disclosure may reflect a patient's misunderstanding or fear about their use. Figure 7.2 offers a protocol for the nurse to follow in completing this type of assessment.

CONCLUSION

Numerous factors make it likely that end-of-life decision making will continue to raise difficult issues for health care professionals, patients, and patients' families. The reasons that people do not complete advance directives and discuss end-of-life care, even after educational interventions, seem much more compelling than the reasons for completing them. Health care providers often do not have enough regular ongoing contact with patients, so patients do not feel comfortable discussing end-of-life issues or completing advance directives.

FIGURE 7.2   Protocol for Nurses: Asking Patients about Advance Directives

Have you ever written down any of your thoughts or choices about future medical treatment, for example, in a power of attorney for health care, a living will, or some other type of advance directive?

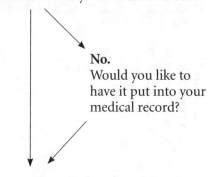

If the answer is yes:
Is this document in your medical record?

No.
Would you like to have it put into your medical record?

Yes.
Would you want anyone to review the document to make sure it is up-to-date?

If the answer is no:
Have you ever considered or thought about these issues for yourself?

Would you like to receive some education materials besides this information card (point out card to patient) or would you like to talk with someone about advance directives? (Check resource list for options.)

Is there anything you would like the staff to know about your thoughts or values regarding your medical care?

From "Protocol for Unit Nurses: Asking Patients About Advance Directives," 1999 (January-February), *Innovations in End-of-Life Care, 1*(1). Reprinted with permission.

Instead of focusing on the actual number of advance directives completed, we should look at whether our activities are encouraging discussions of end-of-life care with patients and families. The evidence to date indicates that simply providing information encourages patients to talk about their preferences with family members and friends—, that is, the people who will be making decisions in the event the patient loses decision-making capacity. Anything that encourages such conversations enhances patient autonomy and self-determination.

Advance directives, Do Not Resuscitate orders, court and legislative actions are all important mechanisms for nurses to consider when seeking ways to resolve the ethical dilemmas that exist when caring for patients at the end of life. Nurses must have oppor-

tunities to think critically and articulate their views and positions on the dilemmas they face as individuals and as professionals. Ethics rounds, grand rounds, ethics colloquium, courses in basic nursing education, continuing education offerings, and conferences all provide forums for nurses, students, faculty, and clinicians to enhance their ethical and legal awareness. The American Nurses Association Center for Ethics and Human Rights is one rich resource for nurses who seek consultation and ethics information.

RESOURCE

Aging with Dignity
P.O. Box 1661
Tallahassee, Florida 32302-1661
www.agingwithdignity.org

EDUCATION PLAN 7.1   Plan for Achieving: Legal Competencies Legal Aspects of End-of-Life Care

Knowledge Needed	Attitudes	Skills	Undergraduate Behavioral Outcomes	Graduate Behavioral Outcomes	Teaching/Learning Strategies
Dilemmas in health care can be ethical or legal issues that must be addressed by nurses	★Appreciate the difference between ethical and legal issues at the end of life. ★Acknowledge nurses' role in legal aspects of end-of-life care.		★Discuss the relevant laws related to end-of-life decision-making. ★Apply legal principles in end-of-life decision-making. ★Collaborate with patients and health professionals in examining and resolving bioethical issues.	★Shape public policy regarding patient and surrogate participation in end-of-life decision-making.	★Review the ethical/legal issues of the Karen Ann Quinlan and Nancy Beth Cruzan cases. Discuss the rulings and the implications for nursing care at the end of life.
The law and end-of-life care: The right to die —Purpose of advance directives —Types of advance directives.	★Affirm the patient's right to refuse life-sustaining treatments. ★Emphasize the value of advance directives.		★Educate patients, families, and other health professionals regarding the purpose and value of advance directives, types of advance directives (including the type recognized by the state), the formalities for executing an advance directive, and limitations in honoring advance directives.	★Guide patients and families in implementing advance directives.	★Invite a guest speaker knowledgeable about the legal aspects of end-of-life care to discuss such issues. ★Encourage students/nurses to complete advance directives, reviewing with them the completion of the forms.

The Patient Self-Determination Act: —Right to participate in medical decision-making and formulate advance directives —Provisions of the legislation	*Acknowledge the key provisions of the Patient Self-Determination Act.	*Inform patients about the provisions of the Patient Self-Determination Act.	*Insure compliance of the institution in informing patients regarding the provisions of the Patient Self-Determination Act.	*Review the Patient Self-Determination Act with students/nurses. Discuss how the act influences nursing practice.
Nurses' responsibilities regarding Do Not Resuscitate orders	*Acknowledge nurses' responsibilities regarding Do Not Resuscitate orders. *Acknowledge that slow or partial codes are unethical.	*Seek a DNR order when resuscitation would be medically futile. *Institute CPR as a full code unless a DNR order has been written. *Communicate to other health professionals that a "slow or partial" code is unethical. *Advocate on behalf of the patient if the physician is unable to comply with the patient's request for a DNR order.	*Assist patients, families, and other health professionals in determining the appropriateness of a DNR order. *Educate health professionals of unethical behavior in performing a partial or slow code. *Review with health professionals the institutional policies and laws governing the use of DNR directives.	*Review the completion of the various forms for DNR orders recognized within institutions and in the community with students/nurses. *Explore students'/nurses' feelings and attitudes regarding DNR orders. Discuss the implications to palliative care.

EDUCATION PLAN 7.1   *(continued)*

Knowledge Needed	Attitudes	Skills	Undergraduate Behavioral Outcomes	Graduate Behavioral Outcomes	Teaching/Learning Strategies
			*Confirm which patients have DNR orders and patient's preferences regarding DNR.		Based on case studies, determine those factors that positively or negatively influence the completion of advance directives. *Invite a panel of guest speakers to class to discuss the completion of advanced directives from a personal perspective and professional perspective.
Factors influencing the completion of advance directives: —Communication with health professionals —Age —Cultural values —Concern about withholding of care or treatment —Socioeconomic factors —Education of nurses and health professionals regarding advance directives	*Appreciate the emotional issues and factors influencing the completion of advance directives. *Acknowledge the responsibility of nurses and other health professionals in discussing advance directives with patients.		*Discuss the completion of advance directives with patients through multiple conversations and in advance of a life-threatening illness.	*Examine the institutional policies or professional and patient behaviors related to the completion of advance directives. *Resolve conflicts among staff with different values and beliefs regarding end-of-life treatment. *Collaborate with members of the interdisciplinary team to implement strategies that will increase the completion of advance directives.	

Informed consent	*Acknowledge the legal responsibility of nurses in obtaining informed consent. *Consider the difference between competency and capacity in determining patient's decision-making ability.	*Demonstrate competence in assessing the decision-making capacity of patients.	*Insure that the informed consent process is accurately met in the provision of care. *Actively participate in discussions with other members of the health care team when determining decisional capacity of a patient	*Coordinate interdisciplinary efforts to determine patient's decisional capacity. *Educate other health professionals regarding the difference between patient competency and capacity in determining decision-making ability.	*Role-play patient caregiving situations to determine patient's decision-making capacity. Have students play the roles of interdisciplinary team members in determining capacity.
Intractable pain legislation	*Affirm the responsibility of nurses in alleviating intractable pain.	*Discuss intractable pain legislation. *Advocate for effective pain management for patients with intractable pain. *Seek referrals to specialists for the management of intractable pain.	*Participate in the development of institutional policies that support adequate pain management, including situations of intractable pain. *Educate health professionals regarding statutes, which encourage physicians and nurse practitioners to treat patients with intractable pain.	*Review case studies of patients experiencing intractable pain. Discuss pain assessment, and interventions in accordance with intractable pain legislation.	

REFERENCES

Ajaj, A., Singh, M. P., & Abdulla, A. J. (2001). Sh ould elderly patients be told they have cancer? Questionnaire survey of older people. *British Medical Journal, 323,* 1160.

American Medical Association Council on Ethical and Judicial Affairs. (1991). *Guidelines for the appropriate use of DNR orders. Journal of the American Medical Association, 265,* 1868–1871.

Anderson, G. C., Walker, M. H., Pierce, P. M., & Mills, C. M. (1986). Living wills. Do nurses and physicians have them? *American Journal of Nursing, 86,* 271–275.

Annas, G. (1997). The bell tolls for a constitutional right to physician-assisted suicide. *New England Journal of Medicine, 337,* 1098–1103.

Applebaum, P. S., & Grisso, T. (1988). Assessing patient's capacities to consent to treatment. *New England Journal of Medicine, 319,* 1635–1638.

Burt, R. (1997). The Supreme Court speaks. Not assisted suicide but a constitutional right to palliative care. *New England Journal of Medicine, 337,* 1234–1236.

Caralis, P. V., Davis, B., Wright, K., & Marcial, E. (1993). The influence of ethnicity and race on attitudes toward advance directives, life-prolonging treatments, and euthanasia. *Journal of Clinical Ethics, 4,* 155.

Collins, F. J., Lombard, J., Moses, A., & Spitler, H. (1994). *Durable powers of attorney for health care directives* (3rd ed., 3.01). Colorado Springs, CO: McGraw-Hill.

Conn. Gen. Stat. Ann. '19A-571.

Cooney, L. M., Kennedy, G. J., Hawkins, K. A., Hurme, S., & Balch, J. D. (2004). Who can stay at home? Assessing the capacity to choose to live in the community. *Archives of Internal Medicine, 164,* 357–360.

Covinsky, K. F., Landefeld, S., Teno, J., Connors, A. F. Dawson, N. Youngres, S. et. al (1996). For the SUPPORT Investigators. Is economic hardship on the families of the seriously ill associated with patient and surrogate care preferences? *Archives of Internal Medicine, 156,* 1737–1741.

Covinsky, K. E., Goldman, L., Cook, E. F., Desbiens, N., Reding, D., Fulkerson, W. et. al (1994). The impact of serious illness on patients' families. *Journal of the American Medical Association, 272,* 1839–1844.

Cruzan v. Director, Missouri Dept. of Health, 497 U.S. 261 (1990), 110 S. Ct. 2841 (1990).

Danis, M., Garrett, J., Harris, R., & Patrick, D.L. (1994). Stability of choices about life-sustaining treatments. *Annals of Internal Medicine, 120,* 567–573.

Davidson, R. W., Hackler, C., Caradine, D. R., & McCord, R. S. (1989). Physician attitudes on advance directives. *Journal of the American Medical Association, 262,* 2415–2419.

Davis, A. J. (1989). Clinical nurses: Ethical decision making in situations of informed consent. *Advances in Nursing Science, 11*(3), 63–69.

Davis, A., Aroskar, M., Liaschenko, J., & Drought, T. (1997) *Ethical dilemmas & nursing practice* (4th ed.). Stamford, CT: Appleton and Lange.

Elder, N. C., Schneider, F. D., Zweig, S. C., Peters, P. G., & Ely, J. W. (1992). Community attitudes and knowledge about advance care directives. *Journal of the American Board Family Practice, 5,* 565–572.

Elpern, E. H., Yellen, S. B., & Burton, L. A. (1993). A preliminary investigation of opinions and behaviors regarding advance directives for medical care. *American Journal of Critical Care, 2,* 161–167.

Emanuel, L. L., von Gunten, C. F., & Ferris, E. D. (Eds.). (1999). *The EPEC curriculum: Education for Physicians in End-of-Life Care.* The EPEC Project. Retrieved 12/3/04 from http://www.EPEC.net

Emanuel, E. J., & Weinberg, D. S. (1993). How well is the patient self-determination act working: An early assessment. *American Journal of Medicine, 95,* 619–627.

Emanuel, L. L., Barry, W., & Stoeckle, J. D. (1991). Advanced directives for medical care—A case for greater use. *New England Journal of Medicine, 324,* 889–895.

Emanuel, L. L., Emanuel, E. J., Toeckle, J. D., Hummel, L. R., & Barry, M. J. (1994). Advance directives: Stability of patient's treatment choices. *Archives of Internal Medicine, 154,* 209–217.

Fins, J., Miller, F., Acres, C., Bacchetta, M., Huzzard, L., & Rapkin, B. (1999). End-of-life decision-making in the hospital: Current practice and future prospects. *Journal of Pain and Symptom Management, 17*(2), 6–15.

Foley, K. (1991). The relationship of pain and symptom management to patient requests for physician-assisted suicide. *Journal of Pain and Symptom Management, 6,* 289.

Frankl, D., Oye, R. K., & Belamy, P. E. (1989). Attitudes of hospitalized patients towards life-support. A survey of 200 medical inpatients. *American Journal of Medicine, 86,* 645–648.

Furrow, B., Greaney, T., Johnson, S., Jost, J. T., & Schwartz, R. (2001). *Hornbook on Health Law* (2nd ed.): Eagan, MN: West Group.

Gamble, E. R., McDonald, D. J., & Lichstein, P. R. (1991). Knowledge attitudes and behavior of elderly persons regarding living wills. *Archives of Internal Medicine,151,* 277–280.

Garger v. New Jersey, 429 U.S. 922 (1976).

Garner, H. C. (Ed.). (2004). *Black's law dictionary* (8th ed.). Barrister Books.

Gazelle G. (1998). The slow code—Should anyone rush to its defense? *New England Journal of Medicine, 338,* 467–469.

Ghusn, H., Teasdale, T. A., & Jordan, D. (1997). Continuity of do-not-resuscitation orders between hospital and nursing home settings. *Journal of the American Geriatric Society, 45,* 465–469.

Gordon, G. H., & Dunn, P. (1992) Advance directives and the Patient Self-Determination Act. *Hospital Practice, 27*(4A), 39–40, 42.

Greco, P. J., Schulman, K. A., Lavizzo-Mourey, R., & Hansen-Flaschen, J. (1991) The Patient Self-Determination Act and the future of advance directives. *Annals of Internal Medicine, 115,* 639–643.

Greenberg, J. M., Doblin, B. H., Shapiro, D. W., Linn L. S., & Wenger, N. S. (1993). Effect of an educational program on medical student's conversations with patients about advance directives. *Journal of General Internal Medicine, 8,* 683–685.

Haas, S., Weissman, J. S., Cleary, P. D., Goldberg, J., Gatsonis, C., Seage, G. R., III, et al. (1993). Discussions of preferences for life-sustaining care by persons with AIDS. *Archives of Internal Medicine, 153,* 1241–1248.

Haidet, P., Hamel, M. B., Davis, R. B., Wenger, N., Reding, D., Fulkerson W, Connors, A. F., et al.(1998). For the SUPPORT Investigators. Outcomes, preferences for resuscitation, and physician-patient communication among patients with metastatic colorectal cancer. *American Journal of Medicine, 105,* 222–229.

Hall, J. (1996). *Nursing ethics and law.* Philadelphia: Saunders.

Hamel, M. B., Phillips, R. S., Davis, R. B., et al. (1997). For the SUPPORT Investigators. Outcomes and cost effectiveness of initiating dialysis and continuing aggressive care in seriously ill hospitalized adults. *Annals of Internal Medicine ,127,* 195–202.

Hamel, M. B., Phillips, R. S., Teno, J. M., et al. (1996). For the SUPPORT Investigators. Seriously ill hospitalized adults: Do we spend less on older patients? *Journal of the American Geriatric Society, 44,* 1043–1048.

Hamel, M. B., Teno, J. M., Goldman, L., et al. (1999). Patient age and decisions to withhold life-sustaining treatments from seriously ill hospitalized adults. *Annals of Internal Medicine, 130*(4), 116–125.

Hare, J., & Nelson, C. (1991). Will outpatients complete living wills? *Journal of General Internal Medicine, 6,* 41–46.

High, D. M. (1993). Advance directives and the elderly: A study of intervention strategies to increase use. *Gerontologist, 33,* 342–349.

Hoffman, D. (1998). Pain management and palliative care in the era of managed care: Issues for health insurers. *Journal of Law, Medicine and Ethics, 26,* 267–289.

Hopp, F., & Duffy, S. (2000). Racial variations in end-of-life care. *Journal of the American Geriatrics Society, 48,* 658–663.

Hyman, C. (1996). Pain management and disciplinary action: How medical boards can remove barriers to effective treatment. *Journal of Law, Medicine and Ethics, 24,* 338–343.

Field, M., & Cassel, C. (Eds.) (1997). Approaching death: Improving care at the end of life. Washington, DC: National Academies Press. IOM (Institute of Medicine). (1997). Committee on End of Life Care.

In re Westchester County Medical Center (O'Connor), 72 N.Y.2nd 517, 531 N.E.2d 607, 534 N.Y.S.2d 886, rev'g 139 A.D.2d 344, 532 N.Y.S.2d 133 (1988). In re Farrell, 108 NJ 335, 529 A.2d 404 (N.J. 1987).

Jacobsen, J. A., White, B. E., Battin, M. P., Francis, L. P., Green, D. J., & Kasworm, E. S. (1994). Patients' understanding and use of advance directives. *Western Journal of Medicine, 160,* 232–236.

Johnson, S. (1998) Introduction: Legal and regulatory issues in pain management. *Journal of Law, Medicine and Ethics, 24,* 265–266.

Kayser-Jones, J. (1990). The use of nasogastric feeding tubes in nursing homes: Patient, family and health care provider perspectives. *Gerontologist, 30,* 469–479.

Knaus, W. A., Harrell, F. E., Lynn, J., et. al (1995). For the SUPPPORT Investigators.

The SUPPORT prognostic model: Objective estimates of survival for seriously ill hospitalized adults. *Annals of Internal Medicine, 122,* 191–203.

Kristjanson, L. (2001). Establishing goals of care: Communication traps and treatment lane changes. In B. R. Ferrell & N. Coyle (Eds.), *Textbook of palliative nursing* (pp. 331–338). New York: Oxford University Press.

Larson, D. G., & Tobin, D. R. (2000). End-of-life conversations: Evolving practice and theory. *Journal of the American Medical Association, 284,* 1573–1578.

Lee, M., Brummel-Smith, K., Meyer, J., Drew, N., & London, M. R. (2000). Physician orders for life-sustaining treatment (POLST): Outcomes in a PACE program. Program of all-inclusive care for the elderly. *Journal of the American Geriatric Society, 48,* 1219–1225.

Lo, B. (1995). *Resolving ethical dilemmas: A guide for clinicians.* Baltimore: Lippincott Williams & Wilkins.

Lo, B., Rothenberg, K., & Vasko, M. (1996) Appropriate management of pain: Addressing the clinical, legal and regulatory barriers. *Journal of Law, Medicine & Ethics, 24,* 285–286.

Louw, S. (2004). Cultural issues in end-of-life decision making. *Age & Ageing, 33,* 212–213.

Luptak, M. K., & Bould, C. (1994). A method for increasing elders' use of advance directives. *Gerontologist, 34,* 409–412.

Mackie, F., Sheridan, A., Alvaro, C., & Garlick, J. (2004) Organ donor potential and missed donors in NSW. *Immunology and Cell Biology,82,* A15.

McKay v. Bergstedt, 106 Nev. 808, 801 P.2d 617 (Nev. 1990).

Meisel, A., & Cerminara, K. L. (2001). *The right to die: Vols. 1 and 2: 2001 Cumulative Supplement.* New York: Aspen Law & Business.

Mezey, M., Mitty, E., Bottrell, M., Ramsey, G., & Fisher, T. (2000). Advance directives:

Older adults with dementia. *Clinics in Geriatric Medicine, 16,* 255–268.

Mezey, M., Leitman, R., Mitty, E., Bottrell, M., & Ramsey, G. (2000). Why hospital patients do and do not execute an advance directive. *Nursing Outlook. 48*(4), 165–171.

Mezey, M., Ramsey, G., Mitty, E., & Rappaport, M. (1997). Implementation of the Patient Self-Determination Act (PSDA) in nursing homes in New York City. *Journal of the American Geriatrics Society, 45,* 43–49.

Mezey, M., Mitty, E., & Ramsey, G. (1997). Assessment of decision-making capacity: Nurse's role. *Journal of Gerontological Nursing, 23*(3), 28–35.

Miller, T. (1995). Advance directives: Moving from theory to practice. In P. R. Katz, R. L. Kane, & M. Mezey (Eds.), *Quality care in geriatric settings* (pp. 68–87). New York: Springer.

Mitty, E. L., & Mezey, M. D. (2004). Advance directives: Older adults with dementia. In M. Matzo and D. Sherman (Eds.). (2004). *Gerontological palliative care nursing* (pp. 118–131). St. Louis, MO: Mosby.

Mitty, E., Mezey, M., Ramsey, G., & Rappaport, M. (1996). Ethics committees and PSDA implementation in 100 nursing homes: Nursing home medicine. *Journal of the American Medical Directors' Association, 12,* 23–28.

Morrison, M. F. (1998). Obstacles to doctor-patient communication at the end of life. In M. D. Steinberg & S. J. Youngner (Eds.). *End-of-life decisions: A psychosocial perspective* (pp. 109–136). Washington, DC: American Psychiatric Press.

Murphy, D. J. (1990). Improving advance directives for healthy older people. *Journal of the American Geriatrics Society, 38,* 1251–1256.

Murphy, P., Kreling, B., Kathryn, E., Stevens, M., Lynn, J. & Dulac, J. (2000). Description of the SUPPORT Intervention. *Journal of the American Geriatrics Society, 48,* S154–S161.

New York State Task Force on Life and the Law. (1995). A message about the Family Health Care Decisions Act of 1995. New York: Author.

Norton, S. A., & Talerico, K. A. (2000). Facilitating end-of-life decision-making: Strategies for communicating and assessing. *Journal of Gerontological Nursing, 26*(9), 6–13.

Olson, E. (1993). Ethical issues in the nursing home. *Mt Sinai Journal of Medicine, 60,* 555–559.

Orentlicher, D. (1997). The Supreme Court and physician assisted suicide. Rejecting assisted suicide but embracing euthanasia. *New England Journal of Medicine, 337,* 1236–1239.

Pain Relief Promotion Act of 1999 (HR 2260).

Patel, R.V., Sinuff, T., & Cook, D. J. (2004). Influencing advance directive completion rates in non-terminally ill patients: A systematic review. *Journal of Critical Care, 19*(1),1–9.

Phillips, R. S., Hamel, M. B., Covinsky, K. E., & Lynn, J. (2000). Findings from SUPPORT and HELP: An introduction. *Journal of the American Geriatrics Society, 48*(5), S1–S5.

Phillips R. S, Hamel, M. B., Teno, J. M., et al (1996). For the SUPPORT Investigators. Race, resource use, and survival in seriously ill hospitalized adults. *J Gen Intern Med;11*:387–396.

Phipps, E., True, G., Harris, D., Chong, U., Tester, W., Chavin, S. I., & Braitman, L. E. (2003). Approaching the end of life: Attitudes, preferences, and behaviors of African-American and White patients and their family caregivers. *Journal of Clinical Oncology, 21,* 549–555.

Prendergast, T. J., & Puntillo, K. A. (2004). Withdrawal of life support: Intensive caring at the end of life. *Journal of the American Medical Association. 288,* 2732–2740.

President's Commission for the Study of Ethical Problems in Medicine and Biomedical and Behavioral Research. (1982, March). Deciding to forego life-sustaining treatment. Washington, DC: U. S. Government Printing Office.

Protocol for unit nurses: Asking patients about advance directives. (1999, January-February). *Innovations in End-of-Life Care, 1*(1). Retrieved 12/31/04 from *http://www2.edc.org/lastacts/archives/archives-Jan99/decisiontree.asp*

Pub.L.No. 101–508, '4206, 4751 [hereinafter OBRA], 104 Stat. 1388–115 to 117, 1388–204 to 206 (codified at 42 U.S.C.A. '1395cc(f) (1) & id. '1396a(a) (West Supp. 1994).

In re Quinlan, 70 N.J. 10, 355 A.2d 647 (N.J. 1976).

Robinson, M. K., DeHaven, M. J., & Koch, K. A. (1993). Effects of the patient self-determination act on patient knowledge and behavior. *Journal of Family Practice, 37,* 363–368.

Roth, Y. L., Meisel, A., & Lidz, C. W. (1977). Tests of competency to consent to treatment. *American Journal of Psychiatry, 134,* 279–284.

Rubin, S. M., Strull, W. M., Fialkow, F., Weiss, S. J., & Lo, B. (1994). Increasing the completion of the durable power of attorney for health care. *Journal of the American Medical Association, 271,* 209–212.

Sachs, G. A., Stocking, C. E., & Miles, S. H. (1992). Failure of an intervention to promote discussion of advance directives. *Journal of the American Geriatrics Society, 40,* 269–273.

Schneiderman, L. J., Pearlman, R. A., Kaplan, R. M., Anderson, J. P., & Rosenberg, E. M. (1992). Relationship of general advance directive instructions to specific life-sustaining treatment preferences in patients with serious illness. *Archives of Internal Medicine, 152,* 2114–2122.

Schloendorff v. Society of New York Hospitals, 211 N.Y. 125, 105 N.E. 92 (1914).

Schonwetter, R. S., Walker, R. M., Kramer, D. R., & Robinson, B. E. (1993). Resuscitation decision making in the elderly: The value of outcome data. *Journal of General Internal Medicine, 8,* 295–300.

Shapiro, J., & Bowles, K. (2002). Nurses' and consumers' understanding of and comfort with the Patient Self-determination Act. *Journal of Nursing Administration, 32,* 503–508.

Shapiro, R. (1996). Health care providers' liability exposure for inappropriate pain management. *Journal of Law, Medicine and Ethics, 24,* 360–364.

Smith, S. A., & Davis, A. J. (1980). Ethical dilemmas: Conflicts among rights, duties, and obligations. *American Journal of Nursing, 80,* 1462–1466.

Solomon, M. Z., O'Donnell, L., Jennings, B., Guilfoy, V., Wolf, S. M., & Nolan, K. (1993). Decisions near the end of life: Professional views on life-sustaining treatments. *American Journal of Public Health, 83*(1), 14–23.

Stetler, K. L., Elliott, B. A., & Bruno, C. A. (1992). Living will completion in older adults. *Archives of Internal Medicine, 125,* 954–959.

Stiller, A., Molloy, D. W., Russo, R., Dubois, S., Kavsak, H., & Bedard, M. (2001). Development and evaluation of a new instrument that measures barriers to implementing advance directives. *Journal of Clinical Outcomes Management, 8*(4), 26–31.

Swidler, R. (1989). The presumption of consent in New York State's do-not-resuscitate law. *New York State Journal of Medicine, 89,* 69–72.

Teno, J., Lynn, J., Phillips, R.S., Murphy, D., Youngner, S. J., Bellamy, P., et al. (1994). For the SUPPORT Investigators. Do formal advance directives affect resuscitation decisions and the use of resources for seriously ill patients? *Journal Clinical Ethics, 5,* 23–30.

Teno, J., Lynn, J., Wenger, N., Phillips, R. S., Murphy, D. P., Connors, A. F., et al. (1997). For the SUPPORT Investigators. Advance directives for the seriously ill hospitalized patients: Effectiveness with the patient self determination act and the SUPPORT Intervention. *Journal of the American Geriatrics Society, 45,* 500–507.

Teno, J. M., Licks, S., Lynn, J., et al. (1997). For the SUPPORT Investigators. Do advance directives provide instructions that direct care? *Journal of the American Geriatrics Society, 45,* 508–512.

U.S. Department of Health and Human Services, Office of the Inspector General. (1993). *Patient advance directives: Early implementation experience* (OEI 06–91–01130). Washington, DC: Author.

Vacco v. Quill, 521 U.S. 793, 117 S.Ct. 2293 (1997).

Valente, S. (2004). End-of-life challenges: Honoring autonomy. *Cancer Nursing, 27,* 314–319.

Virani, R., & Sofer, D. (2003). Improving the quality of end-of-life care: Making changes at every level. *American Journal of Nursing, 103*(5), 52–60.

Washington v. Glucksberg, 117 S. Ct. 2258 (1997).

Wenger, N., Phillips, R., Teno, J., Oye, R., Dawson, N., Liu, H., et al. (2000). Physician understanding of patient resuscitation preferences: Insights and clinical implications. *Journal of the American Geriatrics Society, 48*(5), S44–S51.

Section III

Psychosocial Considerations

June 18

Candy had a friend from the neighborhood over when I arrived today. This woman was so eager to be of help to Candy and her family; apparently the whole neighborhood had rallied and were offering support by grocery shopping, preparing meals, house cleaning, and offering to watch the children. Candy's 5-year-old son was at his first sleepover and she was both pleased and sad that he felt comfortable leaving her to stay with a friend. She talked about how involved her husband was with her and the situation that they were in. She said they laughed about the sounds that came from her colostomy and how she could talk to him about the decisions she had to make regarding her care. Her therapist had talked with the children to determine their feelings and ideas about what was happening and helping them to deal with their

mother's illness. Candy did say that she has not talked to them about dying because she was not ready to talk about it herself. She was still struggling with her loss of function and role changes, now that she did not have the energy to care physically for her children.

Yet, Candy was still hoping for a cure. As a nurse, I knew that at some point the hope would change from a hope of cure to the hope for a comfortable death, free of pain and surrounded by those who loved her. I could only imagine her feelings of loss and grief. I, too, pushed the thoughts of death from my mind. Because I was close to her age, I became increasingly aware of my own mortality. As Candy told me how her children snuggled close to her in bed, I felt incredibly saddened by the thought of her death, and the idea that her children would lose their mother. I imagined the pain of my children, if I were to die.

8

Communicating with Seriously Ill and Dying Patients, Their Families, and Their Health Care Providers

Kathleen O. Perrin

AACN Competency

#3: Communicate effectively and compassionately with the patient, family, and health care team members about end-of-life issues.

> *Mitch*, he continued softly now, *you don't understand, I want to tell you about my life. I want to tell you before I can't tell you anymore.* His voice dropped to a whisper. *I want someone to hear my story. Will you?*
> —Mitch Albom (*Tuesday's With Morrie*)

Seriously ill or dying patients and their families want their health care providers to communicate with honesty (Furukawa, 1996) and caring (Czerwiec, 1996) prognoses and treatment options. The Study to Understand Prognoses and Preferences for Outcomes and Risks of Treatment (SUPPORT, 1995) demonstrated that this discussion does not occur as often as families and hospitalized patients would prefer. Because most Americans still die in hospitals; the absence of such discussion is a major shortfall in the care of dying Americans. Moreover, even for patients who are cared for at home and referred to hospice, discussion and preparation for death are often avoided until hospice referral. Because most patients are not referred to hospice until the last weeks of their lives, this means that discussion of end-of-life care is often postponed until it is unavoidable.

According to Servaty, Krejci, and Hayslip (1996), health care providers with less anxiety about death are more likely to talk meaningfully with dying patients. In their study, nursing students were less anxious and more willing then other college students and beginning medical students to communicate with dying people. Thus, they reasoned, nursing students may be responsive to educational endeavors to promote honest, caring communication with patients and families at the end of life. This chapter will explore ways in which educators might encourage both undergraduate and advanced practice nursing students to facilitate communication with dying patients, their families, and their health care providers.

In addition to patients and their families benefiting from communication with nurses at the end of life, the nurses may also benefit. Stiles (1990) described seven types of personal growth that nurses dealing with dying patients felt they experienced as "gifts" from their patients. These included learning to confront their own mortality, learning about self, developing a faith in self and in a higher being, transcending their limitations, learning realistic expectations, and clarifying personal responsibility. Although experienced nurses perceived these opportunities for personal growth as gifts from their patients, undergraduate nursing students may be more distressed by them. Ways in which nursing faculty members might assist undergraduate nursing students to enrich themselves by working with dying patients will also be explored in this chapter.

This chapter will be organized according to the phases of the therapeutic relationship because in many ways the phases of the therapeutic relationship—introductory, working, and termination—parallel the dying trajectory. When appropriate in the phases, distinctions will be made between the roles and educational needs of the undergraduate nursing student, the nurse with an undergraduate degree, the advanced practice nursing student, and the nurse with an advanced practice degree.

INTRODUCTORY PHASE

During the introductory phase of the therapeutic relationship, the nurse and patient open the relationship, begin to clarify and define the problem that has brought the patient in contact with the nurse, and begin to define their relationship.

Opening the Relationship

For the undergraduate nursing student, the components of this phase include conveying respect for the dying patient and his or her family as well as establishing a trusting relationship. These constituents are no different from their establishment in any therapeutic relationship. The student should introduce herself or himself to the patient and identify how the student will be involved in the patient's care. The nursing faculty member ought to note if the student caring for a dying patient seems unusually reluctant to engage in care of that patient. If the student appears hesitant, the faculty member might demonstrate by introducing himself or herself to the patient that this portion of the relationship is no different merely because the patient is dying. At this very early stage in the relationship, the student, or any health care provider, probably ought to avoid discussing the subject of death and dying unless the patient brings up the topic (Byock, 1997).

In contrast to the undergraduate nursing student or the nurse with an undergraduate degree, it may be the responsibility of the advanced practice nurse to explain to a patient that the patient is severely ill and may be dying during one of their initial meetings. It would always be preferable that the advanced practice nurse and patient have had an opportunity to establish a trusting relationship before the advanced practice nurse is required to deliver such bad news to the patient. However, in today's fast-paced health care environment, especially in emergency departments and critical care units, that is not always possible.

Conveying bad news requires thought and preparation. When preparing for the discussion, Buckman, Lipkin, Sourkes, and Tolle (1997) recommend that the health care provider locate a private place for the discussion, ask the patient to have a family member or friend present, have all information available to explain to the patient, and practice what she or he is planning to say. Buckman and colleagues (1997) suggest that after any introductions are made to the patient and family the patient be asked if it would be permissible to tape the interview. They state that taping the interview and providing the tape to the patient when the interview is finished enhances the patient's long-term adjustment. The steps recommended by Buckman (1992) for breaking bad news are listed in Table 8.1.

TABLE 8.1   Breaking "Bad News"

- Get the context right.

- Find out what is already known.

- Find out how much information the patient and/or family wants to know.

- Share the information, starting from their viewpoint and step by step bring their understanding closer to the medical facts.

- Respond to their reactions using an empathetic approach.

- Explain the treatment plan and prognosis, summarize, and make a contract.

From *How to Break Bad News: A Guide for Health Professionals* by R. Buckman, 1992.

Buckman et al. (1997) recommends starting the interview by finding out what the patient knows or suspects. Often the patient has a preconception of the problem and it may be necessary not only to convey bad news but to counter the patient's and family's misconceptions of the situation. Not all patients want to know the extent of their illness, so it is also important for the advanced practice nurse to determine at this point in the interview how much information the patient desires. Kagawa-Singer and Blackhall (2001) note that people from other cultures may not emphasize autonomy as much as Americans do. In some cultures, it is the family and not the individual who learn the prognosis and agree to a plan of care. To uncover the desires of such patients and families, Kagawa-Singer and Blackhall suggest utilizing the following question: "Some patients want to know everything about their condition, others prefer that we talk with their families. How would you like to get information?" (p. 2995).

Before actually stating the problem, Buckman et al. (1997) suggests foreshadowing the news in simple language such as "I'm sorry I have some bad news for you." They suggest that the situation then be explained in simple terms that are understandable to the patient. At this point, Buckman et al. (1997) recommends something that can be very difficult for the beginning practitioner—silence. During the period of silence, the patient will have an opportunity to absorb the information, react, and ask questions.

After the information is conveyed to the patient and the patient has had a chance to react, Buckman et al. (1997) suggest an empathetic approach. This implies that the advanced practice nurse should first identify the emotion that the patient is experiencing and identify the origins of the emotion. Then, the nurse should respond in a way that tells the patient that the nurse understands what the patient is experiencing. This means the nurse should "reflect, name, and legitimize the patient's feelings" (Buckman et al., 1997 p. 63). For example, the nurse might say, "I can see that this has really upset you. Was that something that you weren't expecting" (Radziewicz & Baile, 2001, p. 952).

The final step in breaking bad news is providing an initial explanation of potential treatments and prognoses. Later in the therapeutic relationship, the advance practice nurse may become involved in empowering the patient to be an active participant in the decision-making process about treatment and developing an agreement about care. At this stage, the possibilities are usually just described to provide the patient and family with an opportunity to begin thinking about goals of treatment. Before the interview is complete, the advanced practice nurse should summarize the discussion for the patient.

Tulsky, Chesney, and Lo (1996) recommend that a new practitioner (such as a resident or advanced practice nurse student) be observed several times and offered feedback before being allowed to discuss bad news without supervision. Emanuel (1998) suggests the new practitioner be provided with talking points so that all of the appropriate information is covered. Latimer (1998) describes criteria for ethical communication of information that might be used to evaluate the communication skills of a beginning practitioner. To be ethical, according to Latimer, the communication should be timely and desired by the patient. The information must be accurate. The words should be understandable to the patient and family and the information must be conveyed in a gentle, respectful, and compassionate manner.

There is developing awareness that an individual health care provider should not confront a patient and family with bad news without informing other members of the health care team of the details of the discussion (Davis, Kristjanson, & Blight, 2003; Fallowfield & Jenkins, 2004; Larson & Tobin, 2000; Pattison, 2004). Unfortunately, more than 80% of physicians in a study by Ptacek, Ptacek, and Ellison (2001) did not have another health care provider accompany them when they delivered bad news. When individual providers provide bad news to patients and families without informing the other members of the health care team, the lack of communication can be a significant barrier to quality end-of-life care (Yabroff & Mandelblatt, 2004). Patients and families who are anxious often do not hear or understand bad news the first time they hear it. Nurses describe feeling caught "in the middle" or "going in blind" when they don't know what a patient has been told and the patient or family is requesting further information or explanations (Davis et al., 2003). In order to improve communication and develop an alliance among health care providers, patient, and families, Pattison (2004) suggests a policy change requiring that a senior or primary nurse be present when such discussions are initiated in the hospital.

Clarifying the Problem

There are several components to the phase of clarifying the problem. They include facilitating the patient's expression of emotions, identification of what the patient and family believe are problems, and identifying and responding to the patient's and family's concerns about care. Nurses at all levels should be expert in assisting patients to clarify what they believe are their significant health-care-related concerns.

When the health care provider delivering the bad news has not informed the other members of the health care team about the discussion, it is often difficult for a nurse to identify if a patient has received bad news or when the patient is prepared to discuss such news. May (1995) suggests that if the nurse was present at the interview when the bad news was delivered, the patient will feel free to initiate a conversation when the patient is ready. If the nurse was not present during the interview, but suspects such an interview has occurred, the nurse might say to the patient, "I noticed the physician [or advanced practice nurse] was speaking with you. What did she have to say?" Larson and Tobin (2000) suggest asking a more general question such as, "How is this hospitalization going for you and your family?" or "What has been the most difficult thing about this illness for you?" (p. 1574). May (1995) emphasizes that the nurse should not initiate such a discussion unless the nurse is able to sit down and actively listen to the patient. Initiating a discussion of patient concerns or problems requires that the nurse have strong facilitative communication skills and be able to put aside other competing demands for her or his time.

May (1995) warns that when a nurse asks a patient how the patient feels, the patient usually responds by describing her or his physical condition. Thus, if a nurse wants information about the person's psychological concerns, the question will need to be phrased somewhat differently. Byock (1997) began using the phrase, "How are you feeling within yourself?" after he had noticed that hospice workers in England successfully cut though defenses and learned how the patient was feeling when they were asked that question. He suggests it as a way of getting immediately to the heart of the patient's concerns. Emanuel (1998) recommends several questions including the following: "During the last few weeks how often have you felt downhearted or blue?" "What do you believe is bothering you?" "Who are you able to confide in?"

Wilkinson (1991) examined factors that influenced how nurses communicated with cancer patients. She concluded that in general, nurses had difficulty employing facilitative communication with patients with cancer. She noted that nurses frequently used blocking techniques when dealing with patients who had had a recurrence of their cancer. Because these blocking techniques prevented the nurses from identifying patient concerns, the nurses obtained only a superficial nursing assessment and planned nursing care based on assumptions rather then on actual patient concerns.

Wilkinson (1991) identified three groups of nurses who used different methods to block patient communication. These were ignorers, informers, and mixed responders. *Ignorers* ignored patient cues to talk about specific problems or issues throughout the interview. These nurses changed the subject, engaged in conversation with the patient's relative, or began social chitchat to avoid emotionally laden conversations. *Informers* were nurses who gave elaborate explanations of procedures, offered inappropriate advice, or stated their opinions without being asked. These nurses indicated that providing such detailed, unasked for information allowed

them to maintain control of the situation and avoid difficult or emotionally laden conversations (Wilkinson, 1991). *Mixed responders* were the largest group of nurses in Wilkinson's study. They utilized both facilitative and blocking responses, attempted to understand patient problems, and were more aware of their blocking behaviors when questioned about them.

Although they had been taught facilitative communication, most of the practicing nurses in Wilkinson's 1991 study were unaware that they were blocking their patients' attempts to communicate important needs and concerns until they listened to an audio tape and discussed their responses. Undergraduate nursing students need experiences in communicating with dying patients, with opportunities to have their interactions evaluated by a nursing faculty member in order to develop proficiency in communication with seriously ill patients. An audiotape allows the faculty member a complete, accurate record of the verbal component of the communication between the student and patient. The patient's consent for taping must be obtained and in some circumstances the Institution Review Board (IRB) of the facility may also need to provide approval. The faculty member then may use the tape as a tool to discuss the student responses as well as possible facilitative alternatives. Heaven and Maquire (1996) noted that demonstration with audiotaping and feedback improved the facilitative communication skills of nurses with an undergraduate degree. However, since the improvement was not to a statistically significant extent, further study of this approach is warranted.

Moreover, taping is often not possible. On occasion, the faculty member may be present during the student's interview with the patient. This has the advantage of allowing the faculty member to observe the nonverbal behavior of the student and patient as well as the verbal. In many circumstances it permits the faculty member to provide immediate feedback to the student. If direct observation is not possible, then student journals or verbatim process recordings can be used to allow faculty to help students develop an ability to facilitate rather then block communication with seriously ill patients.

Slightly less then a quarter of the nurses in Wilkinson's 1991 study used primarily facilitative communication techniques when interviewing cancer patients. Nurses who used these techniques were able to do so no matter how ill the patient was or how emotionally laden the material to be divulged. By employing such standard facilitative communication techniques as active listening, use of open-ended questions, reflection or clarification of patient concerns, and empathy, they were able to obtain a more in-depth understanding of their patients' problems and concerns. In "An Interview with Dr. Stuart Farber," (1999) Farber states that patients and families most welcomed and remembered interactions with nursing staff that were personalized to the needs of the individual patient and family.

Yabroff and Mandelblatt (2004) emphasize that it is not only health care providers who may establish barriers to good communication and optimal patient care. Patients and families may also establish such barriers by their inability to confront death and their utilization of defense mechanisms like disbelief, anger, and denial. Radziewicz and Baile (2001) describe ways that the nurse with an undergraduate degree might recognize and respond therapeutically to each of these behaviors. They define disbelief as "the patient or family's attempt to make sense of what they have heard" (p. 952). They recommend the nurse respond to the patient's disbelief by saying something like, "Accepting such a serious illness must be hard because you have taken such good care of yourself" (p.

952). They believe that anger can be one of the most difficult emotions for an inexperienced nurse with an undergraduate degree to deal with especially since it may be targeted at health care providers. Radziewicz and Baile recommend that the nurse realize the anger is often masking another strong emotion such as fear or disappointment. So, the nurse might respond to the angry patient or family member by saying, "I can see how frightening this is for you. Do you want to tell me more about it?" (p. 952).

Radziewicz and Baile (2001) define denial as the patient's refusal to believe bad news, saying that the news is a mistake and not real. Block (2001) notes that denial is a natural response that may be helping the patient to deal with the illness and should be respected. Radziewicz and Baile believe the nurse should not argue with the patient or family who is expressing the denial, should acknowledge the difficulty in accepting the truth, suggest a possible reason for the difficulty, but avoid continuing any blaming or feeling of mistake (Radziewice and Baile, p. 953). For example, a family member might say, "The doctors don't know what they're talking about. My father is going to be fine! He's going to walk again. I don't want anyone to tell me otherwise." The nurse might respond, "It must be difficult believing something so unimaginable could be happening when everything was fine a few days ago." Block agrees with this approach unless the patient is one of the 10% of patients who is in severe denial and the denial is likely to cause problems. In such a circumstance, Block recommends challenging the patient's denial to achieve a greater good. The nurse with an undergraduate degree might say, "I know that making a decision about this is extremely painful, yet if we don't make plans now, we may lose that chance" (Block, 2001, p. 953).

Rosenbaum and Kreiter (2002), Farrell, Ryan, and Langrick (2001), and Ambuel,

(2003) have demonstrated that health care providers can learn to respond to such patient and family behaviors by role-playing case studies. Some authors suggest scripted case studies, others establish a general style of patient/family behavior and allow the health care participants to practice a variety of responses. In either instance, after role-playing, health care providers indicate more confidence in their abilities and greater willingness to communicate with patients who have received bad news. Nursing faculty members can incorporate case studies in undergraduate or graduate nursing education programs that require nursing students to role-play responses to patient and family defense mechanisms of disbelief, anger, or denial.

It is also important to realize that just because the topic is dying and the problems are serious, the talk does not always need to be solemn. Langley-Evans and Payne (1997) noted that lighthearted talk about illness, symptoms, bereavement, and personal mortality was quite valuable to outpatients in a palliative day-care center. What was important was the nursing staff created an atmosphere that facilitated rather then blocked patients' disclosure of their concerns. Table 8.2 lists essential nursing communication behaviors for both the undergraduate and graduate nurse.

Advance practice nurses can do a great deal to encourage nurses with an undergraduate degree to communicate with dying patients. Studies by Wilkinson (1991) and Booth, Maguire, Butterworth, and Hillier (1996) found the major predictor of nursing staff's use of facilitative communication with patients with cancer or in hospice was the supportiveness of the nurses' supervisor. In the study by Wilkinson, the ward sisters (unit managers) who took assignments, cared for patients, and demonstrated facilitative communication with patients to their staff had staff who were more likely to communicate therapeutically with their patients. These same ward sisters

TABLE 8.2   Essential Behaviors

BASIC	ADVANCED
Interpreting "bad" news	Conveying "bad" news
Listening to clients' and families' concerns about EOL care	Initiating the discussion of EOL treatment options
Reviewing EOL treatment options	Promoting a supportive unit environment
Assisting patients, families, and HCPs to make EOL decisions	Determining with other HCPs that patient is dying
Advocating for patient's choices at EOL	Initiating discussion of EOL treatment withdrawal
Implementing EOL treatment withdrawal	Establishing palliative care contract
Preparing patient and family for physical signs of impending death	Dealing with families in crisis after a sudden unexpected death
Smoothing the passage	Presenting organ donation options
Being with patient and family during the dying process	
Consoling the bereaved family	

also encouraged their nurses to work autonomously and make decisions about nursing care. They had negotiated with the physicians who admitted patients to their units to obtain permission for the nurses to talk truthfully with any patient who requested information about her or his prognosis or treatment.

Advanced practice nurses need to have excellent facilitative communication skills. They must be able to communicate with patients individually but they must also be able to demonstrate to staff members ways to communicate with difficult patients and families. The advance practice nurse's efforts to create an environment where communication between patient and nurse is valued is essential to developing the communication skills of the nurse with an undergraduate degree. Although theory is important, practice with evaluation or supervision by a skilled practitioner is what allows an advanced practice nurse to develop such a level of mastery of facilitative communication skills.

Structuring and Formulating the Care Agreement

There are several components to this phase of the therapeutic relationship. In any therapeutic relationship, the nurse and patient should be continuing to develop trust during this phase, coming to an agreement about the frequency of meetings, and developing goals for care and the relationship. At this point in a dying patient's care, the advanced practice nurse might initiate a discussion of the patient's treatment goals. Murphy and Price (1995) emphasize that the nurse should avoid using any phrase that resembles "There is nothing more that we can do." Although the phrase may be intended by the health care provider to convey that the patient's disease will progress and the patient will eventually die, it often implies to the patient and family that the health care team will abandon the patient.

Instead of focusing on what will not be done, the advanced practice nurse, patient, family, and other members of the health care team should begin to identify goals for patient care.

Farber ("Interview," 1999) identified a number of possible goals that a dying patient might choose. These included living to the last possible second, living until the burden becomes too great, living at home with family, avoiding medical interventions, living as comfortably as possibly until death, and avoiding medical treatments unless they will have meaningful outcomes. Once a goal has been identified, the health care team, patient, and family can begin to identify interventions that will achieve that goal.

Cotton (1993) noted that many physicians avoid initiating discussions about end-of-life treatment with their patients for fear the patients will become depressed or distrustful of the physicians' willingness to care for them. Often physicians of dying patients will delay the conversation until the patient is unresponsive and the family must be consulted (Shmerling, Bedell, Lilienfeld, & Delbanco, 1988). In fact, patients, especially elders, want to identify goals and interventions for end-of-life care and are relieved when the subject is broached. Most Americans do not have an advance directive, yet as long as they are competent, it is their right to have the deciding voice in the type of health care they receive. When the physician or advanced practice nurse avoids discussing the goals of end-of-life care until the patient is unresponsive, the patient is deprived of the right to determine appropriate end-of-life care.

The role of the nurse with an undergraduate degree is to interpret the medical information into terms the patient can understand and repeatedly explain the end-of-life treatment options to the patient. Patients and families often indicate that listening to the health care provider's explanation of a patient's prognosis and possibilities for treatment is like trying to understand a foreign language. In addition, most patients and their families experience stress when they receive bad news. Thus, they are unable to hear or retain much of what the physician or advanced practice nurse explained to them. Being able to repeatedly replay the taped information is one of the reasons a tape recording of the initial interview may be beneficial for some patients and families (Buckman et al., 1997). However, most of the time, it is the responsibility of the nurse with an undergraduate degree to translate medical jargon into language the patient can comprehend and to reinforce the information regularly.

WORKING PHASE

During the working phase of the therapeutic relationship, the nurse explores and understands the patient's feelings and expectations, elaborates on the goals of treatment developed in the previous phase, and facilitates or takes actions that the patient desires. In this case, the feelings and expectations explored relate to the dying process and the goals include defining what the patient believes constitutes dying well.

Exploring and Understanding Patient's Feelings and Expectations About Death and Dying

Both the advanced practice and undergraduate nursing student should be able to assist a patient to define what she or he believes constitutes dying well or represents a good and timely death. Quill (2000) recognizes that health care providers often do not agree about appropriate indications to begin a discussion with patients and families about end-of-life care. Although be believes the discussion should begin sooner, he states it is urgent to have such a discussion with patients who

are facing imminent death, are talking about wanting to die, are inquiring about hospice, have been hospitalized for a severe progressive illness, or are suffering out of proportion to the prognosis. Quill suggests beginning the conversation with a question such as "What would be undone if you were to die sooner rather than later?" (p. 2504). Quill believes this question subtlety conveys the message that time may be short and plans ought to be made now.

Nurses at all practice levels should be involved in helping to identify with the patient which issues would be most important to address so the patient might die well. Some of the issues that may be important to patients at the end of life include participating in those end-of-life rituals that provide meaning to the patient and family, completing unfinished business, resolving relationship concerns with family and friends, and carrying out a life review. Once the issues are identified, members of the health care team may assist in addressing them.

The nurse will need to inquire of the patient and family about any end-of-life customs or rituals that provide meaning to them. Because a range of responses occurs within cultural and religious groups (Kagawa-Singer & Blackhall, 2001; Mazanec & Tyler, 2004), it is imperative that the nurse not assume specific rituals will be of significance to a patient and family simply because they are members of a particular ethnic or religious group. The nurse might want to inquire: "What is your faith or belief? "Is there a religious or ethnic community that is a source of support for you? Would you like me to notify the community or arrange for something for you?" Once these customs or rituals have been identified, Mazanec and Tyler (2004) state they should be integrated into the plan of care for the dying patient.

Patients may have a wide variety of unfinished business. Often these issues are related to the patient's age and developmental level. For example, a teenager might want to graduate from high school or an older adult might want to witness the arrival of a first grandchild. To identify what business, if any, the patient would like to complete, the nurse might ask, "If you were to die soon, what would be left undone?" or "Is there some event that would add a great deal of meaning to your life? What do we have to do so that event can take place?" Once the issue has been identified, rules might need to be bent (e.g., a child be allowed to participate in graduation ceremonies without completing required coursework, a grandchild or pet allowed into an intensive care unit), resources expended, or help mobilized to permit the event to happen.

Patients may need both time and assistance to resolve relationship problems with their family and friends. Byock (2004) advocates that patients and their families make every effort to say four things to each other as they prepare to say farewell: "Please forgive me; I forgive you; Thank you; and I love you"(p. 5). He believes that saying these four things "offers essential wisdom for completing a lifelong relationship before a final parting." When dying people "can reach out to express love, gratitude, and forgiveness . . . they consistently find that they, and everyone involved, are transformed for the rest of their lives, whether those lives last for decades or just days" (p. 7).

Emanuel (1998) notes that some patients seem to be able to postpone dying so that they can complete their family business. Often, deaths occur after important events such as birthdays or holidays. One woman who was dying from respiratory failure asked to have her life prolonged by whatever means necessary until her estranged daughter, whom she had not seen in 10 years, arrived from across the country. After the daughter's arrival, arrangements were made for counseling ses-

sions for the mother and daughter. Two days later, the mother died with the daughter present, holding her mother's hand.

Life review is another important part of both the aging and the dying process. According to Butler ("Roundtable discussion," 1996),

> life review is a normal developmental task of the later years characterized by the return of memories and past conflicts. In some cases, this can contribute to psychological growth, including the resolution of past conflicts, reconciliation with significant others, atonement for past wrongdoing, personality integration, and serenity. (p. 42)

Mazanac and Tyler (2004) encourage nurses to participate in patients' life reviews. They believe that when patients are encouraged to tell their life stories, the patients are often able to recognize meaning and purpose in their lives. Being present with the patient while the patient begins a life review means a commitment on the part of the nurse to listen actively and devote time to the patient. This is a skill that all nurses ought to have, although it does not require the presence of a nurse or even a professional for the patient to conduct a life review. Life review can provide the patient with a powerful way to work out family relationships and gain a sense of inner peace.

Talking with Patients Across the Life Span and Their Families About Death

A nurse caring for a dying child must establish a trusting relationship with the child and its parents. Novice nurses should be especially aware of their emotions and though empathizing with the family should avoid burdening them with their own emotions (Buckman et al., 1997). Children want to know varying amounts of information about their illness. However, most children want to have an appreciation of how the illness will affect the way they will be able to live their lives. Like adults, however, children vary in how much information they are able to understand and absorb even when it is presented at an appropriate level. Young children's verbalization about their potential death can vary across a continuum and may be fluid over time (Buckman et al., 1997). At one end of the continuum, children will state that they are very sick or have a bad disease but will not mention death. Often, children younger than 7 or 8 years of age view death as temporary and reversible, happening only to others and perhaps caused by previous thoughts and actions (Freyer, 2004). Other children may mention an uncertainty about living but will not allude to dying. At the far end of the continuum, usually when the child is older than 7 or 8, the child may understand the central aspects of death and may state that she or he could die from this illness. Freyer believes that children today are more insulated from death than in the past and are more likely to learn about death from television and video games than from real-life occurrences. In order to understand children's concerns, the advance practice nurse might utilize play therapy or drawing with various colors to help children express their emotions, fears, and realizations about death.

Adolescents, especially ones who have been chronically ill, usually have an accurate understanding of death and are able to verbalize its personal significance as well as it its effect on others. Freyer (2004) notes that adolescents "who are medically experienced often demonstrate remarkable insight into their illnesses, prospects for survival, and preferences for how they wish to spend their remaining time" (p. 383). Due to this insight, "adolescents older than 14 are usually assumed to have functional competency to make binding medical decisions for themselves, including decisions relating to the discontinuance of life-sustaining therapy and end of life issues" (Freyer, 2004, p. 383). Freyer emphasizes it is essential that a truthful, honest relationship be established with the adolescent from the very beginning. He believes this can be accomplished if health care providers establish an agreement with the adolescent to share all relevant information with the adolescent as soon as it is available and the adolescent agrees to ask all questions, no matter how trivial. In order to assure that the adolescent feels free to ask all his or her questions, the nurse will want to assure that the nurse has time to spend speaking with the adolescent alone, without either parent present.

Freyer (2004) notes that because most adolescents really do not believe they can ever die, they may talk about death and plan for their eventual death in ways that seem contradictory. At one moment they may be making plans for termination of chemotherapy and a few moments later they may be talking about attending an event that is years in the future. The nurse may want to help the adolescent arrange to attend important life events (e.g., school prom or graduation) in the near future while helping the adolescent recognize and accept his or her deteriorating condition.

Parents of seriously ill, possibly dying children may have difficulty making sense of what is being said or experienced (Anderson & Hall, 1995). They may feel unable to make decisions, especially if they believe that both minor and major decisions are needed simultaneously. At times, according to Anderson and Hall (1995), the parents may feel they cannot differentiate between decisions that merely involve personal preference and ones that have grave implications. They may need help from nurses untangling these concrete issues but also in dealing with more philosophical ones such as how to determine the line between what is best or right for their child and what is best or right for them.

Nurses can help these families by reminding them that "forced or hasty decision making may cause them to abrogate responsibility because they have not had an opportunity to understand the issues, their feelings or their roles" (Anderson & Hall, 1995, p. 16). Experienced nurses with an undergraduate education can assist the parents to understand the issues, express their feelings, and delineate their roles so that the parents can be actively involved in the decision-making process for their children.

Young or middle-aged adults who are dying may feel they have a great deal of unfinished business or many unresolved relationships. The dying patient may need professional assistance in dealing with anger at leaving so much undone. A parent who is dying and leaving young children behind may need assistance from a nurse to find ways to leave mementos or lasting words of wisdom for the children. Some dying parents pick out special Christmas mementos in July for their children. One mother made 12 audiotapes with words of love and encouragement for her only child, one for each year until he would reach age 21.

Older adults are often perceived by health care providers as having lived a full life and being prepared to die. Yet, according to Cavendish (1999), nurses should assess all elders' quality of life prior to the illness and realize that many have the potential for additional healthy, happy years. Farber ("Interview," 1999) states that adults over the age of 70 usually do not believe they have a choice in health care treatment. When asked how they had made decisions, they answered, "What do you mean? The doctor told us what to do and we did it." Nurses, especially advance practice nurses, need to assist elders in participating in their treatment decisions whenever they appear to desire a decision-making role. Finally, life review is particularly important for the dying elder ("Roundtable discussion," 1996), so time and a compassionate listener should be allotted to this important activity. The nurse with an undergraduate degree might be this compassionate listener or the nurse might delegate another individual for this task.

Facilitating and Taking Action

There are several components of this phase. The first part is determining that the patient will die soon. The nurse with an undergraduate degree may be involved with other health care providers in deciding when the patient is entering the active dying phase, while the advanced practice nurse, in some circumstances, may participate in the decision that further treatment is futile when the patient is clearly dying. According to Cassem (Stein, 1999), nurses are the people who guide patients along the path to a peaceful death by recognizing when the patient is suffering needlessly because of inappropriate aggressive treatment. The physician, in some settings, may be the last to realize the patient is dying. Therefore, it becomes incumbent on nurses to relay their impressions to the physician and possibly to the family. The SUPPORT (1995) study indicates that there are problems in the way such information is communicated in hospital settings. Ways to improve the communication between nurses, physicians, and patients or their families when the patient's life is about to end are still under investigation (Jezewski, 1996).

Determining and agreeing that the patient is dying is extremely important, because most deaths in the United States occur in hospitals and all patients in hospitals must receive cardiopulmonary resuscitation (CPR) unless the physician or advance practice nurse has written a Do Not Resuscitate (DNR) order. Once there is a determination that the patient is dying, the physician or advanced practice nurse should discuss a DNR order with the patient, family, and other health care providers.

There are two common mistakes that inexperienced practitioners make when discussing a DNR order. The first is to ask "Do you want everything done?" Most laypersons do not assume "everything" means compressing the chest of a person who has already died. They assume it means comfort, care, and support. So, they often answer yes when they really would not want CPR. The second mistake is to use the words "There is nothing more we can do." Although the patient is dying and medical interventions will not prevent the death, there is much that health care providers can do to help the patient die well. The role of the advanced practice nurse is to initiate this discussion using Latimer's (1998) criteria for ethical communication described earlier and listed in Table 8.3. However, Tulsky et al. (1996) stress that new practitioners, such as residents and advanced practice nursing students, should be evaluated by skilled professionals before being allowed to attempt such a discussion on their own.

The nurse with an undergraduate degree is usually the staff member to whom the patient and family turn to discuss exactly what

a DNR order is and what the ramifications are likely to be for the patient (Peel, 2003). If that nurse was not present for the discussion, he or she might use the question, "I noticed the physician [advanced practice nurse] was speaking with you. What did she say?" The nurse might follow that with, "Many people have questions about what this means for them. What questions do you have?" Most people want reassurance that they are not forgoing an intervention that is likely to offer them benefit. Because only about 12% of all patients survive from CPR to hospital discharge, this reassurance is easy to provide.

As noted previously, the nurse is often the guide on the path to a peaceful death (Stein, 1999). This role is important because the decision to forgo CPR is merely the first of many decisions the patient and family may need to make about end-of-life care. After deciding to forgo CPR, the patient and family might choose to forgo any further curative therapy or might opt to have only comfort measures provided for the patient. Palliative care decisions may need to be made that involve the amount of pain medication the patient desires and whether the patient wishes to receive medical interventions for hydration and nutrition or even to continue eating and drinking. Nurses with an undergraduate degree who are caring for a dying patient should be able to describe the benefits and burdens of each of these therapies to the patient. They should also be able to facilitate patient and family decision-making about these choices through effective communication.

The nurse may be responsible for advocating for the patient's wishes for end-of-life care and communicating them to the family and other health care providers. This is easier if the patient has verbally expressed a preference to the nurse and is willing to state that preference to the physician and family. It may be more difficult when the nurse, physician,

---

TABLE 8.3   Criteria for Ethical Communication of Information

- The communication should be timely and desired by the patient

- The information must be accurate

- The words should be understandable to the patient and family

- The information must be conveyed in a "gentle, respectful, and compassionate manner"

From *Ethical Care at the End of Life*, by E. Latimer, 1998.

and family are trying to interpret an advance directive that does not fit the patient's situation precisely, when the person who has the durable power of attorney for health care purposes is not clear about the patient's wishes, or when there is no advance directive. Harlow, in "Family letter writing" (1999), recommends that the family or proxy consider the following:

1. What type of person was the patient?
2. Did the patient ever comment on another person's situation when they were incapacitated or on life support?
3. Did the patient relate those experiences to his or her own personal views for herself or himself?
4. What vignettes can you recall from the patient's life that illustrates her or his values and beliefs?

In "Family letter writing" (1999), Harlow then asks the family to write a letter incorporating the answers to these questions. He believes that the process is almost a spiritual one for the families that often brings them closer together. It helps them to review and clarify the person's life and understand what was meaningful to the person. Harlow notes that family letter writing may be "experienced by the family as a last act of commitment and caring toward their loved one." The nurse may be the person who encourages the family to begin such an activity. However, the ultimate decision on how to respond to the patient's and family's wishes rests with the physician or advance practice nurse.

Once a decision is made to limit further aggressive, curative treatment, the advance practice nurse may be involved in establishing a palliative care understanding with the patient and family. This is an understanding of what the health care team will do for and with the patient and family. Byock (1997) offers the following version of a commitment between the health care team and a dying patient:

> We will keep you warm and we will keep you dry. We will keep you clean. We will help you with elimination, and your bowels and your bladder function. We will always offer you food and fluid. We will be with you. We will bear witness to your pain and your sorrows, your disappointments and your triumphs; we will listen to the stories of your life and remember the story of your passing. (p. 247)

Although the advance care nurse or physician may be the person who establishes this palliative care understanding, it is the nurse with an undergraduate degree who is responsible for assuring that it is carried out. It is imperative that the nurse demonstrates by words and deeds that the health care providers will not abandon the patient after end-of-life choices are made; that instead, nurses and other health care workers will provide the care the patient needs or will teach and assist family members or friends to provide the care and support the patient requires while dying.

TERMINATION PHASE

During this phase in the therapeutic relationship, the nurse, family, and patient prepare for the end of the relationship, accept the feelings of loss, and review or evaluate what has occurred. As a patient is dying, this phase may entail withdrawing medical interventions, preparing the patient and family for the physical signs of impending death, smoothing the passage, consoling the bereaved family, exploring personal reactions, and evaluating nursing responses.

Withdrawing Medical Interventions

During the termination phase, medical interventions, such as ventilators, IV fluids and nutrition, or dialysis may be withdrawn. The nurse reassures the family that withdrawing such aggressive medical interventions from the dying patient is acceptable to most of the major religious and ethical traditions. The nurse demonstrates that despite the withdrawal of curative measures, the health care team will remain present and will provide aggressive comfort measures and respect the patient's individuality.

Preparing the Patient and Family for Physical Signs of Impending Death

Both the nurse with an undergraduate degree and the advanced practice nurse will need to be able to explain the final stages of the dying process to the patient and family. A family that does not understand the dying process may become anxious and feel unable to cope with the patient's care. The nurse may initiate the discussion by stating, "There are some common signs and symptoms that identify when a person's life is coming to an end. Not all of the signs occur in every person nor do they happen in the same sequence in each person. But it might be helpful if we talk about what may be occurring soon and what you may need or want to do."

Smoothing the Passage

As death approaches, patients may display a variety of typical behaviors. Nurses educated at the undergraduate and graduate levels should be able to explain these behaviors to family members and assist families and dying patients to communicate with each other during the patient's last days and hours. According to Callanan (1994), when a patient is approaching death, she or he may begin to speak in symbolic language. The patient might say, "Oh, here are my mother and brother-in-law, they've come to get me. We have to catch the train." Or, "It's a beautiful place that I'm going to now." Callanan cautions that the family may fear the patient is "losing his mind" or believe she or he is reliving the past. In actuality, it is believed that the patient is preparing to detach from this life. Callanan suggests that nurses should help the family listen to the patient's statements and respond with gentle open-ended questions such as, "When does the train leave?" The family should be discouraged from trying to reorient the patient ("Your mother died years ago") or contradicting the patient ("You're not going anywhere!").

Close to the moment of death, the patient may appear more withdrawn, almost detached from the surroundings. The nurse should inform the family that although the patient may appear unresponsive, they should still communicate verbally with the patient because the patient can probably still hear what people in the room are saying. The family may want to say Good-bye or one of the four things that Byock (2004) believes matters most—"Please forgive me; I forgive you; Thank you; and I love you"—if they have not done so already. This might be a time for the family to recount some favorite memories that illustrate what the dying person meant to them. A member of the family might say, "We will miss you, but we will always love you and we understand that it is time for you to go." Or, a family member or close friend might simply be present with the dying person, sitting nearby, holding the person's hand or lying next to the person and embracing him or her.

It is the role of the nurse to help the patient and families find an appropriate way to express their feelings and to smooth the patient's passage from this life. Individuals take their own time dying, and each death occurs at its own pace. The nurse may need to help the patient's family understand how idiosyncratically and sometimes how slowly the final moments may pass.

Consoling the Bereaved Family

Nurses educated at all levels of practice will need to be able to console families through the bereavement process. If the family has not been present during the death, the nurse will want to prepare the body and attempt to create a peaceful environment for the family to view the deceased. Because the nurse is often the professional present at the death or the one who views the body with the family, the nurse will need to demonstrate an acceptance of death and display respect for the deceased. If the family was not present for the death, the members may want a description of the patient's last moments. The nurse should respond both tactfully and truthfully. If it is true, saying to the family, "She was not alone" or "He seemed to be at peace" may be a great source of comfort to the family.

Although students in undergraduate programs and recent graduates of these programs often are worried about what they ought to say to the family at this time, bereaved families usually are more in need of someone to listen to them. Thus, one of the major roles of the nurse at this time is active, compassionate listening. Short statements like "I'm sorry" and "I'll keep you in my thoughts or prayers" may be helpful but the nurse usually does not need to say much. Trivializing statements such as "She is better off now" or "I know just how you feel" are inappropriate. Depending on the nurse's relationship with the family, a hug might be helpful to both the family and the nurse. The nurse's expression of emotion through tears is not unprofessional when it is an expression of the attachment between the nurse and the patient.

When the death is sudden and unexpected, it is often more difficult for both the health care providers and the family to understand. It is usually the physician or the advance practice nurse who conveys the fact of the death to the family. Buckman et al. (1997) recommend a simple unequivocal statement that the patient (her or his name should be used) has died and the cause stated. Then the health care provider should remain silent and allow an opportunity for the family to respond and ask further questions. A truthful statement that the advance practice nurse is sorry helps some families. Though some people prefer a human touch at this point, others may withdraw in grief. When the initial response has subsided, Buckman recommends focusing on the needs of the family, determining if they need to phone anyone or if they would like an opportunity to view the body. If there is a possibility of organ donation, the advance practice nurse would broach the subject at this time.

Review of the Relationship, Exploration of Personal Feelings, and Evaluation of Nursing Responses

Although not a specific step in the therapeutic relationship, it is always wise following the termination of a relationship for the nurse to review the process to explore her or his feelings and evaluate her or his behavior. An undergraduate nursing student encountering his or her first experience with death may need to explore it with the faculty member or preceptor after the patient and family has been cared for. Ambuel (2003) suggests that a faculty member or preceptor who is debriefing a student should include questions such as, What went well? What was difficult? What did you learn from this experience that will influence your work with patients and families in the future? In most circumstances, it is helpful for the student to be involved in preparing the body and talking with the family. For the first experience with death, it is helpful if a nursing faculty member or an experienced nurse prepares the body with the student. While preparing the body, most undergraduate nursing students find it helpful if the faculty member provides simple factual statements of how the body changes after death. Many students will remark how different the deceased seems once the suffering is over and life has departed.

Undergraduate nursing students often state that listening to the family helps them to find some meaning in the dying experience. If the death has been anticipated, the family will frequently discuss how the patient felt in the last few days and weeks and will often convey a sense of relief that the patient is no longer struggling. The family may review the person's life and help the student to realize that it had reached its natural end.

When the death is sudden and unexpected, undergraduate nursing students often are distraught. This is especially true if the patient was close to their own or their parents' ages. A review of what happened to the patient with an emphasis on how the health care team responded may at least help the student realize there was no way in which the health care team could have prevented the death. Later, many undergraduate nursing students and new graduate nurses question why the person had to die at this time in his or her life. Active listening by the nursing faculty member or perhaps the hospital chaplain is most likely to assist the student to come to some understanding of the death.

Undergraduate nursing students may idealize death; they may want each experience to be mystical and transcendent. However, death, like birth, is both messy and difficult as well as beautiful and transcendent. Learning to live and care within the realm of what is possible for people at the end of their lives is often difficult for the undergraduate nursing student and the new graduate of an undergraduate nursing program. Nursing faculty should help the student recognize the realities that shaped the way in which this particular patient died and identify factors that the student would want to modify when caring for future patients.

CONCLUSION

When nurses communicate with their dying patients and the families, they have a clearer understanding of their patients' needs and goals at the end of life. Once these goals are established, the nurse may assist the patient in dying well. That death might include limited technology, symptom relief, life review with resolution of past uncompleted business, and the presence of loving family and friends. Or it might involve fighting for the last breath, remaining alive until the last possible second, using the latest medical technology. However, without thoughtful communication with the patient and family, the nurse cannot be sure which course to take to help the patient die well.

KEYPOINTS

1. Conveying or discussing "bad news" requires preparation–locating a private place for the conversation, asking the patient or family to have a significant other present, having as much information available as possible, and practicing what will be said.

2. Patients and their families may respond to "bad news" with disbelief, anger, or denial. Nurses and nursing students should practice their reactions to these defense mechanisms.

3. Nurses may inappropriately block patient or family communication by ignoring what the patient or family member has to say, offering elaborate explanations or inappropriate advice, and providing their opinions without being asked.

4. Nurses may assist patients and their families to decide what is important to them while the patient is dying by asking the patient, "What would be left undone if you died sooner rather than later".

5. Byock believes that it is essential that patients, their families, and significant others find time before the patient dies to say to each other "Please forgive me; I forgive you; Thank you; and I love you".

6. It is imperative that nurses demonstrate to patients and their families by their words and deeds that health care providers will not abandon the patient after a decision has been made about end-of-life care.

EDUCATION PLAN 8.1   Plan for Achieving Competencies: Communication With Patients, Families, and Health Care Providers

Knowledge Needed	Attitude	Skills	Undergraduate Behavioral Outcomes	Graduate Behavioral Outcomes	Teaching/Learning Strategies
Importance of communication for patients, families, and health care providers at the end of life.	★Affirm the value for communication at the end of life, for patients, family, and health care provider. ★Appreciate the benefits of communicating honestly with the dying patient and family. ★Acknowledge own level of death anxiety.	★Communicate with the dying patient and family in an honest and empathic manner.	★Effectively and compassionately communicate with patients and families at end of life. ★Clarify information presented by health care providers to the patient and family. ★Communicate patient/family wishes and preferences to members of the interdisciplinary team.	★Serve as a role model for effective and compassionate communication with patients and families at the end of life. ★Create an environment where effective and compassionate communication is a goal of care.	★Use a death anxiety instrument to measure nurses' own level of death anxiety, and discuss their death experiences in post-conference or seminar. ★Have students describe experiences of personal or professional growth related to end-of-life discussions. ★Have students write a letter to a member of their family, describing their end-of-life wishes (not to be shared in class).

(*continued*)

EDUCATION PLAN 8.1 *(continued)*

Knowledge Needed	Attitude	Skills	Undergraduate Behavioral Outcomes	Graduate Behavioral Outcomes	Teaching/Learning Strategies
Phases of a Therapeutic Relationship: Introductory Phase: —Opening the relationship; —Breaking or reinforcing bad news; —Clarifying the problem by effective communication skills; —Structuring and formulating the care agreement and goals of care.	*Convey respect for the dying patient and family. *Recognize the patient's right to participate in and determine end-of-life care and treatment goals. *Appreciate the need for information based on personal preference and culture.	*Demonstrate effective and compassionate communication skills. *Demonstrate by words or actions that the patient/family will not be abandoned. *Initiate discussion with patient and family regarding end-of-life issues.	*Develop a trusting relationship with dying patients and families. *Facilitate patient/families expression of feelings, needs, and concerns. *Assist the patient/family to discuss what he/she believes is dying well. *Facilitate the completion of unfinished business.	*Convey bad news, including diagnosis, prognosis, or death using an empathic approach. *Guide patients and families in determining the goals of care. *Communicate effectively and compassionately in complex and difficult family systems. *Assist patients and families in resolving interpersonal conflicts/issues.	*Role play and critique communication in the following situations: —Delivering bad news; —Reinforcing bad news; —Determining goals of care; —Clarifying information; —Reassessing previous decisions; —Individuals presenting interpersonal conflicts.

Working Phase: *Exploring and understanding patients feelings and expectations about death and dying —dying well —unfinished business; —life review —talking with patients and families about death as it is experienced throughout the life cycle.	*Acknowledge the difficulty of patient and family in making end-of-life decisions. *Accept the patient/family's level of readiness for information related to decision making. *Acknowledge the patients' and families' feelings as valid. *Value nursing presence during the dying process for patient and family and the importance of compassionate care.	*Use effective and compassionate communication skills to deliver information, establish a plan of care, and console the patient, family, and other health professionals. *Act in accordance with state statutes and institutional policies regarding end-of-life decision making. *Teach families impending signs of death.	*Provide the opportunity for patients to conduct a life review. *Describe the benefits and burdens of various treatments at the end of life. *Provide patient and family with assurance of aggressive palliative care to provide comfort during the dying process. *Interpret medical information to patient and family in terms that they can understand. *Convey a change in patient's status to APN, MD, and family.	*Facilitate patient, family, and health care provider communication to determine the goals and plan of care, and affirm end-of-life decisions. *Coordinate health care team activities aimed at achieving the patient's goals and wishes. *Prepare the family and staff for patient's imminent death. *Convey the fact of death to the family. *Present organ donation options to the family, when appropriate.	*Use video taped interviews with patients and families, exemplifying therapeutic communication skills, i.e., "Before I Die," and "Cancer Evolution or Revolution." *As faculty, model therapeutic communication for student in introductions to patients and families. *Conduct an exercise in which one student actively listens to another student regarding a transition in their life without speaking for 5 minutes.

(continued)

EDUCATION PLAN 8.1 *(continued)*

Knowledge Needed	Attitude	Skills	Undergraduate Behavioral Outcomes	Graduate Behavioral Outcomes	Teaching/Learning Strategies
*Facilitating and taking Action: —DNR orders and other advanced directives. —Family letter writing —nurses' reassurance of comfort and non-abandonment. Termination Phase: Withdrawing medical interventions; Preparing patient and family for signs of death; Aggressive comfort measures at the end of life; Consoling the bereaved.	*Express an acceptance of death. *Express respect for the deceased. *Acknowledge feelings of loss and grief expressed by patient, family, and health care providers. *Consider patients' and families' values and beliefs related to the end-of-life care.	*Explain the detachment of the patient in the dying process. *Assist families in expressing their feelings to the patient.	*Console the bereaved. *Seek support and an opportunity for exploration of students'/nurses' feelings and responses related to caring for a dying patient and their family.	*Provide a supportive environment for review of nurses' feelings and behaviors in caring for the dying patient and family.	Discuss the experience of active listening, and the experience of being heard. *Perform a life review with a selected patient in a clinical setting. Describe the initiation of life review, the strategies that enhanced communication and barriers to communication as it relates to the patient, nurse, and environment. *Reconstruct a conversation that the nurse found difficult.

Reviewing the relationships for personal feelings and evaluation of nursing responses.

Evaluate the communication skills, and recommend an alternative communication strategy. *Critique a case study of communication with patient and family at the end of life. *Have students attend a support group for bereaved families to identify bereavement issues, observe the role of the group leader, and identify barriers or facilitators to effective and compassionate communication.

REFERENCES

Ambuel, B. (2003). Delivering bad news and precepting student/resident learners. *Journal of Palliative Medicine, 6,* 263–264.

Albom, M. (1997). *Tuesdays with Morrie.* New York: Doubleday.

Anderson, B., & Hall, B. (1995). Parents perceptions of decision making for children. *Journal of Law, Medicine and Ethics, 23*(6), 15–19.

Block, S. (2001). Psychological considerations, growth, and transcendence at the end of life: The art of the possible. *Journal of the American Medical Association, 285,* 2898–2904.

Booth, K., Maguire, P. M., Butterworth, R., & Hillier, V. F. (1996). Perceived professional support and the use of blocking behaviors by hospice nurses. *Journal of Advanced Nursing, 24,* 522–527.

Buckman, R. (1992). *How to break bad news: A guide for health professionals.* Baltimore: Johns Hopkins Press.

Buckman, R., Lipkin, M., Sourkes, B., & Tolle, S. (1997, June 15). Strategies and skills for breaking bad news. *Patient Care, 6,* 61–66.

Byock, I. (1997). *Dying well: Peace and possibilities at the end of life.* New York: Riverhead Books.

Byock, I. (2004). The four things that matter most: A book about living. New York: Free Press.

Callanan, M. (1994). Farewell messages. *American Journal of Nursing, 94*(5), 19–20.

Cavendish, R. (1999). Improving care for the elderly. *American Journal of Nursing, 99*(3), 88.

Cotton, P. (1993). Talk to people about dying—They can handle it, say geriatricians and patients. *Journal of the American Medical Association, 269,* 321–323.

Czerwiec, M. (1996). When a loved one is dying: Families talk about nursing care. *American Journal of Nursing, 96*(5), 32–36.

Davis, S., Kristjanson, L. J., & Blight, J. (2003). Communicating with families of patients in an acute hospital with advanced cancer. *Cancer Nursing, 26,* 337–345.

Emanuel, E. J. (1998). The promise of a good death. *Lancet, 351* (9114, Suppl.), S1121–1126.

Fallowfield, L., & Jenkins, V. (2004). Communicating sad, bad, and difficult news in medicine. *Lancet, 363,* 312–319.

Family letter writing: An interview with Nathan Harlow. *Innovations in end of life care: An international on-line forum for leaders in end of life care.* (1999). Retrieved 6/12/2000 from http://www2.edc.org/lastacts/featureinn.asp

Farrell, M., Ryan, S., & Langrick, B. (2001). Breaking bad news within a paediatric setting: An evaluation report of a collaborative education workshop to support health professionals. *Journal of Advanced Nursing, 36,* 763–775.

Freyer, D. (2004). Care of the dying adolescent: Special considerations. *Pediatrics, 113,* 381–388.

Furukawa, M. M. (1996). Meeting the needs of the dying patient's family. *Critical Care Nurse, 16*(1), 51–62.

Heaven, C. M., & Maguire, P. (1996). Training hospice nurses to elicit patient concerns. *Journal of Advanced Nursing, 23,* 280–286.

Interview with Dr. Stuart Farber, Living with a serious illness: A workbook for patients and families. *Innovations in end of life care: An international on-line forum for leaders in end of life care* (1999). [on-line] Available: http://www2.edc.org/lastacts/feature inn. asp

Jezewski, M. A. (1996). Obtaining consent for Do-Not-Resuscitate status: Advice from experienced nurses. *Nursing Outlook, 44*(3), 114–119.

Kagawa-Singer, M, & Blackhall, L. J. (2001). Negotiating cross-cultural issues at the end of life: "You got to go where he lives."

Journal of the American Medical Association, 286, 2993–3000.

Langley-Evans, A., & Payne, S. (1997). Light-hearted death talks in a palliative day care context. *Journal of Advanced Nursing, 26,* 1091–1097.

Larson, D. G., & Tobin, D. R. (2000). End of life conversations: Evolving practice and theory. *Journal of the American Medical Association, 284,* 1573–1577.

Latimer, E. (1998). Ethical care at the end of life. *Canadian Medical Association Journal, 158,* 1741–1745.

May, C. (1995). To call it work somehow demeans it: The social construction of talk in the care of the terminally ill patients. *Journal of Advanced Nursing, 22,* 556–661.

Mazanec, P., & Tyler, M. K. (2004). Cultural considerations in end-of-life care: How ethnicity, age, and spirituality affect decisions when death is imminent. *Home Healthcare Nurse, 22,* 317–324.

Murphy, P. A., & Price, D. M. (1995). ACT: Taking a positive approach to end of life care. *American Journal of Nursing, 95*(3), 42–43.

Pattison, N. (2004). Integration of critical care and palliative care at the end of life. *British Journal of Nursing, 13(3),* 132–139.

Peel, N. (2003). The role of the critical care nurse in the delivery of bad news. *British Journal of Nursing, 12,* 966–971.

Ptacek, J. T., Ptacek, J. J., & Ellison, N. M. (2001). "I'm sorry to tell you. . . ." Physicians' reports of breaking bad news. *Journal of Behavioral Medicine, 24,* 205–217.

Quill, T. E. (2000). Initiating end-of-life discussions with seriously ill patients: addressing the elephant in the room. *Journal of the American Medical Association, 284,* 2502–2507.

Radziewicz, R., & Baile, W. F. (2001). Communication skills: Breaking bad news in the clinical setting. *Oncology Nursing Forum, 28,* 951–953.

Rosenbaum, M. E., & Kreiter, C. (2002). Teaching delivery of bad news using experiential sessions with standardized patients. *Teaching and Learning in Medicine, 143*(3), 144–149.

Roundtable discussion: Part 2. (1996). A peaceful death: How to manage pain and provide quality care. *Geriatrics, 51*(6), 32–42.

Servaty, H. L., Krejci, M. J., & Hayslip, B. (1996). Relationships among death anxiety, communication apprehension with dying and empathy in those seeking occupations as nurses and physicians. *Death Studies, 20,* 149–161.

Shmerling, R. H., Bedell, S. E., Lilienfeld, A., & Delbanco, T. L. (1988). Discussing cardiopulmonary resuscitation. *Journal of General Internal Medicine, 3,* 317–321.

Stein, C. (1999). Ending a life. *Boston Globe Magazine, 13,* 24, 30–34, 39–42.

Stiles, M. K. (1990). The shining stranger: Nurse-family spiritual relationship. *Cancer Nursing, 13,* 2235–2245.

SUPPORT Principal Investigators (1995). A controlled trial to improve care for seriously ill, hospitalized patients: The study to understand prognoses and preferences for outcomes and risks of treatments (SUPPORT). *Journal of the American Medical Association, 274,* 1591–1598.

Tulsky, J. A., Chesney, M. A., & Lo, B. (1996). See one, do one, teach one? House staff experience discussing do-not-resuscitate orders. *Archives of Internal Medicine, 156,* 1285–1289.

Wilkinson, S. (1991). Factors that influence how nurses communicate with cancer patients. *Journal of Advanced Nursing, 16,* 677–688.

Yabroff, K. R., & Mandelblatt, J. S. (2004). The quality of medical care at the end of life in the USA: Existing barriers and examples of process and outcome measures. *Palliative Medicine, 18,* 202–216.

9

Caring for Families: The Other Patient in Palliative Care

Suzanne K. Goetschius[1] and Marianne LaPorte Matzo

AACN Competency

#5 Demonstrate respect for the patient's views and wishes during end-of-life care.

> *Death forever changes the world of those who experience the loss of the person dying.* [2]

The nursing care of any patient is planned with an understanding of the system or family in which the person functions. Family can mean direct blood relatives, relationship through an emotional commitment, or the group or person with which someone feels most closely connected (Field & Cassel, 1997). Family can be brothers, sisters, parents, children, cousins, nieces, nephews, aunts, uncles, or grandparents. Family can be spouse, partner, or significant other. Family can be best friends, colleagues, neighbors, or even caregivers. A nursing assistant who gives personal care everyday may have a significant personal tie with a patient. Understanding these roles and relationships is critical to thorough assessment and to effective care planning in nursing. Knowing who is providing home support for a patient is key to developing a successful discharge plan. Knowing who prepares meals is key to teaching nutrition. Knowing whose presence is the most comforting to a patient is key to maintaining their sense of well-being during stressful times. This is especially true in end-of-life care (EOLC), and yet takes on even greater importance. Nurses must consider not only how the family can help the patient, but also how the nurse must help the family—the other patient—face what may be their most difficult challenge: the death of a loved one.

As families struggle to be caregivers of the one who is dying, they must also struggle with their impending loss, their changing roles and relationships, watching a loved one suffer physically and emotionally, and dealing with their own concerns about their ability to be a caregiver. Key nursing competencies in end-of-life care include assisting families to develop skills in effective communication, identifying their roles, coping with all that is happening emotionally, using available resources, and providing direct care (American Association of Colleges of Nursing [AACN], 1998). Teaching nursing students the how-to of the palliative care of families is a challenge. Undergraduate students are overwhelmed with their own issues around death and dying, their limited knowledge base about

---

[1]This chapter is written in the memory of Albert T. Tremblay, RN, MSN who died in 1999. The lessons I learned from him and his family would fill a thousand pages.

[2]Benner, Kerchner, Corless & Davies, 2003, p. 558

"how-to" themselves, and the incredible fear of saying the wrong thing. They are in the position of needing to let the family "do for" and at the same time empowering the family in their own role development when their focus is on "doing" themselves. Advanced practice nursing students may have to correct concepts learned from their undergraduate programs and their own experiences with patients, families, and death: leaving families alone or not getting involved in EOLC.

In this chapter, the interventions and suggestions for palliative care for families will include care in a variety of settings and along the continuum of care that adults may traverse as they approach the end of life.

FAMILIES AND END-OF-LIFE CARE

One of the fundamental principles of palliative care is that the patient and family together are the unit of care (Andershed & Ternestedt, 2001; Reimer, Davies, & Martens, 1991). As the health care system and society have shifted their expectations about EOLC from an institutional setting where professional caregivers are in charge to a home setting where the family is in charge, so must nursing refocus its efforts in addressing the needs of families in EOLC. Each family is unique and will want to be involved in EOLC in its own way (Andershed & Ternestedt, 2001). Family has been the focus of much research both in terms of how family members are affected by the EOLC process and in terms of how their needs can be met.

Joanne Lynn (1997) notes that suggested domains for measuring quality at the end of life should include patient and family satisfaction and family burden, including financial and emotional burden. Patient and family satisfaction should include the patient's piece of mind, the family's perception of the

patient's care and comfort, the decision-making process, the care received both by the patient and the family, and the extent to which opportunities were provided to complete life in a meaningful way. The time spent together by patient and family should be treasured and not simply tolerable. According to Donaldson (1998), assessment of quality in EOLC is focused on patient and family caregivers, but could also include a social network and their support. Survivors' memories of a loved one's death are important in their own right because dying is not only what the patient experiences but also what the survivors remember (Jacobson, 1998). The survivor's experience of EOLC is examined to assess quality and outcome of interventions in EOLC. If the family is essential to measuring quality and positive outcomes in EOLC, then what do nurses who provide EOLC need to know to meet their needs?

Field and Cassel (1997) noted that general nursing curricula should address the variations in dying related to clinical conditions and family circumstances, mental states, and other factors that may require alternate nursing strategies. They also noted that students receive limited exposure to dying patients and limited guidance in handling their personal reactions to the dying and their bereaved families. In textbooks, the most neglected area of content was the needs and roles of family caregivers (Ferrell, 2001). Of the 45,683 pages of textbooks reviewed, only 42 pages (or .1% of content) related to families; 71% of texts reviewed had no content at all related to family caregivers (Ferrell, 2001). Curricular foci should include clinical knowledge, interpersonal skills, ethical awareness, and other aspects of care with case-based learning, role-playing, and experiences in different settings.

A study by Emanuel and colleagues (1999) found that 96% of primary caregivers of terminally ill individuals are family members and 72% are women. Less than 3% of all patients received any volunteer assistance and paid caregivers are used less than 20% of the time. Patients with cancer seemed to fare better than others, having fewer unmet needs, fewer caregiving needs, and less reliance on paid caregivers than those with an illness like heart disease or emphysema. The researchers noted that more attention has been focused on the terminal care needs of cancer patients than on those with other disease processes. Support services may exist for cancer patients and their families that do not exist for others.

Families experience both physical and emotional distress while experiencing the death of a loved one. According to Sherman (1998), there is a "reciprocity of suffering" that can occur for family members. Family members may suffer physical, psychosocial, emotional, and spiritual distress during EOLC. They are not only experiencing their own pain as they deal with the impending death but they also suffer as they try to fulfill new roles as caregivers. They fear being unable to relieve the suffering and pain of their family member. It is necessary to cope with the disruption of their lives, abandonment by friends, and with anticipatory grief. They face financial burdens, loss of employment, and loss of their major source of income. Patients may fear their own suffering and death less than they fear being a burden to their families.

Reimer and colleagues (1991) noted that the EOL process for cancer families could be seen as a passage the researchers referred to as "fading away." The process of fading away starts with "ending," when the family perceives the final decline of the patient is occurring. Families have two tasks during this time: redefining themselves and dealing with burden. Nursing interventions during this phase include being aware that each person will process the change differently and that change will take time. Nurses can provide opportunities for discussion, assist with keeping the patient as independent as possible, provide resources, and tailor interventions to the individual's need to process change. Once the ending has been realized, the family moves from their old way of living with cancer into a neutral zone, where they struggle with the change from their pre-decline life, contend with change, and search for meaning. Here, nurses can serve as a sounding board to validate feelings, to help the family explore options, and to identify the limits of their tolerance. Nurses must also be aware of their own feelings, recognizing the importance of their response to the well-being of the family. Finally, the family moves to their new beginning of living day-to-day in the present and preparing for death. The nurse needs to be able to discuss the inevitability of death and all its implications. By focusing not only on death but also on the life that will go on, nurses can affirm for families their ability to manage and grow from the experience by encouraging life review and the completion of unfinished business. How the family copes with these changes is colored by past coping styles and past experiences with death and loss.

Several authors have noted that families want a few basic interventions from nurses (Briggs & Colvin, 2002; Curtis, 2004; Heyland, Rocker, O'Callaghan, Dodek, & Cook 2003; Hull, 1989; Lewandowski & Jones, 1988; Sherman, 1999; Waltman, 1990). First, families want honest, open communication and the sharing of accurate, straightforward information about the patient's condition and the process their loved one is to undergo. False reassurances, false sympathy, and overzealous attempts to show empathy are not welcomed by families. Second, they want skilled nursing interventions aimed at the care and comfort of the patient. They want to be physically near and sometimes alone with their family member, but not abandoned. Research with 40 families by Lewandowski and Jones (1988) showed that families tend to stay focused on the needs of the family member who is dying and fail to consider their own needs. Assurances that a loved one is comfortable and cared for and having access to information were cited as essential nursing interventions. According to Lewandowski and Jones (1988), families go through three phases of living with cancer: initial, adaptation, and terminal. Families in the initial phase were interested in information and hope. In the second phase, they continued to focus on information. In the third phase, they no longer focused on hope but expressed a need to ventilate feelings, spend time alone, and continue to receive information. Across all three phases, families felt the need for the focus of nursing care to be the patient's care and comfort and not the family. The authors felt it was important for nurses to be knowledgeable about family dynamics and that care planning must focus on the patient as a part of the family system. They emphasized that the family is capable of change and growth even during a terminal illness. Key to family growth was teaching and giving the family information.

Nursing has begun to look at what could be provided to families once basic patient care needs are met. Johnson and Bourgeois (2003) write that assessing support needs of families is complex because they often have a hard time expressing themselves in terms of their own needs. The nurse must assess the family members as well as the patient, and an interdisciplinary team should provide EOLC. The family should be taught about the physical EOL process, the completion of relationship issues, and how to begin letting go. Information regarding the physical, emotional, and spiritual signs of impending death such as withdrawal, visions, unusual communica-

tions, and saying good-bye should also be included in the teaching plan.

Based on interviews with 10 nurse educators and 10 experienced palliative care nurses, Degner, Gow, and Thompson (1991) noted seven critical behaviors in the care of the dying, including responding to the needs of the family. The critical behaviors included responding to the family's need for information, reducing the potential for future regrets, and including them in the care or relieving them of the responsibility depending on their needs. Negative behaviors towards families included not providing information, refusing to discuss dying or spiritual issues even when the family indicated they wished to, and passing judgment on family decisions and behaviors.

Cutillo-Schmitter (1996) recommends four strategies for managing the "ambiguous loss," that is, a loss that accompanies decline from a terminal or a dementing illness and in which the patient's and family's roles and relationships have changed. The path to EOL may be prolonged and uncertain. Family members may have a wide range of responses from denial to anger, helplessness, and guilt. Nursing strategies with ambiguous loss include being present and acknowledging what can and cannot be done, identifying the loss as ambiguous, and clarifying what is lost and what remains of relationships. The nurse can provide family with the opportunity to share their perceptions of the loss, and educate and support the family regarding disease progression and resources.

The five relationship completion tasks of EOL as identified by Byock (1997) are important to explore with family and patient. Such tasks include saying forgive me; I forgive you; I love you; thank you; and good-bye. Knowing where the caregiver is in completing these tasks with the patient may help them to define ways to achieve some of the personal growth and sense of mastery that can occur at the end of life (Byock, 1997).

Czerwiec (1996) interviewed families who experienced death in hospitals. She found that actions directed at patient comfort were important to families, as well as the nurse's attitude while performing the action. The families saw the nurse's actions directed towards their needs as a sign of extraordinary caring. Presence—the time the nurse spent with them—was noted as influential. She recommended assessing how long and how well the family and patient have been coping with the illness, the family members' status as caregivers and their health, how well they understand the illness, and their relationship with the health care team. Recommended interventions included being able to discuss difficult issues, providing for the physical needs of the family, creating a safe environment for the family, offering spiritual care, and learning about the person who is dying. Nursing diagnoses associated with families and EOLC included "hopelessness, anticipatory grieving, spiritual distress, fear, caregiver role strain and altered family processes" (Czerwiec, 1996, p. 35).

Wilson and Daley (1999) found the following aspects for families experiencing EOLC in the institutional long-term-care setting to be important: caring staff behaviors, participation in the dying process, presence at the time of death, and provision of spiritual support. A study by Furukawa (1996) revealed that families in critical care have similar needs from nursing such as assurance that the patient is cared for, proximity or access to their loved one, and information. Implications for nursing care of the family in the critical care setting included unrestricted, flexible visiting policy; early social service intervention; realistic hope; facilitation of communication between families and physicians; and sending sympathy cards to families.

CARING FOR FAMILIES ACROSS THE HEALTH CARE CONTINUUM

Nurses interact with families in a variety of settings from primary through palliative care. Despite evolving societal expectations of where EOLC should occur and increasing numbers of persons who choose to die at home, the majority of people in the United States still die in an institutional setting, though this varies somewhat regionally (Meier & Morrison, 1999). Although the demographics of where nurses' practice continues to change, it is likely that many nurses will experience a patient's death for the first time in an institutional setting. In acute care, the opportunity to develop rapport with families is fleeting and events can occur quickly. A hospitalized patient whose heart failure was stable yesterday may be actively dying today. Nurses must learn palliative care skills to use not just in a hospice setting, but also in these fast-paced settings where they are likely to find themselves dealing with dying patients and their grieving families. The family of a patient who dies in the ICU should have the same opportunity to experience a "good death" despite the limitations the setting may impose. It is important to improving *all* end-of-life experiences to teach nurses how to help families across diverse health care settings.

Understanding why death occurs and the dying process is important in preparing students for EOLC. Much of what we teach about EOLC is based on experiences with oncology patients and their families. However, cancer is not the most common fatal illness in this country. Heart disease continues to be the number one cause of death in this country (Smith, Martin, & Ventura, 1999). In fact, the majority of people who die are older adults dying of chronic illnesses such as heart disease, cancer, cerebrovascular disease, chronic obstructive pulmonary disease, and Alzheimer's disease (Brock & Foley, 1998). The trajectory of illness and decline is different for most progressive fatal diseases when compared to cancer. The SUPPORT study (SUPPORT Investigators, 1995) found the common course at the end of life is a seemingly sudden, unpredictable change in a chronic fatal illness. Yet, we still have very little evidence-based information about meeting the EOLC needs of anyone but cancer patients and their families (Meier & Morrison, 1999). Nurses need palliative care experience and education to provide care to patients and families who are coping with all fatal illnesses and to assist them in making end-of-life decisions.

Nurses can begin to develop the skills needed for more intensive end-of-life care in every setting from the doctor's office to the long-term-care setting. It is critical for nurse educators to use these opportunities as they arise. For instance, a nurse may encounter a woman in a well-baby clinic, and in the course of her assessment find out that this patient is also the caregiver for her dying father. The educator could support the nurse in identifying the issues the woman may have and assessing how they influence her other roles—such as being a new mother—and what interventions may be necessary. Perhaps the family could benefit from a hospice program and the nurse could discuss this option and provide a referral. The new mother may also need referral to a counseling service, some extra assistance with child care at home, referral to a home-care agency's maternal child health services to offer in-home support, or other holistic interventions.

Advanced practice nurses in a long-term-care setting may offer support to the nursing assistant during the death of a favorite patient; a situation where the patient and the nursing assistant may have a true "family" relationship (O'Hara, Harper, Chartrand, & Johnston, 1996). Advanced practice nurses (APN) may also be in the position of having

to tell, or be a partner in telling, a patient and family about a poor prognosis. This may be the true beginning of a family's education about end-of-life care and can set the tone for the rest of the family's and patient's experience. APNs often bring with them a great deal of experience with EOLC and can begin to answer questions for the family and patient. A nurse's skills in therapeutic communication are critical at those moments and may make the APN the best person to have such a discussion, especially if a sound relationship exists.

Nurses will be caring for patients and families when they are diagnosed, admitted with an acute exacerbation of a chronic problem, during their active treatment, and during palliative care. The need for components of palliative care can occur at any time over the course of an illness. Joanne Lynn (personal communication, October 22, 1999) noted that trying to identify an exact point when palliative care should be initiated might not be appropriate:

> Quite simply, I think that such a transition is largely a social construction made to keep us all more comfortable, and it neither serves the patient well nor helps us structure our care system optimally. It would be better, generally, to develop new models of care that combine palliation, treatment (and rehabilitation, prevention, informing, etc.)—in the mix that regularly serves patients of certain sorts. AND [sic] to be able to tailor the fine points of such systems of care to the individual circumstances and preferences of the patient.

Assessing the family and patient over the course of an illness trajectory can be an opportunity to educate nurses about the changes that occur in relationships as the family tries to cope. With a new terminal diagnosis, for example, the patient may be keeping details from the family to protect them, or vice versa.

As a family struggles with the impact of treatment on their lives, the nurses can examine how the roles and values within the family may be changing and how to facilitate skill development for a new role. A nurse in home care may observe that a husband needs assistance with learning how to prepare meals if his elderly wife is no longer able. The nurse may develop a plan of care that begins to examine with the husband other roles that are going to change as the illness progresses and how to begin to prepare. A patient and family choosing palliative care may need education about physical care and also about the changes associated with the dying process. Spiritual support or respite information is also important. The nursing student will need to have the resources to deal with these deficits. Gaining experience in these areas can facilitate managing the more intense clinical needs of an actively dying patient.

ASSESSING FAMILIES DURING END-OF-LIFE CARE

Palliative care is a holistic approach to care for patients and their families during life-threatening illness. The focus of care is the entire family unit as it is altered by the illness of one of its members. Assessing the family as a system and determining appropriate interventions are important in EOLC. As a system, the family is made up of elements (family members) with their own separate traits, who are interdependent, but who also function as a whole. The system/family and the individual elements are constantly impacted by changes from inside the system or by outside influences such as nursing care. Systems strive to achieve equilibrium and stability. When that stability is threatened by an impending loss of a member, the family/system may need some assistance to return to or maintain its stability.

Nurses can assess the individuals and relationships within the family system. The nurse can then begin to develop interventions to counter the influences that have upset the balance of the family system. Families are capable of learning, evolving, and developing through the course of a loved one's illness (Lewandowski & Jones, 1988). In the case of families, understanding how the dying and death of one member affects individuals and their relationships to each other, as well as the family as a whole, allows the nurse to plan interventions to meet the needs of the family. Families identify the care and comfort of their family member as their number one priority (Lewandoski & Jones, 1988). Nurses must also help family members identify what their *own* needs are in EOLC.

Assessing the family is the first step in developing a plan of care. The important areas for assessment include family structure, roles and relationships, modes of communication, strengths and weaknesses, knowledge deficits, and available resources (Cutillo-Schmitter, 1996; Czerwiec, 1996; Lewandowski & Jones, 1988; Sherman, 1998). The care setting can be a barrier in the EOLC assessment process. In an acute care setting, the student may have very little time to gather information from the family. In long-term care, the student may have the time, but little access to family. In hospice, time may or may not be short and access to family may be occurring at a time when they are feeling the burden of care already.

Educators will need to be creative in providing the student assessment opportunities with an EOLC focus. If time is an issue, interdisciplinary assessments by social workers, counselors, pastoral care providers, or nursing staff may give the student access to the information needed or provide validation. Case studies are valuable in developing skills and communication techniques, and they promote an opportunity for discussions about difficult issues the students may encounter when caring for patients and families during EOLC. Conducting home visits also may be of benefit in following a family over the course of the dying process and across various settings.

Family assessment requires an adjustment of the perspective from the patient alone to the system the patient functions in and its components in relation to one another. Families are reluctant to see their needs as vital and may resist any focus on them. It is important to assure them that their loved one's needs are being met and that addressing their needs is equally important in promoting their health and well-being. Through the assessment process, family members and the patient may be able to identify their goals, expectations, and preferences and share what outcomes are critical to them. These outcome measures can assist the nurse in identifying measurable goals and objectives and the appropriate interventions to achieve them. Important points in assessing families include the following (Field & Cassel, 1997; McCracken & Gerdson, 1991; Sherman, 1998):

1. Family structure
   a. Names, sex, and age of each family member
   b. Relationship to the patient
2. Roles and expectations about roles
   a. Pre-EOLC roles if known
   b. Patient's roles and EOLC goals
   c. Members roles at present and EOLC goals
   d. Cultural/ethnic/spiritual influences on roles and goals
   e. Lines of communication and how they share information
   f. Life span issues
   g. Gender issues
3. SWOT Analysis (strengths, weaknesses, opportunities, and threats)

Identify factors that may enhance or inhibit family system
   a. Issues related to the site of care
   b. Family members who have health care training
   c. The frail health of the spouse
   d. Other family members to call on
   e. Dependent care benefits at work
4. Knowledge Deficits
   a. Past death experiences, positive and negative
   b. Understanding the terminal state and prognosis
   c. Awareness of disease progression
   d. Knowledge of caregiving skills
   e. Legal/financial choices
   f. Resources available such as palliative care consultation in acute care, hospice programs in the community, spiritual resources, and respite care

FAMILY STRUCTURE

Family structure includes all members of the family as identified by the patient and may include informal family such as friends or coworkers who provide care or support. Identifying roles may come from interviews and observations of a family over time. The assessment can be documented using a narrative or a family genogram with data filled in beside each individual's name.

If possible, the nurse should identify how the family functioned before the illness. This information can be helpful in understanding problems or planning interventions. A man whose wife had made all of her treatment decisions before her illness progressed may be unsure and hesitant when the role of decision maker becomes his. Without knowing why he was hesitant, the nurse might assume he did not understand the treatment plan. The intervention based on this information might be to talk with the husband about how his wife made decisions and to identify her priorities. This intervention may help him develop confidence in his new role.

ROLES AND EXPECTATIONS

Both family structure and roles will evolve over time as family members' abilities and experiences determine their degree of involvement in EOLC. The nurse may have the greatest impact in supporting or educating a family member who wishes to have a role he or she does not feel prepared for; or finding ways to support the family member's usual roles while the family member is focused on the EOLC role. Family members may not know how to support an ill loved one or what they can do to be a part of the process. For example, in one family, the son was withdrawn and uncommunicative when visiting his father. The nursing student learned that he did not know what to do when he was visiting and felt as if he had nothing to offer. The student showed him how to get his father ice chips and fluids from the kitchen and invited him to go there as needed to help his father. The son was able to offer this service to his father independently and felt relieved to have something concrete to do that helped his father.

Some roles are long-standing and historical like the authority figure of a father. It is difficult for family members to change roles, for instance, for a mother to allow a daughter to be her caregiver. The concept of role reversal is often used to describe changes in role, but this can be a harmful way to frame the switch in tasks that are occurring. Clarifying this is sometimes important in helping families adjust. Although some parents are comfortable being cared for by their child, they may express concern about the discomfort of losing that role and relationship as parent and child. In the film *One True Thing*, a man and his daughter are caring for their terminally ill wife and mother. In a moment of anguish that makes this issue clear, the woman shouts at her caregivers, "I'm still the mother in this house!" The nurse can reframe these "role reversals" as something more positive, for instance, as an opportunity for the children to honor their mother and her role and perhaps to experience some of the joy she felt when she cared for them.

Other roles may be brought about by EOLC situations. In one family, the son had difficulty being in the room while his mother was dying and spent most of his time pacing the halls, telling the nurse how bad he felt that he could not "be in there." He became the family chauffeur for all the relatives who could not drive, bringing them back and forth to visit. Although he could not be there himself, he made sure there was someone who could be. He developed a role that helped the family but was within his comfort zone. The nursing intervention in this case may have been to help him and the rest of the family see his role and its value to the system.

Roles may be altered artificially by the environment of care. Caregivers may unwillingly relinquish their role as physical caregivers if an unobservant nurse takes over these tasks. The nurse needs to assess whether this is the wish of the caregiver before intervening. The authority figure of the nurse, even a student, may intimidate the caregiver and weaken his or her confidence in his or her caregiving abilities.

The well-being of primary caregivers must also be carefully assessed. The success of a given plan of care often rests on the shoulders of this individual and the ability of the family system to support the caregiver's role. The health and functional ability of the caregiver may be compromised by caregiving; knowing the caregiver's limitations in advance can allow the nurse to address potential problems. The primary caregiver's coping skills and support systems are also important. What are the caregiver's needs in the process of EOLC? Does he want to be present at all times? Is she counting on other family members to take on certain tasks and roles, which need to be communicated? Perhaps caregivers see their role as it has always been, as a loving partner or spouse, but they do not want to take on the physical caregiver role. It is important to have the significant other's goals and expectations identified, especially as it relates to the patient.

Knowing patients' roles and goals is critical for planning family interventions because the patient has a significant impact on the family as a whole and on each person in it. For the most part, the patient's preferences and wishes become the outcomes that direct the plan of care and guide family decisions. Assessment should also include how patients fit in the family traditionally and currently; how they handle the role as patient; whether they are still making their own decisions; and whether they are worried about being a burden to the rest of the family. If being a burden is a concern, they may resist the family's attempts to care for them, thwarting the family's role as caregivers. Roles of other family members may be impacted when patients are unable to fulfill their usual roles. When a patient who has been the financial support for the family can no longer work, someone else may have to start working to support the family or maintain insurance coverage. If this someone is also the primary caregiver, it may sabotage a plan for home caregiving.

Understanding cultural, ethnic, and religious influences may help define family roles in EOLC (Pickett, 1993). For example, current American culture espouses that a good death occurs at home with loved ones as caregivers (Jacobson, 1998; Pickett, 1993). A woman who feels she must care for her husband at home in order to be a "good" wife may experience great distress at the prospect of bringing him home if she is not able to provide his physical care. How will she feel if she makes the choice to care for him in a nursing home? Is she still a "good" wife? The guilt and dissonance may be too painful for her to reveal and cause great issues if it is not resolved. If the focus of the nursing care plan was on caregiving skills without identifying and addressing the wife's concerns, the EOLC experience could be a painful one for the wife. In assessing roles, it is important for the student to maintain a culturally sensitive approach in dealing with all potential caregivers. Even dominant cultural beliefs may be the source of issues for family so it is critical that nurses carefully identify subtler or less well-known cultural influences during assessment.

Lines of communication are often related to role. Knowing how information is shared within a family both before and during an illness is important, especially as it pertains to planning interventions. The family spokesperson may be the only one who talks to health care providers while the others wait for feedback from the spokesperson. Clear communication is the key to avoiding role conflicts and confusion. For example, in one family, the daughter asked all the questions about her mother's physical care because she was planning to be the primary caregiver. The father sat quietly by and asked no questions. Rather than assume a lack of concern by the husband, the nurse spoke to him to assess how he felt about what was occurring. From this discussion, she recognized that he was going to continue his role as husband and supportive partner while his daughter did the physical care. Their communication style gave clues as to how they were defining their roles.

Gender and developmental stage may also influence roles and relationships. Older women are more likely to have a limited support network. Often, their spouse has already died, they are living alone, and they may be reluctant to impose on their adult children (Administration on Aging, 1999). They already may have endured significant loss or change of many roles. Older persons are less likely to have a large network of coworkers and friends who can offer tangible support because of their own health problems or limited resources. In these instances, the student may want to look for other types of "family": paid caregivers, religious affiliations, social groups, and so forth. The number of friends and family who want to be involved in EOLC may overwhelm a younger adult. The student may help them identify which roles and relationships are critical and help the family find ways for others to be involved more appropriately. The developmental tasks of all family members need to be assessed. Providing EOLC may alter certain developmental tasks: completing an education, marriage, starting a family, or job-related advancement.

SWOT ANALYSIS

Strengths, weaknesses, opportunities, and threats (SWOT) can be traits of either the family or the environment that potentially imperil or enhance the EOLC process. Strengths might be a facility that has a palliative care consultation service, or a family that has a dependent-caregiver benefit at work. Weaknesses may be a community with no respite services, or a family caregiver who is an alcoholic. Opportunities may be the presence of three grown children who will take turns providing care for their mother at home, or an ICU that has developed a new family-centered care policy for the families of terminal patients. Threats may be a health care provider with limited experience in EOLC, or the declining health of the spouse who is the primary caregiver.

KNOWLEDGE DEFICITS RELATED TO EOLC

Assessing knowledge deficits in EOLC is extremely important. Nurses should understand that after seeing to the comfort and care of the patient, adequate information is the next major issue for families (Andershed & Ternestedt, 2001). The disease process and its variable trajectory will influence what families need to know and when they want to know it. A patient who has been diagnosed recently may not be ready to discuss terminal care in detail. In diseases like congestive heart failure, it may be difficult to identify a time frame for initiating palliative care. The more rapid the illness trajectory, the greater the coping challenge is to patients and their families (Andershed & Ternestedt, (2001). As Benner, Kerchner, Corlis, and Davies, (2003) state,

> In the case of unexpected and untimely death, the patient and family may require more time and guidance in coming to terms with an imminent death. Consequently, the timing and context of the person's dying alters the patient's and significant others' meanings, decision making, and approach to death and loss. (p. 559)

In order to develop a plan of care, the nurse must be attuned to the goals of the patient and family rather than to the process of the illness itself.

Assessing the family's understanding of EOLC will require a more direct discussion and strong therapeutic communication skills, because talking about death directly is still a taboo among many people. Fear of upsetting someone, causing them to cry, and not knowing what to do are often concerns nurses bring up when beginning to work in EOLC. Often nurses want to avoid any discussion of death or terminal illness directly for fear of saying something wrong.

Framing discussions about EOLC as therapeutic offers a different perspective. Anxiety about the unknown and the mysteries that surround the end of life add to the impending loss of a loved one and can be overwhelming. Families need to have a "safe place" to begin discussions regarding end-of-life care. The nurses can model for the family that it is appropriate to talk about this process and ask questions. The nurse educator may take the lead in beginning some of these discussions for novice nurses; pairing them with APNs or staff nurses may be helpful. Working with other care providers such as social workers and chaplains may also give guidance to nurses.

Asking about past death experiences can also elicit valuable information. Nurses can glean information about what the person understood about the experience and process at the time, what the overall impression of the experience was, and what the family might have wanted to be different. Do they have regrets about past choices? What is the one thing they would like to change? Was there a role they wish they could have fulfilled or managed differently? This is often a good starting place for developing a teaching plan.

Skills in fostering therapeutic communication about past death experience should be practiced in advance. The nurse educator may do this as a group exercise to help nurses develop comfort with the process. Interviewing each other and presenting what they gleaned may offer the educator an opportunity to model interviewing techniques. It is also important to receive feedback from one another. It is important for nurses to use discretion in sharing their own experiences with death and dying with families, though it

may serve a critical function in establishing rapport. Nurse educators might also arrange for a panel of family members to share their experiences with the students—what went well, what they disliked, what nursing interventions helped, and what interventions were not helpful. Support groups may be an excellent resource for this type of group and may be helpful for a family member who wants to have an impact on the care of others because of their experience.

Due to their nursing experience, advanced practice nurses probably are best able to assess a family's understanding of the terminal state and prognosis. Nurses should develop an understanding of the specific disease process before meeting with families. Understanding how each disease progresses toward death is important in preparing families for what is to come. A diagnosis of Alzheimer's disease may involve a disease trajectory of 8 to 20 years before death and can be unpredictable in its progression. Cancer is more predictable but varies from type to type. Information about what a family understands about prognosis and disease progression may be obtained from both questioning and observations. Nurses may learn from role-playing some of the difficult situations that might arise during this part of an assessment. Questions about how much time is left, the efficacy of experimental treatments, use of alternative therapies in symptom relief, and telling or not telling the family or the patient about a poor prognosis could be used to stimulate discussion and identify supportive interventions. It may be within the scope of the APN to discuss options for care with the family and patient, such as pursuing further therapy or clinical trials. The level of information needed is most likely beyond an undergraduate student because of the various factors involved in making treatment choices.

Many families focus on physical care skills as their first learning objective. Their key concern is their ability to manage comfort and pain. Experiences with EOLC may reinforce the need to learn technical care skills, especially if family members felt unable to relieve suffering in previous experiences. The role family members feel comfortable with may depend on their confidence in physical caregiving. Often, what a family knows and what they can learn determines the options for where care at the end of life can occur. Nurses can reassure family members that they will be taught the skills needed and explain how support will be provided while skills are developed. Nurses need to validate their knowledge and skills to insure they are current and up-to-date. This is especially true for pain medication and issues such as hydration in EOLC.

The nurse should also address a family's accurate understanding of legal and financial implications of EOLC. Novice nurses as well as APNs should assess a family's understanding of the implications of the presence or absence of an advance directive or a Do Not Resuscitate order. Johns (1996) found that patients might hesitate in discussing advance directives. They prefer that health care providers begin such discussions and often wish to have family members as their surrogates. The trusting quality of nurses' relationships with patients and families may facilitate discussions about advance directives. Johns notes, "Nurses, because of their insights into patients' preferences and their role as patient advocates, have a legitimate role in monitoring compliance of treatment with patient's preferences as expressed in advance directives "(p. 152). For their own sakes, the patient's and family's, nurses should also know how to access resources such as an ethics consult if issues are identified during an assessment of the family.

A nurse's personal issues may also threaten assessment. Although nurses may have had limited exposure to death in their personal lives, they are not immune to its impact. Other nurses may have had a variety of both personal and professional experiences that influence their perceptions and observations regarding death and patient and family responses. It is the nurse educator's role to prepare nurses to achieve clinical competency in EOLC. Experiential exercises such as role-playing may be useful in identifying those students who need extra guidance and clinical support.

There are several barriers to completing a successful assessment of a family that needs EOLC. As mentioned earlier, the site of care may be a barrier, and there may not be enough time to talk with the family. In an acute care setting, the patient's condition may be deteriorating so quickly that nurses have limited time to intervene in all aspects of care. Limited options for family involvement may be a source of frustration. In this case, nurses should identify what would be needed to meet the family's and patient's needs.

The issue of care versus cure may also arise. It may be unclear to the family or staff what the goals of care are. Some family members may be working towards a cure while others are preparing to care; nurses may need some guidance with this type of family discord. Advanced practice nurses may be able to work with the family to help identify gaps in communication and facilitate resolution.

SITE OF CARE

It is important to avoid provider bias in developing any care plan, and this is true with patients and families at the EOL. The prevailing sentiment today seems to be that all good deaths occur at home and any death in a hospital is a "bad death." This belief can lead to great distress if families are led to believe that they are *expected* to care for their family member at home. Care at home needs to be presented without attaching a value to it as a choice in a continuum of care that is available at the end of life. Good deaths do occur in institutions and nursing care is a vital part of any positive EOL experience. What is critical is that a sound assessment be used to match the patient, the family, and its resources to the care that best meets their goals. With our current culture's emphasis on families taking loved ones home for care, families who cannot—or who try and then have to revert to a formal care setting—often experience guilt and a sense of failure. Rather than expecting all families to provide EOLC at home, nurses must assess the family and identify their strengths and weaknesses in order to identify the setting and resources that fit the family. Arblaster, Brooks, Hudson, and Petty (1990) found that patients and families want responsive nursing care that enables them to bring their own resources to the dying process, rather than having nurses impose care that they decide is appropriate. Nurses should be encouraged to provide quality end-of-life care independent of the setting where the care is provided.

Long-term Care

For the patient who is dying in a long-term care setting, it is the nurse who has primary responsibility for documenting the EOL issues and care plan, supporting the families of dying residents, and communicating with other members of the team (Hall, Schroder, & Weaver, 2002). In a review of 185 charts, Hall and colleagues found a higher rate of EOL symptoms in the last 48 hours of life for patients living in long-term-care settings than for cancer patients. In this study, nurses were found to be responsible for initiating discussions with families about changes in conditions and played a crucial role in insuring good symptom management, support

to families, communication with other team members, and objective documentation.

Home Hospice Care

Early discharge, increased acuity of illness, and technology in the home places additional pressure on families as they attempt to provide palliative care in the home. The role of the nurses is less well defined in family care than in direct patient care (Johnson & Bourgeois, 2003). In an interview with 47 families receiving palliative care in their homes, Hudson (2004) documented that the challenges of care in the home include the caregivers' own ill health, unsupportive family circumstances, insufficient skills to manage the patient's symptoms, limited time for themselves, and inadequate support from the health care professional. Dying persons often want to maintain their role within the family while interfacing with newly acquired roles, being unwell, and dealing with impending mortality. The quality of life of patients and caregivers is enhanced when the family is willing to receive external support from outside agencies. Rapport with the nurse is essential to building family relationships that allow entry into the family home (Johnson & Bourgeois, 2003).

Intensive Care Units

Of the patients who die in the hospital, approximately half are cared for in an ICU within 3 days of their death; one third spend at least 10 days in the ICU during their final hospitalization (Curtis, 2004). The majority of deaths in the ICU involve withholding or withdrawal of life support, and families typically are asked to make these decisions in consultation with the medical team (Kirchoff, 2004). The families of these patients typically have not had a prior relationship with the ICU clinicians before having intense life and death discussions. Families reported communication with the physician and nurse as the most important part of their experience of having a loved one die in the ICU (Curtis, 2004). Heyland and colleagues (2003) reported that overall satisfaction with EOLC in the ICU was significantly associated with the completeness of information received by family members, respect and compassion shown to the patients and their family, and satisfaction with the amount or level of health care received. Courtesy, compassion, and respect shown by the ICU staff were correlated with a completely satisfactory experience in the ICU by the family. Adequate communication, good decision making, respect, and compassion shown to both the patient and the family are key determinants of satisfaction. To achieve high-quality care when it is evident the patient is going to die, the shift of more supportive care and compassion to the family is important (Heyland et al., 2003).

Kirchoff (2002) documents six key points related to families' experiences with death in the intensive care unit:

1. Uncertainty pervades the end-of-life experience of patients' families in the intensive care unit.
2. Family members are torn between technology and individual choice.
3. Family members experience a responsibility to protect the patient.
4. Families' information about the patient's prognosis is often lacking or inadequate.
5. Effective communication with the staff is the best antidote for uncertainty among patients' family members.
6. Families need an adequate opportunity to say good-bye.

Prognosis and hope are critical aspects of information that are relayed to patients and their families. There is a need for sensitivity and respect for individual wishes in the communication process with families whose loved ones are dying in the ICU (Kirk, Kirk, & Kristjanson, 2004).

Assessing what the family knows about community or institutional resources is critical in planning care. The presence or absence of resources will influence where EOLC is delivered. A family may be unsure about what resources are available to them in making care decisions, which may limit what they can do for their family member. If families believe they have only one option for care, they can be forced into a decision they may regret.

GOALS AND PLANS FOR CARE

The process of assessment can delineate a number of possible goals and objectives. Validating the goal that family members view as most important is the first step in developing a plan of care that is family-centered and collaborative. Based on the assessment of family roles and knowledge about EOLC, nursing diagnoses can be made and measurable objectives can be developed for short-term goals. Often, the family member's most important goal is identified from past experiences and something they wanted to change. Some examples may be, "I don't want her to die alone," "I want him to be home in his own bed," "I don't want him to be in pain," or, "He wants to have the family with him." Objectives can then be developed to meet that goal. For instance, if the family's goal is to have their loved one die at home, the student may need to teach them how to administer medications, involve other family members in providing respite for the primary caregiver, and educate them about the hospice program available in their community.

It may be difficult for a nurse to distinguish between the family's needs and the patient's needs in care planning. It is valuable to write two separate care plans based on the assessment, one for the family and one for the patient. Comparing the goals and objectives can reveal areas of overlap or conflict that need to be addressed. The nurse can begin to see how each intervention influences the family system and its members. The pain management plan for the patient supports the family's objective of keeping the patient comfortable. For example, a plan to teach a daughter physical care may fulfill the patient's wish to have some time alone with her daughter. Conversely, the patient may be interested in pursuing a clinical trial yet the family wants to take the patient home to die. The nurse may have learned from the assessment that the patient felt it important to do one last good thing for others through a clinical trial, whereas the family wanted to spend as much time with the patient as possible before dying. With this information, interventions can be developed to resolve this difference and lead to a positive outcome.

BARRIERS TO DEVELOPING AN EFFECTIVE PLAN OF CARE

In helping nurses plan care for families at the end of life, it is important to be aware of how values and assumptions influence practice. First, this experience may be the nurse's first close contact with death and dying. It can be as traumatic for the nurse as for the patient and family. The nurse educator must assess the nurse's skill level and prior experiences with EOLC. They need to prepare nurses for how it may feel not to be able to fix everything for the family. Death is ultimately unavoidable despite the best care plan. It will be important for the educator to frame the

outcomes of care so that the student can see successes.

Death is a painful experience, under the best of circumstances. Cutillo-Schmitter (1996) notes that although we cannot take away a family's grief, we can provide our caring presence. Listening is a difficult but valuable way of being present with families. What to say to families after death is even more challenging. Role-playing in advance may be helpful in identifying therapeutic verbal and nonverbal behaviors. Practicing responses and actions may be helpful, such as how you would greet them, whether you would hug them, what to do if you feel like crying, and what to do about contact with the family after the death. Miles (1993), Brown (1994), and Czerwiec (1996) offer simple, straightforward information about how to speak with families and loved ones. Examining what has been learned in the past is beneficial. Interviewing surviving family members on a panel may be useful to nurses. Family members who are comfortable with their experiences may be good speakers with undergraduate students.

The educator must be cognizant of the nurse's own end-of-life experiences and their effect on interaction with the family. In undergraduate and graduate nursing education, knowing student concerns about the clinical assignment to provide EOLC may be useful in planning orientation or pre- and postconference discussions. The students can write a paragraph early in a clinical rotation about their concerns. The nurse educator could ask questions that may help students verbalize their concerns:"What do you worry might happen during this rotation?" "Do you have any concerns about talking with families?" "What worries you most?" "What are you looking forward to?" "What are your strengths in this setting?"

Although understanding a family member's experiences is useful to nurses in developing appropriate goals of care, it is important that nurses understand they cannot wholly compensate for the past. If a family member has significant issues around past EOLC, the nurse may need to refer the person to another member of the interdisciplinary team to assist in resolving the issues, such as a pastoral counselor, a social worker, or a bereavement counselor.

The reality of EOLC is that sometimes even the best plan must be abandoned and rewritten for any number of reasons. If the family's crucial goal was to send someone home to die, nurses may need support if the plan does not occur. Though any care plan can fail, EOLC carries such emotional overtones that the failure to execute a plan can be devastating. It is important to consider an alternate plan—at least in discussions—to prepare patients, family, and staff for the possibility that their plan may not work out.

Debriefing time is critical in formal EOLC clinical settings. The issues of death and dying effect nurses on both a personal and professional level. It can be stressful for less experienced nurses to have a patient who reminds them of their mother; facing the family after a patient dies within minutes of being medicated for pain; or providing postmortem care. It is critical to explore student's thoughts and feelings before and after clinical experiences. In addition, it is important to be aware of resources available to assist the nurse in continued learning regarding palliative care.

INTERVENTIONS: FACILITATING ROLE DEVELOPMENT FOR FAMILY

After assessing the family and developing goals and objectives, the nurse can begin to plan interventions to assist family members in achieving the roles they desire in EOLC. First, the nurse should validate roles desired by the family member. Communication is directed at encouraging the family member to describe what they want. Questions about how they see their role, what their concerns are about the role, what they need to do it, and what barriers exist will help the nurse decide what interventions are necessary. For example, if a daughter has children, a job, and a husband, yet wants to care for her dying mother in her home, the nurse will need to find out what resources are available to help her with child care, what her home is like, what experience she has in providing care, what her fears are, what resources are available in her workplace, and if she is aware of her family-leave program at work. From these answers, the nurse can begin to help plan interventions.

Access to information about available resources to meet the family's needs is critical. and nurses' participation in interdisciplinary teams assisting the family will be important. Nurses can benefit from spending time with other team members as they interact with family members, if appropriate. Collaborative efforts can be initiated with pastoral care staff, social services, mental health counselors, respite providers, and support groups. Although planning for a goal of home care can be largely a staff issue, the nurse should work with the care team and family to achieve some of the objectives needed to facilitate care at home. For instance, the nurse could begin to teach the daughter about physical care, nutrition, or medications.

The nurse should be assessing how the family's plan coincides with the patient's plan. If the nurse notes the mother is uncomfortable with the daughter's providing the physical care, the nurse might want to validate the mother's perceptions and then discuss how to proceed with the interdisciplinary team. It is important for the nurse to communicate the plans to staff so they do not inadvertently interfere with the family's plan. If a family member wants to do the bathing, the nurse needs to be sure that the staff member who is responsible for the task knows the plan and can support it. Documenting objectives and clear interventions in the patient's care plan often is overlooked because the interventions are actually family focused.

Primary caregivers may have clearly defined roles and responsibilities and have received much guidance in developing their role. The nurse can then reinforce teaching and provide support and positive feedback. In addition, the nurse can focus on other family members whose role may be undeveloped. Developing roles for other family members may be subtler, but blends well with the novice nurse's limited technical knowledge base in EOLC. The nurse's intervention of showing the son how to get ice and fluids for the father helped a family member without a role to identify something he could do independent of everyone else. The nurse can encourage family members to teach others the skills they learn as a means of developing possible respite resources.

One source of conflict for less experienced nurses can be their need to learn new tasks at the same time the family is learning. In this scenario, the use of an APN, nurse educator, or staff to teach a task while the nurse and family observe might be best. Sometimes, family members feel better about their relative inexperience when they see that novice nurses have to start with the basics. This has to be assessed carefully because some families may experience more anxiety because of this knowledge. Feedback is necessary for family members to develop their role successfully. The nurse can offer positive feedback to the family as they acquire new skills and explore new knowledge.

Nurses must be as supportive of families who continue to serve in their traditional family roles as they are of those who choose new roles in EOLC. A son who can visit the nursing home and hold his mother's hand for a few hours at a time is fulfilling the role he has always had as a loving son. The nurse can acknowledge his role and provide encouragement to continue. Clarifying how the son wants to be involved when death seems imminent, identifying other family members who may be available to keep vigil and support the son, and documenting the information for the staff is important nursing interventions. The nurse can attempt to provide more information about EOLC and the dying process, reassure the son about all that is being done to care for his mother, and ascertain his understanding about any further interventions.

TEACHING PLANS

Teaching families about EOLC includes education about community or institutional resources, the skills they need to perform their roles, what they can expect from the health care team, and what the process of EOL entails. A complete education plan for families in EOLC may be beyond the experience of the novice nurse. The role of the novice nurse may be to identify the knowledge deficits and then obtain the resources to address them. More advanced nurses may be comfortable with teaching skills. Experienced APNs may have had experience in all areas but should validate that their current knowledge base is appropriate, especially regarding topics such as hydration, pain management, and ethical and legal issues.

Teaching plans need to be considered in light of the urgency of the impending death. A nurse working with a patient newly diagnosed with a terminal prognosis will need to focus on one set of priorities, whereas a nurse in an ICU with a family who has just chosen to stop treatment will have a very different focus. In the first setting, the nurse may need to teach the family about support systems, community resources, and any treatments needed, such as pain management, nutritional support, wound care, and so forth. In the second setting, the nurse must assess quickly the family's understanding of the plan of care and their expectations. The nurse could provide information about the support the team will offer; provide them with privacy if they desire it; and describe what the EOL process will be like and what types of care will be provided, such as pain management, mouth care, skin care, and so forth. At this point, the nurse may ascertain what roles the family wants to play and begin to facilitate this. The nurse may invite a spouse to provide or participate in the patient's personal care if the spouse seems hesitant; help the spouse arrange to be contacted within the hospital so that the spouse can go to get food or rest as needed; and arrange for pastoral care if desired.

The trend of dying in institutions means that the average person has never seen death personally. Many families believe death will be as it is on television, with the patient talking one minute and quietly dying in the next. Novice nurses themselves may believe this. The reality that death is not likely to follow this scenario and the lack of correct information can make it difficult for family to cope with the terminal process. Rather than focusing on the technical aspects of dying, the nurse can relate the process of EOL as "sharing what I see." The phrase "I might see" or "I might expect" followed by a description of a finding or change can help the family to begin to assess the process for themselves.

Nurses can further assess the family's potential needs at the time of death. The death process can be difficult to experience. Some

families want to be alone; others prefer the presence of someone, a nurse, minister, or other family. Nurses will need to determine if they or someone else can provide this caring presence when the time comes. It may be simply being in the room during the last minutes, talking actively with the family about how the process is progressing and what the various symptoms indicate, or checking in at predetermined intervals as requested by the family. The plan should be documented and communicated with other staff to assure continuity. As noted earlier, the novice nurse may not be able to intervene alone and may need support from the interdisciplinary team. The nurse should be clear about what her level of involvement will be with the family. Nurses should let family know when they will be available, when they will return, and how any plans will be communicated and carried out when the nurse is not available.

CONCLUSIONS

The value in preparing nurses to meet the needs of families during end-of-life care seems as obvious as preparing them to manage pain or provide skin care. As outcome tools are developed and tested, the impact of educational preparation on the ability of the nurse to meet those needs will be delineated. Until then, the words of Dr. Joanne Lynn (1993, p. 42) offer a humanistic outcome measure:

> How can this work be other than rewarding? This family so obviously thrived, and this patient had so many good times in our care.... This family can look back on the good time that they shared under the shadow of death. The experience will illuminate and deepen their experiences over each lifetime. The caregivers involved can be confident that lives were made better by their efforts. What more can we ask of our work?

EDUCATION PLAN 9.1   Plan for Achieving Competencies: Caring for Families

Knowledge Needed	Attitude	Skills	Undergraduate Behavioral Outcomes	Graduate Behavioral Outcomes	Teaching/Learning Strategies
Identifying family structure and relationships.	*Accept as family, all individuals identifed by patient as family.	*Elicit a family history to identify members and relationships.	*Document a history that identifies family structure and relationships.	*Communicate family structure and relationships to interdisciplinary team.	*Create a genogram to identify family members' relationships. *Assign students to interview a patient to obtain a family history and compare data to chart documentation. *Present a family history at an interdisciplinary team meeting.

Research relevant to family caregiving.	*Value research related to family care giving in developing evidence-based practice.	*Use research findings to establish plans of care for family members.	*Critique family care giver research. *Utilize research findings in practice. *Identify needs for research in the area of family caregiving at the end of life.	*Collaborate in research related to family caregiving at the end of life.	*Critique 5 research articles relevant to family caregiving at the end of life and present the findings for future research to peers in post-conference or seminar. *As a class, document future areas of research in family caregiving.

(continued)

EDUCATION PLAN 9.1 *(continued)*

Knowledge Needed	Attitude	Skills	Undergraduate Behavioral Outcomes	Graduate Behavioral Outcomes	Teaching/Learning Strategies
The need for family care across the health continuum and health care settings.	*Perceive the need to provide care to family members across the health continuum and health care settings.		*Provide care to family members across the health care continuum and health care settings.	*Educate other health professionals regarding the needs of family caregivers across the health care continuum and health care settings.	*Develop a case history that identifies the changing needs of family members across the illness trajectory and health care settings. *Analyze a selected case history to determine unanticipated or unmet family caregiver needs.

| Family assessment | *Value the importance of a comprehensive family assessment. | *Assess a family using comprehensive assessment guide lines to identify roles, functions, and expectations of family members. | *Perform a comprehensive family assessment to determine basic family care giver needs. | *Perform a comprehensive family assessment to determine complex family caregiver needs. | *Select a patient in the clinical setting or role play to conduct a family assessment. Report assessment findings in post-conference or seminar.
*Use a movie or video to assess family caregiver needs at the end of life and discuss the assessment in class or seminar, i.e., "Fried Green Tomatoes" or "Philadelphia." |

(continued)

EDUCATION PLAN 9.1   *(continued)*

Knowledge Needed	Attitude	Skills	Undergraduate Behavioral Outcomes	Graduate Behavioral Outcomes	Teaching/Learning Strategies
Goals and Plans of Care	*Value the difference between families and patients' needs at the end of life. *Recognize students'/ nurses' own attitudes, beliefs, and past experience in developing a plan of care.	*Separate families' vs. patients' needs and provider bias in developing a plan of care.	*Develop a separate plan of care for family members.	*Develop an interdisciplinary plan of care for family members.	*Utilizing the family assessment above, identify family members' goals of care, and develop a plan of care to address their needs.
Interventions: Facilitating Role Development for Family	*Be respectful of diverse feelings and attitudes toward end of life caregiving by family members.	*Guide the family in determining their roles and way of performing them. *Teach family members related tasks.	*Assist family members in the performamce of caregiving roles.	*Collaborate with members of the interdisciplinary team to facilitate role identification and performance of family caregivers.	*Analyze a family caregiving situation, where roles are unclear or conflicts exist. Role play interventions to facilitate role acceptance and development. *Develop a teaching plan based on identified feamily needs.

REFERENCES

Administration on Aging. (1999). Profile of older Americans: 1999. Retrieved 9/4/2000 from http:// www.aoa.dhhs.gov/aoa/stats/profile/profile99.html

American Association of Colleges of Nursing. (1998). Peaceful death: Recommended competencies and curricular guidelines for end-of-life nursing care. Retrieved 9/4/2000 from http://www.aacn.nche.edu/education/ deathfin.htm

Andershed, B., & Ternestedt, B. M. (2001). Development of a theoretical framework describing relatives' involvement in palliative care. *Journal of Advanced Nursing, 34,* 554–562.

Arblaster, G., Brooks, D., Hudson, R., & Petty, M. (1990). Terminally ill patients' expectations of nurses. *Australian Journal of Advanced Nursing, 7*(3), 34–43.

Benner, P., Kerchner, S., Corless, I., & Davies, B. (2003). Attending death as a human passage: Core nursing principles for end-of-life care. *American Journal of Critical Care Nursing, 12,* 558–562.

Briggs, L., & Colvin, E. (2002). The nurse's role in end-of-life decision-making for patients and families. *Geriatric Nursing, 2,* 302–310.

Brock, D. B., & Foley, D. J. (1998). Demography and epidemiology of dying in the U.S. with emphasis on deaths of older persons. In J. K. Harrold & J. Lynn (Eds.), *A good dying: Shaping health care for the last months of life* (pp. 49–60). Binghamton, NY: Haworth Press.

Brown, M. A. (1994). Lifting the burden of silence. *American Journal of Nursing, 94*(9), 62–63.

Byock, I. (1997). *Dying well: The prospects for growth at the end of life.* New York: Riverhead Books.

Curtis, J. (2004). Communicating about end-of-life care with patients and families in the intensive care unit. *Critical Care Clinics, 20*(3), 363–370.

Cutillo-Schmitter, T. A. (1996). Managing ambiguous loss in dementia and terminal illness. *Journal of Gerontological Nursing, 22*(5), 32–39.

Czerwiec, M. (1996). When a loved one is dying: Families talk about nursing care. *American Journal of Nursing, 96*(5), 32–36.

Degner, L. F., Gow, C. M., & Thompson, L. A. (1991). Critical nursing behaviors in care for the dying. *Cancer Nursing, 14,* 246–253.

Donaldson, M. S. (1998). The importance of measuring quality of care at the end of life. In J. K. Harrold & J. Lynn (Eds.), *A good dying: Shaping health care for the last months of life* (pp. 117–138). Binghamton, NY: Haworth Press.

Emanuel, E. J., Fairclough, L., Slutsman, J., Alpert, H., Baldwin, D., & Emanuel, L. L. (1999). Assistance from family members, friends, paid caregivers, and volunteers in the care of terminally ill patients. *New England Journal of Medicine, 341,* 956–963.

Ferrell, B. (2001). Pain observed: The experience of pain from the family caregiver's perspective. *Clinics in Geriatric Medicine, 17,* 595–609, viii-ix.

Field, M. J., & Cassel, C. K. (Eds.) (1997). *Approaching death: Improving care at the end of life.* Washington, DC: National Academies Press. Retrieved 9/4/2000 from http://www.books. nap.edu/books/0309063728/html/R13HTML

Furukawa, M. M. (1996). Meeting the needs of the dying patient's family. *Critical Care Nursing, 16*(1), 51–57.

Hall, P., Schroder, C., & Weaver, L. (2002). The last 48 hours of life in long-term care: A focused chart audit. *Journal of the American Geriatrics Society, 50,* 501–506.

Heyland, D. K., Rocker, G. M., O'Callaghan, C. J., Dodek, P. M., & Cook, D. J. (2003). Dying in the ICU: Perspectives of family members. *Chest, 124,* 392–397.

Hudson, P. (2004). Positive aspects and challenges associated with caring for a dying relative at home. *International Journal of Palliative Care, 10*(2), 58–65.

Hull, M. M. (1989). Family needs and supportive nursing behaviors during terminal cancer: A review. *Oncology Nursing Forum, 16*, 787–792.

Jacobson, A. F. (1998). Can hospital patients have a "good death"? *American Journal of Nursing, 98*(9), 24.

Johns, J. (1996). Advanced directives and opportunities for nurses. *Image, 28,* 149–153.

Johnson, A., & Bourgeois, S. (2003). Essence of caring for a person dying. *Nursing and Health Science, 5,* 133–138.

Kirchoff, K. T. (2002). Promoting a peaceful death in the ICU. *Critical Care Nursing Clinics of North America, 14,* 201–206.

Kirchoff, K. T. (2004). Caring for the family of the critically ill patient. *Critical Care Clinics, 20,* 453–466.

Kirk, P., Kirk, I., & Kristjanson, L. J. (2004). What do patients receiving palliative care for cancer and their families want to be told? A Canadian and Australian qualitative study. *British Medical Journal, 328,* 1343–1350.

Lewandowski, W., & Jones, S. L. (1988). The family with cancer: Nursing interventions throughout the course of living with cancer. *Cancer Nursing, 11,* 313–321.

Lynn, J. (1993). Travels in the valley of the shadow. In H. Spiro, M. G. McCrea Curnen, E. Peschel, & D. St. James (Eds.), *Empathy and the practice of medicine* (pp. 40–53). New Haven, CT: Yale University Press.

Lynn, J. (1997). Measuring quality of care at the end of life: A statement of principles. *Journal of the American Geriatric Society, 45,* 526–527.

McCracken, A. L., & Gerdson, L. (1991). Sharing the legacy: Hospice care principles for terminally ill elders. *Journal of Gerontological Nursing, 17*(12), 4–8.

Meier, D. E., & Morrison, R. S. (1999). Old age and care near the end of life. *Generations, 23,* 611.

Miles, A. (1993). Caring for the family left behind. *American Journal of Nursing, 93*(12), 34–36.

O'Hara, P., Harper, D., Chartrand, L., & Johnston, S. (1996). Patient death in a long-term care hospital: A study of the effect on nursing staff. *Journal of Gerontological Nursing, 22*(8), 27–35.

Pickett, M. (1993). Cultural awareness in the context of terminal illness. *Cancer Nursing, 16,* 102–106.

Reimer, J. C., Davies, B., & Martens, N. (1991). Palliative care: The nurse's role in helping families through the transition of "fading away." *Cancer Nursing, 14,* 321–327.

Sherman, D. W. (1998). Reciprocal suffering: The need to improve family caregivers' quality of life through palliative care. *Journal of Palliative Care, 1,* 357–366.

Sherman, D. W. (1999). Training advanced practice palliative care nurses. *Generations, 23*(1), 87–90.

Smith, B. L., Martin, J. A., & Ventura, S. J. (1999). *Births and deaths: Preliminary data for July 1997–June 1998* (DHHS Publication No. PHS 99–1120). Hyattsville, MD: National Center for Health Statistics.

SUPPORT Principle Investigators (1995). A controlled trial to improve care for seriously ill hospitalized patients. *Journal of the American Medical Association, 274,* 1591–1598.

Waltman, N. L. (1990). Attitudes, subjective norms, and behavioral intentions of nurses toward dying patients and their families. *Oncology Nursing Forum, 17*(Suppl.3), 55–62.

Wilson, S. A., & Daley, B. J. (1999). Family perspectives on dying in long-term-care settings. *Journal of Gerontological Nursing, 25*(11), 19–25.

10

Loss, Suffering, Bereavement, and Grief

Mertie L. Potter

AACN Competency

#11: Assist the patient, family, colleagues, and one's self to cope with suffering, grief, loss, and bereavement in end-of-life care.

> *. . . weeping may endure for a night, but joy cometh in the morning.*
> —Ps. 30: 5 KJV

LOSS AND SUFFERING

Two deaths stand out in my mind from early childhood: my grandmother's and a little bird's. I was 6 years old. My sister and I were doing our nightly routine. My mother came into our room and sat down on my bed. Mom was crying. She had just received a phone call from "way far away" (my 6-year-old mind's concept of distance) that my grandmother had died. Although I only had seen my grandmother a few times in my young life, I felt very connected to her. I loved her very much, because I felt cherished by her. I also knew my mom and dad loved her greatly, and that Grammie had been sick for a long time. Mom answered our questions and prayed with my sister and me. After my mom and big sister left the room, I remember that I "talked to" Grammie out my bedroom window. I said, "I don't know if you can hear me,

but I love you a lot and will miss you." I felt sad and cried. I waited, half expecting to hear an answer from her; it was okay when I did not. It was our little good-bye with one another. I felt secure that she was in Heaven and that Heaven seemed like a good place for her to be if she were dead and no longer on earth. I felt at peace.

The other striking memory I have related to death occurred at the same period of time. My sister and I were playing in one of our favorite pine-needle-laden spots on our farm. We came upon a dead robin. We were horror-struck to see this beautiful creature lifeless on the ground. We ran and got a dustpan and gently scooted the bird onto it with a little pine branch. We dug a hole, wrapped the bird in a paper towel, respectfully placed it in a shoebox, and laid the bird to rest in its grave. We read Scripture, sang a hymn, and prayed for the bird. I was very grateful I had an older sister who knew how to conduct a proper funeral service for this dear little creature. We were both sad and cried. That also was the first time I remember questioning if animals have souls and where they go when they die.

Loss and suffering are major experiences along life's journey. How one learns to accept, adapt to, and advance through these experiences determines how the individual will move through life itself. Are loss and suffering perceived as natural, functional, growth-promoting, and normal dimensions in, and transitions through, life or are they perceived as unnatural, dysfunctional, harmful, and abnormal circumstances to be avoided?

LIVING WITH AND DYING FROM LIFE-THREATENING ILLNESS

"Losing, leaving, and letting go" are normal processes that help individuals grow (Viorst, 1987, p. 3). Loss and suffering, in fact, are inescapable dimensions of life. How an individual transitions through loss and suffering is what remains variable.

When planning the patient's care, it is important for the nurse to note how the patient with a life-threatening illness and significant others view loss, suffering, and living with and dying from such an illness. It also is important for nurses to examine their own beliefs related to these life experiences. Developing awareness of each person's perspective is key to formulating successful interventions.

Having an awareness of a patient's cultural background is important. Variations within specific cultures exist so it is important to discern with a patient and significant others what specific customs and rituals around death and grief are important and preferred (Clements et al., 2003; Mystakidou, Tsilika, Parpa, Katsouda, & Vlahos, 2003; Shuzman, 2003).

The living-dying interval often is a time of great uncertainty and questioning. Patients may question, Why? Why me? Why now? Patients often seek answers to questions related to the meaning of life, the meaning of suffering, the meaning of death, and the meaning of loss. This may be a time of opportunity for the patient to grow and sense a greater wholeness than ever before in spite

of an acute awareness of loss, suffering, and grief. Patients living with and dying from a life threatening illness need to focus on what they are able to do rather than on what they cannot do.

The Nurse's Role

Nurses meet individuals across the life span and often at the crossroads of their suffering and loss. Regardless of the setting, nurses are in a unique position to help individuals and their significant others who may be in physical, emotional, social, and spiritual pain related to suffering and loss. The nurse has a broad-based background in providing competent nursing care to individuals across the health/illness continuum. The breadth and depth of each nurse's skills in the specific area of giving care to those living with and dying from terminal illness will be dependent upon numerous factors. Some of these include the nurse's personal beliefs and values, life experiences (professional/nonprofessional), level of comfort with death and dying, educational level, licensure, and interest in this area.

Every nurse must be committed to providing patients, either directly or indirectly, quality care at the end of life. Critical to helping the nurse fulfill this obligation is a degree of comfort in dealing with death and dying. Student nurses need experience and support coping with dying and deceased patients. A student nurse shared how traumatic it was for her during her senior preceptorship to be left alone while providing her first postmortem care; the staff member assisting her had to step out of the room temporarily. The student nurse expressed frustration with herself that she felt "frozen" and "scared" until the staff member returned. Processing this experience with her faculty member helped her.

Knowledge of the process of dying and the degree of comfort in dealing with others who are experiencing death and dying are two important areas in which the advanced practitioner's education, experience, and expertise will provide more depth in discerning the special needs of the patient. Furthermore, the advanced practice nurse's skill level is more appropriate for dealing with high-risk and complicated situations.

A number of endeavors have been supported to enhance end-of-life care and further education around death, grief, and bereavement. One project is the End of Life Nursing Education Consortium (ELNEC) funded by the Robert Wood Johnson Foundation. Nurses involved with the ELNEC project developed a curriculum to improve end-of-life nursing care. Nurses are taught interventions that assist patients and families experiencing loss, grief, death, and bereavement, particularly effective and supportive communication strategies (Matzo et al., 2003).

Communication may be impaired or even unintelligible in the dying patient. In such circumstances, the nurse needs to inform the patient that the nurse is attempting to understand. It also is important that the nurse convey an understanding of how difficult it must be for the patient not to be able to communicate and that the nurse will make every effort to meet the patient's needs.

Each patient must be allowed to live and die in his or her own way. The nurse may assist patients to express what this way is. Nurses must be educated to promote holistic care, recognizing that quality-of-life issues that are important to dying patients are more apt to be peace of mind, comfort, and spiritual understanding rather than functional ability and psychological well-being (Stewart, Teno, Patrick, & Lynn, 1999).

Fostering patterns that are health-promoting and positive for individuals is the ideal in nursing care. Unhealthy patterns need to be identified and interventions provided to promote health and healing even as death approaches.

EXPERIENCE OF LOSS AND SUFFERING ACROSS THE LIFE SPAN

At birth, an infant is thrust or pulled into a new environment through expulsion and separation from the mother's womb. The infant has no control over this experience. A fairly traumatic transition takes place; one no longer is in the safe and warm environment that provided nourishment and protection during this critical developmental stage. The infant now has to adjust to a new home. This new environment includes the experiences of suffering and loss.

Nearing the sixth month, the infant usually develops an acute awareness of separation from the mother or mother-figure. This state is referred to as separation-anxiety. This keen awareness of loss may initiate a rudimentary development of death awareness (Backer, Hannon, & Gregg, 1994). This hypothesis is based on Bowlby's (1980) model of attachment between mother and infant and the infant's experience of separation from the mother. As the individual continues to develop, suffering and loss continue to occur. Generally, this occurrence causes the individual to move from a dependent state to an interdependent state and then to an independent state. In some cases, usually due to more loss and suffering, the individual may return to a dependent or interdependent state prior to death. Thus, life often involves a rhythm of change, interfacing with suffering and loss, from the time an individual is born.

Children under the age of 2 usually have a sense of separation but little understanding of the concept of death. For children between 2 and 5 years of age, death is seen as a transient state but not a permanent event.

TABLE 10.1   Developmental Views of Death

Age	Stage of development	Task/Area of resolution
Birth–2 years	Infancy	Sense of separation; no concept of death
2–5 years	Early childhood	Death is transient, not permanent state
6–10 years	Late childhood	Beginning awareness of the reality of death
13–25 years	Adolescence—young adulthood	Similar to adult view—realization of mortality and eventual death; death anxiety more evident; death perceived as a future event
26–65 years	Middle-aged and older adults	More aware and accepting of death

Adapted from McIntier, 1995, and Rando, 1984.

Between 6 and 10 years of age, children begin to grasp the reality of death (McIntier, 1995). Adolescents conceptualize death in a way similar to adults; namely, they are mortal and will eventually die. As the adolescent comes to terms with his or her individuality and increasing independence, there is an increasing awareness of one's own mortality. Although death is considered a future event to adolescents and young adults, death anxiety is more evident than at earlier ages. Middle-aged adults and older adults are more aware and accepting of death. However, no assumptions can be made concerning any age group, and the previous remarks are generalizations. Each individual's response to death is unique (Rando, 1984) (see Table 10.1 for developmental views of death).

THEORETICAL UNDERPINNINGS AND THEORIES ON DEATH AND DYING

As will be reviewed, Freud (1957), Lindemann (1944), Engel (1964), Glasser and Strauss (1965), and Kubler-Ross (1969) developed classical work related to dying and death. Pattison (1977), Bowlby (1980), Worden (1991), and Rando (1984) broadened knowledge in the field with their work. More recent writings by Corr (1992), Buckman (1993), Evans (1994), Copp (1997), and Mallinson (1999) have challenged, as well as added to, previous theoretical information. New information relevant to theories on death and dying is expanding rapidly. Contemporary research on death and dying views the time frame for grief resolution in a less restrictive way than earlier writings. Although different in some ways, most of the authors demonstrate a similar thread and core knowledge related to grief work that is helpful to both the beginning clinician and the advanced practitioner.

Freud (1957) brought the concept of grief work to the forefront after examining his personal feelings and societal observations following the mass losses brought about by World War I. Freud saw grief as a necessary process to assist an individual in adapting to loss. He also felt an individual needed to free himself or herself from attachment to the "lost object."

Lindemann (1944) studied bereavement in individuals who were survivors of the Coconut Grove Hotel fire in Boston (as well as their close relatives); patients who lost a relative while in treatment; relatives of members of the service; and relatives of patients who died while in the hospital. He determined that common physical symptoms, affective symptoms, behavioral manifestations, and physiological changes accompanied each grief experience. Lindemann also first alluded to anticipatory grief in relation to women anticipating the potential death of significant males in their lives during World War II.

Engel (1964) cited three stages through which one progresses in uncomplicated bereavement: shock and disbelief; developing awareness; and restitution and recovery. Engel pointed out that denial predominates initially and helps prevent the individual from being totally overwhelmed. During the second stage, the individual may express guilt and cry. Finally, thoughts and memories of the deceased are discussed and behaviors of the deceased may be displayed by the bereaved.

Glasser and Strauss (1965) examined different contexts related to caregivers and patients in relation to knowledge about a patient's dying. They suggested that there are four states of awareness related to dying: closed awareness, suspicion awareness, mutual pretense awareness, and open awareness. In the first context, closed awareness, caregivers are aware that the patient is dying but keep that information from the patient. In suspicion awareness, the caregivers know that the patient is dying, but the patient only suspects he is dying. The patient is ambivalent about wanting to know and not wanting to know that he is dying. In the mutual pretense context, both the caregiver and the patient act as though they do not know the patient is dying, but both know that the patient is. Within the context of open awareness, there is a sharing of knowledge, information, and communication about the patient's dying between the caregiver and the patient (Glasser & Strauss, 1965; Rando, 1984).

Kubler-Ross (1969) studied more than 200 patients diagnosed with terminal cancer. Her work was pivotal in theorizing that individuals move through (not necessarily sequentially) five phases when trying to cope with pending death. These five stages are: denial and isolation, anger, bargaining, depression, and acceptance. In the denial and isolation phase, an individual experiences shock and disbelief. A comment such as "I don't believe this is happening" may be made. During the anger phase, the individual questions "Why me?" Anger often is displaced. The individual may try to rationalize during the bargaining phase by pleading or regretting, "Yes, me, but . . . "; bargaining is an attempt to postpone death and extend life. It involves self-imposed deadlines. During the depression phase, the individual may express feelings of guilt or sadness, such as "Yes, this is happening to me." There often is an awareness of great loss for the patient. In the acceptance stage, the struggle is over. The individual has come to accept his imminent death and is ready to let go and move on. A comment such as "My time is close; it's all right now" may be made.

Pattison (1977) was the first to focus on a model that examined the "living-dying interval." Pattison defined that interval as existing between knowing that death was imminent and the actual point of death. He incorporates three clinical phases within the living-dying interval: acute crisis phase, chronic living-dying phase, and the terminal phase. During the acute crisis phase, the patient is confronted with the knowledge that a process beyond his control influences his death. The chronic living-dying phase involves an acute awareness of living and dying simultaneously. Last, the terminal phase commences when the patient starts withdrawing from the outside world. There is an internal awareness that he must conserve his energies for himself.

Bowlby (1980) described four phases of bereavement: numbness; yearning and searching; disorganization and despair; and reorganization. His theory is based on an attachment model in which the child must separate from the mother. The process includes (1) shock and disbelief related to the loss (numbness); (2) protest involving an attempt to regain the lost object (yearning and searching); (3) an intense sense of despair in which the individual tries to regain the lost object (disorganization and despair); and (4) completion of the mourning when the individual stops searching and develops new relationships (reorganization) (Evans, 1994).

Worden (1991) refers to four tasks of mourning: accepting the reality of the loss; experiencing the pain of grief; adjusting to an environment in which the deceased is not there; and emotionally relocating the deceased and moving on with life. Mourning may become maladaptive if an individual's response is to avoid, distort, amplify, or prolong grief (Kissane & Bloch, 2002).

Rando (1984) cites six processes of mourning or grief work: recognizing the loss; reacting to the separation; recollecting and reexperiencing the deceased and the relationship in a realistic way; relinquishing old attachments to the deceased and the assumptive world; readjusting to move adaptively in the new world without forgetting the old; and reinvesting. Rando (1984) considers that complicated grief may exist if there is compromise, distortion, or failure of one or more of the six "R" processes occurring after consideration of the amount of time since death.

As mentioned, Corr (1992), Buckman (1993), and Copp (1997) developed more contemporary theories. Corr expanded the theoretical premise of task work postulated by Pattison (1977) and Kalish (1979) to include four major areas of task work in coping with dying, specifically physical, psychological, social, and spiritual loss. Addressing physical tasks involves meeting bodily needs satisfactorily and minimizing the individual's physical distress. Working through psychological tasks maximizes the individual's psychological security, autonomy, and richness of living. In order to meet social tasks, interpersonal attachments of significance must be sustained and enhanced, as well as assisting the individual to explore social implications of dying. In addition, spiritual task work involves determining and affirming sources of spiritual energy that, in turn, stimulate hope.

Buckman (1993) promoted the concept that grief is more characteristic of the individual than of the individual's progression through particular grief stages. The second major point made by Buckman is that an individual's movement during the grieving process is dependent upon resolution of various issues related to emotions rather than changing from one emotion to another, as in Kubler-Ross's model. Additionally, Buckman addressed other responses to dying, such as fear of dying, guilt, hope, despair, and humor (Buckman, 1993).

Copp's (1997) work with dying individuals and the nurses caring for them examined two additional dimensions that seem to occur within the dying individual: readiness to die and a body-person split. Copp observed many direct and indirect actions between patients and nurses: protecting and letting go, watching and waiting, and holding on and letting go. Copp further noted a distinct reference by nurses and patients to the body as separate from the self in relation to patients who were nearing death. A dying individual's personal acceptance of imminent death and physical condition determined the individual's readiness to die. The states of readiness included: (1) person ready, body not ready; (2) person ready, body ready; (3) person not ready, body ready; and (4) person not ready, body not ready). One major thrust of Copp's (1998) work is that the dying experience impacts everyone who is involved with the dying patient.

DIMENSIONS OF LOSS, SUFFERING, GRIEF, AND BEREAVEMENT

Definitions

Loss

Loss is defined as "the condition of being deprived or bereaved of something or someone" (*American Heritage Dictionary*, 2000, p. 1034). Losses can be actual, potential, physical, or symbolic. Loss related to health, function, roles, relationships, and life itself is the central focus of this book. Losses other than the death of the loved one are referred to as secondary losses (Rando, 1984).

Mitchell and Anderson (1983) describe six types of loss: materialistic, relational, intrapsychic, functional, role, and systemic. Material loss involves separation from a physical object or surroundings. In relationship loss, an individual no longer has the ability to relate to another individual. Intrapsychic loss impacts an individual's self-image through loss of what might have been, changed perceptions, lost emotions (i.e., faith, hope, or courage), or emotions that result when a major task has been completed successfully. Functional loss occurs through bodily decline or deterioration in illness or aging. Role loss results when an individual changes or loses (e.g., healthy person to terminally ill person) a customary role or acquires a new role (e.g., patient). Systemic loss involves the loss of contact with customary behaviors or functions within a system, such as absence from a usual work environment or home environment.

Loss can be primary or secondary. Primary loss refers to the initial loss (whether of health for the patient or possibly loss of the patient through death for the significant others). Secondary losses stem from the initial loss. As a result of being diagnosed with a terminal illness, the patient also may experience secondary losses of roles, job, income, etcetera. Significant others may experience secondary losses of roles, income, their own health, and so forth.

Suffering

Suffering is defined as "the condition of one who suffers: the bearing of pain or distress" (*American Heritage Dictionary*, 2000, p. 1730). Suffering impacts a patient's body, mind, and spirit. Cassell (1991) defines suffering as "the state of severe distress associated with events that threaten the intactness of person" (p. 33). Cassell recognizes the importance of human suffering within any of the human dimensions, such as body, mind, and spirit. He also advocates asking individuals about the presence or absence of suffering because suffering is a very individualized experience and may result from treatment, as well as from the disease process or a number of other events.

According to Georgesen and Dungan (1996), the presence of pain compounds suffering and results in spiritual distress. Pain is a frequent companion of terminal illness. Suffering can be present with or without the presence of pain. Suffering, however, cannot be treated or managed like pain. Suffering is a personal experience. Framing suffering in a religious, philosophical, or personally meaningful perspective can help patients endure it better (Rando, 1984).

Suffering can be acute or chronic. Acute suffering occurs when the patient is in crisis and confronted with an immediate loss. Chronic suffering results from the longer-term realization and impact of a loss that carries a great deal of significance for, and meaning to, the patient. The patient with a terminal illness may experience only one type of suffering, both types at different times, or both simultaneously. Intervention involves trying to understand the patient's suffering and trying to help the patient cope effectively with suffering. Key to helping the suffering patient is attempting to understand the meaning of the suffering and attempting to comfort and sustain the individual through it.

Similar to chronic suffering is the middle-range nursing theory of chronic sorrow introduced by Eakes, Burke, and Hainsworth (1998). Chronic sorrow is viewed as normal in response to the recurrent experience of ongoing, significant loss that may be actual or symbolic or both. Major concepts within this theory relate to the following: losses, disparity between reality and idealism, trigger events or milestones, and an individual's internal and external means of managing reoccurring grief that accompanies chronic sorrow. One of the key antecedents to chronic sorrow, namely disparity between the individual's current reality and idealized reality, is what differentiates chronic sorrow from chronic suffering. An individual experiencing chronic suffering does not necessarily face disparity with chronic suffering.

Grief

Grief is defined as "deep mental anguish, as that arising from bereavement" (*American Heritage Dictionary*, 2000, p. 772). Rando

TABLE 10.2   Grief Responses

Physical	Psychological	Spiritual/Sociocultural
• Shortness of breath • Insomnia • Loss of appetite • Loss of sleep • Energy loss • Greater susceptibility to illness • Sighing • Nervousness and restlessness • Sensation of something in the throat • Feelings of emptiness or heaviness[1] • Heart palpitations • Crying • Psychomotor retardation • Decreased libido or hypersexuality • Weight loss[2]	• Depression • Anxiety • Guilt • Anger and hostility • Anhedonia • Self-reproach • Low self-esteem • Helplessness and hopelessness • Sense of unreality • Suspiciousness • Interpersonal problems • Imitation of the deceased's behaviors • Idealization of the deceased • Ambivalent feelings about the deceased[1]	• Spiritual pain and suffering • Spiritual loneliness • Fear of God, the unknown, and/or the future • Feelings of failure and guilt • Feelings of unfairness and anger • Loss of transcendence • Hopelessness[1] • Search for meaning • A need for love and hope • A sense of forgiveness[2] • Participation or lack of participation in formal religious group • Views related to use of "extraordinary" life-prolonging measures • Beliefs related to afterlife • Handling of the body after death • Rituals performed after death[3]

Physical—[1]taken from Lindemann (1944); [2]taken from Rando (1984)

Psychological—[1]taken from Lindemann (1944)

Sociocultural—[1]taken from Stuart & Sundeen, 1991, p. 154; [2]taken from Pritchett & Lucas, 1997, p. 203; [3]taken from Kazanowski, 1999, p. 176

(1984) describes grief as a normal reaction to the perception of loss. Grief is generally a transitory, acute state in response to loss with the possibility that the individual's ability to function may be disrupted temporarily. In addition, the individual may be distracted, disoriented, distressed, or all of these (Mallinson, 1999). Feelings that may accompany grief include anger, shame, helplessness, sadness, guilt, despair, relief, peacefulness, calm, and release (McCall, 1999). Charleton (2003) asserts that current stages of grieving might include any or all of the following: "distress, shock, denial, anger, feeling 'low in spirits,' depression, resignation, acceptance, resolution" (p. 671).

Common grief responses are listed (see Table 10.2). These responses may involve physical, psychological, and spiritual responses. The impact of grief can be extensive and pervasive. Anticipatory grief—feelings of grief experienced prior to an expected loss—has been thought to assist individuals in working through depression related to the upcoming death, rehearsing of the death, attempting to adjust to the consequences of the death, and having an increased concern for the terminally ill (Fulton & Fulton, 1971). Rando (1984) views anticipatory grief as also allowing for gradual absorption of the reality of the loss, helping resolve unfinished business, changing assumptions about life and identity, and making future plans.

Evans (1994) challenges the belief that anticipatory grief experienced prior to death is the same process as the conventional grief experienced in the postdeath period. Evans proposes use of the label "terminal response" to describe the process that occurs between diagnosis of terminal illness and death. Differences noted between pre- and postdeath grieving include the following: (1) anticipatory grieving ends at the time of death, whereas conventional grieving can go on indefinitely; and (2) anticipatory grieving

increases as death draws nearer, but conventional grieving usually diminishes in intensity with time.

Bereavement

Bereavement is defined as the state of being bereaved, which is to be left "desolate or alone, especially by death" (*American Heritage Dictionary*, 2000, p. 170). Rando (1984) describes bereavement as the state of having suffered a loss. McCall (1999) describes bereavement as the "overall reaction to the loss of a close relationship" and sees it as a description of various "patterns, phrases, and/ or stages that an individual goes through when grieving" (p. 42). Mallinson (1999) depicts bereavement as the long-term process of the survivor's accommodating his or her life without the loved one. Bereavement is a major life event that can result in an individual's having impaired health (Charleton, 2003).

Mourning, grief, and *bereavement* often are used interchangeably. Mourning often encompasses a sociocultural dimension and involves customs and rituals that are influenced by sociocultural and religious beliefs and values. Rando (1984) differentiates among the three in the following ways: (1) grief is the response to the perception of loss and is a transitional phase in the overall process of mourning; (2) mourning is the intrapsychic processes initiated by loss; and (3) bereavement is the state of having suffered a loss (pp. 15–16).

SIGNIFICANCE AND MEANING OF THE RELATIONSHIP TO LOSS AND SUFFERING

The intensity of loss for the dying patient and their significant others relates directly to each individual's perceptions of how close the relationship is and how great the loss of this relationship will be. The significance of the relationship impacts how the individual will interpret the loss and the accompanying suffering. The meaning that the patient, significant others, and nurse assign to loss and suffering also will determine how each individual faces the patient's dying and death. Interpretation of loss and suffering is unique to each individual and to each individual's particular circumstances.

Relationships fall into three categories: social, intimate, and therapeutic (Brady, 1997). Social relationships incorporate the everyday contacts individuals have, such as work colleagues and casual friends. Both individuals in this type of relationship are attempting to have their needs met. There is no particular goal within this relationship. Intimate relationships imply commitment by both individuals to one another. Therapeutic relationships involve goal-directed interaction with the purpose of helping one individual obtain an anticipated outcome to meet an identified need and facilitate growth.

The degree of intimacy and involvement within a relationship is not necessarily dependent upon the relationship's being a long-term one versus a short-term one or a blood relationship versus a non-blood relationship. Many factors determine how an individual will view his or her relationship with another individual. Some of these factors include respect, responsibility, commitment, compatibility, values, biases, beliefs, and time.

The stage of growth and development of the individual with terminal illness influences his or her ability to cope with the loss, suffering, and grief related to terminal illness. The stage of growth and development of significant others and the nurse also determine their ability to cope with the loss, suffering, grief, and bereavement related to the patient with a terminal illness. In addition, the stages of growth and development for all three groups (patient, significant others, and nurse) significantly impact how each will deal with the other.

Two of the most difficult aspects of a terminal illness are the accompanying uncertainty and unpredictability. These two factors may stress the relationships between the patient, the significant others, and the nurse. For some individuals, not knowing what is going to happen to the patient and when it might happen are difficult and unbearable aspects of coping with the patient's terminal illness.

Balancing the aspects of "getting through it" and "accepting that it will take time and a lot of hard work" were critical in a study involving 39 families who each had a child diagnosed with cancer; in addition, support from the family unit was considered most important for helping maintain one's spirit and keeping the family together (Woodgate & Degner, 2003, p. 117). Families wanted to share the entire experience of their children's having cancer and not focus on symptomatology.

Some terminal conditions, such as HIV/AIDS, may not be discussed by the patient or significant others because of fear of stigma or repercussions. In such situations, it is imperative that the nurse accept, understand, and be ready to assist the patient and significant others in sharing the pain associated with these conditions.

Nurses, patients, and caregivers assigned similar meaning to pain in a study of patients with cancer (Ferrell, Taylor, Sattler, Fowler, & Cheyney, 1993). Although both nurses and patients viewed pain as a challenge, nurses saw the challenge to eliminate pain, whereas patients saw the challenge to live with the pain in order to obtain vitality. Caregivers greatly empathized with the patient's pain and experienced persona l suffering and grief. Grief was triggered by pain, as it represented death to the caregivers.

Furthermore, an individual's view of change itself will help determine how that individual will accept loss and suffering related to their terminal illness. Has the individual's pattern been to welcome and embrace change or resist and fear change? The answer to that question can assist the nurse in implementing care that will help the patient and significant others to grow through the loss and suffering associated with the patient's terminal illness. Knowledge of change theory can help the advanced nurse facilitate acceptance of, and growth through, loss and suffering for the patient, significant others, and the nurse. Knowing the benefits and risks of change, change strategies, and resistance to change can help the nurse maximize the many changes within the patient's life.

ASSESSMENT—WHERE AM I (THE NURSE) ON THE JOURNEY?

In order to be an effective caregiver to the dying patient and the significant others, nurses must come to terms with their own mortality and views on dying and death. Death is an inevitable outcome of life for each individual. The death of a patient with a terminal illness forces the nurse to acknowledge that a cure cannot always be achieved. Fear related to death and dying is normal. Likewise, issues related to grief and bereavement during the death and dying process also are normal and even necessary for healthy adaptation to the preceding loss and suffering.

In American culture, individuals generally believe that explanations for dying always should be given. Furthermore, Americans feel that options to deal with the dying process always should be available (Kazanowski, in press). This widely held belief impacts the nurse, as well as the patient and signifi-cant others, in relation to high expectations of cure, treatment, care, and avoidance of a painful death. This approach is considered by some to be the "medicalization of human mortality;" this approach has limitations, however, because it cannot address psychological and spiritual factors associated with the suffering related to dying (Kissane & Bloch, 2002, pp. 78–79).

Nurses are encouraged to maintain composure when caring for patients. However, professionalism for the nurse within this context does not require that the nurse deny emotional engagement with the patient and significant others during the dying process and bereavement period. It does require, however, that the nurse's needs be subordinate to the needs of the patient and significant others. Constructive self-disclosure of feelings by the nurse may role-model to others a healthy process of acknowledging and resolving the suffering of loss. The nurse may or may not actually cry with the patient and significant others. If crying occurs, the nurse needs to be able to direct this situation into a meaningful and positive one for the patient and significant others. Empathy appropriately shared in this manner may well be described as a "therapeutic tear."

Lewis (1998) describes a strategy used to assist nursing students in working with patients and significant others who are experiencing loss and grieving. The learning activity is called Culture and Loss: A Project of Self-Reflection. Student nurses are requested to examine how their culture handles loss, to prepare a creative presentation for a small group of peers on how their culture responds to loss, and to describe to their class the meaning of their project and how it connects to their culture. Goals for implementing this strategy are identifying personal responses to loss; recognizing differing responses to loss and the influence of individual and cultural factors; and learning skills related to supporting individuals who are grieving.

Spencer (1994) examined which strategies were helpful to nurses in dealing with their own grieving. The most significant strategy noted was the nurse's informal network of peer group support. In addition, the nurses recommended formal group support and increased grief resolution training. When a team is involved, it is helpful to provide an opportunity for staff members to have open communication and to sustain and care for one another (Leichtling, 2004). There are numerous other health-promoting strategies to help the nurse cope with caring for dying patients. These include regular exercise, good nutrition, diversional activities, focus on caring rather than curing, emphasizing the positive dimensions of the nurse's role, and recalling positive experiences with families (Pritchett & Lucas, 1997).

Advances in technology have prolonged dying and death in our culture. As a result, advance directives have taken on greater significance in relation to end-of-life care. Studies have indicated that patients who have prepared advance directives select palliative care more frequently, are more accepting of death, and have less expensive care and less aggressive treatment (Danis, 1998).

There are incongruences between the ideal and reality in end-of-life care. First, clinicians are expected to be able to predict the expected time of death for a terminally ill patient; however, this involves a great deal of uncertainty. Goals of care may need to change quickly as the patient's condition changes or therapeutic trials fail. Second, it is expected that the patient's clinicians know the patient's wishes concerning dying and death. In reality, organizational factors may impact the patient's care more than the patient's wishes during the end-of-life process. Third, it is thought that the patient's care is well coordinated. Often this is not the case because some intensive care facilities are staffed with their own primary care providers who may not know the patient admitted with a terminal illness. Therefore, it is important for the nurse to work closely with the patient and the significant others concerning the patient's priorities and wishes. Finally, the measurement of goals and outcomes may not be congruent. Measures of care for dying patients usually focus upon frequency of Do Not Resuscitate orders and lengths of time a patient spends on life support or in a coma. It may be more important to patients and significant others to examine issues related to pain management and satisfaction with care (Danis, 1998).

Confronting death with a terminal illness is difficult, painful, and complex. Nurses need to be strong advocates for satisfactory pain management. Keeping abreast of the patient's treatment wishes (which may change during the dying process) and coordinating care between facilities and providers also are important.

Personal Experiences with Death

Personal experiences with dying and death influence how nurses give care to those who are dying and their significant others. For example, examining personal experiences can help nurses understand their own fears and anxieties related to dying and death. Understanding the meaning and significance of relationships helps put the loss in perspective. The nurse's ability to articulate feelings regarding a good or bad death is important when working with individuals who are dying. Exploring individual values and biases can enhance the nurse's competence; this helps the nurse better understand individual's health care attitudes and behaviors (Warren, 1999).

Use the following exercises to help you expand your self-understanding in relation to loss and suffering, dying and death, and grief and bereavement.

Self-Reflective Questions

- What experiences have you had with death? Describe your earliest memory of death. Was anything positive about it? Was anything negative about it? Have you experienced what you would call a "good death?" Have you experienced what you would describe as a "bad death?"

- Can you picture yourself helping someone who is dying? How? What do you have to offer that is special and unique?

- Relate what you believe happens when someone dies. What do you fear about death? What do you fear about your own death?

- Assume you have just received news that you have been diagnosed with a terminal illness. What would be the most difficult things for you to have to give up during this time?

- How do you feel about cultural attitudes or behaviors that may be different from your own?

ASSESSMENT—WHERE IS THE PATIENT ON THE JOURNEY? THE LIFE CYCLE CONTINUUM—ACROSS THE LIFE SPAN ON THE JOURNEY

Living with and dying from a terminal illness can be best understood within the context of a continuum. One generally does not remain on a fixed point along the continuum. Like one's view of health and illness, living with and dying from terminal illness is a dynamic and fluid experience in which the individual moves back and forth across the continuum.

Reactions to dying and death vary across the life span. They also are dependent upon physical, psychological, spiritual, and sociocultural factors that impact the individual's sense of wellness. Physiological change can lead to a sequelae of loss: function, body image, self-esteem, sexuality, and role competence. Furthermore, interfacing of the various factors has the potential to result in grief over lost health (Talerico, 2003). The living-dying interval occurs from the time death is acknowledged as imminent to the point of the actual death. A difficult task during this period is continuing to treat the individual as still living and as a person and not just a patient. Tasks that the individual needs to attend to are arranging his or her affairs; coping with loss (loved ones and self); attending to future care needs; planning remaining time; confronting loss of self and identity; facing one's own death encounter; deciding whether to succumb to or resist the dying process; and struggling with the psychosocial problems of dying. Some of the issues for the individual during this period of time include treatment choices, remissions and exacerbations, expression of sexuality, financial pressures, employment concerns, struggle for control, and suffering (Rando, 1984).

Depending on the patient's level of maturity, the patient may be confronted with the meaning of life, relationship with God and others, and the reality of death (Georgesen & Dungan, 1996). In addition, the patient may face losses related to independence, control, work, physical comfort, a sense of normalcy, sexual activity, and usefulness when living with a life-threatening condition (Ferrell et al., 1993). For example, it may be difficult for older adults who have served as caregivers to receive care from another because of loss of independence. An aid to this transition of caregiving may be to enable older adults to focus on ways they can affirm the individuals now serving as caregivers to them (Talerico, 2003).

Once rapport has been developed, the nurse may suggest that the patient and the patient's significant others consider attending a support group. Support groups have been found to be particularly helpful for significant others facing traumatic (e.g., loss of a child) or stigmatized (e.g., acquired immunodeficiency syndrome) deaths, as well as for individuals who themselves are dying (Callanan & Kelley, 1992; Goodkin et al., 1999; McCreight, 2004; Rando, 1984, Vigil & Clements, 2003).

Individual Needs

During the illness/dying trajectory, the nurse needs to assess the patient's immediate and specific needs. Certain simple pleasures may be more important to the patient than a nurse-perceived need for oxygen. For a peaceful death, a patient may need the comfort and joy that a treat, such as food or music, may represent. Asking the patient (or significant others if the patient is unable to respond) what the immediate and specific needs are may bring insight as to what intervention is needed to help the patient be more comfortable.

Maintaining some control is especially important during this time, as the patient may have had to relinquish control in many areas. Moreover, having control over pain is critical. Patients with a terminal illness and their significant others fear lack of pain control during end-of-life care (Danis, 1998).

Having a sense of order and a sense of closure in personal affairs are important aspects to address with the patient also. Sharing what one needs to say to others, through direct contact (e.g., in person or phone) or indirect contact (e.g., written communication), may help the patient have a more peaceful death.

Sensitivity to the patient's leading in this area is critical.

Areas of Assessment

Use the following questions to assess the patient on the journey living with and dying from a terminal illness in relation to loss and suffering, dying and death, and grief and bereavement.

- How do you view your illness?
- What is the meaning of your illness to you?
- What fears or concerns do you have regarding your illness?
- In what ways are you experiencing loss and suffering?
- Are there any unresolved issues or business that need to be resolved?
- Do you have any specific fears about dying and death in general? About your own dying and death?
- What concerns do you have for others now and after your death?
- What helps you maintain a sense of hope during difficult times?
- What specific needs do you have at this time?
- In what ways might I be most helpful to you in meeting those needs?

ASSESSMENT—WHERE ARE THE SIGNIFICANT OTHERS ON THE JOURNEY?

Healthy spouses of terminally ill cancer patients were studied (Siegel, Karus, Raveis, Christ, & Mesagno, 1996). Males were found to be more at risk for depressive symptoms than females if they were parents of school-aged children. Part of this could be due to their having less of a social network than females in general, and part may be due to their having to assume additional parenting responsibilities as the result of their spouse's illness and subsequent death. Overall adjustment was better for well spouses and inversely proportionate to the number of children in the household. Work was perceived as both a stressor due to the demands of the job and as a stress buffer due to the potential emotional support, sense of control, and predictability it may provide for the significant other.

Elderly males have been found to be at increased risk for suicide after the death of a spouse (McCall, 1999). In general, older adults face multiple losses for numerous reasons including declining health with increasing age (Talerico, 2003).

Sherman (1998) refers to the reciprocal suffering inherent in being a family member or significant other of a patient diagnosed with a terminal illness. This suffering results from the expectations and responsibilities placed upon the significant other to care for the patient, the mutual experience of intensified needs brought about by the patient's illness, and the often rapidly changing needs of both the patient and the significant other. Quality-of-life issues arise for the family members and significant others, as well as for the patient.

Koop and Strang (1997) reviewed a number of studies to determine correlates of greater satisfaction in families of patients with a terminal illness. They found higher satisfaction in families in which there had been psychosocial support from the nurse, fulfillment of basic needs, high frequency of home visits, support at night, connection to other services, visits to the bereaved caregiver, choices in treatments, privacy during hospitalizations, treatment of respiratory symptoms, the presence of professional caregivers (especially if the patient is at home), and participation in a hospice program.

There is interdependence between the patient, the significant others, and the nurse in relation to providing optimal care for the patient with a terminal illness. The nurse can maximize the positive aspects of this interdependence by recognizing and affirming the patient's significant others, incorporating them into the patient's care as desired by the patient, and assisting the significant others in their loss, suffering, and grief related to the patient's dying and death. Kissane and Bloch (2002) recognized the influence of family in Reiss' (1990) study on renal disease, claiming, "This research highlights the potential influence of the family on both the course of illness and survival" (p. 26). Woodgate and Degner (2003) note in their research of children with cancer that, "It is important for those involved in the care to recognize that maintaining the family unit was equally important to families as was beating the child's cancer" (p. 117). In addition, the patient's significant others will experience bereavement issues once the patient dies. Research by Jordan and Neimeyer (2003) demonstrates that "With the help of family and friends, apparently most mourners are able to work through and integrate their losses relatively well" (p. 772).

How does one know when the patient is ready to die? Four types or stages of death occur, usually in the following order: social death, psychological death, biological death, and physiological death (Sudnow, 1967). Social death marks the narrowing of the patient's world, as he has known it. This is a highly individualized stage that is dependent upon the patient's level of involvement versus detachment in his social world. Psychological death is a death of the patient's personality. Relationships change. The patient withdraws and distances himself or herself from others. Terminal illness places demands that result in the patient's becoming regressed and dependent. Biological death involves the loss of consciousness and awareness on a self-sustaining basis; the patient may be on life-supports at this point. Finally, physiological death occurs. All vital organs cease to function (Rando, 1984). At this point, a nurse or physician (depending upon state law) pronounces death. The moment of finality has arrived. Life as the patient and the significant others knew it for the patient has ceased.

Relationships

Support from significant others can aid in decision making and acceptance of death for a patient with a terminal illness. Patients and their significant others may determine together if they want to pursue life-sustaining procedures or to forgo them in light of the uncertainty and potential trauma that surround the situation. Close communication with the nurse during end-of-life care is essential because the needs of the patient and care planned for him are apt to change rapidly. Patients and their significant others may change their minds concerning treatments depending upon the patient's level of consciousness, the patient's pain level, both the patient's and significant others' fear levels, additional troublesome symptomatology for the patient, failure of therapeutic trials, and the level of support and contact between the patient and his significant others (Danis, 1998).

Significant others who care for a terminally ill patient are faced with increased feelings of powerlessness, anger, and grief when the patient's pain is unrelieved (Ferrell et al., 1993). Danis (1998) found that families of deceased patients indicate that more attention should be given to analgesia and communication in end-of-life care. Significant others may or may not provide direct care to the patient. They may have other resources, hired or voluntary, to provide caregiving to the patient. If significant others are providing care, they will be at risk for burnout or fatigue. A proactive approach in order to prevent this should be in place in the patient's care plan.

Areas of Assessment

- Determine with significant others what they perceive as the patient's needs.
- Provide education in pain assessment and pain management strategies.
- Assess how the significant others feel they are doing and what degree of loss and suffering they are currently experiencing.
- What types of secondary losses are being experienced or anticipated as a result of the primary loss (i.e., anticipatory death or actual death of the patient)?
- Determine the level of emotional support needed.
- Ascertain if spiritual support is desired.
- Assure significant others that they are not an imposition to professionals who also are providing care for the patient.
- Identify available resources to help significant others care for the patient.
- Encourage significant others to grieve in whatever ways are best for them.

Normal Grief

Grief is a normal response to loss. Grief may become manifest in feelings, physical sensations, cognition, and behaviors (see Table 10.2). Psychological, sociocultural, and physical factors influence the grief reaction. The nurse needs to assess which factors are influencing the significant others. Rando (1984, pp. 43–57) addresses these influences as follows:

Psychological factors:

- Significance of the loss.
- Attachment level.
- Family role of the deceased.
- Individual coping behaviors, such as avoidance, distraction, preoccupation,

impulsivity, rationalization, intellectualization, prayer, and connection with
others.

- Intelligence and maturity levels.
- Previous experience with death and
  loss.
- Conditioned sex-roles.
- Age of the individual grieving.
- Age and characteristics of the deceased.
- The death of a parent represents loss of
  the past.
- The death of a spouse represents loss of
  the present.
- The death of a child represents loss of
  the future. The death of a child may be
  the most difficult death to handle.
- Unattended business between the griever
  and the deceased.
- Perception of fulfilled life for deceased.
- Circumstances related to death including
  location, type, reason, and preparedness.
- Timing of the death. (Is the death psy-
  chologically acceptable?)
- Perception of death's prevention.
- Sudden or anticipated death.
- Chronic versus acute illness.
- Impact of anticipatory grief on the rela-
  tionship with the dying patient.
- Impact of secondary losses.
- Additional stresses or crises.

Social factors:

- Level, acceptance, timing, and duration
  of support.
- Religious, sociocultural, ethnic, and
  philosophical backgrounds.
- Bereaved's educational, economic, and
  occupational status.
- Positive or negative funeral rituals.

Physiological factors:

- Positive and negative impact of medications.

- Need for nutrition, sleep and rest, exercise, and physical health.

In addition, grief may be mistaken for un-
diagnosed depression. A way to distinguish
between the two is to note if the individual
in question is able to experience pleasure.
Grieving individuals can experience pleasure;
depressed individuals often have difficulty
experiencing pleasure and may lose morale
and hope (Kissane & Bloch, 2002).

CHILD'S EXPERIENCE OF LOSS

The death of a parent impacts a child greatly.
Family life and daily routine are disrupted
permanently. A child may have a depressed
mood, cry, be sad or irritable, withdraw, or
have sleep disturbances during the first 4
months after the loss of a parent. Physical,
behavioral, and emotional responses occur
immediately for young children. Although
infants and toddlers are not at a developmental stage to be able to comprehend loss or
death, they are distraught that someone important to them is absent (Hames, 2003). A
child's reaction may be impacted by individual personality factors, sociocultural factors,
the child's age, child's history, child's religious
beliefs, family dynamics, family's socioeconomic status, sex of the child and the remaining parent, additional stress in the child's life,
parental substitutes, nature of the death, and
how the child was notified (Geis, Whittlesey,
McDonald, Smith, & Pfefferbaum, 1998).

Caregivers must recognize the importance
of age in relation to a child's ability to experience loss and grief. Saldinger, Cain, and Porterfield (2003) note that children may have
a very difficult experience with anticipatory
grief if they are expected to demonstrate levels of "self-sacrifice" that exceed their "levels
of maturity" (p. 175). The ELNEC curricu-

lum provides a table of children's ages and grief reactions that is valuable to caregivers (see Table 10.3).

Degree of attachment also impacts how a child will respond to the loss of a parent. Stroebe (2002) found that individuals who had a more secure attachment to the lost figure had a more fluid movement between loss and restoration orientations and experienced less complications with grieving. Children often experience separation anxiety after the death of a parent. Coming to terms with surviving in a world without the presence of the deceased parent can be traumatic for the child. Secondary to that trauma may be the additional stress of observing a surviving par-

TABLE 10.3   Grief and Bereavement in Children

Birth to Six Months		
Characteristics of Age	View of Death & Response	What Helps
Basic needs must be met, cries if needs aren't met.	Has no concept of death.	Progressively disengage child from primary caregiver if possible.
Needs emotional and physical closeness of a consistent caregiver.	Experiences death like any other separation;—no sense of "finality."	Introduce a new primary caregiver.
Derives identify from caregiver.	Nonspecific expressions of distress (crying).	Nurturing, comforting.
View of caregiver as source of comfort and all needs fulfillment.	Reacts to loss of caregiver. Reacts to caregiver's distress.	Anticipate physical and emotional needs and provide them.
		Maintain routines.

Six Months to Two Years		
Characteristics of Age	View of Death & Response	What Helps
Begins to individuate.	May see death as reversible.	Needs continual support, comfort.
Remembers face of caregiver when absent. Demonstrates full range of emotions.	Experiences bona fide grief. Grief response only to death of significant person in child's life.	Avoid separation from significant others.
Identifies caregiver as source of good feelings and interactions.	Screams, panics, withdraws, becomes disinterested in food, toys, activities.	Close physical and emotional connections by significant others.
	Reacts in concert with distress experienced by caregiver.	Maintain daily structure and schedule of routine activities.
	No control over feelings and responses; anticipate regressive behavior.	Support caregiver to reduce distress and maintain a stable environment.
		Acknowledge sadness that loved one will not return—offer comfort.

(continued)

TABLE 10.3   Grief and Bereavement in Children (*continued*)

Two Years to Five Years		
Characteristics of Age	View of Death & Response	What Helps
Egocentric	Sees death like sleep: reversible.	Remind that loved one will not return.
Cause-effect not understood.		
Developing conscience.	Believes in magical causes.	Give realistic information, answer questions.
Developing trust.	Has sense of loss.	Involve in "farewell" ceremonies.
Attributes life to objects.	Curiosity, questioning.	
Feelings expressed mostly by behaviors.	Anticipate regression, clinging.	Encourage questions and expression of feelings.
Can recall events from past.	Aggressive behavior common.	Keep home environment stable, structured.
	Worries about who will care for them.	Help put words to feelings; reassure/comfort.
		Reassure child about who will take care of them; provide ways to remember loved one.

Five Years to Nine Years		
Characteristics of Age	View of Death & Response	What Helps
Attributes life to things that move; may fear the dark.	Personifies death as ghosts, "bogeyman."	Give clear and realistic information. Include child in funeral ceremonies if he or she chooses.
Begins to develop intellect.	Interest in biological aspects of life and death.	
Begins to relate cause and effect; understands consequences.	Begins to see death as irreversible.	Give permission to express feelings and provide opportunities; reduce guilt by providing factual information. Maintain structured schedule, individual and family activities; needs strong parent.
Literal, concrete.	May see death as punishment; may feel responsible.	
Decreasing fantasy life, increasing control of feelings.	Problems concentrating on tasks; may deny or hide feelings, vulnerability.	
		Notify school of what is occurring, gentle confirmation, reassurance.

TABLE 10.3   Grief and Bereavement in Children *(continued)*

Pre-Adolescent through Teens		
Characteristics of Age	View of Death & Response	What Helps
Individuation outside home.	Views death as permanent.	Unambiguous information.
Identifies with peer group; needs family attachment.	Sense of own mortality; sense of future.	Provide opportunities to express self, feelings; encourage outside relationships with mentors.
Understands life processes; can verbalize feelings.	Strong emotional reaction; may regress, revert to fantasy.	
Physical maturation.	May somaticize, intellectualize, morbid pre-occupation.	Provide tangible means to remember loved one; encourage self-expression, verbal and non-verbal.
		Dispel fears about physical concerns; educate about maturation; provide outlets for energy and strong feelings (recreation, sports, etc.); needs mentoring and direction.

Source: Processes to Optimize Care During the Last Phase of Life by P. Fine (Ed.). (1998). Copyright Vista Care Hospice. Reprinted with permission.

ent cope with the loss or the anticipated loss if such were the case (Saldinger et al., 2003). Nurses can help a dying parent communicate with children who will be left behind; this can enhance meaning and comfort to the dying by making a contribution to their child's journey with grief. Likewise, a surviving parent inadvertently becomes a role model for grieving to children left behind by a deceased parent (Hames, 2003).

If the child loses a sibling, other issues, such as, guilt, ambivalence, denial, increased vulnerability, and fear for his own well-being may arise. Parental response to the surviving siblings helps determine the child's adjustment. Similar responses may occur for adolescents with possible reframing of the adolescent's self-concept, self-identity, and family role (Geis et al., 1998). Tasks that occur for all siblings of a deceased child, regardless of age, include grieving the deceased sibling, coping

with family changes, realigning relationships, and attempting to understand the meaning of the tragedy within the family (Kiser, Ostoja, & Pruitt, 1998).

Areas of Assessment

- How is the child functioning socially according to his or her developmental level? What is the child's involvement in relationships, recreation, and routines?
- Is the child exhibiting any changed behaviors?
- What is the child's predominant mood (sad, withdrawn, hyperactive, angry)?
- How does the child express his or her suffering or "pain" related to the loss?
- What does the child feel might help make the "pain" better (besides the return of the lost loved one)?

Family Caregiving— Parental Experience of Loss

Living with dying can tax a patient and his significant others economically, as well as physically, spiritually, and psychologically. Often the patient or his significant others lose work time due to the patient's care requirements. Additional expenses may arise with treatments, hospitalizations, or other hidden expenses, such as transportation, child care, out of home food purchases, lodging, and so forth. Dying patients often experience much stress because of the financial burdens that fall upon the significant others (Rando, 1984). If the nurse feels unprepared to counsel the patient and significant others in this area, it is imperative to refer them to someone who can.

The loss of a child often is devastating to the parents and to the family. Parents feel responsible for their child's health, well-being, and safety. In the case of a newborn with a serious condition, there is accompanying parental blame and guilt for the infant's condition. Parents must grieve the healthy, "normal" child they lost in addition to the anticipated death of the infant.

Parents usually do not expect their child to die. This is true even in the case of adult children who die before parents. Older adults may experience "survivor guilt, powerlessness, and loss of religious faith"; the deceased child may be idealized which can complicate grief resolution (Talerico, 2003, p. 14).

Grief related to the loss of a child is apt to be severe and complicated. Anniversary events and developmental milestones for the deceased child reopen the grief experience throughout the parents' lifetime (Kiser et al., 1998). Acknowledging that their lives have changed forever is part of the grief resolution that takes place for parents; however, recovery from the death of a child is a lifelong process (Geis et al., 1998). For the single parent, aloneness may be magnified (Backer et al., 1994). Controversy exists about parents' viewing prenatally deceased infants and stillborn infants; in general, viewing the body is thought to help with grieving (Haas, 2003). Nurses must be sensitive to family members' readiness and wishes related to viewing the body of their deceased loved one.

Areas of Assessment

- How has your loved one's illness impacted your life?
- In what ways will you remember your child who died?
- What is the most significant type of suffering you are experiencing right now?
- What are your specific needs at this time and how can I help you meet them?

RISK FACTORS FOR COMPLICATED GRIEF

Predicting bereavement outcomes is difficult because the subjects are considered to be a vulnerable study population. A balance between the need for protection and the benefits of participation must be attained. Studies increasingly suggest that the greatest predictor of well-being during bereavement is prior well-being (Koop & Strang, 1997).

Although each individual's grieving is unique, the bereavement process may be functional or dysfunctional, adaptive or maladaptive. The time for grief resolution has varied from peaks at 4 months to as long as 3 years (Lev & McCorkle, 1998). Prolonged reactions occur in approximately 15% of the ber eaved. These prolonged reactions range from exaggerated normal reactions to abnormal grief reactions. Furthermore, grief may be unresolved or compounded if a loss or losses occur within a community of individuals where the losses are minimized or ignored; this may result in further complications with subsequent losses (Talerico, 2003).

Backer and colleagues (1994) describe three basic types of complicated grief reactions: delayed, inhibited, and chronic grief. In delayed grief, the grief is triggered by the loss of someone or something else. There is minimal impact in this situation. For example, someone whose father has recently died may experience delayed grief related to the death of the individual's mother 10 years prior to the father's death. The individual has never experienced full grief for the death of the mother until the death of the father. His death triggers the deeply felt but unexpressed loss of the mother. Inhibited grief occurs when an individual never grieves. It also may occur if the individual feels great distress related to a lost relationship. This type of grief becomes complicated if another condition develops related to the unfelt grief. Last, chronic grief exists when the grieving is unending, and the intense yearning for the lost relationship continues. A cause for this type of grief could be unspeakable deaths, such as those due to AIDS or suicide.

Rando (1984) addresses delayed, inhibited, and chronic grief reactions but also includes absent grief, conflicted grief, unanticipated grief, and abbreviated grief in her list of complicated grief types. Absent grief is characterized by a total lack of grief emotions and processes of mourning. Conflicted grief involves an amplification of the characteristics of normal grief partnered with a suppression of other manifestations of normal grief. Unanticipated grief takes place after an unexpected loss that the individual cannot grasp. Abbreviated grief is normal grief that lasts a short period of time because of swift replacement of the lost individual or lack of attachment to the lost individual. One study (Prigerson et al., 1997) identifies grief involv-

ing trauma and separation as traumatic grief and indicates that psychiatric sequelae, such as traumatic grief, puts bereaved individuals at risk for complicated grief.

Families grieve in a unique way. Family members all fill unique roles. A lost family member means the family must reassign the lost role. Likewise, families may distort circumstances through idealization, blame, anger, or despair. Families who do not share their grief may experience poor coping or breakdown (Kissane & Bloch, 2002).

There are a number of individuals at risk for complicated grief after the death of an individual with a terminal illness. These include spouses, parents, those experiencing the loss of loved ones through unspeakable deaths, and those with a psychiatric history. Male spouses are more at risk than female spouses because of more limited social networks. Men often feel responsible to be the stronger partner (McCreight, 2004). In her study related to pregnancy loss, McCreight (2004) also found that men did not experience bereavement through "an intellectualization of the process of grief" (p. 346), but rather experienced loss on an emotional level. Furthermore, single parents are at higher risk because of less support. In addition, those diagnosed with depression are at the highest risk for complicated grief (Kurtz, Kurtz, Given, & Given, 1997).

Work done by Pennebaker, Mayne, and Francis (1997) indicates that language usage can help to impact bereavement outcomes in a positive way. Encouraging individuals to talk about traumatic events forces a disorganized event and emotions to become more organized, coherent, and insightful. Over time, the use of insight and causation words in relation to the event and its accompanying emotions helps cognitively reframe the experience that results in more adaptive outcomes.

Frank, Prigerson, Shear, and Reynolds (1997) postulate that individuals experiencing elongated periods of distress (for several months) and exhibiting criteria for major depressive episodes are undergoing traumatic grief reactions. They advocate treatment interventions that involve reexperiencing the moment of death, saying good-bye to the deceased while still retaining special memories of the person, and gradually being exposed to situations that the bereaved has avoided since the deceased's death. The outcome of this traumatic grief treatment has been reduced subjective distress. They do not advocate for pathologizing or treating brief periods of bereavement-related distress.

A number of factors were examined in a study attempting to predict depressive symptomatology in the postbereavement period (Kurtz et al., 1997). Prebereavement depressive symptomatology scores, levels of support from friends, and caregiver optimism, were most predictive of postbereavement depressive symptomatology. The link between prebereavement and postbereavement depressive symptomatology scores was anticipated. The role of optimism is important for nurses to capitalize on and strengthen when working with significant others. The connection between high social support in the prebereavement period from friends and postbereavement depressive symptomatology was strong. This phenomenon could be caused by altered or lost relationships due to the dying and death of the spouse. Possibly friends experience a social death before the physical death of the bereaved's spouse.

Poor bereavement outcomes are apt to occur if the death is unexpected, untimely, or traumatic for the bereaved, such as with homicide or suicide (Vigil & Clements, 2003). Moreover, maladaptive grieving may occur if the significant other had an ambivalent or dependent relationship with the deceased,

perceives their social networks as unsupportive, and is experiencing concurrent loss. Family coping styles that negatively impact outcomes are (1) hostile (high conflict, low cohesiveness, and poor expressiveness); (2) sullen (limited but less in comparison with the hostile group); and (3) intermediate (intermediate cohesiveness and low control and achievement orientation). Additional correlates for poor outcome include use of medications or alcohol, concern for self, level of contentment, and not viewing the deceased's body. Positive bereavement outcomes are more apt to occur in families who are supportive (high cohesion) and resolve conflict well (Kissane, Bloch, & McKenzie, 1997).

In more dysfunctional grieving situations, the advanced nurse practitioner must treat symptoms of pathological grief. Three major symptom categories of pathological grief would be intrusion, denial, and dysfunctional adaptation (Horowitz, Bonanno, & Holen, 1993). Spending long periods of time idealizing the memory of the deceased is a sign of an intrusive thought process. Living as if the deceased were still alive for more than 6 months is evidence of denial. Minimal dysfunction is evidenced in having difficulty making decisions, whereas major dysfunction is evidenced in more severe impairments. Such severe dysfunctional parameters would involve extreme fatigue or somatic symptoms that last more than 1 month; inability to resume work, other interests, routines, and other responsibilities after more than 1 month; and reluctance to develop new relationships after 13 months of grieving (Lev & McCorkle, 1998, p. 147).

Use the following exercises to expand your understanding of helping the patient's significant others on their journey with the patient who is living with and dying with a terminal illness in relation to suffering and loss, death and dying, and grief and bereavement:

Exercise I—Discuss how you might feel and what you might do if you were the nurse who walked into a patient's room just as he has died and his family or significant others are there.

Exercise II—A family member who has been estranged from the dying patient on your floor is in the room as you come in to check on the patient who is unconscious. The family member says, "He wasn't a very good father. He abused my sister and me. I'll be glad when he's dead." How would you respond to this family member?

Exercise III—You are the clinical nurse specialist heading up the first meeting of nursing staff since a patient on your floor died from cancer. What would be your objectives for the meeting?

CONTEXT OF CAREGIVING AND RELATED INTERVENTIONS

Working with the patient who is living with and dying from a terminal illness and that person's significant others requires compassion, skill, energy, sensitivity, and patience. Compassion promotes a positive connection between the nurse and the patient and the significant others. Skill gives the nurse credibility in working with them. Energy, often in the form of providing hope for the moment, moves the patient and significant others forward when they feel like giving up. Sensitivity enhances understanding and rapport in the relationships. Patience allows individuals the time needed to face and plan for an uncertain and unpredictable future.

The nurse attempts to help meet the needs of the patient and the significant others. Addressing immediate needs may take on greater significance with the patient experiencing a terminal illness than addressing either short-term or long-term needs. Values, control issues, and goals of both the patient and significant others need to be taken into consideration, addressed directly, and handled tactfully and sensitively.

The nurse has a unique window into the patient's circumstances. Depending on the setting, nurses may provide 24-hour care. Even if nursing coverage is not for 24 direct-care hours, nursing care may be accessible for that period of time. Generally, it is the nurse who gets the most consistent, current, and constant view of what is actually happening with the patient and significant others. With few exceptions, the nurse usually is the most readily available and informed team player to help coordinate the patient's care.

Developing goals with the patient and family provides some stability and security during this time. It can empower the patient and the significant others to take an active role in planning the patient's remaining earthbound journey, uncertain and unpredictable as it may be. Furthermore, it helps set the stage for the continuing connection between the nurse and the patient's family in the bereavement period following the patient's death.

Nurse

Nurses care for themselves by seeking support from colleagues, assuring time for themselves by maintaining healthy boundaries with the patient and significant others, and tending to their own physical, emotional, sociocultural, and spiritual needs. After a patient's death, nurses may work through their grief by attending the memorial service or funeral for the deceased patient if this is deemed acceptable by the nurse's employing agency policy and the deceased patient's family. Sending a sympathy card to significant others, doing follow-up bereavement work with significant others, and reminiscing about the deceased patient with empathic colleagues usually help nurses in dealing with their own grief.

Nursing Interventions

Nurses are accustomed to action-oriented, "doing for" interventions. However, when intervening with the patient with a terminal illness, the nurse's role may be less action-oriented. At the end of life, nursing interventions involve more "being with" the patient and "caring" instead of "doing for" the patient and "curing" (Rando, 1984).

Given that so many American deaths occur in hospitals, the nurse is most apt to be with the patient and significant others at the exact time of death. Becoming comfortable with viewing the dying and death process, touching the deceased's body, talking with significant others about the death and their feelings, and dealing with the patient's death among staff are important aspects with which the nurse will be confronted.

The nurse's relationship with the patient will be critical in determining how she or he handles grief and bereavement in relation to the patient's dying and death. Was it a short-term nurse-patient relationship or did the nurse have a professional relationship with the patient for an extended period of time? In addition, how comfortable does the nurse feel sharing feelings, and how appropriate is it to share feelings with the patient? Nurses need to answer for themselves what the goal is of sharing their feelings and what the expected outcome is of doing so before proceeding.

Level of intervention by the nurse will be based on professional skills, theoretical background, and clinical setting. The nurse will develop therapeutic relationships; ensure the patient's physical comfort to maintain function; explore the meaning of physical suffering and loss with the patient and significant others; reframe the patient's limitations to identify areas of value that will enhance the patient's quality of life; encourage patient and significant others' attendance at support groups; and identify and maximize prior coping skills of the patient and the significant others. Advanced practice nurses will offer more intensive and extensive interventions for grieving and bereavement needs and be involved in conducting or participating in research studies. For example, the advanced practice nurse may prescribe various medications, offer individual or family counseling, lead a bereavement group, or conduct research on quality of life and quality of dying outcomes.

Patient

Each patient who is living with and dying from a terminal illness is unique. His or her experiences living with and dying from terminal illness also are unique. A critical factor in promoting good nursing care of this patient and significant others is affirming this uniqueness. Affirming the individual's growth and wholeness during this difficult living-dying interval is critical (Georgesen & Dungan, 1996; Talerico, 2003). Empowering patients to integrate the living-dying experience and optimize their quality of life will affirm the patient further.

For example, the patient is affirmed when the nurse acknowledges the patient's level of acceptance of dying and death. The patient's acceptance or denial may seem selective at times. In reality, varying levels of acceptance or denial may serve an adaptive function in which only specific aspects of dying are tolerable at a given point in time. The patient is aided when the nurse accepts and supports the patient's coping in this way to deal with the extensive and intensive challenges during the living-dying interval (Kastenbaum, 1997).

False reassurances prevent patients from accepting reality; the nurse must be honest and not foster false pretenses (Matzo et al., 2003).

Medical science has limitations, and often patients feel dehumanized during some medical procedures. In addition to addressing comfort needs, patients need assurance that their humanity will be respected and valued. The nursing profession has reawakened to the importance of integrating spiritual care within total patient care. Patients have indicated that their spiritual needs are best met through nurses' listening to, talking with, supporting religious practices of, and being with them (O'Neill & Kenny, 1998). Even in the midst of suffering through the loss of physical well-being, patients may sense spiritual well-being. Buckwalter (2003) refers to "moments of ministry" or "ministry of the moment" as those times when nurses or others assist patients in a "holy moment of connection," especially for someone who may be experiencing profound memory loss (p. 22). If a nurse feels inadequate or uncomfortable assisting dying patients in this area in any way, a pastoral care referral may be indicated. In addition, the patient may desire to have clergy closely involved even if the nurse is comfortable meeting the patient's spiritual needs.

Saying good-bye is painful for the patient with a terminal illness, for his significant others, and for the nurse. Discerning when (timing) and how (tone) to say and facilitate others' saying good-bye takes sensitivity (touch, emotional, and, physical) and skill (training/technique) on the nurse's part. This intervention can be illustrated as follows:

Discernment of readiness to facilitate
good-byes = nurse sensitivity (touch) +
skill (training/technique) +
when (timing) + how (tone)

An important question to ask when caring for the patient who is dying from and living with a terminal illness is "What type of patient has the disease, rather than what type of disease does the patient have?" (Harris, 1991, p. 111). Respecting and affirming the patient as a unique and valuable human being will help promote wholeness during a time of brokenness. As the individual is faced with imminent death, she or he must reorient her or his life to adapt to this realization and the accompanying losses. Minimizing losses due to isolation, rejection, and loss of control can decrease the individual's suffering (Rando, 1984). Optimizing patients' strengths is essential in helping them achieve the quality of life they would like to pursue in this living-dying interval.

Chronic sorrow is the "periodic recurrence of permanent, pervasive sadness or other grief related feelings associated with a significant loss" (Eakes et al., 1998, p. 179). Chronic sorrow may be triggered if the individual senses a disparity with norms. For example, the individual may feel different from others. Situations such as hospitalization accentuate this discrepancy to the individual. Both patients and significant others may experience chronic sorrow.

Counseling can assist individuals with chronic sorrow by helping the individual anticipate trigger events and reinforce effective internal and external management strategies. Internal strategies would be continuing involvement in interests and activities, having a positive attitude, focusing on one day at a time, and emphasizing the positive aspects in the individual's life. External strategies are those provided by health care professionals that view chronic sorrow as a normal experience for individuals dealing with chronic, life-threatening illness. Interventions found to be helpful by patients and their significant others include listening, being supportive and reassuring, addressing feelings, and affirming the uniqueness of each patient and significant other (Eakes et al., 1998).

The nurse may advocate for a patient with a terminal illness by employing the following interventions: advancement of grief work, encouraging health-promoting strategies despite a compromised health state, making referrals, meeting with significant others, utilizing cognitive reframing of negative patterns, and engaging the patient in individual or group therapy to work through unresolved situations. The nurse may be asked to work with support staff and significant others to help them accept, support, and devise strategies to work with a patient or significant other who has a dysfunctional approach to suffering and loss.

Family

The family of a patient dying from and living with a terminal illness experiences great turmoil and disequilibrium. Often, the illness becomes the focal point of family activity and organization. If the patient is a child and has siblings, the family struggles at maintaining life within the household, as well as preparing for the death of one of its members. The child simultaneously may be growing in many ways while dying in others. Treatment programs and appointments may consume much of the family's energy, possibly for extended periods of time. Helping the family maintain a sense of normalcy and balance throughout this period will be an important task for the nurse. Keeping the family as involved as possible in the patient's care applies to the patient with a terminal illness of any age (Matzo et al., 2003; Rando, 1984).

The question of where the patient and family would like the anticipated death to occur must be answered. With shortened hospital stays, families have been forced to assume extended and at times intensive care responsibilities for the dying patient in addition to their usual role expectations and demands. Helping the patient and family decide where and when care will take place becomes an important goal (Lev & McCorkle, 1998). The patient may wish to die at home, in a hospice setting, in a hospital, or another setting. Assisting the patient and family to communicate what they each can handle at different stages of the patient's dying will be critical.

A family's response to the patient's death is as unique as the individuals making up the family constellation. A family may seek or need to be referred for counseling if maladaptive symptoms develop. Family bereavement therapy involves assessing the circumstances related to the family member's death; the role of the deceased in the family before and after death; timing of the death in relation to family member's stage of growth and development; previous and current levels of family functioning; the context of the death; and the meaning assigned by the family to the death (Kiser et al., 1998, p. 97). There is little scientific evidence related to the impact of formal interventions with those bereaved; one reason for this may be that uncomplicated grieving resolves on its own (Jordan & Neimeyer, 2003). Jordan and Neimeyer further assert there is more evidence to support relational contexts of therapy (i.e., friends and family) over medical interventions (i.e., psychology or psychiatry) for those bereaved because those aspects promote hope and learning new coping skills.

However, the nurse must now focus attention on helping significant others begin the tasks of bereavement: accepting the reality of the loss, experiencing the pain of grief, adjusting to an environment without the deceased, and reinvesting energy into other relationships (Worden, 1991). Backer and colleagues (1994, p. 165) have identified guidelines for counseling the bereaved as follows:

1. Help actualize the loss by talking about the loss.
2. Identify and express feelings related to the loss.

3. Help the bereaved in decision making.
4. Facilitate emotional withdrawal and development of new relationships.
5. Provide time to grieve and be cognizant of holidays and anniversary dates.
6. Reassure the bereaved that their behavior is normal and that they are not abnormal because of their feelings.
7. Allow for individual differences in the bereavement process.
8. Provide support.
9. Examine individual defenses and coping styles (be aware of problems with alcohol or other substance abuse).
10. Identify pathological behaviors and refer to treatment.

The length of time for intense grief to be resolved varies from individual to individual. As long as the bereaved's grieving behavior does not interfere significantly with their physiological or psychosocial functioning, it is not considered abnormal. In general, intense responses to grief generally subside in about 6 to 12 months (Rando, 1984). Grieving, however, continues throughout the bereaved's life. The loss, in some cases, may be replaced, but in all cases, it is never recovered.

The living-dying interval comes to an end with the death of the patient, yet how does one know when grieving ends for the bereaved? Parkes and Weiss (1983) identified 10 major areas for assessment of recovery:

1. Functioning has returned to a level equal to or better than before bereavement.
2. Outstanding problems are being solved.
3. Acceptance of the loss has occurred.
4. Socialization is as effective as before the death.
5. The future is viewed positively and realistically.
6. General health is at prebereavement level.

7. Anxiety or depression levels are appropriate.
8. Guilt or anger levels are appropriate.
9. Self-esteem levels are appropriate.
10. Coping with future loss is feasible.

Completion of bereavement varies from individual to individual. For some, total resolution may never occur (Rando, 1984). Through appropriate interventions, the nurse can help the bereaved adapt to their loss in a way that will foster their growth and wholeness as well.

CONCLUSIONS

Living with and dying from a terminal illness results in many losses—for the patient, the significant others, and for the nurse. The nurse is both a facilitator and participant in this process. The nurse adds objectivity whereas the patient and significant others resolve the many feelings, issues, and decisions related to the living-dying experience.

This period of time frequently involves suffering in multiple dimensions. The nurse can utilize technical skills to alleviate certain attributes of the suffering, such as the patient's physical pain. When these technical skills are accompanied by the nurse's sensitivity, compassion, and empathy, the patient and significant others are better equipped to face the other attributes of suffering as well. Thus, the nurse, as a caring professional, may contribute meaningfully to the wellness of the patient and his or her significant others through one of life's most challenging and difficult transitions.

ACKNOWLEDGMENTS

The author extends appreciation to Joy L. Potter, BA, for her assistance in updating research for this chapter.

EDUCATION PLAN 10.1   Plan for Achieving Competencies: Loss, Suffering, Bereavement, and Grief

Knowledge Needed	Attitude	Skills	Undergraduate Behavioral Outcomes	Graduate Behavioral Outcomes	Teaching/Learning Strategies
Living with and dying from terminal illness: The nurse's role.	*Express comfort and commitment in caring for individuals who are terminally ill and their families. *Acknowledge personal attitudes regarding dying and death.	*Assure the patient and family that their needs will be meet.	*Communicate effectively and compassionately with terminally ill patient and family. *Provide holistic care that addresses the basic needs of the terminally ill patient and family.	*Provide comprehensive care for the terminally ill patient and family, recognizing complex needs.	*Ask students in post-conference or seminar to remember a significant loss they had in their lifetime and identify what were their attitudes towards loss and death and what was most helpful and least helpful to them during the experience.

(continued)

EDUCATION PLAN 10.1 *(continued)*

Knowledge Needed	Attitude	Skills	Undergraduate Behavioral Outcomes	Graduate Behavioral Outcomes	Teaching/Learning Strategies
					*Complete a death anxiety questionnaire and determine the score. Discuss possible reasons for their score. *Brainstorm as a class euphemisms on death. Discuss their usage and how they reflect their attitudes towards dying and death.

Experience of loss and suffering across the life span.	*Appreciate differences in the interpretation of death across the life span. *Accept diverse responses to loss as normal responses.	*Act in accordance with the developmental age of the individual experiencing loss, bereavement, and grief	*Provide appropriate care to individuals experiencing loss, bereavement, and grief at various developmental stages.	*Educate others as to differences in the needs of individuals experiencing loss, bereavement, and grief at various developmental ages.	*Interview individuals of different age groups who have experienced a loss. Compare their beliefs regarding death and their responses to loss. Present the findings in a written paper, or in a post-conference or seminar presentation.
Theories on death and dying.	*Value theories in developing knowledge regarding dying and death.		*Apply theories about death in providing effective and compassionate care to terminally ill patients and families.	*Evaluate theories about death in the care of terminally ill patients and families.	*Ask students to identify a personal loss and evaluate the experience in light of a given theory regarding dying and death.

(continued)

EDUCATION PLAN 10.1   (*continued*)

Knowledge Needed	Attitude	Skills	Undergraduate Behavioral Outcomes	Graduate Behavioral Outcomes	Teaching/Learning Strategies
Dimensions of Loss, Suffering, Bereavement, and Grief: —Definitions —Significance and meaning of the relationship.	*Appreciate the value of social, intimate, and therapeutic relationships in supporting individuals experiencing loss, bereavement, and grief.	*Demonstrate competence in establishing therapeutic relationships with individuals experiencing loss, bereavement, and grief.	*Provide effective and compassionate care for individuals experiencing loss, bereavement, and grief.	*Role model effective and compassionate care for individuals experiencing loss, bereavement, and grief.	*Using a case study, identify the significance and meaning of various relationships within the context of end of life. *Role play the development of a therapeutic relationship with individuals experiencing loss, bereavement, and grief.

Assessment of the Nurses' Attitudes and Feelings Towards Loss, Bereavement, and Grief.				
*Acknowledge students'/nurses' own attitudes and feelings related to loss, bereavement, and grief.	*Demonstrate constructive self-disclosure of feelings in assisting individuals in acknowledging and resolving loss and grief.	*Utilize the insights gained through personal experiences of loss, bereavement, and grief to offer supportive care to others.	*Assist colleagues in identifying and working toward resolving their own feelings of loss, bereavement, and grief in caring for patients and families at the end of life.	*Conduct a self-reflection exercise in which students/ nurses prepare a creative presentation to examine how people in various cultures handle loss and grief. *Assist students to work through their own issues of loss and grief by establishing a peer support group.

(continued)

EDUCATION PLAN 10.1 *(continued)*

Knowledge Needed	Attitude	Skills	Undergraduate Behavioral Outcomes	Graduate Behavioral Outcomes	Teaching/Learning Strategies
					*Ask students/nurses what unfinished business they would attempt to complete if they knew they would die within a week. Share responses in a small group setting. *Have students/nurses discuss in small groups what they believe would be a good death and bad death. Have two students report to the larger group to consolidate the findings.

*Ask students to imagine their caring for a dying patient and family and answer the following questions:

—What do they fear about death?;

—How would they offer care that is special or unique?

*Ask students to write down what legacy they would like to leave and why this is important to them.

(continued)

EDUCATION PLAN 10.1 *(continued)*

Knowledge Needed	Attitude	Skills	Undergraduate Behavioral Outcomes	Graduate Behavioral Outcomes	Teaching/Learning Strategies
Assessment of Patients and Families Experiencing Life-threatening Illness	*Appreciate the diverse feelings, perceptions, and responses of individuals experiencing loss, bereavement, and grief.	*Perform an assessment related to loss and grief for patients, and families, including children.	*Accurately assess patients' and families' immediate and specific needs related to loss, bereavement, and grief. *Assist patients and families in maintaining control over many areas of their lives as death approaches. *Determine individuals who are at high risk for dysfunctional grieving and the need for appropriate referral.	*Accurately assess patients' and families' immediate and specific needs related to loss, bereavement, and grief in complex caregiving situations.	*Conduct an assessment of a patient and family member in the clinical area who have experienced a loss. Based on the assessment, identify their specific and immediate needs, and indications of those at high risk. Present the assessment findings and diagnoses in post-conference or seminar.

| Normal Grief Reactions and Related Factors | *Consider the various factors that influence normal grief. | *Perform a loss and grief assessment that evaluates the factors influencing the grief reaction. | *Assist patients and families in recognizing normal responses to grief and the factors that influence the grief reaction. | *Educate health professionals regarding normal grief responses and factors that influence the grief reaction. | *Utilizing a case study, identify the physical, emotional, social, and spiritual factors that influence the grief reaction, and the responses to normal grief for individuals of various developmental ages. |

(continued)

EDUCATION PLAN 10.1   *(continued)*

Knowledge Needed	Attitude	Skills	Undergraduate Behavioral Outcomes	Graduate Behavioral Outcomes	Teaching/Learning Strategies
					*Distribute three-by-five cards and have students/nurses identify one physical, emotional, social, or spiritual response they have experienced related to loss and grief. Gather the cards as to the physical, emotional, social, or spiritual responses and review the responses, noting the frequency of symptoms.

Risk Factors for Complicated Grief	*Judge experiences of loss that place individuals at high risk for complicated grief.	*Identify individuals who are experiencing complicated grief and make appropriate referrals.	*Coordinate interdisciplinary initiatives in caring for individuals at risk for or experiencing complicated grief.	*In post-conference or seminar discuss students'/nurses' responses and reactions to the potential or actual death of their patient in the clinical area. Discuss their behaviors and responses in caring for the deceased and their family.

(continued)

EDUCATION PLAN 10.1 *(continued)*

Knowledge Needed	Attitude	Skills	Undergraduate Behavioral Outcomes	Graduate Behavioral Outcomes	Teaching/Learning Strategies
Context of Care-giving and Related Interventions	*Express sensitivity, energy, compassion, and patience in caring for dying patients and their family. *Affirm the need for nurses' self-care within the context of offering end of life care.	*Demonstrate care that is focused more on "being with" the patient and "caring," instead of "doing for" the patient and "curing."	*Establish a therapeutic relationship in which the physical, emotional, social and spiritual needs of patients and families at the end of life are addressed. *Empower patients and family experiencing life-threatening illness to work through unresolved issues, participate in health-promoting activities despite compromised health, and decide on goals of care and death-related plans. * Assist families in the tasks of bereavement.	*Provide intensive interventions to address the physical, emotional, social, and spiritual needs of patients and families in complex care-giving situations and for those experiencing complicated grief. *Lead a bereavement group or conduct individualized counseling. *Participate in or conduct research related to the experience of loss, bereavement, and grief.	* Ask students/nurses to think about someone who had died within their family, and discuss their relationship to the person, the type and duration of the illness, positive and negative interactions they had with health care providers, and suggestions for improving care. *Invite a guest speaker to class to discuss their loss experience and those interventions that were helpful or not helpful to them in their bereavement. *Develop a plan of care for an individual experiencing bereavement. Critique the plan in class, post-conference, or seminar.

REFERENCES

American Heritage Dictionary of the English Language (4th ed.) (2000). Boston: Houghton Mifflin.

Backer, B. A., Hannon, N. R., & Gregg, J. Y. (1994). *To listen, to comfort, to care: Reflections on death and dying.* Albany, NY: Delmar.

Bowlby, J. (1980). *Attachment and loss: Loss, sadness and depression* (Vol. III). New York: Basic Books.

Brady, P. F. (1997). The therapeutic relationship. In B. S. Johnson (Ed.), *Psychiatric-mental health nursing: Adaptation and growth* (4th ed., pp. 49–57). New York: Lippincott.

Buckman, R. (1993). Communication in palliative care: A practical guide. In D. Doyle, G. W. C. Hanks, & N. Macdonald (Eds.), *Oxford textbook of palliative medicine* (pp. 47–61). Oxford, England: Oxford Medical.

Buckwalter, G. (2003). Addressing the spiritual and religious needs of persons with profound memory loss. *Home Healthcare Nurse, 21*(1), 20–24.

Callanan, M., & Kelley, P. (1992). *Final gifts.* New York: Poseidon Press.

Cassell, E. (1991). *The nature of suffering and the goals of medicine.* New York: Oxford University.

Charleton, R. (2003). Managing bereavement. *Practitioner, 247,* 667, 671–674.

Clements, P. T., Vigil, G. J., Manno, M. S., Henry, G. C., Wilks, J., Das, S., et al. (2003). Cultural perspectives of death, grief, and bereavement. *Journal of Psychosocial Nursing, 41*(7), 18–26.

Copp, G. (1997). Patients' and nurses' constructions of death and dying in a hospice setting. *Journal of Cancer Nursing, 1*(1), 2–13.

Copp, G. (1998). A review of current theories of death and dying. *Journal of Advanced Nursing, 28,* 382–390.

Corr, C. A. (1992). A task-based approach to coping with dying. *Omega, 24*(2), 81–94.

Danis, M. (1998). Improving end-of-life care in the intensive care unit: What's to be learned from outcome research? *New Horizons, 6*(1), 110–118.

Eakes, G. G., Burke, M. L., & Hainsworth, M. A. (1998). Middle-range theory of chronic sorrow. *Image: Journal of Nursing Scholarship, 30,* 179–184.

Engel, G. L. (1964). Grief and grieving. *American Journal of Nursing, 64,* 93–98.

Evans, A. J. (1994) Anticipatory grief: A theoretical challenge. *Palliative Medicine, 8,* 159–165.

Ferrell, B. R., Taylor, E. J., Sattler, G. R., Fowler, M., & Cheyney, B. L. (1993). Searching for the meaning of pain. *Cancer Practice, 1,* 185–194.

Frank, E., Prigerson, H. G., Shear, M. K., & Reynolds, C. F. (1997). Phenomenology and treatment of bereavement-related distress in the elderly. *International Clinical Psychopharmacology, 12*(suppl. 7), S25–S29.

Freud, S. (1957). The disillusionment of the war. In J. Strachey (Ed.), *The complete psychological works of Sigmund Freud, Vol. 14 (1914–1916).* London: Hogarth Press and the Institute of Psychoanalysis.

Fulton, R., & Fulton, J. A. (1971). A psychosocial aspect of terminal care: Anticipatory grief. *Omega, 2,* 91–99.

Geis, H. K., Whittlesey, S. W., McDonald, N. B., Smith, K. L., & Pfefferbaum, B. (1998). Bereavement and loss in childhood. *Child and Adolescent Psychiatric Clinics of North America, 7*(1), 73–85.

Georgesen, J., & Dungan, J. M. (1996). Managing spiritual distress in patients with advanced cancer. *Cancer Nursing, 19,* 376–383.

Glasser, B. G., & Strauss, A. L. (1965). *Awareness of dying.* Chicago: Aldine.

Goodkin, K., Blaney, N. T., Feaster, D. J., Baldewicz, T., Burkhalter, J. E., & Leeds, B.

(1999). A randomized controlled clinical trial of a bereavement support group intervention in human immunodeficiency virus type I-seropositive and -seronegative homosexual men. *Archives of General Psychiatry, 56*(1), 52–59.

Haas, F. (2003). Bereavement care: Seeing the body. *Nursing Standard, 17*(28), 33–37.

Hames, C. C. (2003). Helping infants and toddlers when a family member dies. *Journal of Hospice and Palliative Nursing, 5,* 103–112.

Harris, J. M. (1991). Death and bereavement. *Problems in Veterinary Medicine, 3,* 111–117.

Horowitz, M. J., Bonanno, G. A., & Holen, A. (1993). Pathological grief: Diagnosis and explanation. *Psychosomatic Medicine, 55,* 260–273.

Jordan, J., & Neimeyer, R. (2003). Does grief counseling work? *Death Studies, 27,* 765–786.

Kalish, R. A. (1979). The onset of the dying process. In R. A. Kalish (Ed.), *Death, dying, transcending* (pp. 5–17). New York: Baywood.

Kastenbaum, R. A. (1997). *Death, society, and human experience.* Boston: Allyn and Bacon.

Kazanowski, M. (in press). End of life care. In D. D. Ignatavicius, M. L. Workman, & M. A. Mishler (Eds.), *Medical-surgical nursing: Critical thinking for collaborative care* (5th ed.). Philadelphia: Saunders.

Kiser, L. J., Ostoja, E., & Pruitt, D. B. (1998). Dealing with stress and trauma in families. *Child and Adolescent Psychiatric Clinics of North America, 7*(1), 87–103.

Kissane, D. W., Bloch, S., & McKenzie, D. P. (1997). Family coping and bereavement outcome. *Palliative Medicine, 11,* 191–201.

Kissane, D. W., & Bloch, S. (2002). *Family focused grief therapy.* Philadelphia: Open University Press.

Koop, P. M., & Strang, V. (1997). Predictors of bereavement outcomes in families of patients with cancer: A literature review. *Canadian Journal of Nursing Research, 29*(4), 33–35.

Kubler-Ross, E. (1969). *On death and dying.* New York: Macmillan.

Kurtz, M. E., Kurtz, J. C., Given, C. W., & Given, B. (1997). Predictors of post-bereavement depressive symptomatology among family caregivers of cancer patients. *Support Care Cancer, 5*(1), 53–60.

Leichtling, B. (2004). Dealing with dying, death and grief. *Caring: National Association for Home Care Magazine, 23*(1), 38–39.

Lev, E. L., & McCorkle, R. (1998). Loss, grief, and bereavement in family members of cancer patients. *Seminars in Oncology Nursing, 14,* 145–151.

Lewis, M. L. (1998). Culture and loss: A project of self-reflection. *Journal of Nursing Education, 37,* 191–201.

Lindemann, E. (1944). Symptomatology and management of acute grief. *American Journal of Psychiatry, 101,* 141–148.

Mallinson, R. K. (1999). Grief work of HIV-positive persons and their survivors. *Nursing Clinics of North America, 34,* 163–177.

Matzo, M. L., Sherman, D. W., Lo, K., Egan, K. A., Grant, M., & Rhome, A. (2003). Strategies for teaching loss, grief, and bereavement. *Nurse Educator, 28*(2), 71–76.

McCall, J. B. (1999). *Grief education for caregivers of the elderly.* New York: Haworth Pastoral Press.

McCreight, B. (2004). A grief ignored: Narratives of pregnancy loss from a male perspective. *Sociology of Health and Illness, 26,* 326–350.

McIntier, T. M. (1995). Nursing the family when a child dies. *RN, 2,* 50–55.

Mitchell, K. R., & Anderson, H. (1983). *All our losses, all our griefs.* Philadelphia: Westminster Press.

Mystakidou, K., Tsilika, E., Parpa, E., Katsouda, E., & Vlahos, L. (2003). A Greek perspective on concepts of death and expression of grief, with implications for practice. *International Journal of Palliative Nursing, 9,* 534–537.

O'Neill, D. P., & Kenny, E. K. (1998). Spirituality and chronic illness. *Image: Journal of Nursing Scholarship, 30,* 275–280.

Parkes, C. M., & Weiss, R. S. (1983). *Recovery from bereavement.* New York: Basic Books.

Pattison, E. M. (1977). *The experience of dying.* New York: Simon and Schuster.

Pennebaker, J. W., Mayne, T. J., & Francis, M. E. (1997). Linguistic predictors of adaptive bereavement. *Journal of Personality and Social Psychology, 72,* 863–871.

Prigerson, H. G., Bierhals, A. J., Kasl, S. V., Reynolds, C. F., Shear, M. K., Day, N., et al. (1997). Traumatic grief as a risk factor for mental and physical morbidity. *American Journal of Psychiatry, 154,* 616–623.

Pritchett, K. T., & Lucas, P. M. (1997). Grief and loss. In B. S. Johnson (Ed.), *Psychiatric-mental health nursing: Adaptation and growth* (4th ed., pp. 199–218). New York: Lippincott.

Rando, T. A. (1984). *Grief, dying, and death.* Champaign, IL: Research Press.

Reiss, D. (1990). Patient, family, and staff responses to end-stage renal disease. *American Journal of Kidney Disease, 15,* 194–200.

Saldinger, A., Cain, A., & Porterfield, K. (2003). Managing traumatic stress in children anticipating parental death. *Psychiatry, 66,* 168–181.

Sherman, D. W. (1998). Reciprocal suffering: The need to improve family caregivers' quality of life through palliative care. *Journal of Palliative Medicine, 1,* 357–366.

Shuzman, E. (2003). Facing stillbirth or neonatal death: Providing culturally appropriate care for Jewish families. *Association of Women's Health, Obstetric and Neonatal Nurses, 7,* 537–543

Siegel, K., Karus, D. G., Raveis, V. H., Christ, G. H., & Mesagno, F. P. (1996). Depressive distress among the spouses of terminally ill patients. *Cancer Practice, 4*(1), 25–30.

Spencer, L. (1994). How do nurses deal with their own grief when a patient dies on an intensive care unit and what help can be given to enable them to overcome their grief effectively? *Journal of Advanced Nursing, 19,* 1141–1150.

Stewart, A. L., Teno, J., Patrick, D. L., & Lynn, J. (1999). The concept of quality of life of dying persons in the context of health care. *Journal of Pain and Symptom Management, 17*(2), 93–108.

Stroebe, M. S. (2002). Paving the way: From early attachment theory to contemporary bereavement research. *Mortality, 7,* 127–138.

Stuart, G. W., & Sundeen, S. J. (1991). *Principles and practices of psychiatric nursing.* Boston: Mosby Year Book.

Sudnow, D. (1967). *Passing on: The social organization of dying.* Englewood Cliffs, NJ: Prentice-Hall.

Talerico, K. A. (2003). Grief and older adults. *Journal of Psychosocial Nursing, 41*(7), 12–16.

Vigil, G. J., & Clements, P. T. (2003). Child and adolescent homicide survivors: Complicated grief and altered worldviews. *Journal of Psychosocial Nursing, 41*(1), 30–39.

Viorst, J. (1987). *Necessary losses.* New York: Ballantine Books.

Warren, B. J. (1999). Cultural competence in psychiatric nursing: An interlocking paradigm approach. In N. L. Keltner, L. H. Schwecke, & C. E. Bostrom (Eds.), *Psychiatric nursing* (3rd ed., pp. 98–148). Boston: Mosby.

Woodgate, R., & Degner, L. (2003). A substantive theory of keeping the spirit alive: The spirit within children with cancer and their families. *Journal of Pediatric Oncology Nursing, 20,* 103–119.

Worden, J. W. (1991). *Grief counseling and grief therapy: Handbook for the mental health practitioner.* New York: Springer.

Section IV

Physical Aspects of Dying

July 3, 2004

Up until this last week Candy has been relatively independent with her activities of daily living. She was having occasional right sided chest pain, which she rated as a "3" in intensity, but was relieved by 2 Percocet. In the past week, the pain increased in frequency and intensity, and she had dyspnea at rest. In the past three days, Candy became very weak, with no appetite, and she spent most of her time sitting in her "Lazy Boy" chair. Because of her increase in symptoms, I called her daily and visited her every other day. She was extremely lethargic and her husband told me that she became very short of breath on ambulation to the bathroom.

Lethargy and loss of appetite in a person with advanced cancer are common physical symptoms associated with the process of dying. The fact that she was having an increase in symptoms of pain and dyspnea was further evidence that she was nearing death. I called her doctor and asked for a standing order for liquid Morphine and Ativan. I showed Candy and Ron how to administer 5 mg. of the morphine in her cheek and recommended repeating the medication dose in 15 minutes if it wasn't effective, and to take the prescribed rescue dose if she experienced heightened pain or shortness of breath.

Today was the first time in the year that I have known Candy that she mentioned dying. I held her hand while she cried and told me how surprised she was that the end was coming so quickly. I suppose these things are surprising when it is clear that the disease will not be cured. Candy asked me to promise her that she would not suffer at the end; it was such a poignant moment. As I hugged her, I told her I would be with her till the end. With the support of members of the Hospice/Palliative Care team, Candy's pain and symptoms were alleviated, and the emotional and spiritual needs of Candy and her family were being addressed.

July 4, 2004

When I arrived at Candy's house today, I saw that her level of consciousness had significantly declined. She had not had any oral intake for two days, and was only responding occasionally to her name. Her skin was cool and starting to become mottled. Ron said he had given Candy 4 rescue doses of 10mg. of morphine since yesterday. She appeared comfortable and peaceful, with no evidence of grimacing or restlessness, which may indicate pain. Candy did not appear to have difficulty breathing, but her breaths were slow and shallow, and there was a rattle in the back of her throat. I explained that this noise was from secretions in the back of her throat, but that it is usually not distressing to the patient.

I told him that Candy was actively dying and held him as he cried. I suggested to Ron that he get the children if he wanted them to be with her as she died. They came in and crawled into the bed with their mom and lay in her arms for the last time. Ron put his arms around them all, as they prayed together. I was thinking what a good job Candy had done with her kids that they were so comfortable to be with her during this time; I don't know where Ron got his strength to support his family in this way. The love and faith were almost palpable. I stayed at the foot of her bed and did Reiki on Candy's feet, something she had always liked me to do during my visits. She opened her eyes, looked at each of us, stopped breathing, and died.

Ron held the children and told them what had happened. Fortunately, there were family and friends in the house to be with the children, as Ron stayed with me to bathe Candy's body. He wanted to do this final act for her because she never liked to leave the house looking "messy." He talked to her as we prepared her to leave her home for the last time.

As I reflect on this nursing experience, I realize the importance of our relationship that we developed over time. This family allowed me to care for them at one of the most vulnerable times of their lives. I learned so much from Candy about life, living, and ultimately about dying. These are gifts given to us by our patients at the end of life. Palliative care nursing transcends traditional caregiving experiences. In a very intimate way, nurses co-journey with their patients and families experiencing life-threatening illness and helping them to live as fully as possible until death. With the knowledge and skills to alleviate the physical, emotional, social, and spiritual pain and suffering, and by bearing witness to the precious moments of life as patients and their family say their last goodby and express eternal love, nurses experience the joy and rewards of hospice/palliative care nursing. Through competent and compassionate care at the end of life, nurses can make a difference in the quality of life and quality of dying for their patients and their families.

11

Symptom Management in Palliative Care

Mary K. Kazanowski

AACN Competencies

#7: Use scientifically based standardized tools to assess symptoms (e.g., dyspnea, constipation, anxiety, fatigue, nausea and vomiting, and altered cognition) experienced by patients at the end of life.

#8: Use data from symptom assessment to plan and intervene in symptom management using state-of-the-art traditional approaches.

Research regarding care at the end of life validates the knowledge that individuals near death often experience physical symptoms of distress. Recognition and treatment of physical and nonphysical symptoms of distress are essential to achieve and maintain comfort and peace until death.

By virtue of their close proximity to those who are sick, and their commitment to patients throughout the life cycle, nurses play a pivotal role in identifying and treating symptoms of patients who are near death. The provision of quality care near end of life is contingent on nurses receiving adequate education in the treatment of pain and symptoms.

Curriculum content for undergraduates should include signs and symptoms, etiologies, and standard treatment for common symptoms of distress at end of life, such as pain, dyspnea, nausea, vomiting, anxiety, agitation, fatigue, and constipation. Curricula for advanced practice nurses should include this content as well as content related to pathophysiology related to advanced disease states; assessment of the emotional, social, and spiritual components of suffering; effective pharmacologic and nonpharmacologic interventions; measurement issues and assessment tools; and ethical and legal issues related to terminal dehydration, terminal restlessness, refractory symptoms, access to care, barriers to care, and health care policy.

Several studies have defined the most common symptoms experienced by dying patients, with most involving patients with terminal cancer (Lipman, 2000). Studies vary somewhat in identifying which symptoms are most prevalent, but there is consensus that pain, dyspnea, delirium, nausea, vomiting, asthenia (i.e., lack of energy, fatigue, and general weakness) and constipation are often problematic.

As death nears, symptoms of distress may escalate, stay the same, or decrease in intensity. The goals of symptom management for clients near death are to control symptoms, promote meaningful interactions between patients and significant others, and facilitate peaceful death. To achieve these goals, symptoms must be recognized as a threat to client comfort, and therefore be effectively treated and monitored. To decrease suffering, symptoms of distress such as pain, dyspnea, delirium, nausea and vomiting generally require the use of medications such as analgesics, sedatives, and antiemetics and often benefit from access to experts in palliative care. Palliative care services, however, are underutilized, and many individuals lack quality care near death (Field & Cassel, 1997).

ASSESSMENT AT THE END OF LIFE

Clients near the end of life should be assessed comprehensively for any sign or symptom that could potentially cause distress. When first recognized, each symptom should be assessed comprehensively in terms of intensity, frequency, duration, and quality, exacerbating factors, and relieving factors. A method for rating the intensity of that symptom then should be chosen to facilitate ongoing assessments, evaluate treatment response, and assess symptom management over time. Family caregivers and health care providers may need to be taught how to interpret some of these tools. Tools that can be easily explained and interpreted with a minimal amount of time and effort should be used. The use of such tools promotes early recognition of symptoms and changes in symptomatology, and facilitates communication of this change to other providers.

Assessment of symptoms ideally should be based on the patient's perception of the symptom, with the choice of tools based on each patient's understanding. If scales for specific symptoms are not available, a simple flow sheet can be used to prompt health care providers and family caregivers to assess common symptoms of distress. An example of such a flow sheet is found in Table 11.1. Flow sheets such as this are commonly used in palliative care to ensure that priority assessments are consistently performed with each nurse-client encounter.

As one nears the end of life, one commonly grows weak and lethargic, sleeping for longer periods. This lethargy and sleep may progress to the point that the client has a decreased level of consciousness, rousing only to touch. In most cases, the ability of the client to communicate verbally decreases along with a decreased level of consciousness.

This makes it difficult to assess the client's perception of symptoms. When caring for clients who are unable to communicate their distress or needs, it is essential that health care providers identify alternative ways to assess symptoms of distress. Professional caregivers should teach family caregivers to watch closely for objective signs of discomfort such as restlessness, grimacing, or moaning, and identify when these symptoms occur in relation to positioning, movement, medication, or other external stimuli. For example, grimacing when turning from side to side is indicative of pain or discomfort with movement. An increase in respiratory rate and effort when the head of the bed is down may indicate orthopnea. Although the client's point of view is likely to be the most valid indicator of comfort or distress, the perception of symptoms that family members have is also important. Family perceptions of symptoms should be obtained as part of each client's symptom assessment. Research has shown that family caregivers, health care providers, and patients may differ in their perceptions of symptoms, in terms of intensity, significance, and meaning (McMillan, 1996a, 1996b; McMillan & Mahon, 1994a, 1994b; Weitzner, Moody, & McMillan, 1997). Whereas health care providers are often more adept at identifying symptoms of distress, families are often more knowledgeable about client habits and preferences, which often reflects client needs. Health care providers need to incorporate all client-related information into the plan for

TABLE 11.1   Hospice Care Patient Flow Sheet

Date
Respiratory
Dyspnea at rest?
Intensity (0–5)
Dyspnea with activity?
Intensity (0–5)
Episodes/24hr
Treatment
MSIR
Oxygen
Benzodiazepine
Other Med
Repositioning
Air Conditioner
Fan
Cool Cloth to Face
Other (e.g. Reiki)
Treatment Effect
Temperature
Apical Pulse
Respirations
Blood Pressure
Breath Sounds
Left
Right
Sputum
Amount
Color

(continued)

TABLE 11.1   *(continued)*

Anxiety/Agitation
Present?
Episodes/24 hours?
Treatment
Treatment Effect
GI
Nausea?
Episodes of Nausea/24hrs.
Treatment
Treatment Effect
Vomiting?
Episodes of Vomiting/24hrs.
Treatment
Treatment Effect
Last Bowel Movement
Abdominal. Distention
Bowel Sounds

management of symptoms, working with clients and families toward a common goal.

INTERVENTIONS AT END OF LIFE

The literature indicates that unrelieved pain is one of the most common causes of somatic distress in the months, weeks, and days before death (Paice, 1999. Pain is also the most feared symptom near end of life (Brescia et al., 1990. Assessment and interventions for pain near end of life are discussed comprehensively in chapter 12. Assessment and interventions for common symptoms of distress other than pain (e.g., dyspnea, nausea, vomiting, anxiety, and delirium) will be discussed in this chapter. Control and prevention of recurrent symptoms often require administering medication around the clock to maintain comfort and prevent recurrence of symptoms. To facilitate administration of appropriate treatment, a plan for appropriate treatment needs to be in place prior to the occurrence of the symptoms. Any barrier to obtaining or administering medications for symptoms near death can affect the client's comfort at the end of life. The concept of the Symptom Relief Kit (or emergency kits) addresses the need to have appropriate medications readily available in the home, extended care facility, or hospital. With the knowledge that the timing of the dying process cannot consistently be predicted, hospice workers developed the Symptom Relief Kit. These kits generally contain small amounts of a few medications that have been found effective in treating common symptoms of distress in clients near death (see Appendix A).

As is the case with analgesics for pain, the oral route is the preferred route for administration of medications for symptoms of distress near the end of life. However, oral administration of medications can become problematic when clients have a decrease in their level of consciousness. Capsules or sustained-release tablets, which cannot be chewed or crushed, are particularly problematic when a client cannot safely swallow medications. Faced with this situation, the nurse needs to consider alternative routes for medications. The guiding principle for choice of route is to choose the least invasive with the most effective treatment (Coluzzi & Fairbairn, 1998). Identification of appropriate routes and dosages for medications often requires the input of a physician or nurse who is knowledgeable in palliative care. Access to a pharmacist who is able to advise and compound medications for alternative routes is also advantageous.

Sublingual or buccal (cheek or lower lip) administration of certain short-acting medications is often effective, using liquefied small crushed tablets. The volume of medication that can be absorbed from the oral cavity, however, limits these routes. Volumes of 1 cc or less are generally well tolerated. Volumes that are not adequately absorbed should be administered by another route (e.g., rectal, intravenous, or subcutaneous).

The rectal route has the advantage that dosing requirements often remain the same, thus eliminating the need to calculate equianalgesic doses and the need to obtain and purchase new prescriptions. A switch from oral to rectal administration of analgesics not only saves family and health care providers' time and money; it also facilitates ongoing control of symptoms, by avoiding major changes in the treatment plan. Although the rectal route is a good alternative for some dying clients, it is not a good alternative for all. Clients with loose stool, constipation, or rectal bleeding may not adequately absorb medication given rectally. Clients with low platelet counts will be at risk for bleeding from insertion of medication into the rectum. Clients with lesions of the anus or rectum may also experience pain. Rectal administration of analgesics may also pose problems for caregivers who are assuming the responsibility for administration of medications near death. Problems cited by family caregivers include caregiver aversion to touching the rectum, client aversion to having the rectum touched, difficulty turning the client, and inserting the medication in the rectum. It should also be noted that not all oral medications can be administered rectally. Assessment for potential problems related to rectal administration of a medication is necessary to determine the appropriateness and effectiveness of the rectal route.

The transdermal route is an attractive alternative for systemic management of symptoms near death, but its use is limited by the number of medications available for topical use. Few drugs are reliably absorbed through the skin. Use of this route often requires access to pharmacies that compound medications in gel forms that will allow for absorption.

Subcutaneous or intravenous routes may need to be utilized for administration of medications if control of symptoms cannot be achieved via the oral, rectal, or transdermal routes or if rapid titration of medication is necessary. Clients with existing central venous access are the preferred candidates for intravenous medications, because they will not require frequent restarts of peripheral catheters, which can be painful. The subcutaneous route is the preferred route for clients without existing venous access, if the medication can be safely administered by that route.

DYSPNEA NEAR THE END OF LIFE

Dyspnea is a subjective experience described as an uncomfortable awareness of breathing, breathlessness, or severe shortness of breath (Hospice and Palliative Nurses Association [HPNA], 1996) that may be associated with copious secretions, cough, chest pain, fatigue, or air hunger. It is a frequent symptom of distress near the end of life, occurring in 50% to 70% of dying clients (Bruera, Macmillan, Pither, & MacDonald, 1990) and it is thought to be a marker for the terminal phase of life (Escalante et al., 1996). Dyspnea is considered by many patients, families, and health care providers as the worst symptom of distress because it conveys an image of suffering, invoking fear on the part of the patient and the family. Severe dyspnea is also quite difficult to control, which enhances its negative perception.

Causes of dyspnea can be directly related to the client's primary diagnosis (e.g., lung cancer, breast cancer, or coronary artery disease); secondary to the primary diagnosis (e.g., pleural effusion, metastasis to lung or pleura); related to treatment of the primary disease (e.g., congestive heart failure related to chemotherapy or constrictive pericarditis related to radiation therapy; anemia related to chemotherapy); or to an etiology unrelated to the primary disease (e.g., pneumonia). Depending on the cause, the pathophysiology can involve (a) obstructive, restrictive, or vascular disturbances in the airways with tumor or nodal involvement; (b) pulmonary congestion secondary to fluid overload, cardiac dysfunction, or both; (c) bronchoconstriction and bronchospasm as seen with a respiratory infection, COPD, or airway encroachment by a tumor; (d) a decreased hemoglobin carry-ing capacity as with anemia; or (e) hypoventilation secondary to limited movement of the diaphragm as seen with neuromuscular disease.

ASSESSMENT OF DYSPNEA

Research shows that dyspnea near the end of life is inadequately assessed (Escalante et al., 1996). Because of its association with suffering and its resistance to treatment, dyspnea should be routinely assessed in all clients nearing the end of life. The nurse reviews the past medical history of the client for risks of dyspnea related to the primary disease, secondary conditions, or the clinical condition of the client. For example, clients with a history of congestive heart failure or a primary diagnosis of lung cancer or renal failure are at risk for dyspnea because of their primary disease and history. Clients with ascites are at risk for dyspnea related to fluid volume excess.

Symptoms of dyspnea are assessed with particular attention to the client's perception of his or her breathing and the meaning of the dyspnea for the client and family. Assessment is performed using the descriptor that most closely reflects the individual experience of each client. Breathlessness may characterize the experience for some, whereas discomfort, pain, or difficulty breathing may characterize it for others.

Signs of dyspnea are assessed by inspecting the client's respiratory rate and respiratory effort, and auscultating breath sounds. Respiratory rates greater than the client's norm or greater than 20 per minute (for adults), labored respirations manifested by use of accessory muscles and distended neck veins, diminished breath sounds, or auscultation of adventitious lung sounds (e.g., rhonchi or rales) are often associated with dyspnea. Absence of these abnormalities does not refute its existence, because dyspnea, like pain, is a subjective experience, based on primarily the patient's self-report.

Once dyspnea is identified, the nurse obtains information about the frequency, nature, and intensity of the dyspnea, as well as associated factors that trigger, aggravate, and relieve it. Asking the client or family to describe when the dyspnea occurs and how it relates to activity or positioning is often helpful to clients trying to describe the experience. On initial assessment of dyspnea, the nurse also assesses for prior episodes of this symptom, etiologies of prior episodes, treatment, and effect of treatment at that time.

Assessment of the intensity of dyspnea at end of life is most commonly done by determining the presence or absence of the symptom and the relation of the symptom to activity. Ideally, a tool with a visual analog scale should be used to track the symptom over time. Visual analog scales are available with numbers or markers representing "no dyspnea" or "not at all breathless" (= 0) at the low end of the scale and "dyspnea as bad as it can be" or "severely breathless" (= 10) at the high end (Harwood, 1999). Although visual analog scales measure only one aspect (i.e., intensity) of a person's dyspnea, they are useful for evaluating a change in the symptom over time and response to treatment, and they can be utilized with a minimal time commitment.

More comprehensive assessment tools for dyspnea are available that have been found both reliable and valid in client populations with or without malignant disease. Use of these tools, however, is generally reserved for research activities because they require too much time to use in the clinical setting. Examples of more comprehensive tools for assessment of dyspnea include the American Thoracic Society Standardized Questionnaire (American Thoracic Society, 1978); the Pulmonary Functional Status and Dyspnea Questionnaire (Lareau, Carrieri-Kohlman, Janson-Bjerklie, & Roos, 1994); the Modified Baseline Dyspnea Index (Stoller, Ferranti, & Feinstein, 1986); the Shortness of Breath Assessment Tool (Lareau, Carrieri-Kohlman, Janson-Bjerklie, & Roos, 1986); and the Transition Dyspnea Index (Mahler, Weinberg, Wells, & Feinstein, 1984). In addition to measuring intensity, these tools often measure functional ability and impairment related to the symptom.

INTERVENTIONS FOR DYSPNEA

The goals for the client with dyspnea near the end of life are to treat the primary cause and relieve the psychological distress and autonomic response that accompany the symptom (Gavrin & Chapman, 1995). Because diagnostic testing to identify the cause is usually inappropriate, the etiology is determined by physical assessment and knowledge of the underlying condition. If the etiology of dyspnea cannot be successfully treated, interventions are aimed at alleviating the distress.

Dyspnea is a very difficult symptom to control. Because of this, interventions to decrease its intensity and maintain control should be implemented as soon as possible after its occurrence. Use of standard kits, such as Symptom Relief Kit, facilitates prompt treatment of dyspnea at end of life (Appendix A) (Petrin, 1998).

MEDICATIONS

Opioids

Morphine sulfate is highly effective in relieving dyspnea and it is considered the standard treatment for the relief of dyspnea near death (HPNA, 1996). Opioids affect dyspnea by altering the individual's perception of breathlessness, reducing respiratory drive, and reducing oxygen consumption (Harwood, 1999). Although morphine may decrease the respiratory rate, lead to an increase in P_{CO_2}, and a decrease in arterial pH, it generally does not severely compromise one's respiratory status. The primary side effect of morphine is somnolence, which may be managed by decreasing the dose.

Morphine for dyspnea can be administered by mouth, sublingually, per rectum, parenteral via intravenous or subcutaneous boluses or drips, or via nebulizer. Although not intended to be given sublingually, morphine concentrates and soluble tablets can be administered under the tongue or in the buccal mucosa in patients who can no longer swallow. Recent studies of morphine administered in this way have found that the majority of the morphine is actually swallowed, and not absorbed sublingually (Coluzzi, 1998). Nurses need to understand that individuals who are opioid naive (have not been receiving daily opioids) should be initially started on low doses (e.g., 5 mg–10 mg PO or sublingually), which can be repeated if necessary. However, individuals taking opioids for pain will need to have their breakthrough dose of morphine increased by 50% of their usual dose, for effective treatment of dyspnea.

If intravenous access is available, health care providers may give 1 mg–2 mg of morphine to be given every 5 to 10 minutes until relief is obtained. Given the discomfort associated with needle sticks, health providers should not initiate intravenous access in dying clients unless it is necessary to achieve comfort. If clients are unable to swallow safely, effective treatment can also be provided by administering morphine subcutaneously.

Morphine via a facial nebulizer also has been used for dyspnea near end of life, but only a few uncontrolled studies report clinical benefits (Chan, Sham, Tse, & Thorsen, 2004). A review of the literature reported in 2001 did not support use of nebulized opioids for control of dyspnea with terminal illness (Jennings et al., 2001).

Diuretics, Bronchodilators, Corticosteroids, and Antibiotics

Individuals with signs of fluid volume excess manifested by dyspnea, crackles/rales on auscultation of breath sounds, peripheral edema, or signs of heart failure (+ S3) should be given a diuretic such as furosemide (Lasix) to decrease blood volume, reduce vascular congestion, and reduce the workload of the heart. Furosemide can be administered by mouth, intravenously, subcutaneously, or in the muscle (IM). Intravenous administration, which is effective in the pulmonary vascular within minutes, may be preferred for congestive heart failure and pulmonary edema.

Bronchodilators, such as albuterol via metered dose inhalation or nebulizer, may be given for symptoms of bronchospasm (e.g., wheezes on auscultation of breath sounds). Corticosteroids may also be given for bronchospasm and inflammatory problems within and exterior to the lung. Superior vena cava syndrome and lymphangitis carcinomatosis both can cause dyspnea, which may respond to corticosteroids.

A thorough workup for a respiratory infection is not appropriate in clients imminently near death. However, if clients have developed dyspnea along with an elevated temperature, adventitious breath sounds, and a congested cough, it is safe to assume they have an upper respiratory infection. A trial of an appropriate antibiotic should be considered for clients with dyspnea of infectious origin near death, to provide symptom relief and facilitate comfort.

Anticholinergics

Secretions in the respiratory tract and oral cavity may contribute to a client's dyspnea near death. Loud wet respirations (referred to as death rattle) are also disturbing to family and caregivers, even when they do not seem to cause dyspnea or respiratory distress. Anticholinergics such as hyoscyamine (Levsin PO/SL), scopolamine transdermal, and oral atropine drops are used to reduce secretion production (Appendix A). Clients with tenacious secretions may benefit from mucolytic agents. However, steam or nebulized saline will probably be as effective (Levy, 1997).

Oxygen

The use of oxygen for individuals with hypoxemia is recognized as an important part of treatment. However, it has been shown that dyspnea in the terminally ill does not correlate with the degree of hypoxia (Bruera et al., 2000), and the physiological benefits of oxygen in patients with advanced cancer are uncertain. Some health care practitioners believe that oxygen is not necessary near the end of life, that it can actually cause discomfort, and that comfort can be better achieved using morphine. Indeed, many clients with dyspnea near death frequently remove their oxygen and can be kept comfortable without it.

However, the need for oxygen for dyspnea at end of life is dependent on the client's perception of the need, and the perception of its effect. It is imperative that clients with dyspnea who do not promptly respond to morphine (or other medications) be given a trial dose of oxygen to assess its effect, regardless of whether or not they are hypoxemic.

Anxiolytics

Sedatives are commonly used when morphine does not fully control the client's dyspnea. Either benzodiazepines or phenothiazines can be used for their effect on anxiety, fear, and the autonomic responses that accompany dyspnea. The benzodiazepine lorazepam (0.5 mg PO/SL) is commonly given every 4 hours or around the clock, to prevent and control dyspnea or anxiety. Benzodiazepines are more commonly used because phenothiazines have the potential for extrapyramidal side effects. Phenothiazines that have been used for dyspnea include chlorpromazine hydrochloride (Thorazine).

NONPHARMACOLOGICAL INTERVENTIONS

If dyspnea occurs near death, pharmacological interventions should be initiated early. Nonpharmacological interventions are used in conjunction with (not in place of) medications to decrease the impact of the dyspnea on the client. Nonpharmacological interventions include altering the environment to facilitate circulation of cool air, cooling of the body (especially the face), positioning the client to facilitate chest expansion, intervening to conserve client energy, and facilitating the client's rest. An electric fan or air-conditioned room helps decrease the impact of dyspnea. Although dyspnea for many often improves by keeping the head and torso elevated, positions of comfort are individual. If patients have only one lung with limited capacity, they may have less dyspnea lying on their side with the affected lung down (Tyler, 2000). Clients who suffer from dyspnea when exerting to void are offered a Foley catheter, the insertion of which will eliminate the need for exertion to void. This strategy is particularly effective for clients taking diuretics. Research indicates that terminally ill clients are appropriate candidates for urinary catheterization when the goal is comfort, and that the benefit can far outweigh morbidity (e.g., secondary to bacteriuria) (Fainsinger, MacEachern, Hanson, & Bruera, 1992).

Complementary therapies that promote relaxation should also be offered and implemented to reduce the impact of dyspnea. These include imagery, massage, breathing exercises, therapeutic touch, Reiki, music, and aromatherapy.

NAUSEA AND VOMITING NEAR THE END OF LIFE

Although not as common a problem as pain or dyspnea, nausea and vomiting are thought to occur in approximately 40% of terminally ill individuals during the last week of life (Waller & Caroline, 1996). Nausea and vomiting are particularly prevalent in individuals with breast cancer, stomach cancer, and gynecologic cancers and in individuals with AIDS (Dworkin, 1992).

The mechanisms and mediators of nausea and vomiting are complex and remain incompletely defined (Gavrin & Chapman, 1995). Central and peripheral factors both play a role. The chemoreceptor trigger zone and the nucleus solitarius are located in a highly vascular area of the brain stem, which is rich with opioid, dopaminergic, cholinergic, histaminergic, and serotonergic receptors. It is hypothesized that activation of these receptors stimulates an emetic center that produces nausea, vomiting, or both. A vestibular component is particularly prevalent with opioid-induced nausea, and it can be stimulated by movement.

Nausea and vomiting at the end of life are commonly seen with: (1) the initiation of opioid therapy (nausea usually limited to a few days); (2) uremia; (3) hypercalcemia; (4) increased intracranial pressure secondary to brain metastasis; (5) vaginal stimulation secondary to oral candidiasis; (6) stretching of the hepatic capsule; (7) constipation or impaction; and (8) bowel obstruction.

Assessment of Nausea and Vomiting

The client's self-report of nausea is the most reliable way to assess its presence. Clients and family are asked to keep a daily diary, noting the time of each episode of nausea and vomiting, along with associated activities such as movement, coughing, eating, and the frequency of bowel movements. Health care providers can assess and monitor nausea and vomiting using a flow sheet (such as the one shown in Table 11.1). When clients have a decreased level of consciousness, it is very difficult to assess them for nausea. However, if an unresponsive patient is retching or gagging, nausea should be suspected.

Interventions for Nausea and Vomiting

Any client experiencing nausea or vomiting on a daily basis should be given antiemetics around the clock, to control the symptoms and prevent their reoccurrence. There are a variety of antiemetics that can be used for nausea and vomiting occurring near the end of life. The phenothiazine prochlorperazine (Compazine) is commonly administered as a rectal suppository (25 mg) or intravenously (5 mg–10 mg). The antiemetic and gastrointestinal stimulant metoclopramide (Reglan) can be given rectally or parenterally (10 mg every 6 hours), as a single agent or in combination with other antiemetics. Metoclopramide is often the drug of choice with incomplete or high gastrointestinal obstruction or chronic nausea of unknown etiology. This drug, however, should not be used in clients with complete bowel obstruction or clients with colicky abdominal pain.

Clients receiving metoclopramide (Reglan) need to be monitored for signs and symptoms of dystonic reactions, an infrequent but serious side effect of this drug. Dystonic reactions include akathisia (restlessness), anxiety, agitation, and tardive dyskinesia, manifested as muscle rigidity. Dystonic reactions secondary to metoclopramide are more common in individuals under 30 years of age, and are more likely to occur when clients are receiving haloperidol (Haldol) in addition to metoclopramide (Reglan). If dystonic reactions secondary to metoclopramide (Reglan) occur, diphenhydramine (Benadryl) 50 mg is given to reverse the dystonic effect. If metoclopramide (Reglan) needs to be continued, diphenhydramine (Benadryl) 50 mg is given with each subsequent dose (Waller & Caroline, 1996).

A compounded antiemetic known by the mnemonic ABHR—Ativan (lorazepam), Benadryl (diphenhydramine), Haldol (haloperidol), and Reglan (metoclopramide)—is commonly used by palliative care providers for severe cases of nausea or vomiting. It can be compounded into suppositories, troches, or a gel for transdermal use (Petrin, 1998). Although doses of each drug can vary, a common ABHR dose is Ativan 1 mg, Benadryl 12.5 mg, Haldol 1 mg, and Reglan 10 mg. One limitation to the use of ABHR is the need for access to a pharmacist who can compound the medication. ABHR is also associated with significant sedation, which may not be acceptable to clients and their families.

Corticosteroids such as dexamethasone (Decadron) are also used for their antiemetic effects. Decadron is particularly effective in nausea and vomiting related to increased intracranial pressure, gastrointestinal obstruction, hypercalcemia, or uremia. Daily doses range from 8 mg to 60 mg daily, which can be given as single agents or in combination with other drugs such as Ativan (lorazepam), Benadryl (diphenhydramine), and Reglan (metoclopramide). ABDR (Ativan, Benadryl, Decadron, and Reglan) is used when clients do not respond to ABHR or ABCR (Ativan, Benadryl, Compazine, and Reglan) compounds.

ANXIETY AND ALTERED COGNITION

Symptoms of anxiety and altered cognition commonly occur together at the end of life, and the presence of one often relates to the development of the other. Anxiety is defined as a feeling of deep unease without an identifiable cause. Altered cognition is often associated with an acute confusional state or delirium, which represents a disturbance of consciousness with reduced ability to focus or shift attention (March, 1998). Delirium can present as a hyperactive, hypoactive, or fluctuating disorder (Jackson & Lipman, 2000).

There are multiple causes of anxiety and altered cognition near the end of life. Causes of anxiety include poorly controlled pain, altered physiologic states (e.g., hypoxia, septicemia, hypoglycemia, hypocalcemia); medications (e.g., corticosteroids in high doses, metoclopramide in high doses, neuroleptic medications); withdrawal from alcohol, narcotics, or sedatives); psychologic, emotional, or spiritual distress; or a preexisting anxiety disorder (HPNA, 1996).

Etiologies of delirium or altered cognition near the end of life include physiological impairments (e.g., metabolic encephalopathy due to organ failure, electrolyte imbalance, central nervous system abnormalities such as malignancies or opportunistic infections of the brain, hypoxia, dehydration, septicemia, pain, urinary retention, constipation, fatigue, sensory disturbance, sensory alterations, nausea, extreme temperatures, puritis, or immobilization, alcohol or drug withdrawal); and psychological distress, which is often related to spiritual distress.

Delirium associated with restlessness at end of life is often referred to as terminal restlessness or terminal agitation. Terminal restlessness is defined as an observable syndrome characterized by the inability to rest, occurring in clients with varying diagnoses during the last days of life (March, 1998). Observable manifestations of terminal restlessness include frequent, nonpurposeful motor activity, the inability to concentrate or relax, disturbances in sleep/rest patterns, fluctuating levels of consciousness, and cognitive failure or anxiety (HPNA, 1997).

Anxiety and altered cognition are disturbing to clients and families, but terminal restlessness often causes tremendous distress and can put the client and family at risk for injury. Because anxiety and altered cognition often precede terminal restlessness, symptoms should be identified and treated early to obtain and maintain symptom control and facilitate client comfort.

Assessment of Anxiety and Altered Cognition

Assessment of anxiety and altered cognition is initially focused on identifying a physical cause, which may be reversible. The nurse initially assesses for pain, urinary retention, or constipation as the cause. Anxiety that continues in the absence of these problems prompts the nurse to review medications, to identify new additions and recent changes, drug-drug interactions, and consider their anxiety-provoking potential. Withdrawal of benzodiazepines in clients near death is a common cause of delirium near death. Delirium and agitation, however, also can occur secondary to initiation or an increase of a benzodiazepine (Levy, 1999).

If delirium continues despite treatment of reversible causes (e.g., pain, urinary retention, and changes in medications), consideration should be given to the possibility that hypoxemia, hypercalcemia, kidney, or liver failure are contributing causes. It is inappropriate, however, to investigate metabolic causes by invasive means (e.g., laboratory analysis). Invasive procedures often inflict pain and they are usually unsuccessful in establishing the cause (Burke, 1997).

In the absence of a physiological impairment, clients with anxiety and delirium are assessed for their familiarity with the environment, their perceived readiness to die, and their perception of spiritual concerns. Clients in an unfamiliar environment (e.g., a hospital), with unfinished business and spiritual concerns are more likely to be anxious than clients without these stresses (March, 1998).

The Mini Mental Status Exam (Folstein, 1983) is considered the gold standard for evaluating delirium. Spiritual and psychosocial assessment tools are also available for use in clients with social or spiritual concerns. However, clients near death are often unable to respond to questions on these assessment tools because they are obtunded, moribund, or agitated. A systematic assessment for sources of delirium and agitation in clients near death is often unobtainable. If the client is verbal, the nurse and family should listen for statements reflecting client concerns. Clients may want to discuss spiritual matters, beliefs about death, God, or a search for meaning in life. Every effort should be made to discuss areas of concern.

When caring for a client near death, it is imperative that anxiety, delirium, and terminal restlessness be distinguished from movement disorders such as myoclonus and extrapyramidal symptoms. Myoclonus is defined as a sudden, brief, shocklike, involuntary movement caused by active muscular contractions of symmetrical muscle groups (Sjögren, Jonsson, Jensen, Drenck, & Jensen, 1993). A major concern with myoclonic spasms is that the jerking or twitching may progress to convulsions. Myoclonus is often related to rapid increases and high doses of opioids such as morphine and its accumulated metabolites. Myoclonus may also result from a lowered seizure threshold related to medications (e.g., metoclopramide, phenothiazines, antihistamines, haloperidol, tricyclic antidepressants, and anticholinergics), organ failure, brain lesions, hypoxia, dehydration, withdrawal syndromes, and electrolyte or glucose abnormalities (Back, 1992; deStoutz, Bruera, & Suarez-Almazor, 1995).

Extrapyramidal symptoms occur as side effects of neuroleptic medications such as the phenothiazines (e.g., chlorpromazine or prochlorperazine), butyrophenones, and metoclopramide). Examples of extrapyramidal symptoms include muscle rigidity, acute dystonia, akathisia (restlessness), cogwheeling, and akinesia.

Interventions for Anxiety and Altered Cognition

Given that pain is a common cause of anxiety at the end of life, initial treatment of anxiety often involves administration of a fast-acting analgesic such as morphine (solution) PO/SL. If the anxiety is relieved in response to the analgesic, around-the-clock doses should be continued or increased. Clients near death may also experience anxiety secondary to urinary retention, which may occur as a side effect of anticholinergic agents or smooth muscle relaxants. Anxiety in the presence of a distended bladder may resolve with intermittent or indwelling urinary catheterization.

Benzodiazepines

Benzodiazepines are the mainstay of pharmacologic treatment of anxiety in the terminally ill patient (Breitbart, Chochinov, & Passik, 2004) and the drugs of choice for anxiety, restlessness, or myoclonus near death. Shorter acting benzodiazepines such as lorazepam (Ativan) or alprazolam (Xanax) are considered safest because toxic accumulation is avoided. Lorazepam (Ativan) 0.5 mg–2 mg can be crushed, mixed with a few drops of water, given sublingually, and continued every 3 to 6 hours.

Patients who experience breakthrough anxiety or end-of-dose failure may benefit from switching to a long-acting benzodiazepine such as diazepam or clonazepam. Valium has the added benefit of having a rapid onset, and it can be given rectally when no other route is available, at dosages equivalent to oral regimens. Common dosage regimens include diazepam 2.5 mg–10 mg PO q 3 to 6 hours or clonazepam 1 mg–2 mg PO BID or TID. Midazolam (Versed) is a benzodiazepine that is given subcutaneously or intravenously. Its use, however, is generally reserved for terminal agitation that does not respond to more commonly used benzodiazepines and barbiturates (described in a later chapter). Use of midazolam (Versed) is described in this chapter under "Sedation for Refractory Symptoms."

Neuroleptics

Neuroleptics such as haloperidol are useful in the treatment of anxiety when benzodiazepines are not sufficient for symptom control. When delirium is present, haloperidol is considered by many as the drug of choice (Jackson & Lipman, 2000). Neuroleptics are also indicated when delusions or hallucinations accompany the anxiety. Recommended starting dose of Haldol is 0.5 mg–4 mg PO, PR, IV, SC, BID and every 4 hours prn, with a maximum 24-hour dose of 30 mg.

Chlorpromazine (Thorazine) is another neuroleptic that is routinely used for terminal anxiety. It can be used in individuals who respond to haloperidol, but need more sedation. Recommended starting dose of Thorazine is 10 mg–25 mg PO, SL, PR, IV every 4 to 6 hours prn, with a maximum daily dose of 600 mg.

Sedation for Refractory Symptoms

Refractory symptoms at end of life are defined as symptoms of distress that cannot be adequately controlled, despite aggressive effort to identify therapy that does not compromise consciousness (Levy, 1999). Delirium, myoclonus, pain, and dyspnea are at times refractory to aggressive interventions. The decision to utilize sedation for refractory agitation should be made on a case-by-case basis, by experts in palliative care, ideally with input from the interdisciplinary team. Sedation may be employed when providers are confident that appropriate medications have failed, when standard interventions risk excessive and intolerable morbidity, or when standard interventions are incapable of providing adequate relief in a tolerable period.

An increase in doses of opioids, benzodiazepines, and neuroleptics to the point of sedation is one method of sedation for refractory symptoms. This method is the most routine, and it generally involves increasing medications such as lorazepam, alprazolam, diazepam, haloperidol, or chlorpromazine (Levy, 1999). Infrequently, clients may need sedation for refractory symptoms using barbiturates such as pentobarbital, secobarbital, amobarbital, or phenobarbital. In rare cases of refractory symptoms of distress, clients may need extraordinary medications to relieve distress. Medications recommended for extraordinary situations of refractory distress include the benzodiazepine midazolam (Versed), which is administered by subcutaneous or intravenous routes; thiopental, or propofol.

Protocols for palliative sedation (sometimes referred to as terminal sedation) should be used to guide palliative care staff through the process of selecting and implementing appropriate regimens. Acccording to the American Academy of Hospice and Palliative Medicine (2002),

> As a method of palliative care treatment, the use of sedating medications is intended to decrease a patient's level of consciousness to mitigate the experience of suffering, but not to hasten the end of life. Since this represents both an intention and an outcome that is beneficial, sedation in these cases is ethically justified. It is not analogous to euthanasia or physician-assisted suicide in which the primary intent is death of the patient. (p. 72)

Nonpharmacological Interventions

Individuals suffering from existential anxiety may benefit from visits with a member of the clergy. Patients with financial or legal concerns may benefit from visits from professionals knowledgeable about these matters. Cognitive reframing, distraction, and progressive muscle relaxation may also assist in relieving anxiety (Noyes, Holt, & Massie, 1998).

At the first onset of delirium, patients should be placed in a quiet, safe, and supportive environment. Reiki therapy, therapeutic touch, and aromatherapy, using a combination of essential oils such as lavender, marjoram, or geranium, may promote relaxation. Oils used for aromatherapy can be applied to hands and feet, or in the absence of oxygen, may be vaporized (James, 1998).

CONSTIPATION

Clients near death usually demonstrate a gradual decline in their physical condition, often manifested by a decrease in oral intake and decrease in mobility. These clients also often have risks for constipation related to side effects of medications and metabolic changes such as hypercalcemia and hyperkalemia. Constipation in clients with cancer is primarily due to the colonic effects of opioids, which decrease peristalsis. Although it is not a universal problem, constipation secondary to opioids is so common and so potentially distressing that it warrants prophylactic treatment when opioids are initiated and ongoing monitoring for the remainder of the person's life.

Assessment of Constipation

The nurse assesses the level of activity, intake, medication history, diagnosis, and usual pattern of elimination for all clients, identifying individual risks. Although there are variations in elimination patterns, absence of bowel elimination for 3 or more days should prompt the nurse to assess for other signs and symptoms of constipation (e.g., abdominal distention, nausea, vomiting, or rectal impaction). Evidence of symptoms of discomfort from constipation mandates that a digital rectal exam be performed to rule out impaction.

Interventions for Constipation

Bowel protocols or algorithms are often implemented to prevent and treat constipation. Prophylactic treatment with a stool softener (e.g., docusate sodium) and mild stimulant laxative such as senna is commonly prescribed because of its direct effect on the colon and demonstrated effect in these patients (Nursing Drug Handbook, 2000). Patients are commonly instructed to take 1 to 2 tablets of senna orally at bedtime. If stools are hard, the patient may also take 1 tab of docusate sodium for each tab of senna. Dosages of senna can be increased gradually up to 4 tablets TID as needed to maintain a comfortable elimination pattern.

If the patient has not moved the bowels according to his or her usual pattern, but is comfortable, without nausea, vomiting or impaction, 30 ml of milk of magnesia can be given to stimulate the bowel, with a follow-up assessment within 24 hours. Other more potent oral laxatives such as Lactulose 30 ml–60 ml PO, magnesium citrate 8-oz PO, or Fleet Phospho-Soda PO may be used if the client does not respond to milk of magnesia. Palpation of stool in the rectum calls for Dulcolax suppositories or a Fleet enema by rectum. Disimpaction is required if stool is hard and cannot be evacuated via these methods and the client is in distress. Ideally, disimpac-

tion is preceded by administration of an oil-retention enema (120 cc) several hours or the night before the procedure (Waller & Caroline, 1996). Ten minutes prior to the procedure, the rectum is instilled with 10 ml of 1% lidocaine jelly, and the patient is premedicated with morphine. The nurse should begin the procedure by lubricating the surface of the anus and her or his index finger with lidocaine jelly.

Constipation in the immediate period near death is generally not problematic if clients have been monitored. However, clients with abdominal pain, escalation of their usual pain, anxiety, agitation, nausea, or vomiting, need to be assessed for possible constipation and impaction. Administration of enemas, manual disimpaction, or both, is indicated in the period near death only if constipation is contributing to client discomfort.

Intestinal Obstruction

A potential complication of a fecal impaction is a bowel obstruction. Bowel or intestinal obstructions can also occur in individuals near the end of life because of a primary or secondary malignant tumor or a nonmalignant cause such as adhesions (Waller & Caroline, 1996).

Distinction of a fecal impaction from a bowel obstruction is important to determining treatment. Bowel obstructions are particularly common in clients with primary colon, ovarian, stomach, pancreatic, or renal cancers, and retroperitoneal sarcoma. Obstructions can also occur with metastasis to the abdomen from lung, breast, esophageal, or cervical cancers or malignant melanoma (Waller & Caroline, 1996).

Bowel obstructions in clients with advanced cancer are characterized by abdominal distention and tenderness, which occurs in a slow, progressive fashion. Colicky abdominal pain occurs in approximately 75% of patients (Waller & Caroline, 1996), and is characterized as "crampy" pain that comes and goes with relatively pain-free intervals. Episodes of colicky pain may be associated with audible borborygmi.

Continuous or steady abdominal pain occurs in more than 90% of patients with cancer and bowel obstruction (Waller & Caroline, 1996). Unlike colicky pain, which comes and goes, steady pain is produced by stretching of the liver capsule or abdominal distention. Other signs of obstruction include intermittent borborygmi, absence of bowel sounds, and intermittent or continuous vomiting. A flat plate x-ray of the abdomen can be ordered to rule out bowel obstruction versus constipation.

Interventions for Intestinal Obstruction

Depending on the etiology of an obstruction and the goals for the patient, treatment may include hospital admission, nasogastric suction, and in some instances, surgery to release the obstruction. However, the majority of terminally ill patients with intestinal obstruction can be managed medically without nasogastric suction or intravenous fluids (Waller & Caroline, 1996).

In the presence of colicky abdominal pain and abdominal distention, all laxatives are discontinued. Clients taking metoclopramide (Reglan) should discontinue this medication (a) in the presence of incomplete obstruction with colicky pain, and (b) with complete obstruction, because it can increase colic and vomiting. Haloperidol SC or prochlorperazine PR may be used for nausea and vomiting. Antispasmodics such as glycopyrrolate (Robinul) SC or IV, or hyoscyamines (Levsin) SC, IV, or SL are given for colicky pain, with opioids often given SC by continuous infusion. Corticosteroids (e.g., predni-

sone or dexamethasone are used for their anti-inflammatory and antisecretory activity. Sandostatin (Octreotide) SC or IV may be used to inhibit release of GI hormones, thereby reducing gastric, pancreatic, biliary, and intestinal secretions.

Clients with intestinal obstructions at the end of life may be allowed to drink and eat small amounts as tolerated, because the goal is patient comfort. Care to keep the patient's mouth moist is paramount, in order to avoid dryness caused by dehydration and anticholinergic drugs, used for their antisecretory effect. Intractable vomiting (> 2 episodes/8 hours) that does not respond to pharmacological measures may indicate the need for nasogastric intubation for comfort (Waller & Caroline, 1996).

FATIGUE

Fatigue is the most common symptom reported by patients approaching death (Tyler & Lipman, 2000), and it is a source of tremendous distress. Health care providers, however, have given it inadequate attention.

The diagnosis of fatigue is based on the patient's report. Some patients may volunteer the information, but it often goes unrecognized unless the practitioner specifically asks (Tyler & Lipman, 2000). It is important to acknowledge the negative impact of fatigue and help the patient set realistic goals.

Fatigue is often associated with other conditions such as depression, insomnia, anxiety, pain, infection, fever, dehydration, cachexia, hyperkalemia, hypoxia, and drugs that cause CNS depression. The nurse should assess for signs and symptoms of these conditions, and consider treatment, if appropriate.

If present, therapy for depression, anxiety, pain, and hypoxia should be optimized. When possible, medications that cause sedation may be decreased or discontinued. Dehydration can often be managed with oral hydration. Other causes of fatigue, such as anemia, may not be appropriate to treat near death. Blood transfusions or epoetin are expensive, and they lose effect with repeated use. However, a transfusion may be indicated when it provides the strength needed to attend an important event such as a family wedding.

Controversy exists regarding the role of exercise, but establishing a schedule with a set bedtime, wakeup time, and rest periods may be tried. Patients should be asked what activities they enjoy most, and be given permission to rest or sleep during less enjoyable activities to conserve energy. This may involve limiting or excluding certain visitors and prioritizing others. Music and imagery could also be used to stimulate or relax the client at various times of choice, providing sounds and sights that are pleasant for the patient. A video describing a favorite pastime like golf or football may be an excellent source of diversion and enjoyment.

Some patients may benefit from pharmacologic interventions (Tyler & Lipman, 2000) such as corticosteroids (e.g., dexamethasone or prednisone), hormones (e.g., megestrol), or a stimulant (e.g., methylphenidate).

TERMINAL DEHYDRATION

Dehydration in a healthy individual is generally associated with discomfort related to fluid and electrolyte imbalance, often manifested as fatigue, weakness, muscle cramps, nausea, vomiting, and headaches (Musgrave, 1990). Parenteral hydration is used in nonterminal individuals, with the goal of restoring fluid volume status

Unlike dehydration in nonterminal individuals, dehydration in individuals at the end of life is considered a normal physiologic process that occurs to prepare the body for death. It is generally associated with reduced desire and intake of food and fluids. Although it may be associated with weakness, fatigue and thirst, it is not consistently considered an uncomfortable condition that merits reversal. Moreover, research supporting its use for terminally ill clients is lacking. In fact, dehydration may actually have some beneficial effects in terms of symptom palliation (Musgrave, 1990; Zerwekh, 1983). Zerwekh contended that intake cessation leads to a reduced fluid load, which serves to reduce urinary output, nausea and vomiting, pulmonary congestion, and edema. Printz (1992) described a possible endogenous benefit of intake cessation, citing the effects of ketosis and increased levels of endorphins on the central nervous system in rats. Increased endorphins in humans may lead to a heightened state of well-being.

Many palliative care authors contend that with skilled nursing care, patients with terminal disease can die comfortably without artificial hydration (Morita, Tsunoda, Inoue, & Chihara, 1999). Research also indicates that palliative care providers believe that hydration near the end of life is not only unnecessary and futile, but also potentially harmful and capable of causing discomfort (Meares, 1994). Forcing fluids or food on a person who has little or no appetite risks causing nausea, vomiting, and aspiration. Insertion and maintenance of intravenous catheters or nasogastric feeding tubes is often painful for patients. Fluids from intravenous infusions or nasogastric tube feedings can increase respiratory secretions, which in turn increases pulmonary congestion, cough, and sensations of dyspnea; increases urine output and the need to void; and increases fluid retention in the form of edema, ascites, pleural effusions, or gastric secretions that contribute to nausea and vomiting.

Dry mouth is treated with every-2-hour mouth care including hygiene, lubrication, and if safe, ice chips or popsicles. Salivart, which is artificial saliva, can be given as 1 to 2 sprays in the mouth every hour as needed.

A major problem that terminal dehydration presents for patients, families, and palliative care providers is the emotional impact that withholding fluids and food has on the family. In most cultures, food and eating is equated with love; withholding food and fluids may be perceived as abandonment. Research has shown that the point in time when patients can no longer eat represents a major life transition and loss for family caregivers (Meares, 1995).

It is essential that nurses assess patients and their families' perceptions about terminal dehydration, and discuss the advantages and disadvantages of each, maintaining an open dialogue about the topic. Nurses should provide families with reading materials that explain the normal physiologic process at end of life, and allow families time to absorb the information. If, despite explanations, families continue to be uncomfortable with a decision to withhold food and fluids, the option of intravenous or subcutaneous therapy may be offered (see "Fatigue"). Intravenous or subcutaneous fluid should be given at a rate not to exceed 1 to 1.5 liters per day, using furosemide as needed to control symptoms of overhydration (Waller & Caroline, 1996).

CONCLUSIONS

To prevent suffering near death, clients need to be consistently assessed for signs and symptoms of distress such as pain, dyspnea, anxiety, delirium with agitation, nausea, and vomiting, fatigue, and constipation. Systematic assessment of these symptoms and evaluation of the effect of treatment can be accomplished using a symptom-specific tool, measuring level of intensity on a flow sheet (such as in Table 11.1). Table 11.2 outlines interventions to relieve distressing symptoms that people approaching the end of their life may experience. The occurrence of dyspnea, nausea, vomiting, agitation, and altered cognition requires ongoing treatment to prevent escalation of symptoms and to maintain the client's comfort near death.

Treatment of symptoms near death ideally should be directed at the cause of the symptom. When the cause cannot be identified or eliminated, the goal is to control the symptom, and prevent recurrence. Successful interventions reduce or eliminate symptoms. Algorithms or protocols developed by palliative care providers are used to guide pharmacological treatment of symptoms near death. Protocols should be used in conjunction with input from the palliative care interdisciplinary teams, to ensure that assessments are comprehensive and that all factors contributing to the symptom of distress in each individual have been considered.

Inadequate control of symptoms of distress using standard interventions mandates a consult with a palliative care provider to identify other options for symptom management. Changes in medication management should be made as soon as medications are deemed ineffective. Delays in changing medication regimens can cause unnecessary suffering for clients and families. Client and family suffering at the end of life should be perceived by all as unacceptable.

More research is needed regarding the occurrence of symptoms in clients with advanced malignant and nonmalignant disease, and on treatments. Research should consider the impact of the environment on the symptom (e.g., home, hospital, hospice, and extended-care facility), availability of resources, access to care, and family caregiver experiences treating and experiencing symptoms of distress near death.

TABLE 11.2   Symptom Management

Medications	Indications
Dyspnea	
Step 1	
Opiods –	Sensation Of breathlessness
Morphine sulfate –	Pulmonary congestion
PO/SL/SC/IV	
Starting dose 5mg.–10 mg. PO/SL if patient opiod naive. Repeat q 2 hrs. prn	
For patients taking opiods for pain, increase MS04 by 50% their usual breakthrough dose	
Step 2 as indicated by clinical findings:	
Diuretics	Pulmonary congestion (seen with cardiac
Furosemide (Lasix)	dysfunction and/or fluid volume overload)
IM/IV (20–40 mg. +)	
Bronchodilators	Bronchoconstriction/spasm
Albuterol or Ipratropium bromide	
Inhalation	
Corticosteroids IV/SC	For inflammation within and exterior to lung
Dexamethasone	(e.g., Superior vena cava syndrome;
(Decadron)	lymphagitis carcinomatosis)
Antibiotics	Respiratory distress likely due to infection,
Erythromycin PO	manifested by copious secretions
Anticholinergics Hyoscyamine	Secretions
(Levsin)0.125–.25 mg q 6 hr	
PO/SL prn	
Scopolamine	
(transdermal)	
Atropine 1–2mg. IM/SC/or	
Inhalation	
Anxiolytics	Sense of breathlessness, anxiety, fear
(Sedatives)	
Benzodiazepines – Sedatives of choice	
Lorazepam 0.5mg.	
PO/SL q 4 hours PRN or ATC	
or	
Phenothiazines	
Chlorpromazine hydrochloride	
(Thorazine) or haloperidol (Haldol)	
Mucolytic agents	Thick secretions
Nebulized saline	

(continued)

TABLE 11.2   *(continued)*

Medications	Indications
Nausea/Vomiting	
Phenothiazines	Nausea/vomiting of any etiology
Prochlorperazine (Compazine) PR/IV/PO	
GI Stimulant	Incomplete or high GI obstruction or
Metoclopramide (Reglan)	Chronic nausea of unknown etiology
PR/IV/PO/Trouche	
Compounds	Severe nausea or vomiting
ABHR: Ativan (Lorazepam),	
Benadryl (Diphenhydramine),	
Haldol (Haloperidol), and	
Reglan (Metochlopramide)	
Corticosteroids	Nausea/vomiting r/t increased intracranial
Dexamethasone (Decadron) PO/PR/IV	pressure, gastrointestinal obstruction,
	hypercalcemia, and uremia.
Anxiety	
Opiods	Signs and Symptoms of Discomfort
Morphine sulfate (liquid)	
PO/SL or PR.	
Benzodiazepines	Anxiety, restlessness or myoclonus
Lorazepam (Ativan) SL	
or Alprazolam (Xanax)	
Diazepam (Valium)PR	Anxiety, restlessness or myoclonus
Clonazepam (Klonopin)SC	Myoclonus
Midazolam (Versed)	Reserved for terminal agitation that does
IV/SC	not respond to more commonly used
	benzodiazepines and barbiturates
Barbiturates	When benzodiazepines fail to control
Phenobarbital PR	anxiety.
or Pentobarbital	Myoclonus.
or Secobarbital	Seizures prevention.
Thiopental and Propofol	Reserved for use in extraordinary cases of
	agitation, where sedation is needed for
	comfort.
Neuroleptics	Hallucinations or paranoia
Haloperidol (Haldol) PO/SC	
Chlorpromazine (Thorazine) PO/PR	Terminal restlessness

TABLE 11.2   *(continued)*

Medications	Indications
Constipation	
Oral Laxative	In patient taking opiods
Senna with stool softener PO	
Milk of Magnesia (MOM)	If senna not effective
Lactulose, Magnesium Citrate, or Fleet Phospho-Soda PO	If milk of magnesia not effective
Ducolax suppositories or Fleet enema	Stool in rectum, or if constipation with nausea/vomiting
Oil Retention Enema	Stool Impaction

EDUCATION PLAN 11.1   Plan for Achieving Competencies: Symptoms Management

Knowledge Needed	Attitude	Skills	Undergraduate Behavioral Outcomes	Graduate Behavioral Outcomes	Teaching/Learning Strategies
The need for symptom management at the end of life.	*Accept the pivotal role of nurses in symptom management at the end of life.		*Address symptom management in patients' plan of care.	*Advocate for aggressive symptom management for patients and family at the end of life.	*Evaluate case studies for evidence of effective or in-effective symptom management.
Symptom assessment: —dyspnea —nausea and vomiting —anxiety —altered cognition —constipation —intestinal obstruction —fatigue —terminal dehydration	*Accept that symptoms are what the patient says they are.	*Perform a comprehensive assessment to determine symptoms at the end of life, utilizing various measurement instruments.	*Accurately identifies symptoms and related suffering of patients and family at the end of life.	*Utilize advanced knowledge to diagnose complex symptoms and related suffering of patients and family at the end of life.	*Utilize case studies to identify symptoms and suffering issues at the end of life for patients and family. *Assess patients in clinical setting, and utilize measurement instruments to identify symptoms and suffering experienced at the end of life. Present findings during post-conference or interdisciplinary team meetings.

Pharmacological and nonpharmacological management of symptoms and suffering; —dyspnea —nausea and vomiting —anxiety —altered cognition —constipation —intestinal obstruction —fatigue —terminal dehydration	*Recognize and suspend practitioner bias related to pharmacological and nonpharmacological interventions. *Value the role of the interdisciplinary team and the potential need for consultation with other experts.	*Administer optimal treatment for the management of symptoms and suffering. *Guide pharmacological treatment of symptoms utilizing established protocols and algorithms developed by palliative care providers.	*Provide optimal symptom management and relief of suffering based on prescribed plan of care or through consultation with members of other disciplines.	*Prescribe a plan of care, utilizing pharmacological and nonpharmacological modalities to alleviate symptoms and suffering of patients and family at the end of life. *Collaborate with other disciplines when needed for optimal symptom management.	*Present a clinical experience to peers in postconference or seminar, for critique of the plan of care as related to symptom management. *Evaluate case studies for the effectiveness of interventions. *Using case studies, identify appropriate pharmacological and nonpharmacological interventions.

REFERENCES

American Academy of Hospice and Palliative Medicine. (2002). *Statement on sedation at end-of-life.* Silver Springs, MD: Author.

American Thoracic Society. (1978). Recommended respiratory disease questionnaires for use with adults and children in epidemiological research. *American Review of Respiratory Disease, 14*(7), 53.

Back, I. N. (1992). Terminal restlessness in patients with advanced malignant disease. *Palliative Medicine, 6,* 293–298.

Breitbart, W., Chochinov, H., & Passik, S. (2004). Psychiatric symptoms in palliative medicine. In D. Derek, G. Hanks, N. Cherny, & K. Calman (Eds.). *Oxford textbook of palliative medicine* (3rd ed., pp. 746–771). Oxford, UK: Oxford University Press.

Brescia, F. J., Adler, D., Gray, G., Ryan, A., Cimino, J., & Mamtini, R. (1990). Hospitalized advanced cancer patients: A profile. *Journal of Pain and Symptom Management, 5,* 221–227.

Bruera, E., Macmillan, T., Pither, J., & MacDonald, N. (1990). Effects of morphine on the dyspnea of terminal cancer patients. *Journal of Pain and Symptom Management, 5,* 341–344.

Bruera, E., Schmitz B., Pither, S., Neumann, C.M., Hanson, J. et al. (2000). The frequency and correlates of dyspnea in patients with advanced cancer. *Journal of Pain and Symptom Management 19,* 357–362.

Burke, A. (1997). Palliative care: An update in "terminal restlessness." *Medical Journal of Australia, 166*(1), 39–42.

Coluzzi, P. H. (1998). Sublingual morphine: Efficacy reviewed. *Journal of Pain and Symptom Management, 16,* 187–192.

Coluzzi H., & Fairbairn, B. S. (1999). The management of pain in terminally ill cancer patients with difficulty swallowing. *American Journal of Hospice and Palliative Care, 16,* 731–737.

deStoutz, N. D., Bruera, E., & Suarez-Almazor (1995). Opioid rotation for toxicity reduction in terminal cancer patients. *Journal of Pain and Symptom Management, 10,* 378–384.

Dworkin, B.M. (1992). Gastrointestinal manifestations of AIDS. In G.P. Wormser (Ed.), *AIDS and other manifestations of HIV infection* (2nd ed., pp. 419–432). New York: Raven Press.

Escalante, C. P., Martin, C. G., Eltin, L. S., Cantor, S. B., Harle, T. S., Price, K. J., et al. (1996). Dyspnea in cancer patients: Etiology, resource utilization, and survival-implications in a managed care world. *Cancer, 78,* 1314–1319.

Fainsinger, L., MacEachern, T., Hanson, J. & Bruera, E. (1992). The use of urinary catheters in terminally ill cancer patients. *Journal of Pain and Symptom Management, 7,* 333–338.

Field, M., & Cassel, C. (1997). *Approaching death: Improving care at the end of life.* Washington, DC: National Academies Press.

Folstein, M. F. (1983). The Mini Mental Status examination. In T. Crooke, S. Rerris, & R. Bartus (Eds.), *Assessment in geriatric psychopathology* (pp. 47–51). New Canaan, CT.

Gavrin, J., & Chapman, C. R. (1995). Clinical management of dying patients. Caring for patients at the end of life [Special issue]. *Western Journal of Medicine, 163,* 268–277.

Harwood, K. V. (1999). Dyspnea. In C. H. Yarbro, M. H. Frogge, & M. Goodman (Eds.), *Cancer symptom management* (2nd ed., pp. 45–57). Boston: Jones and Bartlett.

Hospice and Palliative Nurses Association. (1996). *Clinical practice protocol: Dyspnea.* Pittsburgh, PA: Hospice and Palliative Nurses Association.

Hospice and Palliative Nurses Association. (1997). *Clinical practice protocol: Terminal restlessness.* Pittsburgh, PA: Hospice and Palliative Nurses Association.

Jackson, K., & Lipman, A. (2000). Delirium in palliative care patients. In A. G. Lipman, K. D. Jackson, & L. S. Tyler (Eds.), *Evidence-based symptom control in palliative care* (pp. 59–70). New York: Haworth Press.

James, K. (1998). Healing Touch. In M. Snyder & R. Lindquist (Eds.), *Complementary/alternative therapies in nursing,* (3rd ed., pp. 139–147). New York: Springer.

Jennings, A. L., et al. (2001). Opioids for the palliation of breathlessness in terminal illness. *The Cochrane Database Systematic Review, 4,* CD002066.

Lareau, S. C., Carrieri-Kohlman, V., Janson-Bjerklie, S., & Roos, P. J. (1994). Development and testing of the Pulmonary Functional Status and Dyspnea Questionnaire (PFSDQ). *Heart and Lung, 23,* 242–250.

Lareau, S., Kohlman-Carrieri, V., Janson-Bjerklie, S., & Roos, P. J. (1986). Functional levels and dyspnea in patients with COPD. *American Review of Respiratory Disease, 133,* 163A.

Levy, M. (1997). *Symptom control in advanced cancer.* Australia: Pharmacia & Upjohn.

Levy, M. (1999, October). *Sedation in palliative care: Walking an ever-fine line.* Paper presented at 1999 Annual Conference New Hampshire Cancer Pain Initiative and New Hampshire Hospice Organization, Portsmouth, NH.

Lipman, A. G. (2000). Evidence-based palliative care. In A. G. Lipman, K. D. Jackson, & L. S. Tyler (Eds.). *Evidence-based symptom control in palliative care* (pp. 1–9). New York: Haworth Press.

Mahler, D. A., Weinberg, D. H., Wells, C. R., & Feinstein, A. R. (1984). The measurement of dyspnea: Contents, inter-observer agreement, and physiologic correlates of two new clinical indexes. *Chest, 85,* 751–758.

March, P. A. (1998). Terminal restlessness. *American Journal of Hospice and Palliative Care, 15*(1), 51–53.

McMillan, S. C. (1996a). Quality of life of primary caregivers of hospice patients with cancer. *Cancer Practice, 4,* 191–198.

McMillan, S. C. (1996b). The quality of life of patients with cancer receiving hospice care. *Oncology Nursing Forum, 23,* 1221–1228.

McMillan, S. C., & Mahon, M. (1994a). Measuring quality of life in hospice patients using a newly developed Hospice Quality of Life Index. *Quality of Life Research, 3,* 437–447.

McMillan, S. C., & Mahon, M. (1994b). The impact of hospice services on the quality of life of primary caregivers. *Oncology Nursing Forum, 21,* 1189–1195.

Meares, C. J. (1994, May/June). Terminal dehydration: A review. *American Journal of Hospice and Palliative Care,* 10–14.

Meares, C. J. (1995). *The Dinnerhour and other losses: Caring for a hospice patient who ceased nutrition.* (Doctoral dissertation, Boston College, 1995). *Dissertation Abstracts International, 56,* 5420.

Morita, T., Tsunoda, J., Inoue, S., & Chihara, S. (1999). Perceptions and decision-making on rehydration of terminally ill cancer patients and family members. *American Journal of Hospice and Palliative Care, 16,* 509–516.

Musgrave, C. F. (1990). Terminal dehydration: To give or not to give intravenous fluids. *Cancer Nursing, 13*(1), 62–66.

Noyes, R., Holt, C. S., & Massie, M. J. (1998). Anxiety disorders. In J. C. Holland (Ed.), *Psycho-oncology* (pp. 548–563). New York: Oxford University Press.

Paice, J. (1999). Pain. In C. H. Yarbro, M. M. Frogge, & M. Goodman (Eds.), *Cancer symptom management* (2nd ed., pp. 118–147). Boston: Jones and Bartlett.

Petrin, R. (1998). The symptom relief kit for hospice patients. *International Journal of Pharmaceutical Compounding, 2,* 116–117.

Printz, D. (1992). Terminal dehydration, a compassionate treatment. *Archives of Internal Medicine, 152,* 697–700.

Sjögren, P., Jonsson, T., Jensen, N., Drenck, N., & Jensen, T. (1993). Hyperalgesia and myoclonus in terminal cancer patients treated with continuous intravenous morphine. *Pain, 55*(1), 93–97.

Stoller, J., Ferranti, R., & Feinstein, A. (1986). Further specification and evaluation of a new index for dyspnea. *American Review of Respiratory Disease, 134,* 129–134.

Tyler, L. (2000). Dyspnea in palliative care patients. In A. G. Lipman, K. Jackson, & L. Tyler (Eds.), *Evidence-based symptom control in palliative care* (pp. 109–127). Binghamton, NY: Pharmaceutical Products Press.

Tyler, L., & Lipman, A. (2000). Fatigue in palliative care patients. In A. G. Lipman, K. Jackson, & L. Tyler (Eds.), *Evidence based symptom control in palliative care* (pp. 129–141). Binghamton, NY: Pharmaceutical Products Press.

Waller, A., & Caroline, N. L. (1996). *Handbook of palliative care in cancer.* Newton, MA: Butterworth-Heinemann.

Weitzner, M. A., Moody, L. N., & McMillan, S. C. (1997). Symptom management issues in hospice care. *American Journal of Hospice and Palliative Care, 14,* 190–195.

Zerwekh, J. V. (1983, January). The dehydration question. *Nursing,* 47–51.

12

Pain Assessment and Pharmacological Interventions

Nessa Coyle and Mary Layman-Goldstein

Nessa Coyle and Mary Layman-Goldstein

AACN Competency

2: Promote the provision of comfort care to the dying as an active, desirable, and important skill, and an integral component of nursing care.

Few things are of more concern to patients at end of life and to their families than that pain will be well controlled (Ferrell & Whiteman, 2003; Foley, 1991; Ng & von Gunten, 1998). In the words of one patient, "It is not dying that I'm afraid of, but how to get from A to D—alive to dead. I don't want to suffer." Unrelieved pain can consume the attention and energy of those who are dying, and create an atmosphere of impotency and despair in their families and caretakers (Chang, Hwang, Feuerman, & Kasimis, 2000; Coyle, 2004; Hwang, Chang, & Kasimis, 2002). The fear of unrelieved pain expressed by patients and their families is sadly often reflective of what they have or will experience (Coyle, 2004; Lynn, Teno, Phillips, Wu, & Desbiens, 1997; SUPPORT, 1995; Von Roenn, Cleeland, Gonin, Hatfield, & Pandya, 1993). And yet, with the knowledge and art that is now available, we have the ability to relieve the majority of pain including pain at the end of life.

The intent of this chapter is to provide nurses with a basic overview of the principles of pain assessment and pharmacological management at end of life. The needs of special populations who have been identified as "at risk" for inadequate pain control are highlighted including those who are elderly, those who are communication impaired, those with a history of substance abuse, and children. Chapter 13 addresses integration of nondrug interventions into a comprehensive pain management plan.

SECTION 1: PAIN ASSESSMENT AND PHARMACOLOGICAL INTERVENTIONS

The prevalence of pain in those with advanced illness varies by diagnosis and other factors. Pain in the cancer population is highly prevalent, has been widely studied, and is therefore a useful model from which to review pain assessment and management at the end of life. Cancer is the second leading cause of death in the United States after heart disease (American Cancer Society, 2004), and is frequently associated with significant pain at end of life (Chang et al., 2000; Meuser et al., 2001; Morita, Ichiki, Tsunoda, Inoue, & Chihara, 1998; Wells, 2000). The assessment and management of cancer pain will therefore be used as the framework for this chapter. It is recognized that pain associated with a terminal disease may be superimposed on many other chronic pain syndromes, including musculoskeletal pain such as osteoarthritis and low back pain. The principles outlined in this chapter can be applied to any pain situation.

Barriers

Numerous clinician-related, institutional-related, and patient- and family-related barriers have been identified that consistently interfere with adequate pain management.

Clinician related barriers include inadequate knowledge of pain management, incomplete assessment of pain, concern about regulation of controlled substances, fear of causing patient addiction, concern about analgesic side effects, and concern that if strong opioids are used "too early" they will be ineffective later when the need is greatest. In addition, a failure of clinicians to evaluate or appreciate the severity of the pain problem and to appreciate the impact of pain on the patient's day-to-day existence is likely to be a major predictor of inadequacy of relief (Lasch et al., 2002; O'Brien, Dalton, Konsler, & Carlson, 1996; Von Roenn et al., 1993; Weinstein et al., 2000).

Institutional-related barriers include lack of visibility of pain, lack of a common language to describe pain, lack of commitment to pain management as a priority, and failure to use validated pain measurement tools in clinical practice (Bookbinder et al., 1995; Foley, 1998). Economic factors and drug availability are further impediments to adequate pain treatment, especially in underserved and minority communities and when pain is to be managed in the home (Anderson et al., 2002; Foley, 1998; Joranson, Cleeland, & Weisman, 1992; Morrison, Wallenstein, Natale, Senzel, & Huang, 2000).

Patient-related barriers have many similarities to clinician-related barriers and include reluctance to report pain, reluctance to follow treatment recommendations, fears of tolerance and addiction, concern about treatment-related side effects, fears regarding disease progression, and belief that pain is an inevitable part of cancer and must be accepted (Anderson et al., 2000; Gunnarsdottir, Donovan, Serlin, Voge, & Ward, 2002; Paice, Toy, & Shott, 1998; Potter, Wiseman, Dunn, & Boyle, 2003; Ward, Berry, & Misiewicz, 1996). In evaluating these patient-related barriers, Ward and colleagues (1993) found that a higher level of concern was associated with those who were elderly, less educated, and had lower incomes, and was correlated with undermedication of pain.

Family related barriers to pain management at end of life are extremely important to understand (Berry & Ward, 1995; Keefe et al., 2003; Ward et al., 1996). Frequently, it is a family member who is the primary care provider in the home and it is a family member who will be assessing pain and administering the pain medications. An early small descriptive study investigated the experience of managing pain at home from the perspectives of the patient, the primary family caregiver, and the home-care nurse, and it encapsulated many of the important areas that still affect pain management in the home (Taylor, Ferrell, Grant, & Cheyney, 1993). Areas of decision making and conflict mainly centered around the use of medications. Patients were preoccupied with decisions about which pain medication to take and how much of it to take. Negative side effects and meaning in regard to these medications contributed to conflicts in the patient's mind as to whether they were doing the "right thing" in taking the pain medication. Nearly all the patients assumed their pain would increase with impending death. Patient decisions about how to live with and cope with their pain included considerations of how what they did and said affected their health care professionals and family members. Sometimes these factors led the patients to deny the pain (Taylor et al., 1993). Similarly, the decisions and conflicts that arose most frequently for family caregivers also related to pain medication and having to make decisions about which pill to give and when. Compounding these decisions were the concerns related to overdosing, adverse side effects, and addiction.

A variety of approaches and specific programs have been developed to address all of these barriers, for example, making pain visible within an institution by incorporating a pain measurement tool into institutional daily clinical practice and making pain the fifth vital sign (Figure 12.1); and introducing broad educational efforts to change attitudes, behaviors, and knowledge deficits in patients, clinicians, and institutions (Bookbinder et al., 1995). The use of continuous quality improvement (CQI) programs also has been

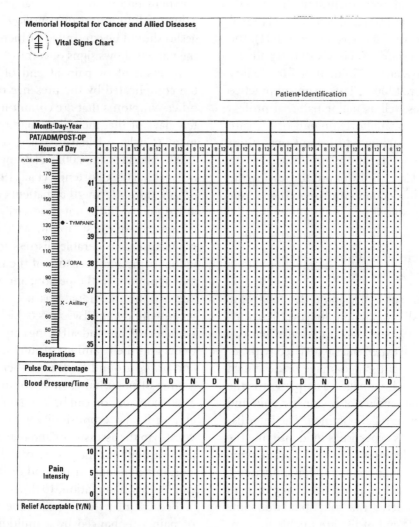

FIGURE 12.1   Pain as the fifth vital sign.

From Bookbinder, M., et al. (1995). Improving pain management practices. In D. B. McGuire, C. H. Yarbro, & B. R. Ferrell (Eds.), *Cancer pain management* (2nd ed., p. 347). Boston: Jones and Bartlett. (Reprinted with permission.)

demonstrated to be effective in providing the framework for initiatives for change (Book-binder et al., 1995). The Joint Commission on Accreditation of Healthcare Organizations (JCAHO) standards on pain management has been helpful in making institutions accountable for assessment and management of pain across care settings (Berry & Dahl, 2000; Cohen et al., 2003). In addition, a variety of professional organizations have developed clinical practice guidelines for the assessment and management of pain including the American Pain Society (APS, 2003), the National Comprehensive Cancer Network (2004), the American Geriatric Society (2002), and the National Consensus Guidelines for Quality Palliative Care (2004). These clinical practice guidelines, as well as major national professional educational efforts on end-of-life care (End of Life Nursing Education Consortium [ELNEC] and Education for Physicians on End of Life Care [EPEC]) are addressing the problem of inadequate control of pain in palliative and hospice care.

Basic Principles of Pain Assessment at the End of Life

Pain is always subjective and is defined by the International Association for the Study of Pain (IASP, 1979) as "an unpleasant sensory and emotional experience associated with actual or potential tissue damage or described in terms of such damage." The patient is the expert on the severity of his or her pain and the adequacy of relief obtained. The interdisciplinary team's expertise is in identifying the different etiologies of the pain and arriving at effective management strategies. Although verbal report of pain and adequacy of pain relief is considered the gold standard, some individuals at end of life are unable to communicate verbally (APS, 2003; Twycross & Lichter, 1998). Other behavioral measures for

assessing pain are therefore required (Herr, 2004; Taylor & Herr, 2003). For example, patients who are semiconscious or in a coma may moan or cry out or exhibit other signs of distress when moved. Although these behaviors are not necessarily associated with pain, the likelihood of pain should be strongly considered. If the decision is made to medicate the patient for pain, subsequent signs of diminished distress on movement would indicate that pain had been present. If such a patient had been on an analgesic regimen prior to diminution of consciousness, analgesics should be continued or increased until the patient shows signs of comfort.

Assessment of pain at end of life is often complicated by the presence of multiple other symptoms that are common in the last few days of life, including cognitive impairment (Coyle, Adelhardt, Foley, & Portenoy, 1990; Miaskowski, 2002; National Institute of Health, 2002; Portenoy et al., 1994). In addition, the suffering that patients experience at the end of life is not necessarily related to the severity of the symptom. Mild symptoms may cause considerable distress to the individual sometimes because of the meaning of that symptom to the person, and sometimes because the individual has not yet come to terms with dying (Twycross & Lichter, 1998). Unrelieved pain and suffering can deprive patients and their families of interaction at the end of life around anything other than pain. A time of potential growth, communication, and reconciliation can be lost. Nurses have an extraordinary responsibility to be patient advocates in the assessment and management of pain throughout the course of a disease process, but especially at the end of life (American Nurses' Association, 1990).

Because of its complexity, the assessment of pain is enhanced by a multidimensional and interdisciplinary approach (Ingham & Coyle, 1997). The tissue damage response leading to the complaint of pain, the suffering component of the pain, and the meaning of the pain to the individuals and their families all need to be addressed. Although this comprehensive pain assessment is usually interdisciplinary, it is the nurse who brings that assessment and plan to the bedside. The assessment of pain is carried out within the framework of goals of care, patient and family values, knowledge of the disease process, and nearness of the individual to death.

Types of Pain—Neurophysiological Mechanisms of Pain

Two major types of pain, *nociceptive pain* (which includes somatic and visceral pain) and *neuropathic pain,* have been described in the cancer patient (Payne & Gonzales, 2004). *Somatic* pain occurs as a result of activating pain sensitive structures, or nociceptors, in the cutaneous and deep musculoskeletal tissues. This pain is typically well localized and may be felt in the superficial cutaneous or deeper musculoskeletal structures. Examples of somatic pain include bone metastases, postsurgical incisional pain, and pain accompanying myofascial or musculoskeletal inflammation or spasm (Payne & Gonzales, 2004). Somatic pain is responsive to the nonsteroidal anti-inflammatory drugs, the opioid drugs, and steroids.

Visceral pain results from infiltration, compression, distention, or stretching of thoracic or abdominal viscera (e.g., liver metastases or pancreatic cancer). This type of pain is poorly localized, often described as deep, squeezing, pressure, and may be associated with nausea, vomiting, and diaphoresis (especially when acute). Visceral pain is often referred to cutaneous sites that may be remote from the site of the lesion, for example, shoulder pain associated with diaphragmatic irritation. Tenderness and pain on touching the refer-ral cutaneous site may occur. Visceral pain is responsive to the nonsteroidal anti-inflammatory drugs, the opioid drugs and steroids (Payne & Gonzales, 2004).

Neuropathic pain results from injury to the peripheral or central nervous systems. In the cancer patient, neuropathic pain most commonly occurs as a consequence of the tumor compressing or infiltrating peripheral nerves, nerve roots, or the spinal cord. In addition, this type of pain may result from surgical trauma and chemical or radiation-induced injury to peripheral nerves or the spinal cord from cancer therapies. Examples of common neuropathic pain syndromes include metastatic or radiation-induced brachial or lumbosacral plexopathies, epidural spinal cord or cauda-equina compression, postherpetic neuralgia, and painful chemotherapy-induced neuropathies. Neuropathic pain is often described as having sharp, shooting, electric-shocklike qualities that are unfamiliar to the patient. It can also be described as a constant dull ache, sometimes with a pressure or viselike quality with episodic paroxysms of burning or electric-shocklike sensations. Neuropathic pain is often severe, very distressing to the patient, and sometimes difficult to control. Although partially responsive to the nonsteroidal anti-inflammatory drugs and to the opioid drugs, neuropathic pain is also responsive to adjuvant drugs such as antidepressants, anticonvulsants, steroids, local anesthetics and N-Methyl-D-receptor antagonists (NMDA) such as ketamine (Elliot & Foley, 1988; Payne & Gonzales, 2004).

Temporal Pattern of Pain

Pain can also be defined on a temporal basis, for example, acute pain and chronic pain. Patients at the end of life frequently have a combination of both acute and chronic pain

(Cherny & Portenoy, 1994b; Foley, 1998; Merskey, 1986).

Acute pain is characterized by a well-defined pattern of onset. Generally the cause of the pain can be identified and the pain may be accompanied by physiological signs of hyperactivity of the central nervous system such as a rapid pulse and elevated blood pressure. Acute pain usually has a precipitating cause, for example, small bowel obstruction, a painful dressing change, or a pathological fracture. The pain tends to be time-limited and responds to analgesic drug therapy, and where possible, treatment of the precipitating cause. Acute pain can be further subdivided into subacute pain and intermittent or episodic types (Foley, 2004). Subacute pain describes pain that comes on over several days, often with increasing intensity, and may be associated with a variety of causes such as a progressive pathological process or an analgesic regimen that has not been titrated upward to accommodate for a progressive painful disease process. Episodic pain refers to pain that occurs during defined periods of time, on a regular or irregular basis (Foley, 2004). Intermittent pain is an alternative way to describe episodic pain. Such pain may be associated with movement, dressing changes, or other activities. Because the trigger for intermittent pain often can be identified, the nurse, through appropriate use of analgesics prior to the pain-provoking event, can have a significant impact on decreasing these painful episodes for the patient. The fear of pain associated with these activities is therefore lessened for the patient.

Chronic pain differs from acute pain in its presentation. These differences are essential for the nurse to understand because patients with chronic pain are at risk to have their pain unrecognized, untreated, or undertreated. Chronic pain is defined as pain that persists for more than 3 months (Foley, 2004). Adaptation of the autonomic system occurs and the patient does not exhibit the objective signs of pain found so frequently in those with acute pain (e.g., there is no rapid pulse or elevated blood pressure). Poorly relieved chronic pain at the end of life can contribute to fatigue, depression, insomnia, general despair, withdrawal from interaction with others, and desire for death (Cherny & Coyle, 1994; Coyle, 2004; Ferrell, Rhiner, Cohen, & Grant, 1991; Foley, 1991).

Breakthrough pain is a more recent classification within the various types of pain. Breakthrough pain is defined as a transient increase in pain to greater than moderate intensity, occurring on a baseline pain of moderate intensity or less (APS, 2003; Foley, 2004; Portenoy & Hagen, 1990). Breakthrough pain has a diversity of characteristics. In some patients, for example, it is characterized by marked worsening of pain at the end of the dosing interval of regularly scheduled analgesics. In other patients, it occurs by the action of the patient or the nurse, for example, when turning or having a dressing change, and is referred to as incident pain. Patients frequently have a combination of these different types of pain; noting the patterns of pain in a particular individual is an essential component of pain assessment. Attention to such details is the essence of symptom control at the end of life. A pain diary or log, kept by the patient or family, can help identify the pattern of pain. The log can indicate, over the course of the day, the patient's rating of pain, medication taken, activity level, and any other pain relief measures tried (McCaffery & Beebe, 1989). Additional information on this intervention is included in Section 2 of this chapter.

Clinical Assessment of Pain

The previously described mechanisms of pain and types of pain that can be experienced by patients with advanced progressive disease are a useful background from which to start a clinical pain assessment. The clinical assessment is based on a process of both observation and interview. The basic principles of a pain assessment are outlined in Table 12.1. Taking a history of the pain complaint involves the following parameters:

Onset

Have the patient describe when the pain first began. Was it associated with a particular activity or known medical event? Did other symptoms accompany the onset of pain such as nausea or vomiting?

Site(s)

Ask the patient to point to the site or sites of pain. Frequently, individuals with pain have multiple sites of pain. Each site needs to be assessed as the management approach may differ depending on the etiology of the pain.

TABLE 12.1   Clinical Assessment of Pain: Basic Principles

- Believe the patient's complaint of pain. The patient is the expert on the pain being experienced. The multidisciplinary staff are the experts in determining the etiology of the pain.
- Take a careful history of the pain complaint and place it within the context of the patient's medical history and goals of care. If the patient is unable to communicate verbally, obtain a history from those most involved in the patient's care, both family and formal health care providers.
- Observe the patient for nonverbal communication regarding pain, for example, guarding, wincing, and moaning, or crying out when turned or moved.
- Recognize that the patient near the end of life may have multiple symptoms complicating pain assessment.
- Assess the characteristics of each pain, including the site, pattern of referral, what makes it better and what makes it worse, and the impact of the pain on the individual's activity of daily living and quality of life; for example, mood, sleep, movement and interaction with others.
- Clarify the temporal aspects and pattern of the patient's pain; for example, acute, chronic, baseline, intermittent, breakthrough, or incident.
- Assess the psychological state of the patient and the meaning of the pain to the patient and their family.
- Examine the site of the pain.
- Facilitate an appropriate diagnostic work-up making sure that the patient's pain is adequately managed during the work-up.
- Provide continuity of care for the patient and family during ongoing pain assessment and management.
- Assess and reassess the effectiveness of the pain management regimen both for baseline pain and breakthrough pain.
- Give a time frame where you would expect to see evidence of patient comfort after the start or adjustment of a pain management approach. If this is not evident, reassess the patient. Ongoing reassessment is essential in the setting of a complex patient with multiple symptoms.
- Assess and reassess for the presence of adverse side effects from the pain management regimen.

Quality of the Pain

Have the patient describe the quality of the pain. Word descriptors used by patients to describe their pain help the clinician to arrive at an inferred pain mechanism. This in turn influences the choice of pharmacotherapy. For example, sharp, shooting, electric-shock-like descriptions of pain, often described by the patient as "unfamiliar," suggests a neuropathic component to the pain (Elliot & Foley, 1988). Such pain may be responsive to the adjuvant drugs as well as to opioid analgesics.

Severity of the Pain

Have the patient describe the severity of the pain. It is particularly important that the nurse recognize the significance of escalating pain within the construct of that particular patient's disease process, value system, goals of care, and nearness to death. Treatment decisions take all of these factors into account. For measuring severity of the pain, a variety of tools are available for use in clinical practice. These include numerical estimates, for example, 0 indicating no pain and 10 indicating the worst pain imaginable; word descriptors such as none, mild, moderate, and severe (Wallenstein, Rogers, Kaiko, & Houde, 1986); visual analog scales where a 10-centimeter line is anchored at one end by no pain and the other end by the worst possible pain (Ahles, Blanchard, & Ruckdeschel, 1983); and happy/sad faces (Wong & Baker, 1995; Wong & Wiffen, 2002).

Although numerical estimates are the most frequently used method of assessing severity of pain and adequacy of pain relief, some patients cannot use a numerical estimate and one of the other tools may be more appropriate. It is important that the staff be consistent in using a particular assessment tool with an individual patient so that communication regarding that patient's pain management is enhanced.

Assess Pain Severity at Times of Different Activity

Pain intensity should be assessed at rest, on movement, and in relation to daily activity and the patient's analgesic schedule. Asking certain questions helps establish if the appropriate drug has been selected, dose efficacy, and if the time interval between doses for this patient is correct: "How much pain is relieved when you take the pain medication?" "How long does the relief last?" and "Are side effects present?" A more global 24-hour assessment of the adequacy of pain management in general includes asking the patient their pain scores—"right now," "at its best," "at its worst," and "on average" (Daut, Cleeland, & Flanery, 1983).

Exacerbating and Relieving Factors

Identifying factors that increase or relieve the patient's pain can be helpful in arriving at a pain diagnosis and in giving the nurse the opportunity to reinforce techniques that the patient has found useful in the past to relieve pain. A patient with cancer who reports rapidly escalating back pain with a bandlike quality that is worse when lying in bed and better when standing is considered to have cord compression until proved otherwise (Posner, 1995). Early recognition of cord compression and treatment, frequently by steroids, radiation therapy, or both, may prevent paraplegia in the last few weeks or months of a patient's life. Escalating back pain may be the only sign of the impending cord compression. To reiterate, it is imperative that the nurse who is caring for a patient at the end of life recognize the significance of escalating pain within the construct of that particular patient's disease process and goals of care.

Impact of the Pain on the Patient's Psychological State

The interface between pain and suffering has been well defined (Cherny & Coyle, 1994,

1999; Cherny & Portenoy, 1994; Coyle, 1995; Foley, 1991; Portenoy, 1991; Saunders, 1967; & Stiefel, 1993). In clinical situations, when patients are asked, "What does this pain mean to you?" and "What do you think is causing the pain?" a flood of suffering and fear is often expressed. Patients are fearful of what their dying will be like, of uncontrolled and excruciating pain, of being a burden on their family, and of being "drugged out." The same questions may be asked by the patient and family time and time again, and need to be responded to in a sensitive, accurate, and reassuring manner. Some clinicians, when meeting a patient in severe pain for the first time, ask if the pain has ever been so bad that the individual has thought of harming himself or herself. Again, the response may indicate that suicide has been considered as an option if the pain is not controlled or if things get "too bad." These are important questions for an experienced clinician to ask, so that the patient's vulnerabilities and anxieties are verbalized, suicide vulnerability factors identified, and education and support from other members of the interdisciplinary pain team including psychiatrists, psychologists, social workers, and chaplains mobilized (Cherny & Coyle, 1994; Cherney & Portenoy, 1994; Foley, 1991). All of the patient's worries and fears must be addressed if the pain is to be adequately controlled (Coyle, 2004; Paice et al., 1998; Ward et al., 1993; Weiner & Rudy, 2002).

Pain Treatment History and Responses to Previous and Current Analgesic Regimens

The patient needs to be asked very specifically about what approaches have been used to manage pain in the past—both pharmacological (including over-the-counter medication) and nonpharmacological—and how effective those approaches have been. Included should be analgesics that have been previously prescribed, dosages, time intervals, routes of administration, effects, side effects, and the reasons why a particular approach was discontinued. Fear of recurrence of previously experienced side effects (e.g., sedation, nausea, mental haziness, and constipation) may make a patient reluctant to start a new analgesic regimen. Focusing attention on their concerns and a clear explanation of how side effects will be managed if they do occur can do much to allay these fears. This is a commitment that will require close monitoring of the patient's response to therapy and a rapid response to the management of any adverse side effects should they occur.

Examine the Patient and the Site of the Pain

Examining the site of the pain and possible referral sites may help identify the source of the pain (Foley, 2004). This is always done within knowledge of the patient's disease process, extent of disease, possible referral sites of pain, and goals of care. The source of the pain may be obvious, for example, a distended abdomen associated with a full bladder, bowel obstruction or liver distention, a prior skin eruption with postherpetic neuralgia, a bony deformity or inability to use a limb due to a pathological fracture, or an open fungating infected wound. Figure 12.2 shows an example of an initial pain assessment tool.

In the advanced cancer patient, the cause of pain is frequently multifactorial requiring a multimodal approach (Ahles, Blanchard, & Ruckdeschel. 1983; Bates, 1987; Foley, 2004; McGuire, 1995). Whenever possible, within the constraints of nearness to death and goals of care, an attempt is made to treat the cause of the pain as well as the pain itself. The extent of the diagnostic workup depends on the goals of care and the likely impact of the results of the diagnostic workup on the patient's treatment plan and overall quality of life. The benefit-to-burden ratio to the patient is of uppermost concern and needs to be discussed fully with the patient and family or the patient's health care proxy (Latimer, 1991).

FORM 3.1 **Initial Pain Assessment Tool**

Date _____

Patient's Name _____ Age _____ Room _____

Diagnosis _____ Physician _____

Nurse _____

1. LOCATION: Patient or nurse mark drawing.

2. INTENSITY: Patient rates the pain. Scale used _____

   Present: _____

   Worst pain gets: _____

   Best pain gets: _____

   Acceptable level of pain: _____

3. QUALITY: (Use patient's own words, e.g., prick, ache, burn, throb, pull, sharp) _____

4. ONSET, DURATION, VARIATIONS, RHYTHMS: _____

5. MANNER OF EXPRESSING PAIN: _____

6. WHAT RELIEVES THE PAIN? _____

7. WHAT CAUSES OR INCREASES THE PAIN? _____

8. EFFECTS OF PAIN: (Note decreased function, decreased quality of life.)

   Accompanying symptoms (e.g., nausea) _____

   Sleep _____

   Appetite _____

   Physical activity _____

   Relationship with others (e.g., irritability) _____

   Emotions (e.g., anger, suicidal, crying) _____

   Concentration _____

   Other _____

9. OTHER COMMENTS: _____

10. PLAN: _____

FIGURE 12.2   Example of an initial pain assessment tool

From McCaffery, M., & Pasero, C. (1999). *Pain: Clinical Manual* (2nd ed., p. 60). St. Louis: Mosby. (Reprinted with permission.)

Components of Pain Management

Pain is a multidimensional experience that involves sensory, affective, cognitive, behavioral, and sociocultural components (McGuire, 1995) Figure 12.3. Although pharmacotherapy is the foundation of pain management, pharmacotherapy alone will not be an effective approach to pain management at the end of life. A multimodal approach is usually required including attention to the suffering and spiritual or existential component to the patient's pain (Byock, 1997; Cherny & Coyle, 1994; Coyle, 1995; Saunders, 1967; Twycross

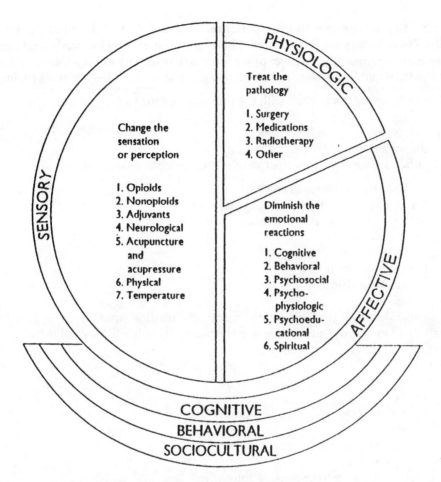

FIGURE 12.3   Multidimensional approach to pain management.

From McGuire, D. B. (1995). The multiple dimensions of cancer pain: A framework for assessment and management. In McGuire, D. B., Yarbro, C. H., & Ferrell, B. R. (Eds.), *Cancer pain management* (2nd ed., p. 12). Boston: Jones and Bartlett. (Reprinted with permission.)

& Lichter, 1998; Twycross & Wilcock, 2001). In addition, the needs of the family must be addressed (Ferrell, Ferrell, Ahn, & Tran, 1994; Ferrell, Grant, Chan, Ahn, & Ferrell, 1995). Table 12.2 illustrates factors that contribute to the concept of "total pain" at end of life and its multidimensional nature.

PHARMACOLOGICAL THERAPY

Inadequate knowledge of analgesic pharmacotherapy is one of the most commonly cited reasons for undertreatment of pain (Lasch et al., 2002; O'Brian et al., 1996; Weinstein et al., 2000). Developing expertise in the use of analgesic drugs is an integral part of nursing care at the end of life.

Over a decade ago, an expert committee convened by the cancer unit of the World Health Organization (WHO) developed a three-step "analgesic ladder" approach to the selection of drugs for the treatment of cancer pain (WHO, 1986). The basic principles of analgesic selection developed by this committee apply to pain management at the end

TABLE 12.2   Factors contributing to a patient's "Total Pain" or "Existential Distress" at end-of-life. These factors are interrelated. Their interrelatedness is dynamic and non-linear. When one factor changes it influences other factors. The impact of each factor varies from patient-to-patient and within one patient at any given time. This list is not all-inclusive:

Tissue Damage Response associated with the disease or its treatment causing pain:
    Nociceptive pain
    Neuropathic pain
    Mixed pain syndrome
    Multiple other disease related or treatment related distressing symptoms

Psychological, Spiritual and Social Distress
    Anxiety, fear and spiritual distresss associated with:
        Uncontrolled pain or other symptoms
        Perceived loss of dignity
        Loss of bodily control
        Uncertainty about the future
        Uncertainty about God
        Fear of death
        Fear of abandonment (by God, family, friends, the medical team)
        Worry about exhausting and burdening the family, friends and medical team
        Worry about how will be remembered
        Worry about finances and financially depleting the family
    Depression associated with:
        Loss of sense of "self"
        Loss of social position and role in the family
        Loss of control
        Sense of helplessness and demoralization
        Perceived loss of dignity
        Loss of meaning and purpose in continued life
        Loss of hope
    Anger associated with:
        Delays in diagnosis resulting in late diagnosis and diminished hope for a cure
        Bureaucratic bungling
        Therapeutic failures
        Insensitive communication
        Friends that don't visit

of life. Three categories of analgesic drugs are included in the three-step analgesic ladder: nonsteroidal anti-inflammatory drugs (NSAIDs), opioids, and adjuvant analgesics. With a focus on end-of-life care, discussion around these groups of drugs will include rationale for selection, dose titration, routes of administration, and side-effect management. For a more in-depth discussion of classes of medications used in pain management, the reader is referred to recent comprehensive review articles (Breitbart & Dibiase, 2002; Bruera & Kim, 2003; Foley & Gelband, 2001; Mantyh, 2002; McCaffery & Pasero, 1999a; Portenoy & Conn, 2003; Portenoy & Lesage, 1999; Ripamonti, 2003).

Nonsteroidal Anti-inflammatory Drugs

The NSAIDs include many subclasses, are frequently used in all steps of the "analgesic ladder" (McQuay & Moore, 2004), and are analgesic, antipyretic, and anti-inflammatory (APS, 2003; Rawlins, 1998). Table 12.3 shows guidelines for selection and use of NSAIDs. Aspirin is the prototype of the NSAIDs. Acetaminophen, although lacking in significant anti-inflammatory effects and with a different side-effect profile, is often classified within this group. Nonsteroidal anti-inflammatory drugs are most effective in treating mild to moderate pain when there is an inflammatory component present and are used in step 1 of the analgesic ladder. When greater relief is needed, they are continued along with the opioid drugs in steps 2 and 3 of the analgesic ladder. The NSAIDs can be extremely effective when combined with an opioid drug in treating bone pain in cancer patients; prostaglandins, which are rich in the periosteum of the bone, are implicated in pain modulation (Paice, 1999). NSAIDs interfere with prostaglandin synthesis and in this way can make a significant impact on the experience of pain. Their mechanism of action is described in more detail below. Unlike the opioid drugs, NSAIDs have a ceiling effect, that is, a dose beyond which added analgesia is not obtained (APS, 2003). These drugs do not produce tolerance or physical dependence, and are not associated with psychological dependence (addiction) (APS, 2003). This class of drugs may also have an opioid sparing effect in some patients.

Mechanism of Action

The nonsteroidal anti-inflammatory drugs impact pain perception in three ways. First, they inhibit the conversion of arachinidonic acid to prostaglandin G2 by inhibiting the enzyme cyclo-oxygenase (Jenkins & Bruera, 1999). There are two known types of cyclo-oxygenase enzymes: COX-1, which is part of normal cells, and COX-2, which is induced in the inflammatory process. Inhibition of COX-2 is responsible for the anti-inflammatory processes of the NSAIDs, whereas COX-1 inhibition is responsible for many of the side effects of the NSAIDs (Jenkins & Bruera, 1999; Rawlins, 1998). A new group of NSAIDs drugs have been developed that selectively inhibit COX-2 cyclo-oxygenase, while leaving the more protective COX-1 cyclo-oxygenase intact. However, new information regarding the relative cardiovascular risks associated with this class of NSAIDs suggests careful patient evaluation is needed prior to recommending their use.

The second way in which NSAIDs affect pain perception is through their action on the cell membranes of neutrophils to inhibit the release of inflammatory mediators. These two mechanisms reduce inflammation in tissues and thus decrease the release of substance P and pain-producing cytokines, thereby reducing nociception (Jenkins & Bruera, 1999). A third way by which the NSAIDs may have impact on pain perception is through mechanisms at the brain and spinal cord level (Yaksh, Dirig, & Malmberg, 1998).

Acetaminophen, although lacking in significant anti-inflammatory effects, is often classified with the NSAIDs. Its mechanism of action is not known (APS, 2003). Acetaminophen has fewer adverse effects than the NSAIDs. Gastrointestinal toxicity is rare, and there are no adverse effects on platelet function or cross-reactivity in patients with aspirin hypersensitivity (APS, 2003). Hepatic toxicity can occur, however, and patients with chronic alcoholism and liver disease can develop severe

TABLE 12.3   Nonsteroidal Antiinflammatory Drugs (limited number of examples) and Acetaminophen*

Drug	Maximum dose	Description	Comments
Acetaminophen (Tylenol)	4000 mg/day	Drug of choice for mild to moderate pain	Adjust dose by 50% in patients with impaired hepatic metabolism
Aspirin	4000mg/day (q4–6h dosing)	Prototype NSAID, non-selective COX enzyme inhibitor	GI, renal and CNS toxicities
Celecoxib (Celebrex)	200mg bid	Selective COX-2 inhibition. Pain and anti-inflammatory activity similar to other NSAIDs	Less gastric toxicity (use under 1-yr), less platelet inhibition. Same renal toxicities as other NSAIDs
Nabumetone (Relafen)	2000 mg qd	Partially COX-2 selective. Gastric toxicity may be less, occasionally requires q 12 h dosing	Avoid maximum doses for prolonged periods
Salsalate (Disalcid)	3000 mg qd (q6–8h dosing)	Hydrolyzed in small intestine to aspirin	Elderly may require dose adjustment downwards to avoid salicylate toxicity.
Ibuprofen (Motrin by prescription; Advil, Nuprin, and others OTC)	2400 mg qd (q6–8h dosing)	Gastric, renal, and abnormal platelet function may be dose dependent; constipation, confusion, and headaches may be more common in older persons	Avoid high doses for prolonged periods of time
Naproxen (Naprosyn by prescription; Aleve and others OTC)	1000mg qd (q8–12h dosing)	Same as ibuprofen. May require a loading dose	Dose may need downward adjustment for the elderly or frail elderly
Diflunisal (Dolobid)	1000 mg qd maximum dose. Loading = 1000mg then 500 mg q12h or 750 mg then 250mg q8h in frail elderly	Relatively good analgesic properties but requires loading dose	Dose may need downward adjustment for frail elderly

TABLE 12.3 *(continued)*

Drug	Maximum dose	Description	Comments
Ketorolac (Toradol)	Only NSAID approved for IM administration. 120mg qd (30–60mg loading dose, followed by half the loading dose, 15–30 mg q6h, limited to not more than 5 days). PO 60 mg qd (q6h dosing limited to not more than 14 days)		Substantial GI toxicity as well renal and platelet dysfunction. May precipitate renal failure in dehydrated patients. Reduce dose by half for those > 65 years of age.

Starting doses should be one half to two thirds recommended dose in the elderly, those on multiple drug or those with renal insufficiency,.

q = every; h = hour.

(Adapted from Ferrell B, Whiteman JE, Pain. IN Morrison RS, Meier DE (eds.). Geriatric Palliative Care. Oxford University Press; Oxford, 2003, p. 216 and American Pain Society, Principles of Analgesic Use in the Treatment of Acute Pain and Cancer Pain, Fifth Edition)

*This Table is to be used as a guide only and not to replace a more comprehensive review.

hepatotoxicity even when the drug is taken in usual therapeutic doses (Whitcomb & Block, 1994).

Adverse Effects and Their Management

Patients, particularly at end of life, are very susceptible to adverse side effects of pharmacotherapy. A careful balance is needed between achieving the desired effect of the selected drug for the patient and the potential for adverse effects. This is particularly important in this group of drugs. Unlike the opioids where the adverse effects are usually dose-dependent and controllable, NSAIDs have a largely "hidden" side-effects profile (Jenkins & Bruera, 1999). Although they occur in a minority of patients, these adverse effects are often "silent," not producing symptoms until a major event occurs such as gastrointestinal bleeding without prior warning. The nurse is an active participant in assessing this risk/benefit ratio for the patient and needs to become familiar with the relative side-effect profile for each of the drugs within this category. The potential adverse effects of the NSAIDs that have been described earlier (excluding acetaminophen) include those affecting the hematologic, gastrointestinal, renal, and central nervous systems. As noted earlier, the selective COX-2 inhibitors differ in their side-effect profile from other NSAIDs in relation to potential for gastric irritation and interference with platelet aggregation. However, renal adverse effects are similar and there is a growing concern about relative cardiovascular risks suggest that they should not be used with cardiac caution in "at risk" patients.

Hematologic Effects

Nonsteroidal anti-inflammatory drugs (with the exception of selective COX-2 inhibitors) inhibit platelet aggregation resulting from inhibition of prostaglandin synthetase. This results in prolonged bleeding time. Single doses of aspirin above 40 mg irreversibly inhibit platelet aggregation (normal platelet function is expressed only by those platelets produced after cessation of aspirin therapy) (Sunshine & Olsen, 1993). Consequently, aspirin may prolong bleeding for many days after administration ceases. In contrast, other NSAIDs produce reversible platelet aggregation inhibition. These drugs render the patient more susceptible to bleeding only for the period during which drug circulates in the plasma (Sunshine & Olsen, 1993).

A bleeding diathesis of any cause is a strong relative contraindication to the use of these drugs. The selective COX-2 inhibitors, however, do not interfere with platelet aggregation, and may be considered for patients at risk for hematologic adverse effects after a careful evaluation of their cardiovascular risk factors. Similar to the nonacetylated salicylates, such as choline magnesium trisalicylate, they do not change bleeding time and also may be a safer NSAID to choose in patients at risk for bleeding (Sunshine & Olson, 1993). To ractirates however, a growing body of evidence suggesting cardiac toxicities associated with COX-2 inhibitors must be taken into account when weighing the benefit burden of a drug in this class for a particular patient, especially with long-term use.

Gastrointestinal Effects

Nonsteroidal anti-inflammatory drugs can cause ulceration throughout the gastrointestinal tract, most commonly in the stomach, but also in the small and large bowel (Hawkey, 1990; Jenkins & Bruera, 1999). Overall the risk of ulceration is threefold in patients using NSAIDs (excluding the selective COX-2 inhibitors) over the general population (Jenkins & Bruera, 1999). This ulceration occurs by two mechanisms. The first is through direct irritation of the gastric mucosa. This is felt to play a minor role in gastric ulceration, and can be overcome by using enteric-coated products or a route other than oral for administration.

The second and more important mechanism is through NSAID-induced decrease in the production of cytoprotective prostaglandins. People with previous ulcer disease and older adults appear to be most at risk (Roth, 1988). Those patients with a relatively high risk for developing ulceration should be considered for the prophylactic use of gastroprotective therapy (APS, 2003; Hawkey & Yeomans, 1998). The NSAIDs should not be used concomitantly with other drugs that have the potential to cause gastric erosion (e.g., corticosteroids).

Renal Effects

In the palliative care population, the renal adverse effect of most concern is NSAID-induced renal failure. Patients at increased risk include older adults and those with congestive heart failure, chronic renal insufficiency, and cirrhosis with ascites. In addition, patients who have a decreased effective circulating volume and are dependent on prostaglandin-mediated renal vasodilation to maintain their renal blood flow are at risk (Jenkins & Bruera, 1999).

Central Nervous System Effects

Tinnitus, deafness, headache, and dizziness, which are well-known manifestations of salicylate toxicity, can also be side effects of other NSAIDs (Goodwin & Regan, 1982). The direct impact of NSAIDs on cognition at end of life has not been studied. Terminally ill patients have a high incidence of delirium, which is multifactoral (Breitbart, Bruera, Chochinov, & Lynch, 1995; Pereira, Hanson, & Bruera, 1997). The adverse effects of NSAIDs on renal function may contribute to end-of-life delirium through the mechanisms previously described.

Hypersensitivy Reactions.

Two subgroups of aspirin-sensitive patients have been reported. One subgroup develops a respiratory reaction with rhinitis, asthma, or nasal polyps. The second develops urticaria, wheals, angiodema, and hypotension (Clissold, 1986; Szczeklik, 1986). Bronchospasm with NSAIDs occurs in 8% to 20% of the population with asthma, nasal polyps, and chronic urticaria (Jenkins & Bruera, 1999). These hypersensitivities usually develop within minutes of ingestion, and almost always within an hour. Patients who are sensitive to aspirin may also develop sensitivities to the other NSAIDs. A history of aspirin intolerance is therefore a contraindication to use drugs within this category.

Principles of Administration of the NSAIDs

Drug Selection

A careful medical and pain history provides the nurse with information about potential benefits and risks for a patient about to receive an NSAID. An analgesic history should illuminate the patient's prior exposure to the NSAIDs, including frequency of administration, analgesic effects, and side effects. Information regarding the timing interval of other analgesics is important so that a prescribed NSAID regimen fits in with the patient's total analgesic plan. For example, if a patient is on an 8- or 12-hour dosing regimen of a controlled release morphine preparation, an NSAID with a similar dosing profile would

be appropriate (refer to Table 12.3). This may aid patient compliance and cut down on the feeling of having to take medication constantly.

Choice of a Starting Dose and Dose Titration

An NSAID is combined with an opioid drug in step 2 and step 3 of the analgesic ladder. Doses are often started at the lower end of the recommended scale in these medically fragile individuals who are coming to the end of their lives and are increased as needed (refer to Table 12.3). Although several weeks are needed to evaluate the efficacy of a dose, when NSAIDs are used in the treatment of grossly inflammatory conditions such as arthritis, clinical observation suggests that a shorter time period, usually a week, is adequate for pain relief in a patient with cancer pain. Pain and other symptoms should be monitored before and after starting the NSAIDs to document any improvement or adverse effects. If no benefit is seen or if adverse effects are noted, consideration should be given to discontinuing the drug or switching to an alternate NSAID, as marked variability has been noted in patients' response to different NSAIDs. Indicators of an effective response would be either a significant improvement in pain, or a significant decrease in the opioid use with a subsequent reduction in opioid-related side effects. The degree of monitoring for adverse effects from the NSAIDs should be individualized to the patient. Table 12.4 provides guidelines to the nurse for the selection and use of NSAIDs in the management of pain.

The Opioid Drugs

A clear understanding of the clinical significance of tolerance, physical dependence, and psychological dependence, as these terms relate to the use of opioid drugs, is essential if nurses are to break down the pervasive barri-

TABLE 12.4   Key points in the Selection and Use of NSAIDs in the Management of Pain

- Patients at the end-of-life are very susceptible to adverse side-effects of pharmacotherapy; therefore start low and go slow.
- Always give the patient and family written instructions about their medications that are concise and written in layman's language. Review these written instructions with the patient and family to be sure they are understood and "doable" for the patient.
- Selective-Cox-2 inhibitors differ in their side effect profile from traditional NSAID's in relation to potential for gastric irritation and interference with platelet aggregation *but renal adverse effects are similar*. There are also relative cardiovascular risks with this group of drugs.
- Avoid NSAIDs if possible in patients with gastroduodenopathy, bleeding diathesis, renal insufficiency, hypertension, severe encephalopathy, and cardiac failure; avoid acetaminophen in patients with severe liver disease.
- If NSAIDs strongly indicated in patients with relative contraindications (except severe liver disease) consider acetomenophen; if anti-inflammatory effects are wanted consider gastroprotective therapy, or choline magnesium trisalicylate.
- Consider individual differences (note prior treatment outcomes) and patient preferences.
- Be aware of available routes of administration (e.g., oral, rectal, intravenous).
- Begin with a low dose and adjust weekly if dose escalation is needed.
- Increase dose until adequate analgesia achieved, adverse effects occur, or maximum recommended dose reached.

ers that surround the use of these drugs and result in inadequate pain relief and much unnecessary suffering.

Tolerance is the phenomenon characterized by the need for increasing dose to maintain the same drug effect (APS, 2003). Usually the reason for dose escalation at the end of life occurs in the setting of increasing pain associated with progressive disease (Foley, 1993). Patients with stable disease do not usually require increasing opioid doses (Foley, 1993; Levy, 1989). This observation, integrated with the knowledge that there is no "ceiling" effect to the opioid drugs, implies the following: (1) concern about tolerance to analgesic effects should not impede the use of opioids early in the course of the disease, and (2) worsening pain in a patient on a stable dose of opioids is assumed to be evidence of disease progression until proven otherwise (Coyle & Portenoy, 1995).

Physical dependence is an altered physiologic state that occurs in patients who use opioids on a long-term basis. If the drug is stopped abruptly or an antagonist is given, the patient exhibits signs of withdrawal. Signs of opioid withdrawal include anxiety, alternating hot flashes and cold chills, salivation, rhinorrhea, diaphoresis, piloerection, nausea, vomiting, abdominal cramping, and insomnia (APS, 2003). The time frame of the withdrawal syndrome depends on the half-life of the drug. For example, abstinence from drugs with a short half-life such as morphine and hydromorphone may occur within 6 to 12 hours of stopping the drug and be most severe after 24 to 72 hours. After withdrawal of drugs with a long half-life such as methadone, the symptoms may not occur for a day or longer (Hanks, Cherny, & Fallon, 2004). Gradual reduction of the opioid dose in the physically dependent patient who no longer has pain will prevent the withdrawal syndrome (APS, 2003). Clinical experience suggests that administering 25% of the previous analgesic dose will prevent the withdrawal syndrome (Hanks et al., 2004). Patients must be closely monitored during the tapering process to be sure they are not experiencing symptoms of withdrawal.

The use of an antagonist such as naloxone in the physically dependent patient will precipitate acute withdrawal symptoms unless carefully titrated (Manfredi, Ribeiro, & Payne, 1996). If a drug overdose is suspected in a patient who has received opioids for more than a few days, a dilute solution of naloxone can be used (0.4 mg in 10 ml of normal saline solution) (APS, 2003). This may be administered in 1 ml bolus injections every 1 to 3 minutes until the patient becomes responsive. It is reiterated that the need to use naloxone to reverse opioid-induced respiratory depression at end of life is exceedingly rare (Fins, 1999).

Psychological dependence (addiction) is defined as a pattern of compulsive drug use characterized by a continued craving for an opioid, loss of control, and continued use despite harm. Clinical experience with cancer patients and limited studies suggest that addiction is extremely uncommon in patients without a history of drug abuse who are receiving opioids for pain (Passik & Portenoy, 1998; Perry & Heidrich, 1982; Porter & Jick, 1980; Schug et al., 1992). In patients who do have a history of drug abuse, the data is scant. Concerns about this outcome, however, continue to be a reason for undertreatment of pain (Cleeland, 1989; Hanks et al., 2004). In the setting of poorly relieved pain, "aberrant" drug-seeking behavior such as clock-watching requires careful nursing assessment. The term "pseudoaddiction" has been used to describe drug-seeking behavior reminiscent of addiction that occurs in the setting of inadequate pain relief and is eliminated by improved analgesia (Weissman, Burchman, Dinndorf, & Dahl, 1990). For the most part, this behavior signifies inadequate pain relief. Patients and their families need to be reassured that use of opioid drugs in the amount that is needed to control pain regardless of what that amount is, is unlikely to cause addiction if an individual does not have a history of drug abuse. In a patient who does have a history of previous drug abuse, there is minimal data in this respect; however, pain can still be well managed using this class of drug. The management of pain in patients with a history of drug abuse will be discussed in the section on special populations.

Opioids and the 3-Step Analgesic Ladder

Opioid analgesics are the mainstay of pain treatment at the end of life (WHO, 1986). These drugs are used for moderate to severe pain in step 2 and step 3 of the analgesic ladder. They are frequently used in combination with an NSAID (APS, 2003). When formulated in combination with an NSAID drug, dose escalation is limited by reaching the maximum recommended daily dose of the NSAID. When formulated as a single agent, however, there appears to be no ceiling effect (Hanks et al., 2004). Dose escalation may be limited by adverse effects such as sedation, confusion, nausea and vomiting, myoclonus, and (rarely) respiratory depression (Hanks et al., 2004). Dose escalation is governed by the balance between pain relief and intolerable and unmanageable side effects (Hanks et al., 2004). This balance can be determined only by ongoing assessment and documentation of the effects and side effects produced by the opioid.

Mechanism of Action

Opioids produce their effects through binding to receptors in the brain and spinal cord to prevent the release of neurotransmitters involved in pain transmission (Paice, 1999). Opioids also can have a peripheral site of action in the presence of inflammation (Stein, 1995). In addition, opioid receptors are present in immunocompetent cells that migrate to inflamed tissue (APS, 2003; Sibinga &

Goldstein, 1988). The opioids can be divided into agonists, agonist-antagonists, and antagonists classes based on their interactions with the receptor types. Pure opioid agonists, for example, morphine, hydromorphone, oxycontin, fentanyl, and methadone bind primarily to the mu receptors.

Partial agonists and mixed agonist-antagonists either block or remain neutral at the mu opioid receptors while activating kappa opioid receptors (Jaffe & Martin, 1990). Partial agonists, for example, butorphanol and pentazocine, have limited use in palliative care. Their pharmacology is characterized by a ceiling effect to analgesia and the ability to precipitate withdrawal symptoms in patients who are physically dependent on pure agonist drugs (e.g., morphine) (Hanks et al., 2004). The incidence of psychomimetic effects (agitation, dysphoria, confusion) from the mixed agonist-antagonist is greater than that of pure agonists (morphinelike drugs) (Hanks et al., 2004). The opioid antagonist drugs include nalaxone and naltrexone. These drugs bind to opioid receptors and block the effect of morphinelike agonists. The most commonly used opioids in end-of-life care are briefly reviewed below.

Morphine is the prototype opioid agonist. The WHO placed morphine on the essential drug list and requested that it be made available throughout the world for cancer pain relief (WHO, 1986). Morphine is available in tablet, elixir, suppository, and parenteral form. Various oral controlled-relief preparations provide analgesia with a duration of from 8 to 12 to 24 hours. Alternate routes of drug administration are available for patients who are unable to use the oral or rectal route.

Patients with severe pain are initially titrated with immediate-release morphine tablets, or if in a hospital setting with parenteral opioids, and once stabilized are converted to a controlled-release preparation. To manage breakthrough pain or incident pain, immediate-release morphine should be made available to all patients receiving controlled-release preparations. Absorption of morphine after oral administration occurs mostly in the upper small bowel. The average bioavailability for oral morphine is 20% to 30% (Gourlay, Plummer, Cherry, & Purser, 1991). This explains why there is a need to increase the patient's opioid dose when changing from the parenteral to the oral route of drug administration. In patients with normal renal function, the average plasma half-life is 2 to 3 hours, whereas the average duration of analgesia is about 4 hours (Hanks et al., 2004). Morphine-6-glucoronide (M-6-G), an active metabolite of morphine and a powerful analgesic, may accumulate in patients with impaired renal function. This accumulation may lead to signs of opioid toxicity (Portenoy, Thaler, Inturissi, Friedlander-Klar, & Coyle, 1994; Tiseo et al., 1995), which will be described later in the chapter. Morphine–3-glucuronide is also an active metabolite of morphine and may contribute to myoclonus seizures and hyperalgesia in a dying patient with marked renal impairment (Anderson et al., 2002; Smith, 2000). Because of these and other factors, the nurse must take note of the patient's renal status when administering morphine and monitor accordingly for signs of opioid toxicity.

Hydromorphone and *oxycodone* are synthetic short-half-life opioids that are a useful alternative to patients who tolerate morphine poorly. Hydromorphone is more potent than morphine and can be administered by the oral, rectal, parenteral, and intraspinal routes. The half-life of hydromorphone of 1/2 to 3 hours is slightly shorter than that of morphine, and it has an oral bioavailability of 30% to 40% (Houde, 1986). The comparative potency of the opioid drugs and bioavailability dependent on route of administration underscores the need for nurses to be competent in the use of the equianalgesic table (Table 12.5). The main metabolite of hydromorphone, H-3-glucoronide, may lead to central nervous system (CNS) toxicity including myoclonus, hyperalgesia, and seizure especially in the setting of renal failure (Fainsinger, Schoeller, Boiskin, & Bruera, 1993; Lee, Leng, & Tierman, 2001; Smith, 2000; Wright, Mather, & Smith, 2001). Personal clinical experience suggests that these adverse effects usually occur in the setting of high parenteral doses being administered by continuous infusion. Hydromorphone is no longer available in a controlled-release formulation.

Oxycodone is a synthetic opioid with a better oral absorption than morphine (Davis et al., 2003). The equianalgesic ratio to that of morphine is approximately 20–30:30. It has a half-life of 2 to 4 hours and is mainly excreted by the kidneys. Oxycodone is available in combination with aspirin (Percodan) or acetaminophen (Percocet) or as a single immediate-release or controlled-release tablet. The controlled-release tablet (Oxycontin) provides the patient with analgesia for 8 to 12 hours. Both hydromorphone and oxycodone are used in steps 2 and 3 of the analgesic ladder. Oxycodone is not available in parenteral form.

Fentanyl is a potent short-half-life opioid that is being used with increasing frequency in palliative care. Fentanyl comes in a transdermal, transmucosal, and parenteral form. In the transmucosal and parenteral form it has a rapid onset of action. The transdermal fentanyl delivery system consists of a drug reservoir in the form of a patch that is separated from the skin by a copolymer membrane that controls the rate of drug delivery to the skin surface. This approach provides the means to infuse an opioid drug continuously without the need for needles and pumps (Payne, Chandler, & Einhaus, 1995). Clinical experience with cancer patients suggests that a 100 mcg fentanyl patch is equianalgesic to 2 mg to 4 mg of parenteral morphine (Hanks et

al., 2004). Although most patients maintain satisfactory pain control with a patch change every 72 hours, some patients require the patch to be changed after 48 hours. Careful monitoring of adequacy of pain relief and evidence of end-of-dose failure will guide the nurse in the needs of the particular patient. It is important that the nurse also realize there is a lag in absorbing fentanyl through the skin. It takes 12 to 16 hours for the patient to see a substantial therapeutic effect (Hanks et al., 2004; Payne et al., 1995). Availability of a different route of drug administration is therefore necessary during the 12 to 16 hours following the initial patch placement. An alternate route of drug administration is also required for breakthrough pain medication. Significant concentrations of fentanyl remain in the plasma for about 24 hours after removal of the patch because of delayed release from the tissues and subcutaneous depots. Drug side effects (if present) may persist for that length of time. Fever, cachexia, obesity, edema, and ascites may all have significant effect on absorption predicability of blood levels and clinical effect (Menten, Desmedt, Lossignol, & Mullie, 2002; Radbruch et al., 2001).

Oral transmucosal fentanyl (OTFC) provides a useful mode of delivering a potent, short-half-life opioid to a patient who requires a potent drug with a rapid onset of action and short duration of effect for severe breakthrough pain. Oral transmucosal fentanyl citrate is recommended only to be used in patients who are opioid tolerant and who are receiving the equivalent of no less than 60 mg of oral morphine a day or transdermal fentanyl 50 mcg every 3 days. Oral transmucosal fentanyl differs from other breakthrough pain medication in that there is no relationship between the baseline dose of the patient's pain medication, and the microgram dose of OTFC required to relieve breakthrough pain (APS, 2003; Christie et

TABLE 12.5   Equianalgesic Dose Table: Relative Potencies, Half-lives, and Duration of Action of Commonly Used Opioids for Cancer Pain. Starting doses based on opioid naive elderly patient—dose titration will usually be required

Drug	Half-Life (H)	Equianalgesic Intramuscular Dose (MG)**	Intramuscular Oral Potency (MG)	Starting Oral Dose (MG)	Comment
Morphine-like Agonists					
Morphine	2–3	10	3 (repeated dose)	15–30 (q 4 h)	Standard of Comparison for opioid analgesics. Available in liquid, tablet, suppositories. Controlled-release available. M6G & M-3-G accumulation in patients with renal failure. Lower doses for the elderly.
Oxymorphone		1	—	1	Available in suppository Form as Numorphan
Hydromorphone	2–3	1.5	5	2 (q 4 h)	Useful alternative for Morphine. Active metabolite H-G-3. Available in liquid, tablet, suppositories. NO controlled release
Methadone	15–190	10***	2	2.5 (q12–8 h)	Accumulates with repetitive dosing. Available in liquid and tablet form. Monitor patient closely
Meperidine	2–3	75	4	Not recommended	CNS excitatory toxic metabolite meperidine. Contraindicated for repetitive dosing, for patients with renal failure, or receiving MAO inhibitors.

Drug					Comments
Fentanyl	4–7	—			Short half-life when used acutely. Parenteral use via infusion. Clinical experience suggests 4mg IV morphine sulfate/hr=100ug transdermal patch. Patches available to deliver 25,50,75,100 ug/hr.-Transmucosal delivery system available-200mcg-1600mcg. Only to be used in opioid tolerant patient
Oxycodone	2–3	2	5 (q 4 h)		Available in liquid or tablet preparation. Also in combination with a non-opioid. Controlled-release available.
Codeine	2–3	130	1.5	30–60	Used orally for less severe pain. Usually combined with a non-opioid–limits titration. Constipation limits usefulness
Hydrocodone	4	—	5 (q 4 h)		Usually combined with non-opioid—limits titration

*Table based on a variety of published sources including the American Pain Society, 2003; Hanks et al., 2004; Cherny & Portenoy, 1994; Coyle & Portenoy, 1995; Hewitt & Foley, 1999; & Jacox et al., 1994. This Table is to be used as a guide only and is not to replace a more comprehensive review.

**Dose that provides analgesia equivalent to 10 mg i.m. morphine. These ratios are useful guides when switching drugs or routes of administration (see text). In clinical practice, the potency of the i.m. route is considered to be identical to the IV and subcutaneous routes.

***When switching from another opioid to methadone, the potency of methadone is much greater than indicated on this table (see text). Frequently 5–10% of the equianalgesic dose is used.

al., 1998; Streisand et al., 1998). In all other opioid drugs there is a relation between the two. With OTFC, the smallest available dose is initially chosen (200 mcg) and titrated up depending on the patient's response (available strengths range from 200 to 1,600 mcg per unit).

Methadone is another useful synthetic opioid for the management of pain including pain at the end of life (De Conno, Groff, & Brunelli, 1996; Manfredi, Borsook, Chandler, & Payne, 1997). However, methadone is more difficult to administer than other morphine-like opioids because of its variable long half-life (range 13 hours to over 100 hours) (Hanks et al., 2004) and a discrepancy between drug half-life and the duration of analgesic effect (4 to 8 hours). Patients are at increased risk for drug accumulation and subsequent toxicity when treatment is initiated, the dose is increased, or multiple organ failure develops (Davis & Walsh, 2001). Patients may become confused, increasingly sedated, and progress to a respiratory arrest if not closely monitored especially during the titration period (Fainsinger, Schoeller, & Bruera, 1993; Hunt & Bruera, 1995). Because of this risk, methadone is considered a second-line drug in the treatment of pain at end of life. The risk of delayed toxicity from methadone accumulation can be significantly reduced if the initial period of dosing is accomplished with as-needed administration (Ettinger, Vitale, & Trump, 1979). When a steady state has been approached, a fixed dosing schedule of every 6 to 8 hours can be substituted for most patients, although some individuals require a shorter time interval between doses. An opioid with a short half-life such as morphine or hydromorphone is frequently used for supplementary or "rescue" dosing, although methadone can also be used.

The equianalgesic dose ratio of morphine to methadone has been a matter of controversy and confusing lack of clarity for clinicians. Early studies suggested that the ratio was 1:1 and that still appears to hold true for opioid naïve patients. However, data from more recent studies indicate that the ratio correlates with the total opioid dose administered before switching to methadone, and the ratio increases (that is methadone is more potent) as the previous dose or oral opioid increases (Moryl et al., 2002; Watanabe, Tarumi, Oneschuk, & Lawlor, 2002). For example, among patients receiving low doses of morphine before switching to methadone the ratio is approximately 4:1. In contrast, for patients receiving more than 300 mg of oral morphine the ratio is approximately 10:1 or 12:1 (Ripamonti et al., 1998).

Meperidine is rarely indicated for the management of chronic pain either at the end of life or earlier in the disease process. Meperidine has an active metabolite, normeperidine, that is twice as potent as a convulsant and half as potent as an analgesic as its parent compound (Kaiko, 1983). The half-life of normeperidine is 3 to 4 times that of meperidine, and accumulation of the metabolite with repetitive dosing can result in central nervous system excitability characterized by tremor, myoclonus, agitated delirium, and seizures (Szeto et al., 1977). Naloxone does not reverse meperidine-induced seizures and potentially could precipitate seizures by blocking the depressant effects of meperidine and allowing the convulsant effects of normeperidine to become manifest (Kaiko, 1983; Umans & Inturrisi, 1982).

Principles of Opioid Selection and Administration

Numerous factors, both patient-related and drug-related, must be considered in the selection of an appropriate opioid for a patient (Hanks et al., 2004). The opioid should be compatible with the patient's pain severity, age, dosing and route requirements, underlying illness, and metabolic state. Selection of an opioid that is available as a controlled-release formulation, such as morphine or oxycodone, may be an important consideration for some patients. For the older adult or those who have major organ dysfunction, an opioid with a short half-life, such as morphine, hydromorphone, or oxycodone, may be preferable. Patients with marked renal insufficiency must be monitored closely for signs of opioid toxicity.

The potential for additive side effects and serious toxicities from drug combinations must be recognized by the nurse each time a new drug is added to a patient's regimen (Portenoy, 1994). Patients frequently have many distressing symptoms and are receiving multiple drugs. The impact of each new drug added to the patient's regimen must be carefully weighed for benefit versus burden.

Opioid rotation

Sequential trials of opioid drugs may be needed to find the most favorable balance for the patient between pain relief and adverse effects (Galer, Coyle, & Pasternak, 1992). The patient and family should be warned that this is a possibility so that they do not become discouraged during the process. Usually if one or two side effects are present and pain control is good, an attempt is made to treat the side effects and maintain the current opioid. If more than two side effects are present (excluding constipation), opioid rotation is probably warranted. The steps followed when rotating opioids are based on the following assessment:

1. Is the pain control good but significant side effects present? If so reduce the equianalgesic dose of the new opioid by 50% (to accommodate for cross-tolerance) and continue to monitor the patient for resolution of adverse side effects and adequacy of pain control.

Frequent rescue doses should be available to the patient.

2. Is the pain control poor and are significant side effects present? If so reduce the equianalgesic dose by 25% to 50% and continue to monitor the patient closely for resolution of adverse side effects and improvement in pain control. Frequent rescue doses should be available to the patient.

3. Is the plan to convert the patient to methadone? If so, the around-the-clock equianalgesic dose of methadone should be decreased by 90%, with provision for frequent rescue doses and careful monitoring of the patient for signs of drug accumulation and toxicity, especially sedation. Because of the large inter-patient variability, in all instances when an opioid dose is decreased or the drug is changed the patient must be closely monitored for adequacy of pain relief or presence of adverse side effects (Hanks et al., 2004).

This monitoring is a critical nursing function.

Choice of a Starting Dose and Dose Titration

A patient who is relatively opioid-naive should generally begin treatment at an opioid dose equivalent to 5 mg to 10 mg of parenteral morphine every 4 hours (Cherny & Portenoy, 1994a,b). Titration of the opioid dose is usually necessary at the start of pain therapy and at different points during the disease course. At all times, inadequate relief should be addressed with dose escalation until relief is reported or until intolerable and unmanageable side effects occur. Integration of around-the-clock (ATC) dosing with supplemental rescue doses provides a rational stepwise approach to dose escalation and is appropriate to all routes of drug administration. Patients who require more than four to six rescue doses

TABLE 12.6   Principles of Opioid Use in the Management of Pain

- Patients at the end-of-life are very susceptible to adverse side-effects of pharmacotherapy; therefore start low and go slow.
- Always give the patient and family written instructions about their medications that are concise and written in layman's language. Review these written instructions with the patient and family to be sure they are understood and "doable" for the patient.
- Select a drug from step 2 or step 3 of the analgesic ladder appropriate to the patient's level of pain and analgesic history.
- Take into consideration patient's age, metabolic state, presence of major organ failure (renal, hepatic, or respiratory), and presence of coexisting disease.
- Consider pharmacologic issues (e.g., potential accumulation of active metabolites, effects of concurrent drugs, and possible drug interactions).
- Know the drug class (e.g., agonist, agonist/antagonist), duration of analgesic effects, and pharmacokinetic properties.
- Be knowledgeable about the various drug formulations (e.g., controlled release, immediate release, liquid transmucosal).
- Be aware of the available routes of administration (e.g., oral, rectal, transdermal, transmucosal, subcutaneous, intravenous, epidural) and equianalgesic dosages among drugs and between routes.
- Select the least invasive route appropriate to the patient's needs.
- Consider issues in patient compliance (e.g., convenience, ease for home management, and cost).
- Administer the analgesic on a regular basis. Make sure that supplemental or "rescue" doses are available.
- Titrate to achieve a favorable balance between good pain relief and minimal adverse side effects.
- Use drug combinations, if appropriate to provide added analgesia (e.g., NSAIDs and adjuvants).
- Avoid drug combinations that increase sedation without enhancing analgesia.
- Anticipate and treat side effects.
- If one or two side effects present treat the side effects and continue on the current opioid. If more than two adverse side effects (excluding constipation) consider opioid rotation.
- Prevent precipitating an acute withdrawal syndrome in the patient who is physically dependent on an opioid drug (e.g., taper opioids if a patient has a neuroablative procedure and is pain free; do not abruptly stop the opioid).
- Systematically evaluate effectiveness of analgesic regimen (e.g., amount of relief, duration of relief, frequency of breakthrough pain, frequency and pattern of "rescue" use, presence of adverse effects, and satisfaction with mode of therapy).
- Teach the patient and family the principles of analgesic therapy. Address their fears about addiction and tolerance.

per day should generally undergo escalation of the baseline dose. In all cases, escalation of the baseline dose should be accompanied by a proportional increase in the rescue dose so that the size of the supplemental dose remains a constant percentage of the fixed dose. Nursing assessment of the patient's pattern of pain, rescue use, and level of pain relief is essential for appropriate dose titration. Table 12.6 summarizes the basic principles in the use of opioid drugs to manage pain.

Selecting a Route

Opioids should be administered by the least invasive and safest route capable of producing adequate analgesia. Clinical experience indicates that the majority of patients can use the oral route of drug administration throughout the course of most of their disease. However, at times some patients become unable to use this route and require an alternate approach (Coyle et al., 1990; Foley, 2004). Nurses need to be skilled in selecting among the alternate routes to meet the needs of a particular patient. The most commonly used alternate routes include rectal, sublingual, transmucosal, transdermal, subcutaneous, intravenous, epidural, and intrathecal.

A switch in route of opioid administration requires that the nurse have knowledge of relative potencies, to avoid overdosing or underdosing (refer to Table 12.5). These times of transition from one drug or route to another place patients at risk for pain escalation or the development of adverse effects. Frequent assessment is therefore required during the transition period. The equianalgesic dose table provides a guide to dose selection when these changes are made. The calculated equianalgesic dose is usually reduced 25% to 50% when switching drugs to account for incomplete cross-tolerance. As noted previously, a much larger reduction (sometimes as much as 80 to 90%) is necessary when switching to methadone.

Dosing Interval

Patients with continuous or frequently occurring pain generally benefit from scheduled around-the-clock (ATC) dosing. This provides a more stable plasma level of the drug and helps prevent pain from recurring. A rescue dose is offered on a PRN basis and provides a means to treat pain that breaks through the fixed analgesic schedule. The drug used for breakthrough pain is usually the same as that administered on a regular basis. An alternative short-half-life drug is recommended when using methadone or transdermal fentanyl (Hanks et al., 2004). However, some clinicians prefer to use methadone as the rescue drug if a patient is already on methadone. Clinical experience suggests that the rescue dose should be calculated as about 25% to 50% of the hourly dose, or 5% to 15% of the 24-hour baseline dose (Hanks et al., 2004; Jacox et al., 1994). For example, a patient receiving 60 mg of a controlled-release oral morphine preparation every 12 hours should have a rescue or supplemental dose of 10 to 15 mg of immediate-release morphine available on a 1- to 2-hour basis.

Patient-Controlled Analgesia

Patient-controlled analgesia (PCA) in the palliative care arena is a method that refers to parenteral drug administration in which the patient controls a pump that delivers analgesics according to parameters set by the nurse or physician. These parameters include concentration of the drug, basal infusion rate, and bolus dose with permitted intervals between doses for breakthrough pain. Use of a PCA device is fairly common in palliative care patients who require a parenteral route of drug administration. This technique can be managed safely at home for most patients, providing a system of education, monitoring, and support is in place (Coyle, Cherny, & Portenoy, 1994).

Opioid Side-Effects and Their Management

Constipation

Constipation in the palliative care setting is common and usually multifactorial (Bruera et al., 1994; Hanks et al., 2004; Portenoy, 1994; Walsh, 1990). It is the most frequently encountered side effect experienced during opioid therapy and the one to which patients rarely develop tolerance. Opioid binding to peripheral receptors in the gut prolongs colon transit time by increasing or decreasing segmental contractions and decreasing propulsive peristalsis (Sykes, 1996). Because the likelihood of constipation is so great in palliative care patients who are receiving opioid therapy, laxative medications should be prescribed in a preemptive manner (Walsh, 1990). Table 12.7 outlines a nursing approach to the assessment and management of constipation for patients receiving chronic

---

TABLE 12.7   Guidelines in Assessment and Management of Constipation in the Patient Receiving Chronic Opioid Therapy

Anticipate that a daily bowel regimen will be needed by all patients' receiving ATC opioid therapy for pain. Implement a preemptive bowel regimen.

- Identify patient's present bowel pattern and how it varies from their norm.
- Identify factors that may be contributing to this patient's constipation for example:
  - Potentially constipating drugs in addition to the opioids (e.g., antidepressants).
  - Decreased mobility associated with generalized weakness.
  - Inability to get to the toilet because of weakness or neurological impairment so has to use a bedpan.
  - Lack of privacy when toileting.
  - Dehydration, fever.
  - Metabolic abnormalities (e.g., hypercalcium, hypokalemia).
  - Lack of bulk and fiber in diet.
- Address those factors that may be amenable to change in this particular patient.
- Disimpact patient if necessary (give analgesic rescue dose beforehand).
- Establish a bowel-management program appropriate to the patient.
- Consider combination of stool softener with drug that increases peristalsis as a first-line management approach (e.g., ducusate plus senna).
  - Use bulk agent to supplement fiber in the diet if appropriate; avoid in severely debilitated patients and those with partial bowel obstruction. May increase flatulence, distention, bloating, and abdominal pain in patients with intra abdominal disease.
  - Have "backup" agents available for episodes of refractory constipation (e.g., lactulose, magnesium citrate, rectal suppositories, enema).
- In patients with persistent refractory constipation consider:
  - A prokinetic agent to improve colonic transit (e.g., metoclopramide).
  - Oral administration of Naloxone to produce "bowel withdrawal" without concurrent systemic withdrawal. Treatment with oral Naloxone should always incorporate dose escalation (e.g., starting at a dose of 0.8 mg daily [0.4 mg BID], and doubling the dose every 2 to 3 days until a favorable response or any signs of systemic withdrawal occur).

opioid therapy. In cases of refractory opioid-induced constipation, naloxone—an opioid antagonist with an oral bioavailability of only 3%—can be given orally to produce "bowel withdrawal" through local action on opioid receptors in the gut without causing systemic opioid withdrawal. Because of individual variability, however, patients in whom this therapy is tried must be watched for symptoms of withdrawal (Sykes, 1996; Yuan et al., 1997). Treatment should always start with a low dose such as 1mg mg by mouth once or twice daily, followed by dose escalation every few days. Clinical experience suggests doses such as 12 mg to 14 mg by mouth may be needed to reverse opioid-induced constipation.

Sedation

Some level of sedation is experienced by many patients at the initiation of opioid therapy and during significant dose escalation. Patients usually develop tolerance to this effect in days to weeks (Bruera, Macmillan, & MacDonald, 1989; Bruera, Miller, McCallion, Macmillan, & Hanson, 1992; Hanks et al., 2004; Portenoy, 1994). Should sedation persist, at a level that is unacceptable to the patient, a careful assessment by the nurse is needed. Confounding factors such as other sedating drugs, metabolic disturbances, sleep deprivation, and the somnolence that may occur at end of life must be identified. Nursing evaluation and management of persistent unwanted sedation in patients receiving opioid therapy is outlined in Table 12.8. Management steps include elimination of nonessential drugs with central nervous system depressant effects, reduction of the opioid dose if feasible, changing to an alternate opioid drug, and if necessary adding a psychostimulant such as modafinil or methylphenidate (Portenoy, 1994; Webster, Andrews, & Stoddard, 2003).

TABLE 12.8   Guidelines in Assessment and Management of Persistent Sedation in the Patient Receiving Chronic Opioid Therapy

- Evaluate potential disease or treatment-related causes for the patient's persistent sedation, including: drugs other than opioids, metabolic abnormalities, sleep deprivation, and closeness to death.
- Evaluate the level of sedation within goals of care for patient, and whether sedation is troublesome to the patient.
- Evaluate if analgesia is satisfactory.
- If level of sedation is unacceptable to the patient:
  - Eliminate nonessential CNS depressant medication.
  - If analgesia is satisfactory, reduce current opioid dose by 25%.
  - If analgesia is unsatisfactory, or dose reduction is not viable, consider rotating to an alternate opioid (see p. 34 of the text), especially if current opioid is one with a long half-life such as Methadone.
  - Consider addition of a NSAID or adjuvant analgesic that may allow reduction in opioid use with compromise to analgesia.
- If sedation persists:
  - Consider addition of a psychostimulant (e.g., caffeine, methylphenidate, modafinil, dextroamphetamine).
  - Consider change to an epidural route to allow dose reduction.
  - Consider use of an anesthetic approach.

TABLE 12.9   Guidelines in Assessment and Management of Confusion in the Patient Receiving Chronic Opioid Therapy

- Establish whether the patient's confusion is long-standing or acute in onset. Identify the pattern (constant, intermittent, worse in the evening and at night).
- Evaluate potential disease or treatment-related causes for the patient's confusion. Treat underlying cause whenever possible.
- Recognize the prevalence of end of life delirium.
- Remember that opioids alone rarely cause persistent confusion.
- Review patient's drug therapy. Eliminate nonessential centrally acting medication.
- If analgesia is satisfactory, reduce opioids by 25%; reassess.
- If analgesia is unsatisfactory or confusion persists, consider switching to an alternate opioid. Select an opioid with a short half-life.
- Consider a trial of a neuroleptic (e.g., haloperidol).
- If opioids are considered to be a major contributing factor, and opioid rotation is not effective, consider use of an anesthetic approach to allow for opioid reduction.

Confusion

Like sedation, mild cognitive impairment is common after initiation of opioid therapy (Bruera et al., 1989, 1992; Portenoy, 1994). Patients may express this as feeling "mentally hazy" or "not as sharp as before." Patients should be reassured that these effects are transient in most individuals and last from a few days to a week or two. Persistent confusion attributable to opioids alone is uncommon. More commonly, confusion in patients at the end of life is multifactorial including electrolyte disorders, neoplastic involvement of the CNS, sepsis, vital organ failure, and hypoxia (de Stoutz, Bruera, & Suarez-Almazor, 1995; Portenoy, 1994). Table 12.9 guides the nurse in the evaluation and management of persistent confusion in palliative care patients receiving opioid therapy.

Nausea and Vomiting

Nausea and vomiting are not uncommon at the start of opioid therapy (Hanks et al., 2004; Portenoy, 1994). Tolerance to this effect typically develops within days to weeks. Both peripheral and central mechanisms are

thought to be involved. Opioids stimulate the medullary chemoreceptor trigger zone and increase vestibular sensitivity. Direct effects on the gastrointestinal tract include increased gastric antral tone, diminished motility, and delayed gastric emptying (Hanks et al., 2004; Portenoy, 1994). Constipation may also be a contributing factor. Establishing the pattern of nausea may clarify the etiology of the symptom and guide management approaches. Frequently, a combination of cognitive and pharmacological approaches are used, depending on the pattern of the nausea and assumed underlying mechanism. Cognitive techniques might include relaxation training with focused breathing, guided imagery, and distraction (Fishman, 1991). For nausea associated with early satiation and bloating, metoclopramide is often the initial pharmacologic approach. If vertigo or movement-induced nausea are the predominant features, the patient may benefit from an antivertiginous drug such as scopolamine (transdermal) or meclazine. Scopolamine may cause confusion in the patient who is elderly or frail and so must be watched. Other options include trials of alternative opioids, treatment with an antihistamine (e.g., hydroxyzine or diphenhydramine), neuroleptic (e.g., haloperidol or chlorpromazine), benzodiazepine (e.g., lorazepam), or a steroid (e.g., dexamethasone). The role of serotonin antagonists (e.g., ondansetron) has not been established in opioid-induced nausea and vomiting.

Multifocal Myoclonus

Mild and infrequent multifocal myoclonus can occur with all opioids (Hanks et al., 2004). The effect is dose-related and the mechanism is unclear. Pronounced myoclonus is extremely distressing to the patient. The uncontrolled, abrupt, jerking movements of the patient's limbs or torso can increase already existing pain. Myoclonus can be a sign of opioid toxicity and is a reason to switch to an alternate opioid. In addition, a benzodiazepine, for example, clonazepam, can be used to treat the symptom (Twycross & Lichter, 1998).

Urinary Retention

Urinary retention can occur in patients receiving opioid drugs, especially in those who require rapid escalation of the drug, are receiving other drugs with anticholinergic effects such as the tricyclic antidepressants, or have compromised bladder function. Older men with an enlarged prostate are particularly at risk. Opioids increase smooth muscle tone and infrequently cause bladder spasm or an increase in sphincter tone, which may lead to urinary retention (Hanks et al., 2004).

Pruritus

Pruritus can occur with any opioid, is associated with histamine release, and is most commonly seen with morphine use. Fentanyl and oxymorphone may be associated with less histamine release (APS, 2003). Ondansetron has been reported to relieve opioid related pruritus (Larijani, Goldberg, & Rogers, 1996).

Respiratory Depression

Fear of respiratory depression is a frequently cited concern among medical and nursing staff when initiating opioid therapy or when rapidly increasing opioid drugs to control pain or dyspnea in a debilitated patient at the end of life. Giving sufficient opioid dosages to a patient who is dying, hypotensive, and in pain in order to control the pain is good palliative care and not euthanasia (Coyle, 1992).

Clinically significant respiratory depression is always accompanied by other signs of central nervous system (CNS) depression, such as sedation and mental clouding, and is unusual in the patient receiving chronic opioid therapy unless other contributing factors are present. Pain antagonizes CNS depression, and respiratory effects are unlikely to occur in the presence of severe pain. With repeated administration of an opioid, tolerance develops rapidly to the respiratory depressant effects of the drug (Foley, 1991). Unwarranted fears of respiratory depression should not interfere with appropriate upward titration of opioid drugs to relieve pain (APS, 2003; Brescia, Portenoy, Ryan, Drasnoff, & Gray, 1992; Lipman & Gauthier, 1997).

Occasionally, staff unfamiliar with the dying process and the altered breathing pattern that so frequently occurs at this time become concerned that continued use of opioids will hasten death, especially in the higher doses sometimes required to control pain at the end of life. The input and mentoring by a nurse who is knowledgeable in pain and palliative care will help refocus the more inexperienced staff on appropriate dosing strategies in the symptomatic dying patient.

Adjuvant Analgesia

Adjuvant analgesics are those drugs that have a primary indication other than pain but are analgesic in certain pain states (Walsh, 1990). These drugs can be used at any step of the analgesic ladder. As with the institution of any analgesic regimen, their use is based on a careful assessment of the pain, inferred pain mechanism(s), and analgesic history. Adjuvant drugs in the palliative care setting are typically used to enhance the effects of the opioid drugs, or to allow for dose reduction because of adverse opioid side effects (Lussier & Portenoy, 2004). In the palliative care setting, it is useful to classify the adjuvant anal-

TABLE 12.10   Adjuvant Analgesics for Pain and Some Opioid Related Side Effects*

Drug	Description	Comments
Tricyclic antidepressants (amitriptyline, desipramine. Nortriptyline, others	Anticholinergic effects may outweigh benefit in many older patients; desipramine or nortriptyline is a better choice than amitriptyline. Used for continuous neuropathic pain. Benefit of anti-depressant properties and aids sleep	Adjunct to other therapies for neuropathic pain. Start low and increase slowly every 2–3 days.
Anticonvulsants (e.g., gabapentin, carbamazepine)	Used for lancinating neuropathic pain	Start low and increase slowly
Local anesthetics (lidocaine, intravenous or transdermal patch, EMLA cream)	IV lidocaine associated with delirium	
Oral local anesthetics (e.g., mexiletine)	Common side effects include tremor, dizziness, paresthesias; rarely may cause blood dyscrasias and hepatic damage	Avoid use in patients pre-existing heart disease. Start low and titrate slowly. Monitor EKGs
Muscles-relaxants (baclofen, chlorzoxazone, cyclobenzaprine)	Monitor for sedation, anticholinergic effects. Abrupt withdrawal of baclofen may cause CNS irritability	Monitor for sedation and anticholinergic effects. Taper baclofen on discontinuation
Capsaicin-topical application	Substance P inhibitor. Burning sensation on application limits its acceptability to many patients. Patients may take 2–3 weeks for maximum response	Start with small doses. Can be partially removed with vegetable oil
Alpha-2 Adrenergic Agonists (e.g., Clonodine, Tizanidine)	Clonodine useful for difficult to control pain	Can be used in combination with an opioid epidurally

gesics into three broad groups: multipurpose adjuvant analgesics, adjuvant analgesics used primarily for neuropathic pain, and adjuvant analgesics used for bone pain. Table 12.10 provides a guide to the commonly used adjuvant drugs. As a general principle, low initial doses are suggested with dose titration until symptom relief is achieved.

N-methyl-D-aspartate (NMDA)
Receptor Antagonists

N-methyl-D-receptor antagonists warrant special mention because of their growing use in the management of neuropathic pain. Neuropathic pain includes a large number of diverse pain syndromes, some of which are

TABLE 12.10   *(continued)*

Drug	Description	Comments
NMDA receptor Antagonists (dextromethorphan, ketamine, amantadine)	N-Methyl-D-Aspartate antagonists ketamine potent anesthetic in higher doses	Parenteral Ketamine in lower doses useful for refractory neuropathic pain. Use with caution because of psychmimetic effects. May cause delirium. Consult with anesthesia colleagues
Corticosteroids (dexamethasone; prednisone)	Powerful anti-inflammatory, reduces edema	Useful for pain from infiltration of neural structures; bone pain, pain crisis. Higher doses used in cord compression
Neuroleptics (e.g., haloperidol)		Pain complicated by delirium, nausea. Side effects of opioids
Analeptics (e.g., methylphenidate, modafinil)	Useful to treat opioid related sedation	Methylphenidate also used as a rapid onset antidepressant. May be used in combination with a standard antidepressant while awaiting antidepressant effects
Bisphosphinates (e.g., Pamidronate)	Used for bone pain. Inhibit osteoclast activity	Monitor calcium, phosphate, magnesium and potassium blood levels
Octreotide	Reduces secretions. Useful for conservative management of bowel obstruction causing abdominal pain and nausea	

Q=every hour; h=hour.
(Adapted from Ferrell B, Whiteman JE. Pain. IN Morrison RS, Meier DE (eds). Geriatric Palliative Care. Oxford University Press: Oxford, 2003, p. 216 and American Pain Society, Principles of Analgesic Use in the Treatment of Acute Pain and Cancer Pain, Fifth Edition)

*This Table is to be used as a guide only and is not to replace a more comprehensive review.

thought to be mediated by so-called NMDA receptors in the spinal cord. N-methyl-D-aspartate receptors bind excitatory amino acids, such as glutamate, and it is likely that processes that involve the excitation of these receptors lead to neurophysiologic changes that ultimately result in pain and allodynia (when touch that is not normally experienced as painful is experienced as being extremely painful.) The NMDA receptors are also postulated to be involved in the phenomenon of opioid tolerance (Portenoy, 1998). Drugs that block the NMDA receptor such as dextromethorphan and ketamine have been shown to reduce some types of neuropathic pain and are now in clinical use (Backonja, Arndt, Gombar, Check, & Zimmerman, 1994; Eide, Jorum, Stubhang, Bremners, & Breiril, 1994; Fine, 2000; Persson, Axelsson, Hallin, & Gustafsson, 1995; Portenoy, 1998; Stannard & Porter, 1993).

A trial of parenteral ketamine, either by subcutaneous or intravenous infusion, is justified in the medically frail patient at the end of life in the setting of refractory neuropathic pain (Fine, 2000). However, ketamine can produce psychomimetic effects (delirium, nightmares, hallucinations, and dysphoria). Assessment for these symptoms prior to initiating the infusion and on an ongoing basis is necessary. As with an infusion of local anesthetics, anesthesia members of the pain and palliative care team are usually involved in decisions surrounding a ketamine infusion in palliative care. A ketamine trial can be initiated at low doses of 0.1 to 0.15 mg/kg for a brief infusion or 0.1 to 0.15 mg/kg/hr for a continuous infusion (Portenoy, 1998).

Managing a Pain Crisis

A pain crisis can be defined as pain that is severe, uncontrolled, and distressing to the patient. It may be acute in onset or may have progressed gradually in severity. A pain crisis is considered a medical and nursing care emergency for those at the end of life. At the same time the pain is being managed, the probable etiology of the pain is assessed within the framework of the previous pattern of pain, probable cause of present pain crisis, goals of care, and the most effective long-term management approaches. Refer to Table 12.11 for the pharmacological management of a pain crisis.

In patients who do not respond to opioid titration, or who develop intolerable side effects, the following adjuvants should be considered: (1) A parenteral NSAID, for example, ketorolac, for no longer than 5 days. During this period other longer-term approaches for pain relief should be considered; (2) Parenteral steroids, for example, dexamethasone, with the dose being gradually tapered down to the lowest effective dose for the patient. Anecdotal experience has shown the use of parenteral NSAIDs or steroids to be effective in a pain crisis associated with bone pain and neuropathic pain; (3) If the pain is predominantly neuropathic, intravenous lidocaine or ketamine can be helpful for some patients (Portenoy, 1998). The efficacy of a nerve block or spinal delivery system of drug administration for this particular clinical situation should be considered (Swarm, Karanikolas & Cousins, 2004). The reader is referred to Section 2 of this chapter, "Pain Management in Special Populations," for further information.

Sedation at the End of Life

A proportion of patients at the end of life will experience refractory symptoms, including pain that is not possible to control in the absence of sedation, despite the use of state-of-the-art techniques. The number of patients involved is not clear. Palliative sedation at end of life is always an option

TABLE 12.11   Guidelines to Managing a Pain Crisis-Pharmacological Approach

These are merely guidelines and do not substitute for good clinical judgment. Dose selection is influenced by the patient's age; pulmonary, renal, and cardiac status; and potential for drug interactions.

Managing a pain crisis in the home when the patient does not have access to parenteral drugs

- Evaluate the possible causes of the pain flair. Review the patients use of prescribed pain medication over the past 24-hrs. Were the prescribed doses being taken, were rescue doses being used, if not why not? Were other factors contributing to the pain flare, such as change in activity, a fall, upsetting information? Has anything changed in the home situation or dynamics?
- Instruct the patient to take two times their standard oral PRN "rescue" dose stat.
- Repeat in 1 hour if pain persists > 5–6/10 or relief is unsatisfactory for the patient and there are no limiting side effects such as excessive sedation.
- Monitor the patient closely via telephone for adequacy of pain relief and presence of side effects.
- Once the patient has achieved pain relief, adjust the ATC dose and PRN "rescues" dose to their new requirements.
- If the patient's pain is not controlled despite escalating doses of opioids, the patient must be evaluated that day by the home care nurse or hospice nurse.
- Prepare to admit the patient if that is their choice so that the pain flare can be evaluated, brought under more rapid control with parenteral drugs and the patients then be discharged home.

Managing a pain crisis in the hospital where the patient has access to parenteral drugs

- Evaluate the possible causes of the pain flair. Review the patients use of prescribed pain medication over the past 24-hrs. Were the prescribed doses being taken, were rescue doses being used, if not why not? Were other factors contributing to the pain flair, such as change in activity, a fall, upsetting information? Has anything changed in the home situation or dynamics?
- Convert the patient's rescue dose of pain medication to an IV equivalent
- Administer double that dose intravenously (give same dose subcutaneously if IV route not possible).
- Repeat same dose in 20 minutes if no relief.
- If pain persists > 6/10 with no side effects increase the IV or S/C dose by 50%
- Continue to administer a dose every 20 minutes until the patient experiences pain relief or adverse side effects
- Also consider IV adjuvants such as steroids or parenteral ketorolac (short term).
- Once the patient has achieved adequate pain relief
  - If a patient controlled analgesia (PCA) to be started, determine the total amount of opioid the patient has taken in the past 24-hours (ATC opioid + all rescue doses + all single doses given).
  - Convert into an IV dose equivalent for the past 24-hours.
  - Convert into an hourly dose for PCA basal rate—with rescue doses of 25% to 50% of the hourly basal rate allowed every 20-minutes as needed.
  - If the patient is to be maintained on the oral route—adjust the ATC dose and PRN "rescues" dose to the new patient requirements.

for these individuals. In its position paper on promotion of comfort and relief of pain in dying patients, the American Nurses Association (ANA, 1990) states unambiguously:

> Nurses should not hesitate to use full and effective doses of pain medication for the proper management of pain in the dying patient. The increasing titration of pain medication to achieve adequate symptom control, even at the expense of life thus hastening death secondarily, is ethically justified.

The principle evoked here is the principle of double effect, which distinguishes between the compelling primary therapeutic intent—to relieve suffering—and the unavoidable untoward consequences—likely diminution of consciousness and potential for accelerated death (Cherny & Coyle, 1999; Latimer, 1991). The reader is referred to chapter 6 of this book for a more comprehensive discussion on the principle of double effect. In a study of opioid doses in patients cared for in an inpatient palliative care unit, there was no correlation between the opioid doses and the timing of death (Brescia et al., 1992).

Clear documentation and communication among the team members and with the family is essential when the plan is to provide palliative sedation at end of life to ease intractable symptoms. It should reflect the goals of care, clearly stated in unambiguous terms with resuscitation status established; discussion with the patient or health care proxy with informed consent; symptom being treated and management approach selected; and end point to be achieved and monitoring parameters. Opioid or sedative drug dose escalation without clear indications should not occur. In this way, the integrity of the process is maintained.

SECTION 2: PAIN MANAGEMENT IN SPECIAL POPULATIONS

The principles discussed concerning the assessment of the patient in pain, and the use of pharmacologic interventions in the comprehensive pain management plan, can be applied to all patients. However, there are issues specific to special populations that play a role in their pain assessment and pain management plan at end of life. The Management of Cancer Pain Panel advocates for clinicians to give special attention to the assessment and treatment of pain in special populations (Jacox et al., 1994). The purpose of this section is to highlight briefly end-of-life pain-related issues in four populations as an example of some of the concerns in special populations and is not intended as a comprehensive approach. The following section will look at issues specific to the following four groups: those with a history of substance abuse, those with impaired communication, older adults, and pediatrics. These four groups were chosen because they are frequently encountered. Cultural factors and religious factors play a role in the pain management of certain groups. Sometimes there is a mismatch between the normative values of the patient and the health care provider. It is the practice setting that frequently determines which populations a nurse cares for. It is the responsibility of the nurse to know the needs and special concerns of the populations that he or she cares for most often.

Special Considerations in Those with a History of Substance Abuse

The prevalence of substance abuse (or chemical dependency) in the United States and the association between drug abuse and life-threatening diseases such as AIDS, hepatitis C, and some types of cancer make it likely that nurses caring for patients at the end of life will work with some individuals who have a history of substance abuse (Passik & Portenoy, 1998). As a group, it is very heterogeneous with very diverse clinical problems (Passik, Portenoy, & Ricketts, 1998a). It will include individuals who are living drug-free lives, those in methadone maintenance programs, and those who are currently abusing drugs (Fultz & Sonay, 1975). It is not uncommon to find individuals with addictive disease who also have a concurrent psychiatric illness such as anxiety, depression, bipolar disorder, or schizophrenia (Compton, 1999). Changes in comorbid physical and psychosocial factors, which drugs an individual has abused, and with what frequency, can further complicate issues that clinicians face (Passik et al., 1998a).

The challenge is to provide humane, high-quality care to people at the end of life who have a history of drug abuse in a society context that often views addiction from a moral or criminal perspective (Compton, 1999). The field of addiction medicine is a developing science that is based upon recent neuroscience advances that include identification of the brain mechanisms involved with addiction vulnerability and nociception (Portenoy et al., 1997). Despite this developing scientific understanding of the disease of addiction, individuals with a substance addiction are rarely cared for in an approach that draws upon this knowledge and their pain is frequently undertreated (Compton, 1999). This is true even in the area of palliative care. Recent formal involvements by experts from the fields of pain management and chemical dependency are working to remedy this problem (Portenoy et al., 1997).

The following points are helpful to keep in mind when working with dying persons who have a history of substance abuse:

- In order to maintain an objective, nonjudgmental approach, be aware of one's own reaction when asked to administer an opioid to a patient with a history of substance abuse.
- Individuals with a history of substance abuse, past or present, will be tolerant to opioids and will require higher doses of opioid to effectively treat pain than those with no history of drug abuse (Passik & Portenoy, 1998).
- Staff who may be reluctant to administer opioids in adequate amounts to relieve pain because of concerns of worsening addiction or "readdicting" contribute to the problem of undermedication (Gonzales & Coyle, 1992).
- Identify whether the individual has a far distant history of drug abuse, is in a methadone maintenance program (MMP), or is actively abusing substances (Jacox et al., 1994).
- Patients who have a far distant history of drug abuse or who are in MMP may be reluctant to take opioids because of fear of readdiction (Gonzales & Coyle, 1992).
- Patients who are actively abusing substances are the most challenging of the three groups to work with. An interdisciplinary team that emphasizes clear communication is most effective in addressing the multiple medical, psychosocial, and administrative problems present (Passik & Portenoy, 1998).
- If a patient is currently in MMP, permission must be obtained to contact the program and coordinate therapy. Some MMP providers wish to remain actively involved at the end of life, and others do not (Passik & Portenoy, 1998).
- Many MMP patients at the end of life frequently keep the methadone dose taken for addiction separate from whatever medication they take for pain control. For others, however, it may be useful to incorporate the equianalgesic

daily methadone dose into their analgesic regimen, especially for those who are unable to swallow.

- Although sometimes time-consuming, support of the patient in managing his or her addictions can help support the integrity of the individual patient and in turn help reduce their suffering (Passik & Theobald, 2000).

- Methadone may be stigmatized as an analgesic in patients who have a history of substance abuse. Patients and their families and friends may need education about the effectiveness of methadone as an analgesic.

- Providers need to be aware of the need for more frequent dosing of methadone when given for analgesia, usually at least every 6 hours (Passik et al., 1998b).

- One nurse practitioner or physician should be identified to write all analgesic orders or prescriptions. This needs to be communicated to all caring for the patient.

- Consistent documentation that shows the assessment of the four domains of functioning—pain relief, patient functioning, adverse effects, and drug-related behaviors (Passik et al., 2004)— which is important in the care of all patients receiving chronic opioid therapy is also important in working with those who have a history of substance abuse. Accurate documentation can help to allay fears about the use of opioids in those with a history of chemical dependancy and improve pain control by the use of a systematic evaluation.

- Individuals with a history of substance abuse frequently have difficulties handling stress and will need extra support at the end of life. Psychiatric symptoms and comorbidities such as anxiety, depression, and bipolar disorders are frequently encountered and are to be treated (Passik & Portenoy, 1998).

- Nondrug methods can be employed, as appropriate, in any pain management plan for dying patients, but these methods should not be used as substitutes for medications to treat pain, depression, anxiety, or other symptoms (Passik & Portenoy, 1998).

- Individuals with a history of substance abuse who want to die at home need a careful assessment of their home environment to ensure adequate pain management and safety at home.

Special Considerations in Those with Impaired Communication

Impaired communication can be caused by a language barrier where the patient's primary language is not that spoken by the nurse or caregivers. The impaired communication can also be from an organic or functional etiology. This can include sensory impairment, cognitive impairment, aphasia, and others. This impairment may or may not be a result of the life-threatening illness the patient is experiencing. Because of the difficulties that these patients have with communication, they may not report their pain in an accurate or timely fashion. This may cause their pain to be undertreated. Other factors that can impede the communication of pain is the religious or cultural background of a patient. Cultural or linguistic differences may impair adequate assessment of pain and also may inhibit the patient's willingness to accept treatment for pain (Adelhardt et al., 1995).

The American Pain Society (APS, 1999) recommends that patients who are unable to communicate and who undergo a procedure that would be painful for others are to be treated presumptively for pain. The Acute Pain Management Guidelines Panel (1992) recommends that if pain is suspected, an analgesic trial can be made to diagnose pain as well as to treat it. Terminally ill patients with pain who are unable to speak and who are known to have pain are likely to continue to have pain and should have continuing pain treatment (Levy, 1985).

In caring for dying individuals with impaired communication, the following are useful:

- Identify the communication deficit that is impeding the patient's ability to report pain and pain relief and to comply with the pain management plan.
- Obtain the appropriate pain assessment tools and place at the patient's bedside.
- If the patient and his or her caretakers do not speak the same language, identify the patient's language and identify available translators. Obtain a pain scale in the patient's language and review it with the patient and translator. It is helpful to write key words or phrases in both the patient's language and the corresponding translations in the caregiver's language (Adelhardt et al., 1995).
- Provide more frequent pain assessments if a patient is unable to ask for pain medication or does not reliably ask for pain medication.
- If the patient cannot communicate, it is useful to collaborate with the patient's family and caregivers to determine what behavioral activities may indicate pain for this patient (Adelhardt et al., 1995). These may be grimacing, pacing, restlessness, moaning, lying still, or guarding (APS, 1999).
- Document possible pain behaviors and any tools needed for pain assessment in the patient's record to assist other caregivers in providing continuity of care.
- If the patient is to die at home, issues related to impaired communication need to be addressed in the home setting (Adelhardt et al., 1995). Family members and other caregivers may need extra education and support. In some communities, it may be possible

to obtain nurses or home health aides who speak the patient's language if language barrier is an issue.

SPECIAL CONSIDERATIONS FOR OLDER ADULTS

The probability is high that the older patient will experience pain at the end of life. Pain prevalence increases significantly with age and is due to both malignant and nonmalignant causes (Hewitt & Foley, 1997). Aggressive pain management is as necessary for those who are elderly as it is for younger individuals (Jacox et al., 1994). In elderly patients, pain is frequently undertreated across all practice settings. The dying older patient may be cared for at home, in a nursing home, or in a hospital. In any setting, untreated pain can lead to loss of function and psychological complications in this vulnerable population.

Misconceptions regarding pain in the older adult can interfere with good pain management. Ferrell and Ferrell (1995) reported that common misconceptions may include the following: (a) pain is a normal or expected part of aging; (b) if individuals do not complain of pain, they must not have much pain; and (c) the side effects from opioids make them too dangerous to use with elderly people. Nurses need to reinforce that pain is not an inevitable part of aging. Pain in the older patient is to be evaluated and treated (Hewitt & Foley, 1997).

In treating pain in the older adult, it is important to be aware of the effects of age on the pharmacokinetic and pharmacodynamic responses to analgesic medications including risk of drug accumulation (Hewitt & Foley, 1997; Jacox et al., 1994). The general rule for using medications with the older adult is to "start low and go slow." In her review of the literature, Miaskowski suggests that a starting dose of one half to one third the usual adult dose is appropriate (Hill et al., 1999). The reader is referred to several thoughtful detailed texts on this and other information relevant to the care of the older patient in pain at the end of life (Coyle & Derby, in press; Ferrell, 1998; Ferrell & Ferrell, 1995; Herr & Mobily, 1991; Hewitt & Foley, 1997; Hofmann, Farnon, Javed, & Posner, 1998; Shimp, 1998). Nurses caring for dying older adult patients with pain need to be aware of the following:

- Pain assessment can be disproportionately confounded by cognitive impairment or dysfunction, memory difficulties, depression, and abuse of alcohol (Ferrell et al., 1994).
- The presence of polypharmacy, multiple diagnosis, and complex symptoms from comorbid conditions may further complicate the pain experience (Ferrell et al., 1994).
- The patient's ability to self-medicate independently and participate in the pain management plan may be affected by functional factors, such as impaired vision, impaired fine motor skills of hands, memory problems, and cognitive impairments.
- Identify the caregiver. The caregiver may be an older person, or the patient may live alone with the caregiver living elsewhere. Evaluate the ability, availability, and desire of the caregiver and of other family and friends to assist with care, administer pain medications, and participate in the pain management plan (Adelhardt et al., 1995).
- Assess the role of the dying older patient within their family and community. Because of pain or disease, they may no longer be able to function in roles they had previously performed, such as care of a spouse or family member. The nurse may wish to facilitate discussion of the redistribution of roles and responsibilities.

Special Considerations in Pediatric Patients

Until recently, the dying child with pain was not viewed as a significant problem. Children were not considered to feel pain as intensely as adults and were therefore considered not to need aggressive pain management. Fortunately, the literature on pediatric pain has expanded significantly since the 1970s and pediatric pain is viewed as a specialty in its own right. Nurses have played a significant role in this development (Eland, 1990). The nurse caring for the dying child needs to be well versed in how to manage pain in children, using a multidimensional approach with an awareness of issues specific to the pediatric population. More detailed information on assessment and management of pain in children at the end of life can be found in literature written by Berde and Sethna (2003); Field and Behrman (2003); Finley and McGrath (1998); Frager (1997); Hockenberry, Wilson, Winkelstein, and Klein (2003); Layman-Goldstein, Byrnes-Casey, and Collins (2005); Schechter, Berde, and Yaster (2003); and the World Health Organization (WHO) (1998).

The following pointers are helpful in working with the children with pain at the end of life:

- The child and family are the unit of care.
- Parents and caregivers must be incorporated into the pain management plan as part of the therapeutic alliance, which also includes the child and the health care providers (Layman-Goldstein et al., 2005; Jacox et al., 1994).
- Address family concerns regarding the risk of addiction in the medically ill child (Walco, Cassidy, & Schechter, 1994).
- Pain assessment is dependent upon the child's age and cognitive development stage (Layman-Goldstein et al., 2005).

- A child's self-report of pain is considered the most reliable and valid indicator for estimate of pain location and intensity (Jacox et al., 1994).
- It is helpful to initiate discussions about pain and to learn the individual child's word for pain (Adelhart et al., 1995).
- Developmentally appropriate tools exist to evaluate the child in pain.
- Behavioral observation is the primary assessment measure for preverbal or nonverbal children. Observed pain behaviors may include vocalizations, facial expressions, body movements, autonomic responses, or changes in daily activities, usual behaviors, appetite, or sleep (Jacox et al., 1994).
- The goal of pain management in children is to prevent as much pain as possible and to treat procedural pain aggressively (WHO, 1998).
- It is important to consider the child's age, developmental level, verbal capabilities, past experiences, cultural factors, type of pain, and context when developing a pain management plan (Layman-Goldstein et al., 2005).
- The pharmacologic management principles—by the ladder, by the clock, by the appropriate route, and by the child—are similar to those used with adults with the exception that the starting doses are determined by chronological age and body weight (milligrams or micrograms per kilogram). The child is frequently assessed and doses are titrated to effect (WHO, 1998).
- The oral route is the desired route whenever possible (Jacox et al., 1994).
- Avoid IM injections and utilize the intravenous or subcutaneous route when parenteral administration is necessary

(Miser, Moore, Greene, Gracely, & Miser, 1986).

CONCLUSIONS

The assessment and pharmacologic management of pain in patients with life-threatening, progressive illness underscores the importance of integrating assessment and treatment strategies to address the needs of the individual patient. Nurses are expected to care for those who are seriously ill and dying from the moment the nurses graduate. The delivery of optimal therapy depends on an understanding of the clinical pharmacology of the analgesic drugs and comprehensive assessment of the pain; the patient's medical condition, psychosocial state; and goals of care. Although the nurse will usually be part of an interdisciplinary team, he or she will often be the one responsible for assessing pain, administering analgesics, monitoring for adequacy of pain relief and presence of side effects, communicating with other members of the team, and ensuring continuity of pain management across care settings. These responsibilities cannot be met unless the nurse is knowledgeable in the basic principles of pain assessment and pharmacological management, and in the recognition of patients who are at risk for inadequate pain assessment and control. In addition, recognition and respectful acknowledgment of the central role the family plays in managing pain in the home at end of life has major implications for nurses in their responsibility to educate and support families in this task. In few areas does the advanced practice nurse have a greater potential to impact on quality of life for those who are dying and their families than in facilitating effective pain management.

EDUCATION PLAN 12.1   Plan for Achieving Competencies: Pain Assessment and Pharmacological Management

Knowledge Needed	Attitudes	Skills	Undergraduate Behavioral Outcomes	Graduate Behavioral Outcomes	Teaching/Learning Strategies
The significance of unrelieved pain at the end of life: —Barriers to pain management.	*Acknowledge the fear of patients and families related to unrelieved pain. *Consider students'/nurses' own personal attitudes toward pain management.		*Recognize patient, clinician, and institutional barriers that interfere with adequate pain management. *Educate patients and families regarding the significance of unrelieved pain.	*Educate patients, families, clinicians, and administration regarding the importance of effective pain management to overcome related barriers.	*In the classroom, post-conference, or seminar, ask students/nurses to reflect on a personal experience of pain and its significance to their sense of physical, emotional, social, and spiritual well-being. Compare and contrast responses. *Within the context of a clinical setting, identify patient, clinician/self, and institutional barriers that interfere with adequate pain management.

Basic principles of pain assessment at the end of life: —Definition of pain; —Need for a multidimensional and interdisciplinary approach; —Clinical assessment of pain: *Types of pain; *Temporal patterns of pain;	*Accept the importance of the nurses' role and responsibilities in the interdisciplinary assessment of pain. *Accept that pain is what the patient says it is. *Affirm the importance of pain assessment as a nursing priority. *Consider the multidimensional aspects of pain.	*Obtain a comprehensive pain history to determine the type and temporal pattern of the patient's pain. *Determine the severity of pain using a pain assessment tool. *Conduct a physical examination based on the patient's history and knowledge of the disease process.	*Contribute to the interdisciplinary management of pain through comprehensive history and physical assessment.	*Coordinate the interdisciplinary team efforts related to the comprehensive assessment of pain. *Role model comprehensive assessment skills. *Educate other health professionals regarding the assessment of level of pain and need for pain management prior to their interventions.	*Role play a patient-clinician interaction to obtain a pain history, conduct a physical exam, and utilize a pain assessment instrument. *Analyze a written or videotaped case study to evaluate the comprehensiveness of the pain history and physical examination.

(continued)

EDUCATION PLAN 12.1 *(continued)*

Knowledge Needed	Attitudes	Skills	Undergraduate Behavioral Outcomes	Graduate Behavioral Outcomes	Teaching/Learning Strategies
★Pain history: • onset • location/site • quality • severity • exacerbating and relieving factors • impact of pain on psychological well-being • history of treatment • responses to previous and current analgesic regiments. —Physical examination —Use of pain assessment tools.					★In the clinical setting, complete a health history and physical examination of a patient and document the findings in the clinical record.

Components of Pain Management: • WHO Analgesic Ladder • NSAIDS • Mechanisms of action; • Adverse effects and management; • Drug selection; • Choice of starting dose and titration; • Opioids • Mechanisms of actions; • Principles of opioid administration;	*Affirm the importance of effective pain management. *Emphasize the need to suspend clinician bias related to use of opioids. *Dispel myths related to pharmacological management of pain.	*Demonstrate competence in managing pain using NSAIDS, opioids, and adjuvant therapies. *Set up accurately the equipment needed for parenteral infusions of pharmacologic agents for pain management. *Accurately titrate doses of pharmacological agents to achieve pain relief. *Correctly calculate opioid conversions using equianalgesic dose tables.	*Administer appropriate pharmacological therapies to achieve maximal relief of pain. *Assess for side effects and adverse effects of pharmacological pain therapies. *Administer appropriate therapies to relieve side effects of analgesics. *Educate patients and families regarding the use of opioids and other analgesics as it relates to tolerance, addiction, and physical dependence.	*Determine a comprehensive plan to treat and manage pain and related symptoms. *Coordinate interdisciplinary team efforts to execute comprehensive pain therapies. *Educate other health care providers regarding effective and comprehensive pain management.	In the clinical laboratory, have a faculty demonstration and students'/nurses' return demonstration of the set-up and titration of opioids using a PCA pump, or other infusion equipment.

(continued)

EDUCATION PLAN 12.1   *(continued)*

Knowledge Needed	Attitudes	Skills	Undergraduate Behavioral Outcomes	Graduate Behavioral Outcomes	Teaching/Learning Strategies
• Choice of a starting dose and dose titration. • Managing a pain crisis; • Sedation at the end of life; • Tolerance, physical dependence, and psychological dependence; • Opioid side effects and their management; • Adjuvant analgesia: • Corticosteroids • Benzodiazepines • Antidepressants		*Effectively manages adverse effects of analgesics.			*Based on case studies, determine the appropriate pharmacological management, using the WHO analgesic ladder, and calculate the titration and conversion of opioids. *Based on case studies, evaluate the appropriateness of various pain management plans based on type of illness, etiology of pain, pain history and assessment, patient preference, health status, goals of care, and mechanism of action, and pharmaco-therapeutic properties of pharmacological agents.

- Anticonvulsants
- GABAB Agonists
- Alpha 2-Adrenergic antagonists
- Local anesthetics
- Topical analgesics
- NMDA receptor antagonists
- Radio-pharmaceuticals
- Biphosphonates

*In the clinical setting, implement a plan of care for pain management of a select patient. In postconference, discuss the barriers to effective pain management, the patient's response to pain management, side effects experienced by the patient due to opioid use, and recommended changes, if needed, in the plan of care.

(continued)

EDUCATION PLAN 12.1   *(continued)*

Knowledge Needed	Attitudes	Skills	Undergraduate Behavioral Outcomes	Graduate Behavioral Outcomes	Teaching/Learning Strategies
					*Have students develop pain management protocol or practice guidelines for a specific patient population. Develop the protocol based on empirical evidence through critiquing related research studies and in collaboration with members of the interdisciplinary team.

| Special Populations Concerns at the End of Life: —Patients with a history of substance abuse; —Patients with impaired communication; —Elder patients; —Pediatric patients. | *Consider the special needs of patients who have a history of substance abuse, have impaired communication, are older adults, or children. *Acknowledge personal attitudes and misconceptions toward patients with a history of substance abuse or the older adult and how those attitudes may affect compassionate and effective care, including the relief of pain. | *Demonstrate accurate pain assessment skills for patients from special populations. | *Provide effective pain management for those frequently undertreated for pain, specifically individuals with a history of substance abuse, those with impaired communication, the older adult, and children. *Seek referral from consultants when necessary for appropriate pain management in special populations. | *Educate patients, family, and health professionals regarding the pain assessment and management for individuals of special populations. *Establish protocols and clinical practice guidelines to insure compassionate and effective pain management of special patient populations. | *Explore with students/nurses their assumptions regarding patients with a history of substance abuse, those with impaired communication, older adults, and children. *Have each student/nurse analyze a past clinical experience in which they cared for a patient in a special population described above with regard to the adequacy of pain assessment and management. Discuss the barriers and facilitators to effective pain management in the case. |

(continued)

EDUCATION PLAN 12.1   *(continued)*

Knowledge Needed	Attitude	Skills	Undergraduate Behavioral Outcomes	Graduate Behavioral Outcomes	Teaching/Learning Strategies
					*Select a particular patient scenario with regard to medical diagnosis, discuss how the assessment and treatment would differ if the patient had a history of substance use, had impaired communication, was an elder or a child. *Assign students to care for a patient within the special populations described, and develop a plan of care for effective pain management. Evaluate the plan of care in class or post-conference.

REFERENCES

Acute Pain Management Guidelines Panel. (1992). *Acute pain management: Operative or medical procedures and trauma. Clinical practice guideline.* AHCPR Pub. No. 92–0032. Rockville, MD: Agency for Health Care Policy and Research, Public Health Services, U.S. Department of Health and Human Services.

Adelhardt, J., Byrnes, M., Derby, S., Holritz, K., Layman-Goldstein, M., Racolin, A., & Staniewicz, J. (1995). *Care of the patient in pain: Standard of oncology nursing practice.* New York: Memorial Sloan-Kettering Cancer Center.

Ahles, T. A., Blanchard, E. B., & Ruckdeschel J. C. (1983). The multidimensional nature of cancer-related pain. *Pain, 17,* 277–288.

American Cancer Society Statistics, 2004. Retrived July 28, 2004, from http://www.cancer.org

American Geriatric Society. (2002). Panel on persistent pain in older persons. *Journal of the American Geriatric Society, 50*(6 Suppl.), S205–224.

American Nurses Association. (1990). Position paper on the promotion of comfort and relief of pain in dying patients. Washington, DC: American Nurses Association. Revised December 5, 2003.

American Pain Society. (2003). Principles of analgesic use in the treatment of acute pain and cancer pain (5th ed.). Glenview, IL: American Pain Society.

Anderson, G., Jensen, N. H., Christrup. L., Hansen, S. H., & Sjogren, P. (2002). Pain, sedation and morphine metabolism in cancer patients during long term treatment with sustained–release morphine. *Palliative Medicine, 16,* 107–114.

Backonja, M., Arndt, G., Gombar, K. A., Cjeck, B., & Zimmermann, M. (1994). Response of neuropathic pain syndromes to ketamine: a preliminary study. *Pain, 56,* 51–57.

Bates, M. S. (1987). Ethnicity and pain: A biocultural model. *Social Science Medicine, 24*(1), 47–50.

Berde, C. B., & Sethna, N. F. (2003). Analgesics for the treatment of pain in children. *New England Journal of Medicine, 347,* 1094–1103.

Berry, P. E., & Dahl, J. L. (2000). The new JCAHO pain standards: implications for pain management nurses. *Pain Management Nurses, 1,* 3–12.

Berry, P. E., & Ward, S. E. (1995). Barriers to pain management in hospice: A study of family caregivers. *Hospice Journal, 10,* 19–33.

Bookbinder, M., Coyle, N., Kiss, M., Layman-Goldstein, M., Holritz, K., Thaler, H., et al. (1995). Implementing national standards for cancer pain management: Program model and evaluation. *Journal of Pain and Symptom Management, 12,* 334–347.

Breitbart, W., Bruera, E., Chochinov, H., & Lynch, M. (1995). Neuropsychiatric syndromes and psychological symptoms in patients with advanced cancer. *Journal of Pain and Symptom Management, 10,* 131–141.

Breitbart, W., & Dibiase, L. (2002). Current perspectives in pain in AIDS. *Oncology, 16*(7), 964–968.

Brescia, F., Portenoy, R. K., Ryan, M., Drasnoff, L., & Gray, G. (1992). Pain, opioid use and survival in hospitalized patients with advanced cancer. *Journal of Clinical Oncology, 10,* 149–155.

Bruera, E., Macmillan, K., & MacDonald, N. (1989). The cognitive effects of the administration of narcotic analgesics in patients with cancer pain. *Pain, 39*(1), 13–26.

Bruera, E., Miller, L., McCallion, J., Macmillan, K., & Hanson, J. (1992). Cognitive failure in patients with terminal cancer, a prospective study. *Journal of Pain and Symptom Management, 7,* 192–195.

Bruera, E., Suarez-Almozor, M., Velasco, A., Bertolino, M., MacDonald, S. M., & Hanson, J. (1994). The assessment of constipation in terminal cancer patients admitted to a palliative care unit: A retrospective review. *Journal of Pain and Symptom Management, 9,* 515–519.

Bruera, E., & Kim, H. N. (2003). Cancer pain. *Journal of the American Medical Association, 290,* 2476–2479.

Bruera, E., & Portenoy, R. K. (Eds.). (2005) *Cancer pain: Assessment and management.* Cambridge, UK: Cambridge University Press.

Byock, I. (1997). *Dying well: The prospect of growth at the end of life.* New York: Riverhead Books.

Cancer Pain, National Comprehensive Cancer Network (practice guidelines) (2002). Retrieved July 10, 2004, from www.nccn.org

Chang, V. T., Hwang, S. S., Feuerman, M., & Kasimis, B. S. (2000). Symptom and quality of life survey of medical oncology patients at veterans' affairs medical center: A role for symptom assessment. *Cancer, 88,* 1175–1183.

Cherny, N., & Coyle, N. (1994). Suffering in the advanced cancer patient: A definition and taxonomy. *Journal of Palliative Care, 10,* 57–70.

Cherny, N., & Coyle, N. (1999). Ethical principles in the management of cancer pain. In G. M. Aronoff (Ed.), *Evaluation and treatment of chronic pain* (3rd ed., pp. 643–654). Baltimore: Williams & Wilkins.

Cherny, N. I., & Portenoy, R. K. (1994a). Sedation in the management of refractory symptoms: Guidelines for evaluation and treatment. *Journal of Palliative Care, 10,* 31–38.

Cherny, N. I., & Portenoy, R. K. (1994b). The management of cancer pain. *Cancer Journal* for Clinicians, 44, 262–303.

Christie, J. M., Simmonds, M., Patt, R., Coluzzi, P., Busch, M. A., Nordbrock, E., et al., (1998). Dose titration: A multicenter study of oral transmucosal fentanyl citrate for the treatment of breakthrough pain in cancer patients using transdermal fentanyl for persistent pain. *Journal of Clinical Oncology, 16,* 3238–3245.

Cleeland, C. E. (1989). Pain control: Public and physicians' attitudes. In C. S. Hill & W. S. Fields (Eds.), *Drug treatment of cancer pain in a drug-oriented society. Advances in Pain research* and Therapy (pp. 81–89). New York: Raven Press.

Clissold, S. P. (1986). Aspirin and related derivatives of salicylic acid. *Drugs, 32*(Suppl. 4), 70–77.

Cohen, M. Z., Easley, M. K., Ellis, C., Hughes, B., Ownby, K., Rashad, B. G., et al. (2003). Cancer pain management and the JCAHO's pain standards: An institutional challenge. *Journal of Pain and Symptom Management, 25,* 519–527.

Compton, P. (1999). Substance abuse. In M. McCaffery & C. Pasero (Eds.), *Pain: Clinical* manual (2nd ed., pp. 428–466). St. Louis, MO: Mosby

Coyle, N. (1992). The euthanasia and physician-assisted suicide debate: Issues for nursing. *Oncology Nursing Forum, 19*(7), 41–46.

Coyle, N. (1995). Suffering in the first person. In B. R. Ferrell (Ed.), *Suffering* (pp. 29–64). Boston: Jones and Bartlett.

Coyle, N. (2004). In their own words: Seven advanced cancer patients describe their experience with pain and the use of opioid drugs. *Journal of Pain and Symptom Management, 27,* 300–309.

Coyle, N., Adelhardt, J., Foley, K. M., & Portenoy, R. K. (1990). Character of terminal illness in the advanced cancer patient: Pain and other symptoms in the last four weeks of life. *Journal of Pain and Symptom Management, 5,* 83–93.

Coyle, N., Cherny, N. I., & Portenoy, R. K. (1994). Subcutaneous infusions at home. *Oncology, 8*(4), 21–32.

Coyle, N., & Derby, S. (in press). Assessment and pharmacologic management of pain in the older adult. In Cope D. Reb A (eds.) *An Evidence-Based Approach to the Treatment and Care of the Older Adult with Cancer.* ONS Press.

Coyle, N., & Portenoy, R. K. (1995). Pharmacologic management of cancer pain. In D. B. McGuire, C. H. Yarbro, & B. R. Ferrell (Eds.), *Cancer pain management* (2nd ed., pp. 89–130). Boston: Jones and Bartlett.

Daut, R. L., Cleeland, C. S., & Flanery, R. C. (1983). Development of the Wisconsin Brief Pain Questionnaire to assess pain in cancer and other diseases. *Pain, 17,* 197–210.

Davis, M. P., Varga, J., Dickerson, D., Walsh, D., LeGrand, S. B., & Lagman, R. (2003). Normal-release and controlled-release oxycodone: Pharmacokinetics, pharmacodynamics, and controversy. *Supportive Care Cancer, 11*(2), 84–92.

Davis, M. P., & Walsh, D. (2001). Methadone for the relief of cancer pain: A review of pharmacokinetics, pharmacodynamics, drug interactions and protocols of administration. *Supportive Care Cancer, 9*(2), 73–83.

De Conno, F., Groff, L., & Brunelli, C. (1996). Clinical experience with oral methadone administration in the treatment of pain in 196 advanced cancer patients. *Journal of Clinical Oncology, 14,* 2836–2842.

de Stoutz, N., Bruera, E., & Suarez-Almazor, M. E. (1995). Opioid rotation for toxicity reduction in terminal cancer patients. *Journal of Pain and Symptom Management, 10,* 378–384.

Eide, P. K., Jorum, E., Stubhang, A., Bremners, J., & Breivil, H. (1994). Relief of postherpetic neuralgia with the N-methyl-D-aspartic receptor antagonist ketamine: A double blind, crossover comparison with morphine and placebo. *Pain, 58,* 347–354.

Eland, J. M., Pain in Children *Nurs Clin North Am 25*(4): (1990) 469–475.

Elliot, K., & Foley, K. M. (1988). Neurologic pain syndromes in patients with cancer. *Neurologic* Clinics, 7, 333–360.

Ettinger, D. S. Vitale, P. J., & Trump, D. L. (1979). Important clinical pharmacologic considerations in the use of methadone in cancer patients. *Cancer Treatment Reports, 63,* 457–459.

Fainsinger, R., Schoeller, T., & Bruera, E. (1993). Methadone in the management of cancer pain: A review. *Pain, 52,* 137–147.

Fainsinger, R., Schoeller, T., Boiskin, M., & Bruera, E. (1993). Palliative care rounds: Cognitive failure and coma after renal failure in a patient receiving captopril and hydromorphone. *Journal of Palliative Care, 9*(1), 53–55.

Ferrell, B. A. (1998). Supportive care in elderly people. In A. Berger, R. K. Portenoy, & D. E. Weissman (Eds.). *Principles and practice of supportive oncology* (pp. 853–859). Philadelphia: Lippincott-Raven.

Ferrell, B. A., & Whiteman, J.E. (2003). Pain. In R. S. Morrison & D. E. Meier. (Eds), *Geriatric palliative care* (pp. 205–229). Oxford, UK: Oxford University Press.

Ferrell, B. R., & Ferrell, B. A. (1995). Pain in elderly persons. In D. B. McGuire, C. Henke Yarbro, & B. R. Ferrell (Eds.), *Cancer pain management* (2nd ed., pp. 273–287). Boston: Jones and Bartlett.

Ferrell, B. R., Ferrell, B. A., Ahn, C., & Tran, K. (1994). Pain management for elderly patients with cancer at home. *Cancer, 74*(Suppl.), 2139–2146.

Ferrell, B. R., Grant, M., Chan, J., Ahn, C., & Ferrell, B. A. (1995). The impact of cancer pain education on family caregivers of elderly patients. *Oncology Nursing Forum, 22,* 1211–1218.

Ferrell, B. R., Rhiner, M., Cohen, M. Z., & Grant, M. (1991). Pain as a metaphor for illness. Part 1: Impact of pain and family caregivers. *Oncology Nursing Forum, 18,* 1303–1309.

Field, M. J., & Behrman, R. (Eds). (2003). *When children die: Improving palliative and end-of-life care for children and their families* (Report of the Institute of Medicine Task Force). Washington, DC: National Academy Press.

Fine, P. G. (2000). Low-dose ketamine in the management of opioid non-responsive terminal cancer pain. *Journal of Pain and Symptom Management, 17,* 296–300.

Finley, G. A., & McGrath, P. J. (Eds.) (1998). *Measurement of pain in infants and children. Progress* in pain research and management (Vol. 10). Seattle, WA: IASP Press.

Finns, J. J. (1999). Acts of omission and commission in pain management: The ethics of naloxone use. *Journal of Pain and Symptom Management, 17,* 120–124.

Fishman, B. (1991). The treatment of suffering in patients with cancer pain: Cognitive behavioral approaches. In K. M. Foley, J. J. Bonica, & V. Ventafridda (Eds.). *Advances in pain research and therapy* (pp. 301–316). New York: Raven Press.

Foley, K. M. (1991). The relationship of pain and symptom management to patient requests for physician-assisted suicide. *Journal of Pain and Symptom Management, 6,* 289–297.

Foley, K. M. (1993). Changing concepts of tolerance to opioids: What the cancer patient has taught us. In C. R. Chapman, & K. M. Foley (Eds.). *Current and emerging issues in cancer pain:* Research and practice (pp. 331–350). New York: Raven Press.

Foley, K. M. (1998). Pain assessment and cancer pain syndromes. In D. Doyle, G. W. C. Hanks, & N. MacDonald (Eds.). *Oxford textbook on palliative medicine* (2nd ed., pp. 310–331). Oxford, UK: Oxford University Press.

Foley, K. M. (2004). Acute and chronic pain syndromes. In D. Doyle, G. Hanks, N. Cherny, & K. Calman. (Eds.). *Oxford textbook of palliative medicine* (3rd ed., pp. 298–316). New York: Oxford University Press.

Foley, K. M., & Gelband, H. (2001). Improving palliative care for cancer. Washington, DC: Institute of Medicine and National Research Council.

Frager, G. (1997). Palliative care and terminal care of children. *Children and Adolescent Psychiatric* Clinics of North America, 6, 889–909.

Fultz, J. M., & Sonay, E. C. (1975). Guidelines for the management of hospitalized narcotic addicts. *Annals of Internal Medicine, 82,* 815–818.

Galer, B. S., Coyle, N., & Pasternak, G. W. (1992). Individual variability in the response to different opioids: Report of five cases. *Pain, 49*(1), 87–91.

Gonzales, G. R., & Coyle, N. (1992). Treatment of cancer pain in a former opioid abuser: Fears of the patient and staff and their influence on care. *Journal of Pain and Symptom* Management, 7(4), 246–249.

Goodwin, J. S., & Regan, M. (1982). Cognitive dysfunction associated with naproxen and ibuprofen in the elderly. *Arthritis and Rheumatism, 25,* 1013–1015.

Gourlay, G. K., Plummer, J. L., Cherry, D. A., & Purser, T. (1991). The reproducibility of bioavailability of oral morphine under fed and fasted conditions. *Journal of Pain and Symptom* Management, 6, 431–436.

Gunnarsdottir, S., Donovan, H. S., Serlin, R. C., Voge, C., & Ward, S. (2002). Patient-related barriers to pain management: The Barriers Questionnaire II (BQ-II). *Pain, 99,* 385–396.

Hanks, G. W., Cherny, N. I., & Fallon, M. (2004). Opioid analgesic therapy. In D. Doyle, G. Hanks, N. Cherny, & K. Calman (Eds.). *Oxford textbook of palliative medicine* (3rd ed.) (pp. 316–341) Oxford, UK: Oxford University Press.

Hawkey, C. J. (1990). Non-steroidal antiinflammatory drugs and peptic ulcers. *BMJ,* 3,300(6720):278–84, review.

Hawkey, C. J., & Yeomans, N. D. (1998). Evolving strategies for managing non-steroidal antiinflammatory drug associated ulcers. *American Journal of Medicine, 104*(Suppl. 3A), 1S–96S.

Herr, K. (2004). State of the art review of tools for assessment of pain in nonverbal adults. Retrieved July 1, 2004, from City of Hope Pain Resource Web site: http://www.cityofhope.org/prc/eledrly.asp

Herr, K. A., & Mobily, P. R. (1991). Complexities in pain assessment in the elderly: Clinical considerations. *Journal of Gerontological Nursing, 17*, 12–19.

Hewitt, D. J., & Foley, K. M. (1997). Pain and pain management. In C. K. Cassel, H. J. Cohen, E. B. Larson, D. E. Meier, N. M. Resnick, L. Z. Rubenstein, & L. B. Sorenson (Eds.), *Geriatric* medicine (3rd ed., pp. 865–882). New York: Springer-Verlag.

Hill, C. S., Audell, L. G., Kanner, R., Miaskowski, C., Paice, J., & Rogers, A. G. (1999). A roundtable discussion: The management of pain in special populations of cancer patients. *Primary Care & Cancer, 19*(3), 16, 27, 32–34.

Hockenberry, M., Wilson, D., Winkelstein, M., & Kline, N. (2003). Wong's nursing care of infants and children (7th ed.). St Louis, MO: Mosby.

Hofmann, M. T., Farnon, C. U., Javed, A., & Posner, J. D. (1998). Pain in the elderly hospice patient. *American Journal of Hospice and Palliative Care, 15*, 259–265.

Houde, R.W. (1986). Clinical analgesic studies of hydromorphone. In K. M. Foley, C. E. Inturrisi (Eds.), *Advances in pain research and therapy* (Vol. 8, pp. 129–136).

Hunt, G., & Bruera, E. (1995). Respiratory depression in patients receiving oral methadone for cancer pain. *Journal of Pain and Symptom Management, 10*, 401–404.

Hwang, S. S., Chang, V. T., & Kasimis, B. (2002). Dynamic cancer pain managemen outcomes: The relationship between pain severity, pain relief, functional interference, satisfaction and global quality of life over time. *Journal of Pain and Symptom Management, 23*, 190–200.

Ingham J., & Coyle, N. (1997). Teamwork in end-of-life care: A nurse-physician perspective on introducing physicians to palliative care concepts. In Clark, D., Hockley, J., & Ahmedzai, S. *New Themes in Palliative Care.* Buckingham: Open University Press, pp. 255–274.

International Association for the Study of Pain. (1979). Pain terms: a list with definitions and usage. *Pain*, 6:249.

Jacox, A., Carr, D. B., Payne, R., Berde, C. B., Breithart, W., Cain, I. M., et al. (1994). *Management of cancer pain. Clinical* Practice Guideline No. 9 (AHCPR Publication No. 94–0592). Rockville, MD: Agency for Health Care Policy and Research, U.S. Department of Health and Human Services, Public Health Services.

Jaffe, J. H., & Martin, W. R. (1990). Opioid analgesics and antagonists. In A. G. Gilman, T. W. Rall, A. S. Nies, & P. Taylor (Eds.). *The pharmacological basis of therapeutics* (8th ed., pp. 485–521). New York: Permagon Press.

Jenkins, C. A., & Bruera, E. (1999). Nonsteroidal anti-inflammatory drugs as adjuvant analgesics in cancer patients. *Palliative Medicine, 13*, 183–196.

Joranson, D. E., Cleeland, C. S., & Weissman, D. E. (1992). Opioids in chronic pain and non-cancer pain: A survey of state medical board members. *Federal Bulletin: Journal of Medical* Licensure and Discipline, 79, 15–49.

Kaiko, R. F. (1983). Central nervous system excitatory effects of meperidine in cancer patients. *Annals of Neurology, 13*, 180–185.

Keefe, F. J., Ahles, T. A., Porter, L. S., Sutton, L. M., McBride, C. M., Pope, M. S., et al., (2003). The self-efficacy of family caregivers for helping cancer patients to manage pain at end-of-life. *Pain, 102*, 157–162.

Larijani, G. E., Goldberg, M. E., & Rogers, K. H. (1996). Treatment of opioid-induced pruritus with ondansetron: Report of four patients. *Pharmacotherapy,* 16, 958–960.

Lasch, K., Greenhill, A., Wilkes, G., Carr, D., Lee, M., & Blanchard, R. (2002). Why study pain? A qualitative analysis of medical and nursing faculty and student's knowledge of and attitudes to cancer pain management. *Journal of Palliative Medicine,* 5,(1) 57–71.

Latimer, E. J. (1991). Ethical decision-making in the care of the dying and its application to clinical practice. *Journal of Pain and Symptom Management,* 6, 329–336.

Layman-Goldstein, M., Byrnes-Casey, M., & Collins, J. J. (2005). Pediatric pain: Knowing the child before you. In B. R. Ferrell & N. Coyle (Eds.), *Textbook of palliative care nursing* (2nd ed.). New York: Oxford University Press.

Lee, M. A., Leng, M. E., & Tierman, E. J. (2001). Retrospective study of the use of hydromorphone in palliative care patients with normal and abnormal urea and creatinine. *Journal of Palliative Medicine,* 15(1), 26–34.

Levy, M. (1985). Pain management in advanced cancer. *Seminars in Oncology,* 12, 384–410.

Levy, M. H. (1989). Integration of pain management into comprehensive cancer care. *Cancer,* 63, 2328–2335.

Lipman, A. G., & Gauthier, M. E. (1997). Pharmacology of opioid drugs. In R. K. Portenoy & E. Bruera (Eds.), *Topics in palliative care* (Vol. 1, ch, 7). New York: Oxford University Press.

Lussier, D., & Portenoy, R. K. (2004). Adjuvant analgesics in pain management. In D. Doyle, G. Hanks, N. Cherny, & K. Calman (Eds.). *Oxford textbook of palliative medicine* (3rd ed., pp. 349–377). Oxford, UK: Oxford University Press.

Lynn, J., Teno, J. M., Phillips, R. S., Wu, A. W., Desbiens, N., & Harrold, J. (1997). Percep-tions of family members of the dying experience of older and seriously ill patients. *Annals of Internal Medicine,* 126, 97–106.

Manfredi, P. L., Ribeiro, S. W., & Payne, R. (1996). Inappropriate use of naloxone in cancer patients with pain. *Journal of Pain and Symptom Management,* 11, 131–134.

Manfredi, P. L., Borsook, D., Chandler, S. W., & Payne, R. (1997). Intravenous methadone for cancer pain unrelieved by morphine and hydromorphone: Clinical observations. *Pain,* 70, 99–101.

Mantyh, P. W. (2002). A mechanism based understanding of cancer pain. *Pain,* 96, 1–2. Review.

McCaffery M. & Beebe, A. (1989) *Pain: Clinical Manual.* St. Louis, MO: Mosby.

McCaffery, M., & Pasero, C. (Eds.) (1999a). *Pain: Clinical manual* (2nd ed.). St Louis, MO: Mosby.

McCaffery, M., & Pasero, C. (1999b). Practical nondrug approaches to pain. In M. McCaffery & C. Pasero (Eds.), *Pain: Clinical manual* (2nd ed., pp. 399–427). St. Louis, MO: Mosby, Inc.

McGuire, D. B. (1995). The multiple dimensions of cancer pain: A framework for assessment and management. In D. B. McGuire, C. H. Yarbro, & B. R. Ferrell (Eds.). *Cancer pain* management (2nd ed., pp. 1–17). Boston: Jones and Bartlett.

McQuay, H. J., & Moore, A. (2004). Non-opioid analgesics. In D. Doyle, G. Hanks, N. Cherny, & K. Calman (Eds.). *Oxford textbook of palliative medicine* (3rd ed., pp. 342–349). Oxford, UK: Oxford University Press.

Menten, J., Desmedt, M., Lossignol, D., & Mullie, A. (2002). Longitudinal follow-up of TTS-fentanyl use in patients with cancer-related pain: Results of a compassionate-use study with special focus on elderly patients. *Current Medical Research Opinion,* 18, 488–498.

Merskey, H. (1986). Classification of chronic pain: Descriptions of chronic pain syndromes and definition of pain terms. *Pain, 3*(Suppl.3), S217.

Meuser, T., Pietruck, C., Radbruch, L., Stute, P., Lehmann, K. A., & Grond, S. (2001). Symptoms during cancer treatment following WHO-guidelines: A longitudinal follow-up study of symptom prevalence, severity and etiology. *Pain, 93,* 247–257.

Miaskowski, C. (2002). The need to assess multiple symptoms. *Pain Management Nursing, 3,* 115.

Miser, A. W., Moore, L., Greene, R., Gracely, R. H., & Miser, J. S. (1986). Prospective study of continuous intravenous and subcutaneous morphine infusions for therapy-related pain in children and young adults with cancer. *Clinical Journal of Pain, 2,* 101–106.

Morita, T., Ichiki, T., Tsunoda, J., Inoue, S., & Chihara, S. (1998). A prospective study on the dying process in terminally ill cancer patients. *American Journal of Hospice and Palliative Care, 15,* 217–222.

Morrison, R. S., Wallenstein, S., Natale, D. K., Senzel, R. S., & Huang, L. L. (2000). "We don't carry that"—failure of pharmacies in predominantly non-white neighborhoods to stock opioid analgesics [commentary]. *New England Journal of Medicine, 342,* 1023–1026.

Moryl, N., Santiago-Palma, J., Kornick, C., Derby, S., Fishberg, D., & Payne, R., et al. (2002). Pitfalls of opioid rotation: Substituting another opioid for methadone in patients with cancer pain. *Pain, 96,* 325–328.

National Comprehensive Cancer Network. (2004). NCCN Clinical Practice Guidelines in Oncology—v.1.2004. Retrieved 8/13/05 from http://www.nccn.org

National Consensus Guidelines for Quality Palliative Care. (2004). Retrieved from www.nationalconsensusproject.org

National Institutes of Health State-of-the-Science Statement on symptom management in cancer: Pain, depression, and fatigue.

(2002, July 15–17, 19). *NIH Consensus State-of-the-Science Statements,* 1–29.

Ng, K., & von Gunten, C. F. (1998). Symptoms and attitudes of 100 consecutive patients admitted to an acute hospice/palliative care unit. *Journal of Pain and Symptom Management, 16,* 307–316.

O'Brien, S., Dalton, J. A., Konsler, G., & Carlson, J. (1996). The knowledge and attitudes of experienced oncology nurses regarding the management of cancer-related pain. *Oncology Nursing Forum, 23,* 515–521.

Paice, J., Toy, C., & Shott, S. (1998). Barriers to cancer pain relief: Fear of tolerance and addiction. *Journal of Pain and Symptom Management, 16*(1), 1–9.

Paice, J. A. (1999). Symptom management. In C. Miaskowski & P. Buchsel (Eds.). *Oncology nursing: Assessment and clinical care.* St Louis, MO: Mosby.

Passik, S. D., Kirsh, K. L., Whitcomb, L., Portenoy, R. K., Kats, N. P., Kleinman, L., et al. (2004). A new tool to assess and document pain outcomes in chronic patients receiving opioid therapy. *Clinical Therapeutics, 26,* 552–561.

Passik, S. D., & Portenoy, R. K. (1998). Substance abuse issues in palliative care. In A. Berger, R. K. Portenoy, & D. E. Weissman (Eds.), *Principles and practice of supportive oncology* (pp. 513–529). Philadelphia: Lippincott-Raven.

Passik, S. D., Portenoy, R. K., & Ricketts, P. L. (1998a). Substance abuse issues in cancer patients. Part 1: Prevalence and diagnosis. *Oncology, 12,* 517–521, 524.

Passik, S. D., Portenoy, R. K., & Ricketts, P. L. (1998b). Substance abuse issues in cancer patients. Part 2: Evaluation and treatment. *Oncology, 12,* 729–734.

Passik, S. D., & Theobald, D. E. (2000). Managing addiction in advanced cancer patients: Why bother? *Journal of Pain and Symptom Management, 19,* 229–234.

Payne, R., Chandler, S. W., & Einhaus, E. (1995). Guidelines for the clinical use of transdermal fentanyl. *Anti-cancer Drugs, 6*, 50–53.

Payne, R., & Gonzales, R. G. (2004). Pathophysiology of pain in cancer and other terminal diseases. In D. Doyle, G. Hanks, N. Cherny, & K. Calman (Eds.). *Oxford textbook of palliative medicine* (3rd ed., pp. 288–298). Oxford, UK: Oxford University Press.

Pereira, J., Hanson, J., & Bruera, E. (1997). The frequency and clinical course of cognitive impairment in patients with terminal cancer. *Cancer, 79*, 835–842.

Perry, S., & Heidrich G. (1982). Management of pain during debridement: A survey of US burn units. *Pain, 13*, 267–280.

Persson, J., Axelsson, G., Hallin, R. G., & Gustafsson, L. L. (1995). Beneficial effects of ketamine in a chronic pain state with allodynia, possibly due to central sensitization. *Pain, 60*, 217–222.

Portenoy, R.K. (1994). Management of common opioid side effects during long-term therapy of cancer pain. *Annals of the Academy of Medicine Singapore, 23*, 160–170.

Portenoy, R. K. (1998). Adjuvant analgesics in pain management. In D. Doyle, G. W. C. Hanks, & N. MacDonald (Eds.). *Oxford textbook of palliative medicine* (2nd ed., pp. 361–390). Oxford, UK: Oxford University Press.

Portenoy, R. K., & Conn, M. (2003). Cancer pain syndromes. In E. Bruera, & R. K. Portenoy (Eds.). *Cancer pain assessment and management* (pp. 89–108). Cambridge, UK: Cambridge University Press.

Portenoy, R. K., Dole, V., Joseph, H., Lowinson, J., Rice, C., Segal, S., et al.(1997). Pain management and chemical dependency: Evolving perspectives. *Journal of the American Academy of Medicine, 278*, 592–593.

Portenoy, R. K., & Hagen, N. A. (1990). Breakthrough pain: Definition, prevalence and characteristics. *Pain, 41*, 273.

Portenoy, R. K., & Lesage, P. (1999). Management of cancer pain. *Lancet, 353*, 1695–1700.

Portenoy, Thaler, Inturissi, Friedlander-Klar, & Coyle, 1994.

Portenoy, R. K., Thaler, H. T., Kornblith, A. B., Lepore, J. M., Friedlander, K. H., & Coyle, N. (1994). Symptom prevalence, characteristics and distress in a cancer population. *Quality of Life Research, 3*, 183–189.

Porter, J., & Jick, H. (1980). Addiction rare in patients treated with narcotics [letter to the editor]. *New England Journal of Medicine, 302*, 123.

Posner, J. (1995). *Neurological complications of cancer.* Philadelphia: Davis.

Potter, V. T., Wiseman, C. E., Dunn, S. M., & Boyle, F. M. (2003). Patient barriers to optimal pain control. *Psychooncology, 12*, 153–160.

Radbruch, L., Sabatowski, R., Petzke, F., Brunsch-Radbruch, A., Grond, S., & Lehmann KA. (2001). Transdermal fentanyl for the management of cancer pain: A survey of 1005 patients. *Palliative Medicine, 15*, 309–321.

Rawlins, M. D. (1998). Non-opioid analgesics. In D. Doyle, G. W. G. Hanks, & N. MacDonald (Eds.). *Oxford textbook of palliative medicine* (2nd ed., pp. 355–361). Oxford, UK: Oxford University Press.

Ripamonti, C. (2003). Pharmacology of opioid analgesics: Clinical principles. In E. Bruera & R. K. Portenoy (Eds.). *Cancer pain: Assessment and management* (pp. 124–149). Cambridge, UK: Cambridge University Press.

Ripamonti, C., Groff, L., Brunelli, C., Polastri, D., Stravrakis, A., & DeConno, F. (1998). Switching from oral morphine to oral methadone in treating cancer pain: What is the equianalgesic dose ratio? *Journal of Clinical Oncology, 16,* 3216–3221.

Roth, S. A. (1988). Non-steroidal anti-inflammatory drugs: Gastropathy, deaths and medical practice. *Annals of Internal Medicine, 109,* 353–354.

Saunders, C. M. (1967). *The management of terminal illness.* London: Hospital Medicine.

Schechter, N. L., Berde, C., & Yaster, M. (2003). *Pain in infants, children, and adolescents* (2nd ed.). Philadelphia: Lippincott, Williams, & Wilkins.

Schug, S. A., Zech, D., Grond, S., Jung, H., Meuser, T., & Stobbe, B. (1992). A long-term survey of morphine in cancer pain patients. *Journal of Pain and Symptom Management, 7,* 259–266.

Shimp, L. A. (1998). Safety issues in the pharmacologic management of chronic pain in the elderly. *Pharmacotherapy, 18,* 1313–1322.

Sibinga, N. E. S., & Goldstein, A. (1988). Opioid peptides and opioid receptors in cells of the immune system. *Annual Review of Immunology, 6,* 219–249.

Smith, M. T. (2000). Neuroexcitatory effects of morphine and hydromorphone: Evidence implicating the 3-glucuronide metabolites. *Clinical Experimental Pharmacology Physiology, 27,* 524–528.

Stannard, C. F., & Porter, G. E. (1993). Ketamine hydrochloride in the treatment of phantom limb pain. *Pain, 54,* 227–230.

Stein, C. (1995). The control of pain in peripheral tissues by opioids. *New England Journal of Medicine, 332,* 1685–1690.

Stiefel, F. (1993). Psychosocial aspects of cancer pain. *Supportive Care in Cancer, 1,* 130–134.

Streisand, J., Busch, M. A., Egan, T. D., Gaylord Smith, B., Gay, M., & Pace, N. L. (1998). Dose proportionality and pharmacokinetics of oral transmucosal fentanyl citrate. *Anesthesiology, 88,* 305–309.

Sunshine, A., & Olson, N. Z. (1993). In P. D. Wall & R. Melzack (Eds.), *Textbook on pain* (3rd ed., p. 927). New York: Churchill Livingston.

SUPPORT (1995). A controlled trial to improve care for seriously ill hospitalized patients. *Journal of the American Medical Association, 274,* 1591–1598.

Swarm, R. A, Karanikolas M., & Cousins, M. J. (2004). Anaesthetic techniques for pain control. In D. Doyle, G. Hanks, N. Cherny, & K. Calman (Eds.). *Oxford textbook of palliative medicine* (3rd ed., pp. 278–396). Oxford, UK: Oxford University Press.

Sykes, N. P. (1996). An investigation of the ability of oral naloxone to correct opioid-related constipation in patients with advanced cancer. *Palliative Medicine, 10,* 135–144.

Szczeklik, A. (1986). Analgesics, allergy and asthma: Non-narcotic analgesics today, benefits and risks. *Drugs, 32*(Suppl 4), 148–163.

Szeto, H. H., Inturrisi, C. E., Houde, R., Saal, R., Cheigh, J., & Reidenberg, M. M. (1977). Accumulation of normeperidine an active metabolite of meperidine, in patients with renal failure or cancer. *Annals of Internal Medicine, 86,* 738–741.

Taylor, E. J., Ferrell, B. R., Grant, M., & Cheyney, L. (1993). Managing cancer pain in the home: The decisions and ethical conflicts of patients, family caregivers and homecare nurses. *Oncology Nursing Forum, 12,* 919–927.

Taylor, L. J., & Herr, K. (2003). Pain intensity assessment: A comparison of selected pain intensity scales for use in cognitively intact and cognitively impaired African American older adults. *Pain Management Nursing, 4,* 87–95.

Tiseo, P. J., Thaler, H. T., Lapin, J., Inturrisi, C. E, Portenoy, R. K., Foley, K. M. (1995).

Morphine-6-glucoronide concentrations and opioid-related side effects: A survey in cancer patients. *Pain*, 61(1):47–54.

Twycross, R., & Lichter, I. (1998). The terminal phase. In D. Doyle, G. W. C. Hanks, & N. MacDonald (Eds.), *Oxford textbook on palliative medicine* (2nd ed., pp. 984–992). Oxford, UK: Oxford University Press.

Twycross, R, & Wilcock, A. (2001). *Symptom management in advanced cancer* (3rd ed.). Oxford, UK: Radcliffe Medical Press.

Umans, J. G., & Inturrisi, C. E. (1982). Antinociceptive activity and toxicity of meperidine and normeperidine in mice. *Journal of Pharmacology and Experimental Therapeutics, 223,* 203–206.

Walco, G. A., Cassidy, R. C., & Schechter, N. L. (1994). Sounding board: Pain, hurt, and harm. The ethics of pain control in infants and children. *New England Journal of Medicine, 331,* 541–544.

Von Roenn, J. H., Cleeland, C. S., Gonin, R., Hatfield, A. K., & Pandya, K. J. (1993). Physician attitude and practice in cancer pain management. A survey from the Eastern Cooperative Oncology Group. *Annals of Internal Medicine, 119,* 121–126.

Wallenstein, S. L., Rogers, A. G., Kaiko, R. F., & Houde, R. W. (1986). Crossover trials in analgesic assays: Studies of buprenorphine and morphine. *Pharmacotherapy.* 6(5): 228–35.

Walsh, T. D. (1990). Prevention of opioid side effects. *Journal of Pain and Symptom Management, 5,* 363–367.

Ward, S. E., Berry, P. E., & Misiewicz, H. (1996). Concerns about analgesics among patients and family caregivers in a hospice setting. *Research Nursing Health, 19,* 205–211.

Ward, S. E., Goldberg, N., Miller-McCauley, V., Mueller, C., Nolan, A., & Pawlik-Plank, D., et al. (1993). Patient related barriers to management of cancer pain. *Pain, 52,* 319–324.

Watanabe, S., Tarumi, Y., Oneschuk, D., & Lawlor, P. (2002). Opioid rotation to methadone: Proceed with caution. *Journal of Clinical Oncology, 20,* 2409–2410.

Webster, L., Andrews, M., & Stoddard, G. (2003). Modafinil treatment of opioid-induced sedation. *Pain Medicine, 4,* 135–140.

Weiner, D. K., & Rudy, T. E. (2002). Attitudinal barriers to effective treatment of persistent pain in nursing home residents. *Journal of the American Geriatric Society, 50,* 2035–2040.

Weinstein, S. M., Laux, L. F., Thornby, J. L., Lorimor, R. J., Hill, C. S., & Thorpe, D. M., et al. (2000). Physicians' attitudes towards pain and the use of opioid analgesics: Results of a survey from the Texas Cancer Pain Initiative. *Southern Medical Journal, 93,* 479–487.

Weissman, D. E., Burchman, S. L., Dinndorf, P., & Dahl, J. L. (1990). *Handbook of cancer pain management* (2nd ed.). Milwaukee: Wisconsin Cancer Pain Initiative.

Wells, N. (2000). Pain intensity and pain interference in hospitalized patients with cancer. *Oncology Nursing Forum, 27,* 985–991.

Whitcomb, D. C., & Block, G. D. (1994). Association of acetaminophen toxicity with fasting and ethanol use. *Journal of the American Medical Association, 272,* 1845–1850.

Wong, D., & Baker, C. (1995). *Reference manual for the Wong-Baker FACES pain rating scale,* Tulsa, OK: Wong and Baker.

Wong, R., & Wiffen, P. J. (2002). Biphosphonates for the relief of pain secondary to bone metastases. *Cochrane Database Systematic Review,* CD002068.

World Health Organization. (1986). *Cancer pain relief and palliative care. Report of a WHO Expert Committee* (WHO Technical

Support Series, No. 804). Geneva, Switzerland: World Health Organization.

World Health Organization (1998). *Cancer pain relief and palliative care in children*. Geneva, Switzerland: World Health Organization.

Wright, A. W., Mather, L. E., & Smith, M. T. (2001). Hydromorphone-3-glucoronide: A more potent neuro-excitant than its structural analogue, morphine-3-glucoronide. *Life Science, 69*, 409–420.

Yaksh, T. L., Dirig, D. M., & Malmberg, A. B. (1998). Mechanism of action of non-steroidal anti-inflammatory drugs. *Cancer Investigation, 16*, 509–527.

Yuan, C. S., Foss, J. F., O'Connor, M., Osinski, J., Roizen, M. F., & Moss, J. (1997). The safety and efficacy of oral methylnaltrexone in preventing morphine-induced oral-cecal transit time. *Clinical Pharmacology Therapeutics, 4*, 467–475.

13

Nondrug Pain Interventions

Mary Layman-Goldstein and Nessa Coyle

AACN Competencies

9: Evaluate the impact of traditional, complementary, and technological therapies on patient-centered outcomes.

In addition to the pharmacological approach to pain management at the end of life, there are other approaches that may be useful. These nondrug or nonpharmacological interventions or techniques can complement the treatment of the underlying pain etiology and the mainstay pharmacological approach to pain management. Nondrug interventions cover a broad spectrum of approaches. These types of interventions can modify the pain experience and give individuals an increased sense of control, decrease anxiety, improve mood, and improve sleep.

Some of the nondrug approaches that will be discussed are considered mainstream, traditional Western medicine. Other nonconventional therapies fall under the heading of complementary or alternative. Although complementary and alternative therapies are often grouped together under the heading of complementary and alternative medicine (CAM), they are very different. Complementary therapies are used *in addition to* conventional therapies and in some settings are labeled "integrative." Alternative therapies are used *in place of* traditional, mainstream treatment (Berenson, 2005; Deng, Cassileth & Simon Yeung, 2004). The nondrug interventions that will be discussed here, either traditional or complementary/integrative, are considered a part of the overall pain management plan.

There are a variety of factors that promote and inhibit the use of nondrug techniques. On their own, patients often initiate nondrug interventions such as application of heat or use of vibration. The different methods chosen by patients are often based on previous use of a particular intervention or on home remedies and may or may not be an optimal method to relieve a particular type of pain. Although the inclusion of pharmacologic interventions are usually a well-thought-out part of the plan, the use of nondrug interventions often is not. There may be little input from an individual's doctor or nurse in initiating an intervention (Rhiner, Ferrell, Ferrell, & Grant, 1993).

Patients using nondrug methods may report reduced distress, a sense of control, improved mood, or more bearable pain (Layman-Goldstein & Altilio, 1993). Some patients strongly believe that nondrug interventions should be used instead of analgesics or to increase the time between doses of analgesics. For most patients, the maximum benefit from nondrug interventions is obtained when they are used in addition to analgesics (Layman-Goldstein & Altilio, 1993).

Compared to the extensive studies that support the use of pharmacologic techniques, the strong scientific evidence supporting the use of many of these techniques is just being established (Deng et al. 2004; McCaffery & Pasero, 1999b). In 1999, the Center of Complementary and Alternative Medicine was established under the auspices of the National Institutes of Health to establish an information clearinghouse and to establish data for evaluating the clinical usefulness of various nontraditional interventions (Decker, 2000). It is hoped that as more money and energy goes into the rigorous evaluation of integrative techniques, it will be easier to appropriately add these interventions into an individual's plan of care. Yet, despite the current situation, patients express benefit from these methods and there are reasons to pursue their use (Berenson, 2005; Deng et al., 2004; Jacox et al., 1994).

The five main categories of nondrug approaches to pain management are (1) psychological interventions; (2) physiatric interventions; (3) neurostimulatory interventions; (4) invasive interventions; and (5) integrative interventions. In the following discussion, various techniques will be placed in the context of these catagories. However, there is no common taxonomy and no uniformly accepted classification system for nonpharmacologic interventions (Devine, 2003). Often, an intervention may fall into more than one category or subcategory.

When reviewing the nondrug techniques for use in palliative care, it useful to consider whether a specific intervention will need high or low levels of patient and caregiver involvement, and whether it is noninvasive or invasive. Some of the interventions, such as acupuncture, are invasive and should only be done by skilled practitioners. Because of this

and other factors, it may or may not be possible to facilitate use of some of the nondrug techniques in individuals with advanced disease. The Clinical Practice Guidelines for the Management of Cancer Pain Panel Consensus stated that "with rare exceptions, noninvasive approaches should precede invasive palliative approaches" (Jacox et al., 1994, p. 89).

PSYCHOLOGICAL INTERVENTIONS

A palliative care patient needs a biopsychosocial approach to pain management, one that includes the body, mind, and emotions. Incorporation of these elements into a patient's plan of care can lead to more effective pain management. Psychological interventions can help to do this. These interventions can primarily be classified as psychoeducational, cognitive, behavioral, or psychotherapeutic. They can include such things as patient and family education, distraction, self-statements, relaxation techniques, guided imagery and hypnosis, patient pain diaries, and cognitive-behavioral therapy (CBT). Devine's (2003) recent meta-analysis of the effects on pain of nonpharmacologic interventions, such as educational, psychosocial, and cognitive behavioral interventions in adults with cancer supported the use of the use of these interventions as an adjuvant to analgesic therapy. The Clinical Practice Guidelines for the Management of Cancer Pain Panel (Jacox et al., 1994) and the National Comprehensive Cancer Network (NCCN) Cancer Pain Guidelines both adults (2005a) and pediatrics (2005b) encourage the use of psychosocial interventions for pain management early in the course of disease, as part of a multimodal approach. The nurse who is caring for an individual with a life-threatening illness may find that this person is well versed in using specific psychological approaches and is open to using these techniques to aid in coping with pain and other symptoms. On the other hand, the person whom the nurse may be caring for may be too weak, debilitated, and cognitively impaired to be taught or even to use a simple, previously utilized, relaxation technique. Assessment is key to developing a realistic plan. The intervention must match the specific problem with an appreciation for the patient's abilities and motivations.

Psychoeducational

Patient and family education regarding pain management is an intervention that can increase an individual's sense of control. Ideally, at the end of life, patients, their families, and their caregivers will be well informed about pain management. However, the nurse working with these individuals often will find that this is not the case, especially in individuals who initially present with advanced disease. Whatever the circumstances, it is necessary to maintain ongoing assessment and reinforcement of educational information as the clinical situation and patient's needs change. Lack of knowledge regarding pain management is a well-established barrier to good pain control (McCaffery, 1999).

In the palliative care setting, especially for end-of-life pain management, the inclusion of family, supportive friends, and caregivers is essential. They too have important educational needs and their role in successful pain management cannot be underestimated. A study by Ferrell, Grant, Chan, Ahn, and Ferrell (1995) showed that a structured pain education program improved quality of life outcomes for both elderly patients and their family caregivers.

Knowledge regarding pain management (reviewed in chapter 12) should include pain and its etiology, the principles and methods of pain management, types of analgesics, potential side effects of analgesics and their management, equipment and devices used to deliver analgesics, the concepts of physical

dependence, tolerance, and addiction, non-pharmacologic interventions, and expected participation in pain management (Adelhardt et al., 1995). Recent work suggests that to implement a pain management regimen successfully at home, patients and families will also need other knowledge to assist them in problem solving to improve pain control. Challenges include obtaining and processing further information, obtaining prescribed analgesics, applying prescribed regimens to their very individual situation, managing new or changed pain, and managing side effects and other concurrently occurring symptoms (Schumaker et al., 2002b). Knowledge of how to approach these challenges will enable individuals and their families to be active, informed participants in the plan of care. Knowledge deficits related to pain management encompass all dimensions of learning: cognitive, psychomotor, and affective. It is especially important to allay fears and concerns about opioid use, specifically addiction, tolerance, and physical dependence (refer to chapter 12 for a review of these concepts). Individuals who need equipment to relieve their pain will need special opportunities for their families and them to practice with that equipment management (Adelhardt et al., 1995).

There are several well-developed references that elaborate on teaching pain management information to patients, families, and caregivers which can be useful to nurses (Ferrell et al., 1995; Grant & Rivera, 1995; McCaffery & Pasero, 1999a). Readers are encouraged to review these references for more detailed information. An evaluation of all learners prior to any educational efforts will help to determine priorities and focus efforts. It is best to wait until pain is adequately controlled before giving patients and their families too much information. Teaching sessions may need to be brief with the most important information presented first and continually repeated. A wide variety of written, audio, and CD learning tools on pain management are available to reinforce information. All educational efforts are to be documented. This will improve continuity of care and provide a mechanism for identifying continuing education needs (Grant & Rivera, 1995).

Ideal outcomes of a successful pain management educational intervention will include the patient, family, or caregivers being able to notify the physician, nurse practitioner, physician's assistant, or registered nurse of any new or unrelieved pain; change in pain location, quality, or intensity, and any side effects experienced; identify the cause of pain; state the rationale of the prescribed analgesic regimen; identify the medications, doses, route, frequency, and potential side effects of an analgesic regimen; if indicated, use equipment related to pain management properly (such as PCA pump); comply with the analgesic regimen, using nonpharmacologic methods appropriately; and express understanding of the differences between tolerance, physical dependence, and addiction.

A small study by Oliver, Kravitz, Kaplan, and Meyers (2001) compared standard educational instruction on controlling cancer pain to an individualized education and coaching session in the outpatient setting, and showed an improvement in average pain outcomes for those in the individualized educational and coaching group.

In 2003, Devine performed a meta-analysis on the effect of nondrug interventions such as educational, psychosocial, and cognitive-behavioral interventions on adults with cancer-related pain by reviewing 25 interventional studies published from 1978 through 2001. Six of these studies tested the effect of education. A homogeneous small-to-moderate statistically significant beneficial effect on pain was found. In her discussion Devine pointed out that with the widely accepted strong mandate to educate patients about

their pain and its management, there may not be much of a difference between experimental and control content (Devine, 2003).

A recent study of 64 patients with cancer-related pain and their primary caregivers was conducted to determine whether patients who were given access to continued information—either through a pain hot line or weekly provider-initiated follow-up calls for 1 month following the education program—had improved pain control during a 6-month follow-up period (Wells, Hepworth, Murphy, Wujcik, & Johnson, 2003). The basic pain management program that all study participants received included both structured and tailored components. Following this baseline education, all patient and caregiver study participants showed an improvement in knowledge and beliefs. The long-term outcomes of pain intensity, interference due to pain, analgesic adequacy, and relief from pain were not affected by continued access to pain information. It is important to note that the analgesic regimen of patients who had access to pain information was not adjusted by the nurse making the follow-up calls or by the hot-line respondent.

Education about pain and its management is an important component of any pain management plan. However, additional education without a systematic approach that addresses other barriers, such as inadequate analgesic titration or untreated side effects, may not enhance pain control (Wells et al., 2003). A recently developed program, the PRO-SELF pain control program "uses education along with repeated reinforcement, skill building, and ongoing nursing support to improve self-care pain management in patients with cancer and their family caregivers" (West et al., 2003). It has been successful in improving the management of cancer pain (Miaskowski et al., 2004).

A combination approach may be the wave of the future. The literature reveals four general categories that are useful in assisting patients with pain. These include (1) self-care management; (2) information, decision making, and problem solving; (3) communication with health care professionals; and (4) counseling and support (Given et al., 2004) Future work will evaluate whether this approach that combines education with ongoing nurse coaching and interactive nursing support may prove to be useful to patients and caregivers in other non-cancer pain populations and how to best enhance outcomes for patients and their families.

Cognitive

Cognitive interventions are often discussed under the topic of mind-body therapies, which are techniques whose goal is to enhance a person's mental ability to reduce symptoms and enhance function (Deng et al., 2004; Given et al., 2004). This discussion will cover the areas of distraction, self-statements, relaxation, guided imagery and hypnosis, which can be useful to individuals with pain at the end of their life.

Distraction is an intervention that focuses on the cognitive component of the pain experience, and is sometimes referred to as cognitive refocusing or attention diversion. This technique's goal is to divert attention "away from the sensation of pain to a neutral of pleasant stimulus" (Thomas & Weiss, 2000, p. 161). It is thought that because a person has a limited capacity for processing information, the individual who focuses on something other than the pain pays less attention to the pain and is distracted from the pain. This distraction can be passive or active (Fernandez, 1986). Passive distraction can include such things as listening to music, watching a ball game, or watching a movie. Listening to or watching tapes that are humorous to an individual should be considered. Rhiner and colleagues (1993) promote the use by patients of

a library of various musical and humorous choices when utilizing distraction as a nondrug treatment. Active distraction can include such things as mental problem-solving, singing, playing an instrument, or playing a video game.

Often, for distraction to be effective, its focus must be of interest to the individual. The distraction strategy for a particular individual will depend upon the individual's ability to concentrate and his or her energy level. At the end of life, one's energy level is not predictable. For example, an individual could start listening to recorded music but decide to make it a more active diversion by tapping out the rhythm and singing along. McCaffery and Pasero (1999b) review in-depth ways to assist patients effectively in using distraction. They suggest that effective distraction strategies should stimulate the four major sensory modalities of sound, sight, touch, and movement.

The use of distraction for short periods of time for such things as painful procedures is well established. Its use is thought to increase self-control and pain tolerance, and decrease pain intensity (Jacox et al., 1994; McCaffery & Pasero, 1999b; Rhiner, Ferrell, Ferrell, & Grant, 1993; Spross & Wolff Burke, 1995). It has been associated with positive mood and changes and decreases in pain intensity (McCaffery & Pasero, 1999). The use of distraction for chronic pain is more controversial. McCaffery and Pasero (1999), in their review of the literature, found that after using distraction, patients with chronic pain may experience more intense pain. It is uncertain why this occurs. It may be that distraction prevents the individual from recognizing that certain activities are causing more pain. Following the use of distraction, an individual may be fatigued, irritable, and more aware of the pain. Also, without education, family and caregivers may feel that the individual who is utilizing distraction does not have the pain or the degree of pain that he or she says. This can lead to a variety of negative situations, including a reluctance to administer analgesics.

Self-statements can be helpful in getting one through a painful experience. The use of self-statements is based on Bandura's theory of self-efficacy. This theory focuses on a person's beliefs regarding his or her ability to perform behaviors that will produce certain outcomes. It is hypothesized that a person's expectation of self-efficacy will determine "whether a person will initiate coping behavior, the amount of effort a person will put into it, and how long the person will persist in the face of obstacles" (Dunajcik, 1999, p. 501). Application of this theory involves teaching the patient methods the patient can use to lessen the severity of pain or improve the ability to cope with the pain. Practicing and reinforcement of these methods is important. A health care professional works in "coaching" the patient in the use of self- statements (Given et al., 2004)

All people carry on internal dialogues that both manifest and influence their belief systems. By becoming aware of the ongoing self-statements, one can gain insight into perceptions and appraisals. Once an appraisal is accessed, a determination is made concerning the helpfulness of the belief system. Clinicians can help patients to use cognitive coping statements to enhance adaptations and to counteract the maladaptive thought processes (Loscalzo, 1996).

Coping self-statements are devised to assist the patient in getting through a painful situation (Fernandez, 1986). For example, at the start of a pain flare, instead of focusing on the fear of the pain, a person is taught to say to himself or herself, "I've had this kind of pain before, I can keep it under control. I will do this and this. . . ." Another version of this technique is reframing or cognitive reappraisal. To use this, individuals are taught to be alert to negative thoughts they might be having and to replace them with more positive thoughts and images. Use of reframing can increase a person's sense of control. For example, instead of thinking, "I've had this kind of pain before and it was awful," an individual could say to himself or herself, "I've had this kind of pain before and it has gone away" (Jacox et al., 1994, p. 82).

Relaxation techniques utilize methods designed to produce a "state of relative freedom from both anxiety and skeletal muscle tension" (McCaffery & Pasero, 1999, p. 400) as an adjunct to pain treatment. These techniques are helpful for people whose pain experience causes them to feel out of control, those who will be experiencing procedures or activities that may be stressful or uncomfortable, and those who have successfully used relaxation techniques in the past, including meditation, yoga, and Lamaze. Through the use of relaxation techniques, a person can be taught behaviors to use independently or with other that counteract the physical, emotional, and behavioral changes produced by stressors and to maximize control and cope with stressful situations. The goal is to relax one's physical body and quiet one's mind (Layman-Goldstein & Altilio, 1993).

There are a few relative contraindications to the use of relaxation techniques. These include individuals with a history of posttraumatic stress disorder, or thought disorders such as dementia, delirium, or schizophrenia; heavily sedated individuals or those experiencing respiratory compromise; and individuals who are experiencing a pain emergency (Layman-Goldstein & Altilio, 1993; Schaffer & Yucha, 2004). Only experts who are very experienced and well-trained in the use of these techniques should work with individuals with respiratory compromise. The unavailability of these experts or the presence of contraindicated conditions may be a barrier to the use of relaxation techniques at the end of life for some patients. Also, bear in mind that individuals who never have incorporated relaxation into their lives may find trying to do so during a period of increased stress to be countertherapeutic (Rhiner et al., 1993). During a pain crisis, relaxation will not be effective and the patient will associate the technique with severe pain instead of the desired outcome, pain relief. It is important not to set up a situation where the patient makes the paired association of severe pain and relaxation techniques. To optimize the patient's learning and effective use of this technique, it is better to wait until the pain is under better control. If you are able to stay with a patient during a pain crisis, you could consider having the patient breathe with you (Layman-Goldstein & Altilio, 1993). Also of concern is the use of relaxation techniques in individuals with bradycardia or heart block because of the physiological effects of relaxation. These effects can include decreased pulse, blood pressure, respiratory rate, oxygen consumption, carbon dioxide production, and basal metabolism (Spross & Wolff Burke, 1995). These effects may interact synergistically to cause adverse physiological effects. Spross and Wolff Burke (1995) suggest that in the acute care setting clinicians do a pre- and postrelaxation exercise check on pulse and blood pressure when assisting patients with relaxation techniques.

The National Institutes of Health (NIH) Technology Panel evaluated the effects of relaxation on pain and sleep and provided strong evidence for the use of relaxation techniques to reduce pain. In its review, the panel divided relaxation techniques into brief and deep methods. In general, the brief methods take less time to acquire or practice. Very often brief methods are abbreviated forms of a corresponding deep method. The brief methods include deep breathing, focused breathing, paced respiration, and self-control. Deep methods include such techniques as progres-

sive muscle relaxation (PMR), autogenic training, and meditation. To use autogenic training, one is taught to imagine a peaceful environment and focus on a "heaviness in the limbs, warmth in the limbs, cardiac regulation, centering on breathing, warmth in the upper abdomen, and coolness in the forehead" (NIH Technology Assessment Panel, 1996, p. 314). The use of PMR involves the tensing and then relaxing in sequence of each of the 15 major muscle groups.

Health professionals may benefit from practicing relaxation techniques on themselves before attempting to assist patients in its use. It is useful to have beginning practitioners practice with each other to gain experience and to provide each other with feedback. In learning the technique, consider taping oneself. An exercise that a beginning practitioner can use with patients teaches focused breathing and can be taped so that the patient can use it whenever he or she wants (Layman-Goldstein & Altilio, 1993). In this way, patients and their families also may be conditioned to associate the clinician's voice with support, comfort, and emotional connection in future interactions (Loscalzo, 1996b). The reader is referred to several references that teach in detail the use of relaxation techniques (Benson, 1975; Copley Cobb, 1984; Loscalzo, 1996; Mast, Meyers, & Urbanski, 1987a, 1987b, 1987c; McCaffery & Pasero, 1999; Schaffer & Yucha, 2004, and chapter 2 of this text).

It is important to set the right tone before instructing individuals in relaxation techniques. Ideally, the environment should be as quiet and as calm as possible. This is often challenging, if not impossible, in hospital environments. How one enters the room, what one says, and how one communicates one's sense of competence is important. One may be able to influence a patient's sense of control and ability to cope. It is important when working with patient's families to calm them, increase their confidence, and engage them as collaborators.

Most relaxation techniques necessitate active patient involvement. However, McCaffery and Pasero (1999) describe specific techniques that utilize the patient as a passive recipient. These include superficial massage for relaxation, listening to music pleasing to the patient, and animal companion visits. These latter techniques may be effective when individuals are fatigued or are lacking the mental or physical ability to actively participate in relaxation techniques.

Guided imagery and hypnosis are related cognitive techniques used to manage pain. Spross and Wolff Burke (1995) define imagery as "a mental process that draws on any or all of the senses to create mental representations of reality in order to achieve a specific goal such as reducing pain" (p. 172). Fanning (1988) thinks of imagery as either process or end-result imagery in which one imagines the act of doing something (process) or achieving a desired end result. A state of positive expectancy regarding a problem is created by the belief that a successful solution exists, the confidence that the needed resources are available, and that the use of imagery will promote healing.

Imagery also can be useful when presented as incompatible or transformative (Fernandez, 1986). Incompatible imagery can be incompatible emotive imagery (imagery that evokes emotions such as anger, humor, or self-assertion, which are incompatible with pain) or incompatible sensory imagery (images of "pure" sensations that have no obligatory link to particular emotions, such as imagining a cold winter day while experiencing a "hot, burning" pain). Transformative imagery is designed to alter specific features of the pain experience.

Patients in a variety of situations can use imagery to cope with disease and gain control of their lives (Stephens, 1993). The most familiar use is to enhance treatment effects. Patients can also use imagery to distract themselves from the present, cope with limitations (such as immobility), and anticipate the future. The latter three are perhaps the most useful for patients with pain who can use imagery to regain control of negative thoughts (Spross & Wolff Burk, 1995). Stephens (1993) views imagery as influencing such potential outcomes as improving problem solving and role relations, increasing sense of control, and reducing anxiety. This, in turn, can influence things such as immune response, motor functioning, pain reduction, and wound healing.

Although imagery can be a very useful technique, it may not be helpful for all individuals. Individuals who are not candidates for imagery include those with a history of mental illness such as psychosis or those with dementia or delirium (a common problem at the end of life). Unstructured, free-flowing imagery can bring to the surface "intense, latent feelings and unconscious conflicts" (Stephens, 1993, p. 240). It is imperative to monitor an individual for distress, restlessness, or agitation during the use of imagery. Individuals need to be taught that they are in complete control of the situation at all times. If, for any reason, the imagery is unpleasant or distressing, they can simply open their eyes to stop the situation (Stephens, 1993).

A debriefing after the use of imagery can be helpful to identify what did or did not work and to determine how to proceed. Those who have positive experiences may wish to modify the original script to make it more effective. Some will want the therapist to create an audiotape for future use (Spross & Wolff Burke, 1995). Some clients who experience distress may be open to exploring the source of their feelings, some may not.

It is thought that the techniques of relaxation, imagery, and hypnosis do not differ empirically. For this reason, Syrjala, Donaldson, Davis, Kippes, and Carr (1995) relabeled hypnosis as "relaxation and imagery" in order to facilitate patient acceptance of their study entitled "Relaxation and imagery and cognitive-behavioral training reduce pain during cancer treatment: A controlled clinical trial." In this study, it was found that "relaxation and imagery," or hypnosis, reduced cancer treatment-related pain.

Hypnosis involves "achieving an intense state of relaxation, or trance" that enables one to receive suggestions to alter the individual's thoughts, feelings, sensations or behavior (Thomas & Weiss, 2000, p. 161). This state of being can be used "to manipulate the perception of pain" (Jacox et al., 1994, p. 186). It was found by the Management of Cancer Pain Guideline Panel to have the highest strength and consistency of evidence supporting its use. Historically, hypnosis is well established in the treatment of pain. It both induces deep relaxation and redirects the patient's attention away from his or her pain (Cleeland, 1987). Healthy, intact individuals vary in their ability to utilize hypnosis. Debilitated individuals who are at the end of life may have less than their usual ability to utilize hypnosis, making it suitable for even fewer. Hypnosis should only be done by specially trained professionals and will not be reviewed here in greater depth. It is important that entry into practice and advanced practice students are aware of the value of hypnosis and consider making a referral to a trained professional if hypnosis is something that a patient wishes to explore.

Behavioral

A *pain diary* is a tool that is especially useful for the ambulatory population of patients. Clinicians can review this diary with patients over the phone, at home, or on clinic visits. Its use facilitates pain assessment, evaluation of pain management interventions, and need for further education (Grant & Rivera, 1995). It can be as simple or as sophisticated as the patient using it. The amount of information included often is a reflection of the patient's energy level. Essential information includes date and time of events, medication, dose of medication, and pain intensity before and after interventions. It is helpful if patients include their activities, periods of rest and sleep, pain quality, mood, and other symptoms, but this is up to the individual patient. Some prefer to use preprinted forms provided by pharmaceutical companies or other sources, whereas others prefer to use their computer or a Palm Pilot, or a simple spiral notebook. A pain diary can give a patient a sense of control and puts words to feelings that they can share with the family and others. These diaries have been shown to be helpful in heightening awareness of pain, facilitating communication, guiding pain management actions, and improving sense of control (Schumacher et al., 2002a). A recent randomized crossover study found that patients used an electronic diary more frequently than a paper pain diary. Patients in this study felt using the electronic pain diary led them to a more regular intake of their medicine. The reason for this may be related to the messages they received from the study manager that were generated by each log in, or from the built-in acoustic memory function (Gaertner, Elsner, Pollmann-Dahmen, Radbruch, & Sabatowski, 2004). The impact of technology on the use of patient pain diaries is evolving and merits further study.

Patients with advanced disease at some point may be unable to maintain a pain diary. Often their caregivers can be encouraged to record some of the basic information. Use of a pain diary can help patients or family members identify pain management barriers and successes. Use of this tool can assist some in gaining a sense of control in an over-whelming situation (Grant & Rivera, 1995) and promote communication (Schumacher et al., 2002a). Successful use of this tool requires patient and family education and reinforcement of its use and use of collaborative reviews.

Psychotherapeutic

Fishman (1992) writes of the experience of self-disintegration faced by individuals with advanced disease who are often dealing with the frustration of personal and interpersonal needs and aspirations while dealing with multiple symptoms and aggressive cancer treatments. The experience of total pain can add to an individual's sense of fear, anger, anxiety, hopelessness, and helplessness.

Cognitive behavior therapy (CBT) was originally developed by psychologists to treat anxiety, stress, and depression, using some of the psychoeducational, cognitive, and behavioral techniques previously described. Cognitive behavioral therapy has been used to treat individuals in a variety of situations with the goal of therapy based upon the situation. For the individual with cancer-related pain, the goal of CBT is to enhance the sense of self-efficacy or personal control (Fishman & Loscalzo, 1987).

CBT can be done in a variety of formats, including individual or group sessions (Thomas & Weiss, 2000). It works best in a series of structured sessions that are flexible and modifiable, according to the developing needs of the individual, no matter what the format. Fishman and Loscalzo (1987) suggest that there be clear and explicit goals for both the series of sessions and for each individual session. These goals are to be developed collaboratively by therapist and patient. Together, they will look at the range of problems present and prioritize them. This list will be reviewed on a regular basis and reprioritized as personal, social, and medical changes develop. Based on this list, appropriate interventions to address these problems will be determined. The purpose of the interventions is to resolve specifically defined current problems, not long-term personality and social relations disturbances. Also, the interventions are to be made in a standard and systematic manner. The use of this flexible, adaptive collaboration is designed to enhance the patient's sense of self-control and sense of coherent purpose (Fishman & Loscalzo, 1987; Thomas & Weiss, 2000). Certain individuals and their families are more receptive to CBT than to traditional psychological approaches, which they may view as too intrusive (Loscalzo, 1996). CBT, a psychotherapeutic approach, provides a structure that some clinicians find useful, in which to collaborate with patients and their families to apply the nondrug psychological interventions to a pain management plan.

Ideally, work with CBT occurs early in the treatment phase of an illness. As disease progresses, an individual may experience cognitive impairment from a variety of causes that make it impossible to employ psychology. It may be necessary to focus more on the family and caregivers as the disease progresses. In this situation, the goal still would be to maximize their coping skills and increase their sense of control.

Cognitive behavioral therapy, a pragmatic psychological approach, and its techniques can be taught to interested clinicians who do not have specialized training in psychology or psychopathology. Nurses and social workers often obtain training in the use of some of these techniques. In an article aimed at the non-mental-health clinician, Fishman and Loscalzo (1987) review the principles and application of CBT. Realistically, the beginning staff nurse may be able to learn and apply the specific techniques of relaxation and distraction. More training would be needed for the use of CBT and the techniques of guided imagery and hypnosis and structured support. Often the nurses who have expertise in using these techniques are advanced practice nurses, especially psychiatric clinical nurse specialists. The practice setting dictates what is possible. A busy, noisy inpatient unit may limit use of some techniques. Often the knowledge that a patient may benefit from CBT and a timely referral to a skilled practitioner are the most that can be achieved.

Techniques that tailor cognitive behavioral approaches to individual patients (Dalton & Coyne, 2003; Dalton, Keefe, Carlson, & Youngblood, 2004) and those that combine education with ongoing nurse coaching and interactive nursing support build upon the foundation of CBT. Research that evaluates the effectiveness of these approaches may lead to better assistance to individuals who choose to control their response to pain and suffering.

PHYSIATRIC INTERVENTIONS

Physiatric interventions are another kind of nondrug intervention that can be helpful in the pain management plan. These interventions include positioning and movement, application of modalities such as heat, cold, vibration, and massage, and the use of supportive orthotic devices. Physical rehabilitation professionals are the experts in the use of physiatric interventions. The fact that pain is disabling is well established. Palliation and rehabilitation are not incompatible (Cheville, 1999). No matter what the goals of care are, the input from a physical rehabilitation expert may be useful to help the individual achieve his or her fullest physical, psychological, social, vocational, avocational, and educational potential (Dietz, 1982). The rehabilitation expert looks at an individual with cancer-related disability from four rehabilitation perspectives: (1) preventive, to minimize the effects of predictive disabilities; (2) adaptive, to assist the individual to adapt to definite changes; (3) maintenance, that is, maintaining the individual at the current level of functioning; and (4) palliative rehabilitation, keeping the individual functioning and involved in the environment. For nurses to set realistic, achievable goals with the patient with pain, it is useful to consider these four possibilities.

Positioning and Movement

A debilitated individual with pain may be in static positions for extraordinary lengths of time. This in itself can exacerbate existing pain or produce new pain, including pressure sores and painful joint conditions. Healthy individuals are unconsciously and continuously initiating pain-relieving movements. A nurse can assist patients and their caregivers to promote positions or postures that maintain or facilitate normal physiologic function of the musculoskeletal system. When properly done, positioning places minimal stress on the joint capsule, tendons, and muscle structure (Spross & Wolff Burke, 1995). Basic nursing texts give thorough overviews of the basic principles of positioning and movement that are so essential to good nursing care at the end of life.

Patients who experience pain with movement may need to be premedicated prior to positioning. Care must be taken with patients who have bone disease and a high risk of pathologic fractures. An individual's pain or anxiety should not be increased with positioning. Although repositioning can be a helpful intervention to decrease pain, it may be appropriate to do it less often as death nears if the patient experiences significant discomfort from this activity.

For the palliative care patient who is not so close to death, range of motion (ROM), either active (AROM), active assisted (AAROM), or passive (PROM) can promote comfort and maintain or restore the integrity of muscles, ligaments, joints, bones, and nerves used in movement. It is hoped this will in turn prevent the development of additional complications. An individual who lacks the energy for AROM may attempt AAROM or PROM (for the patient who is neurologically impaired or unconscious). McCaffery and Wolff (1992) have written a useful review of the use of cutaneous modalities, positioning, and movement to facilitate pain relief in the hospice population.

Supportive Orthotic Devices

In attempting to decrease pain and increase functioning, it may be helpful to consult with a physical therapist or rehabilitation-medicine physician to evaluate the possible use of a supportive orthotic device such as a splint, sling, brace, or corset. Their use can immobilize or provide support to painful tissues and maximize the use of weakened tissues to promote functioning. Appropriate use of such a device may decrease incident or mechanical-type pain for certain patients (Dunajcik, 1999; Tunkel & Lachmann, 1998). Also, the use of certain devices for patients with bone metastasis may immobilize areas of potential fractures to prevent this painful complication (Jacox et al., 1994).

Assistive devices such as canes, walkers, and wheelchairs when appropriately used can promote mobility, decrease pain, and prevent injury (Tunkel & Lachmann, 1998). Consulting with a rehabilitative specialist to obtain the correct assistive device for an individual patient and teaching the patient and the caregivers the proper use of such devices can be invaluable. Often, an evaluation of the home situation will be necessary to recommend the most appropriate device to maximize an individual's rehabilitation efforts.

Other modalities, such as the application of heat, cold, vibration, and massage, also fall under the heading of physiatric methods. Some would argue that these techniques actually are neurostimulatory because of their activation of the large diameter nerve fibers. The gate control theory proposed that activation of the large diameter fibers inhibited the smaller "pain" fibers and closed the gate to the transmission of stimuli by smaller nerve fibers. These techniques frequently are referred to as cutaneous stimulation. As more information about the underlying mechanisms of pain has become known, the gate control theory gradually has been replaced. However, the actual mechanisms that affect pain relief from cutaneous stimulation are unclear. Most of the cutaneous interventions are thought to counteract the effects of decreased oxygen and accumulated metabolites associated with musculoskeletal pain and to promote superficial increases in circulation (Spross & Wolff Burke, 1995). These methods are thought possibly to reduce pain, inflammation, and muscle spasm. They are noninvasive, relatively low cost, easy to use, and often can be done by the patients themselves or by their caregivers (Jacox et al., 1994). To provide pain relief, these modalities can be applied directly over the site of pain, proximally to the site of pain, distally to the site of pain, or contralaterally to the site of pain (McCaffery & Pasero, 1999).

Superficial heating or cooling can cause a decrease in sensitivity to pain. There is a lack of well-controlled studies concerning the use of heat and cold. Most of the information discussed is based on clinical experiences presented in the literature. Despite the lack of firm evidence, the Management of Cancer Pain Guideline Panel recommends the offering of cutaneous stimulation techniques, such as applications of superficial heat and cold, to alleviate pain (Jacox et al., 1994). Patients with aching muscles, muscle spasm, joint stiffness, low back pain, or itching may benefit from the use of superficial heating or cooling. Their use seems to be most effective for well-localized pain (McCaffery & Passero, 1999). It is important to consider patient safety and comfort when using these interventions. This method should not be used with patients who have bleeding disorders, or pains such as causalgia (which are characterized by a hypersensitivity to touch); or in areas with recent injury, broken skin, open wounds, or skin where a patient is receiving radiation therapy (Jacox et al., 1994; McCaffery & Pasero, 1999; Spross & Wolff Burke, 1995). Sites proximal, distal, or contralateral should be considered if the area of pain is contraindicated. Cold should not be used if an individual has a history of peripheral vascular disease (such as Raynaud's disease), connective tissue disease, or reports an "allergy" to cold. Often, those who report an allergy to cold may experience an asthma attack upon exposure to cold air (Bailey, 1999). Heat should not be used with topical menthol products because of the potential for tissue damage (Jacox et al., 1994; McCaffery & Pasero, 1999; Spross & Wolff Burke, 1995).

Most hospitalized individuals will need an order or institutional protocol before initiation of superficial heating or cooling. There are several convenient ways of utilizing these modalities for palliative patients. For example, cold application can be done safely using gel packs that are kept in the refrigerator, homemade cold packs (sealed plastic bags filled with 1/3 alcohol and 2/3 water placed in freezer), or 1-lb. bags of frozen peas or corn (which have been hit gently to separate contents). Heat can be administered by heating pad, hot packs, immersion in water, or retention of body heat with plastic wraps. Care must be taken with both modalities to protect the skin with at least a layer of terry cloth or pillowcase. Moisture increases the intensity of the heat or cold. Patients are to be discouraged from lying on heat sources. The skin

must be inspected at regular intervals for irritation, swelling, blistering, excessive redness that does not subside between treatments or bleeding. Some patients develop a "hunting reaction," in which the skin alternatively blanches and turns red after the application of cold. If this occurs, the use of cold should be immediately discontinued. Extreme vigilance is necessary for patients with impaired or decreased sensation, cognitive impairment, or who are unconscious and may be considered a relative contraindication. Treatment should be discontinued if the patient asks or if pain or any form of skin irritation occurs (Jacox et al., 1994; McCaffery & Pasero, 1999; Spross & Wolf Burke, 1995).

Research is lacking concerning the frequency and duration of such treatments. McCaffery and Pasero (1999) suggest a trial and error approach that is individualized to the patient. They suggest that a minimal effective duration for application of hot or cold is 5 to 10 minutes with the usual duration 20 to 30 minutes. The decision to use heat or cold will depend upon the patient's situation. When compared to heat, cold often relieves more pain and relieves it faster. Often, pain relief from cold will last longer. Cold can either relieve or exacerbate joint stiffness. Evaluation of each situation is necessary. It may be useful to alternate between heat and cold. The duration of application may be as short as 5 to 10 seconds or 3 minutes of heat, and then alternating to 1 minute of cold for a period of 20 to 30 minutes (McCaffery & Pasero, 1999; Spross & Wolff Burke, 1995).

Individuals often will need education on the use of superficial heat and cold as a pain-relieving measure. Educational information that is useful in teaching patients and their family members and caregivers about the use of superficial heat and cold for pain relief can be found in several sources (McCaffery & Pasero, 1999; Rhiner et al., 1993).

Although helpful for some painful situations, methods of applying deep heat, diathermy, microwave diathermy, and ultrasound, will not be discussed in detail here. It is thought that they increase blood flow and metabolic rate even more than superficial heat does,. Methods that deliver deep heat must be used with caution in patients with active cancer and are not to be used over areas of active tumor (Jacox et al., 1994; Tunkel & Lachmann, 1998). Also, methods that deliver deep heat may be fairly challenging to use with palliative care patients who have advanced disease. Consultation with a physiatrist would be necessary when considering the use of deep heat.

Massage, another form of cutaneous stimulation, uses touch in the various forms of pressure, friction, and vibration to muscle and connective tissue, potentially to reduce pain and tension, improve circulation, promote relaxation (Deng et al., 2004), and communicate care and concern, especially in patients who have a communication impairment or language barrier. In a nondrug intervention program for pain relief, 63% of cancer patients selected massage/vibration as a nondrug intervention for pain relief (Rhiner et al., 1993). It is thought to decrease pain by increasing superficial circulation and, in some situations, by relaxing muscles. Studies that utilized massage in ill populations showed that brief massages are tolerated and safe (Bauer & Dracup, 1987; Meek, 1993; Tyler, Winslow, Clark, & White, 1990). The National Center for Complementary and Alternative Medicine (NCCAM) recommends massage for refractory cancer pain (Berenson, 2005). A 3-year study of 1,290 cancer patients receiving massage therapy showed a decrease in various symptom severity from pre- to postmassage symptom assessment, including a 40.2% improvement in pain (Cassileth

& Vickers, 2004). A smaller massage study that utilized 41 hospitalized oncology patients also showed statistically significant outcomes for pain (Smith, Kemp, Hemphil, & Vojir, 2002). A meta-analysis of the effects of back-rub effleurage suggests that patient comfort and relaxation is enhanced by a simple 3-minute back rub. Also, positive changes were demonstrated on heart rate, blood pressure, and respiratory rate. Some variables, such as gender, length of massage, and environmental conditions seem to play a role in effectiveness (Labyak & Metzger, 1997). Further research may look at psychological, physiological, and molecular mechanisms that play a role in the central nervous pathways involved (Esch, Guarna, Bianchi, Zhu, & Stafano, 2004).

Massage is contraindicated over sites of tissue damage (such as open wounds or tissue undergoing irradiation), in patients with bleeding disorders or thrombophlebitis, patients uncomfortable with touch, or those who might misinterpret touch as sexual (although this might be acceptable if the massager was a spouse or close partner). In working with cancer patients, light pressure is best and deep or intense pressure is to be avoided (Berenson, 2005; Deng et al., 2004). When considering massage, it is important for the nurse to consider the patient's comfort with touch, previous experiences with massage, and preferred techniques (Spross & Wolff Burke, 1995).

Massage to the site of pain may or may not serve to decrease pain at that site. Palliative care patients may not be up to an extensive massage, but may find massage of limited sites beneficial and not requiring much effort on their part. For example, massage of the neck, back, or shoulders may be sufficient to promote comfort. Some may find this too strenuous. For these patients, the nurse could consider massage to the hands or feet. Massage movements can include rhythmic strok-ing, kneading or circular, distal-to-proximal movements. Effleurage, using slow, smooth, long strokes, is usually done to promote re-laxation. The patient should be involved in choosing the sites and massage movements that provide the most comfort along with how long the massage should last. It may be helpful to try different types of strokes with varying degrees of pressure in an effort to find what is most effective for an individual (Jacox et al., 1994; McCaffery & Pasero, 1999; Spross & Wolff Burke, 1995). The patient may be sitting in a chair, or lying on his or her side, or prone on a bed or table. It is helpful to determine with the individual if the room will be quiet, if music will be played, or if conversation will take place during the mas-sage (McCaffery & Wolff, 1992).

During the actual massage, ideally both the nurse and patient will be as relaxed as pos-sible. The patient should be in a position that is supported and easy to maintain for the du-ration of the massage. The massager should be in a position that utilizes good body me-chanics. Patient comfort and modesty are to be maintained with sheets, blankets, or tow-els. The use of a warmed, alcohol-free lotion will decrease friction. One hand should be on the patient at all times until the massage is over. For example, the right hand could be-gin its stroke as the left hand is completing its stroke. Removing both hands can commu-nicate to the patient that the massage is over. Patients may fall asleep during massage (Mc-Caffery & Pasero, 1999; McCaffery & Wolff, 1992). Feedback from the patient, if possible, is useful for future planning. If patients find massage helpful, it should be scheduled on a regular basis. Massage can be quite comfort-ing to dying patients who are often deprived of human touch at the end of life. Family members and caregivers may wish to be in-structed or included in this pain-relieving in-tervention. They should be taught to use the techniques that the patient found to be most helpful (McCaffery & Pasero, 1999). Others who are overwhelmed may find this a burden, one more thing for them to do.

Vibration is a form of massage that passes fine tremors either electrically (using a vi-brator) or manually (using one's hands) to the skin (Spross & Wolff Burke, 1995). It is thought to increase superficial circulation and stimulate large-diameter fibers (Jacox et al., 1994). It should not be used over sites overlying tumor, where skin has been injured, on areas of thrombophlebitis, with patients who bruise easily, or for migraine headache or headache that is worsened by sound or move-ment (McCaffery & Passero, 1999). Vibration can be used for itching, muscle spasm, neu-ropathic pain, phantom pain, and tension headache. It can be used as a substitute for TENS (McCaffery & Pasero, 1999; McCaffery & Wolff, 1992; Spross & Wolff Burke, 1995). One can vary the effect by varying the pres-sure of vibration. When applied with light pressure, its results are similar to massage. Moderate pressure vibration may act to re-lieve pain by causing numbness, paresthesia, or anesthesia to the stimulated area (McCaf-fery & Pasero, 1999).

Electric vibrators can be either hand-held or stationary. Some are battery powered and some are plugged into an electrical outlet. Many have at least two frequencies, high (100 to 200 Hz) and low (10 to 50 Hz); some have a heat-delivery option. Although the high set-ting is often the more effective frequency, it is advised to try the low frequency initially. De-pending on the site of pain, some patients are able to administer the vibrator themselves. Use of the vibrator, like other cutaneous stimula-tion interventions, is often a trial and error situation with the site and duration of treat-ment up to the patient (McCaffery & Pasero, 1999; Spross & Wolff Burke, 1995). One study looked at the duration of poststimulatory pain relief resulting from brief (1 to 15 minutes) treatments and longer (30 minutes). The relief from the brief intervention was brief whereas the longer treatment resulted in prolonged relief (Lundeberg, Nordeman, & Ottoson, 1984). In most institutional settings, use of a vibrator will require an order from the health care provider (McCaffery & Pasero, 1999).

NEUROSTIMULATORY INTERVENTIONS

Transcutaneous electrical nerve stimulation (TENS) has been defined as "a method of producing electroanalgesia through electrodes applied to the body" (Jacox et al., 1994, p. 188). The TENS system is a small battery-operated device that is attached by cables to electrodes taped to the skin overlying a nerve. Initiation requires an order from the health care provider. Patients with musculoskeletal, arthrogenic, or neurogenic pain may benefit from the use of TENS. It should not be used with patients who are unable to communicate its effects. It is contraindicated in individuals with demand-type pacemakers. Those who have a history of epilepsy, transient ischemia attacks, strokes, epilepsy, or myocardial disease should not have the TENS electrodes placed on the head, neck, or chest. The electrodes should not be placed over the site of tumors, near the carotid sinus, or directly on the eye. The TENS unit should be started by a health care professional who is trained in its use and who will be able to take the time to instruct the patient in its use. Patients should be informed that it may take various adjustments to the TENS settings, electrode placements, and duration of treatment to find the most effective settings. Their feedback is essential in this process. A body chart can be used to document these trials easily (Spross

& Wolff Burke, 1995). Thompson and Filshie (1998) describe the use of TENS in detail.

Use of a *spinal cord stimulator*, a more invasive technique that acts on sympathetic fibers is usually not indicated in an actively dying patient. However, patients with neuropathic pain, such as postherpetic neuralgia pain or postthoracotomy pain, may benefit from this technique. Nurses caring for these individuals who are at the end of life and have permanently implanted spinal cord stimulators may need to become knowledgeable about this technique (Miguel, 2000).

INVASIVE INTERVENTIONS

Invasive interventions can be considered for a small percentage of palliative patients whose pain cannot be adequately controlled by pharmacologic means. This population includes individuals whose pain is localized to one or two areas and is expected to persist, and who cannot achieve an acceptable balance between analgesia and intolerable, dose-limiting side effects from these analgesics.

In evaluating patients for invasive approaches, it is important to clarify that all feasible primary therapies that are likely to improve patient outcomes have been initiated, that the opioid dose has been titrated up to the maximal tolerated dose, that side effects have been treated with appropriate medication therapy or through opioid rotation, that appropriate adjuvant analgesics have been considered or tried, and that the appropriate routes of drug administration have been instituted. Other patient-related factors to assess include presence of active infection, coagulopathy or use of anticoagulant drugs, coexisting medical conditions that increase risks (Cherney, Arbit, & Jain, 1996), functional status (Arbit & Bilsky, 1998), and the potential rapidity of tumor growth in areas unaffected by the neurodestructive intervention (Schroeder, 1986). Also to be considered is "the likelihood and duration of analgesic benefit, the immediate and long-term risks, the likely duration of survival, the availability of local expertise, and the anticipated length of hospitalization" (Cherney et al., 1996, p. 128).

Neurodestructive procedures should be considered irreversible with potentially irreversible side effects (Schroeder, 1986). A dying, bed-bound patient may be willing to accept the possible disabilities of motor weakness, loss of bowel or bladder functions, or loss of position sense as a reasonable exchange for adequate pain relief. However, hope for life, especially a "normal" one, frequently continues in those who are dying. An ambulatory patient is rarely receptive to the possibilities of these side effects (Swarm & Cousins, 1998).

Neural blockade is an anesthetic intervention for either temporary or permanent effect and is commonly called a nerve block. A local anesthetic (usually lidocaine or bupivacaine) is injected into or around a nerve. Nerve blocks can be considered diagnostic, prognostic, therapeutic, or preemptive/prophylactic. A *diagnostic nerve block* is done to determine the specific pain pathway and to aid in the differential diagnosis. A *prognostic nerve block* is one that is done to predict the efficacy of a permanent ablating procedure. A *therapeutic nerve block* is done to provide temporary pain relief in a pain crisis or to treat painful conditions that respond to these blocks (e.g., a celiac block for the relief of pain due to pancreatic cancer). A *preemptive/ prophylactic nerve block* is done proactively to prevent the development of a chronic pain syndrome. Neurolysis is a permanent procedure that interferes with the transmission of a painful stimulus by injection of a chemical substance such as alcohol or phenol to destroy or ablate the nerve (Saberski, 1998).

A successful prognostic nerve block may not always mean a successful neurolysis. This may be due to such things as analgesic and sedating premedications, placebo response, spread of local anesthetic to adjacent neural structures, or systemic absorption of local anesthetics. Also, patients near the end of their lives may be unwilling or unable to undergo two blocking procedures, the prognostic followed by the neurolysis. In this situation, the anesthesiologist may decide on a neurolytic procedure without a preceding prognostic block (Swarm & Cousins, 1998). Contraindications to an individual undergoing a nerve block includes infection, coagulopathies, ineffective prognostic block, inadequate patient and family preparation, patient refusal, inability to understand and sign informed consent, and inability to cooperate during the procedure. The use of ultrasound guidance—a more recent development that allows the anesthesiologist to position the needle more accurately and monitor the distribution of the local anesthetic medication—has improved both safety and efficacy of neural blockade (Marhofer, Greher, & Kapral, 2004; Marhofer, Sitzwohl, Greher, & Kapral, 2004).

General types of neural blockade are peripheral blocks (including brachial plexus, and cranial, intercostal, and sacral nerves), neuroaxial blocks (including epidural and intrathecal), and sympathetic nerve blocks (including celiac plexus block and superior hypogastric block) (Swarm & Cousins, 1998). Specific nerve blocks are identified by the anatomical location where they are performed. Depending on the location of the block, some of the risks or complications include fatigue, oversedation (if analgesics are not decreased in relation to decreased pain), sensory loss, motor weakness, altered bowel and bladder function, altered sexual function, intravascular injection, hematoma, and new pain. If sufficient denervation occurs from a somatic block, for example, a deafferentation pain will result. It is estimated that 14% to 30% of individuals undergoing peripheral neurolytic blockade may develop neuropathic pain as a result (Swarm & Cousins, 1998). Side effects from nerve blocks can include Horner's syndrome, characterized by constricted pupil, ptosis, "and decreased sweating resulting from interruption of the sympathetic pathways to the eye" (Goldberg, 1983, p. 86); numbness, weakness, increased warmth, diarrhea, and lowered blood pressure. These effects are temporary if done with a local anesthetic, or long-lasting or permanent, if done with alcohol or phenol (as with a neurodestructive block). It is the responsibility of nurses caring for individuals undergoing these procedures to be knowledgeable about the side effects and alert to developing complications. Readers are encouraged to review the work of de Leon-Casasola (2000); Miguel (2000); Cherny et al., (1996); Saberski (1998); Schroeder (1986); Swarm and Cousins (1998); and Eisenberg, Carr, and Chalmer (1995) for more detailed information on neural blockade.

Cordotomy is a neuroablative neurosurgical procedure that involves making a lesion in the anterior spinothalamic tract, contralaterally to the pain site, either percutaneously or with an open surgical approach, to destroy the function of a portion of the particular spinothalamic tract that innervates the site of pain. The spinothalamic tract is important in several ways. Pain and temperature for the contralateral side of the body is mediated through the anterior spinothalamic tract. The area for superficial pain is found in the superficial area of this tract and the area for deep visceral pain and temperature is found in the deeper area (Arbit & Bilsky, 1998). Deliberate damage to the spinothalamic tract through a neuroablative procedure will affect the dermatomal area innervated by the selected level. Preservation of proprioception and power is often possible with cordotomy, but the level of analgesia may tend to decrease over time (Cherney et al., 1996).

Cordotomy is most successful in patients with unilateral pain below C-5 (Arbit & Bilsky, 1998; Saberski, 1998). Cordotomy is indicated in pain that is unresponsive to other therapy in patients with a life expectancy of less than 1 year (Saberski, 1998; Sanders & Zuurmond, 1995). Because of a variety of factors, including progressive disease, it is difficult to ascertain its actual success rate. It is thought that in skilled hands, complete pain relief immediately after cordotomy is as high as 60% to 80% (Saberski, 1998). As time progresses, pain relief drops, possibly due to progression of disease and the resulting development of new pain. Saberski (1998) and Sanders and Zuurmond (1995) discuss the possibility of developing a delayed postcordotomy dysesthesia, "a condition in which a disagreeable sensation is produced by ordinary stimuli" following a lesion in a peripheral or central pathway (Stedman, 1995, p. 531, 1995). Arbit and Bilsky (1998) estimate that 1% of patients can develop postcordotomy dysesthesia anytime after the cordotomy, even more than a year later. For this reason, it is advised to avoid this procedure in individuals with an extended life expectancy (Arbit & Bilsky, 1998).

Sometimes the relief of one pain by cordotomy unmasks a new or mirror pain in the ipsilateral side. Prior to the procedure, the patient may not be aware of this pain because of the overwhelming contralateral pain. Sometimes, the nociceptive components of a pain may be successfully relieved but not the neuropathic components (Arbit & Bilsky, 1998; Nagaro et al., 2001). A study by Sanders and Zuurmond (1995) demonstrated the effectiveness and safety of percutaneous cervical cordotomy in terminally ill cancer patients. Complications following cordotomy can include dysfunction of autonomic respiration, sleep apnea,

Horner's syndrome, arterial hypotension, hemiparesis (usually transient), and bladder dysfunction (Arbit & Bilsky, 1998). As with neural blockade, the use of CT for guidance in percutaneous cordotomies can help to increase effectiveness and decrease complications of both unilateral and bilateral percutaneous cordotomies (Yegul & Erhan, 2003). The function of the ipsilateral diaphragm can be impaired by cordotomy (Saberski, 1998). Patients with pulmonary disease on the contralateral side of the cordotomy are at risk for respiratory decompensation. It is recommended that patients undergo pre-operative pulmonary function tests to help identify individuals at increased risk. Bilateral cordotomy is associated with a higher risk of sleep apnea, respiratory compromise, and arterial orthostatic hypotension. These conditions may or may not be transient and self-limiting. Their presence is thought to be a major contributing factor to mortality following bilateral procedures. Because of this, the presence of a low ejection fraction or significant preexisting heart disease contraindicates the use of the bilateral procedure (Arbit & Bilsky, 1998). The unilateral percutaneous cordotomy is the preferred procedure. When bilateral lesions are necessary, the open approach may be indicated (Saberski, 1998). As a safety measure, Arbit and Bilsky (1998) suggest waiting at least 1 week between cordotomies to assess for the development of respiratory compromise from unilateral lesions. Sometimes, open cordotomy is done if the percutaneous procedure is not available, or if a patient is unable to lie supine for a percutaneous procedure (Saberski, 1998). An individual's ability to tolerate the actual procedure plays a role in what is done. Often, patients with advanced disease may be unable to tolerate multiple sessions to alleviate pain. Ideally, the neurosurgeon can make the most of a single opportunity to relieve the pain (Arbit & Bilsky, 1998). In recent years, invasive neurosurgical approaches have been used less frequently and replaced by neuromodulatory approaches; however, for select patients, neurosurgical approaches can be most useful (De Conno, Panzeri, Brunelli, Saita, & Ripamonti, 2003; Meyerson, 2001). A detailed review of other neurosurgical interventions for pain can be found in Giller (2003).

INTEGRATIVE INTERVENTIONS

In reviewing integrative interventions, it may be helpful to consider the five major classifications or domains used by the National Center for Complementary and Alternative Medicine (NCCAM). These are alternative medical systems, mind-body interventions, biologically based therapies, manipulative and body-based methods and energy therapies. The following review will include useful evidence-based techniques for pain management at the end of life from all of the NCCAM classifications except from the biologically based therapies. Acupuncture, mind-body therapy, and massage therapy are shown in studies to have the strongest evidence for their clinical use in pain control (Deng et al., 2004).

Alternative Medical Systems

Acupuncture, a treatment from Traditional Chinese Medicine (TCM), has been shown to treat pain, depression, nausea, and other health problems effectively (Deng et al., 2004; NIH Consensus Conference, 1998). In this holistic, energy-based approach, thin, disposable needles, usually stainless steel, are placed in precise anatomical points (365 specific locations) to balance energy movement along the body's 12 meridians (Berenson, 2005; Decker, 2000). *Acupressure* is the application of finger pressure to the acupuncture points. *Moxibustion* is the stimulation of an acupuncture point by heat. This is done by burning a special compressed combustible substance near the acupuncture point. Other variations in acupuncture stimulation of sites include the use of electrical stimulators or lasers. The NIH Consensus Development Panel on Acupuncture (1998) found that the incidence of adverse effects from acupuncture is substantially lower than for many standard medical procedures or medications used for the same conditions. Adverse effects from acupuncture can include an occasional drop of blood or bruise at the needle insertion site, mild discomfort at site, infection, or, depending on insertion site, pneumothorax. The latter two effects are rare and depend on the experience and training of the acupuncturist (Berenson, 2005).

In TCM, it is thought that good health depends on the balance of energy in the body. Energy—called *chi* or *qi,* is thought to be constantly circulating in the body. Acupuncture acts to promote circulation of chi or qi vital energy. Acupuncture is based on a holistic, energy-focused approach to individuals, not on a disease-oriented, diagnostic treatment approach. The fact that acupuncture causes a multitude of biological responses has been demonstrated clearly. Much work is currently underway to understand better the anatomy and physiology of the acupuncture points (NIH Consensus Conference, 1998). Western medicine considers the proposed mechanisms of action for pain relief by acupuncture to include endorphin release, mediation of pain-producing neurotransmitters, and stress-induced analgesia (Berenson, 2005; Spross & Wolff Burke, 1995).

In their review of the data, the NIH Consensus Development Panel on Acupuncture (1998) stated that at present the "data in support of acupuncture are as strong as those for many accepted Western medical therapies" (p. 1520). At present, there is fairly convincing data showing the effectiveness of acupuncture in postoperative dental pain, and in adult postoperative and chemotherapy nausea and vomiting. Some studies indicate that it may be helpful as an adjunct treatment in painful situations such as headache, menstrual cramps, fibromyalgia, myofascial pain, osteoarthritis, and low back pain. Its effectiveness in relieving musculoskeletal pain remains controversial (Deng et al., 2004). Controlled studies using acupuncture in palliative care patients are in the process of devopment. In this population, it may be both difficult and controversial to implement an acupuncture study comparing acupuncture to placebo or sham under controlled conditions, utilizing standardized outcomes. Ideally, as more research is done and acupuncture is further incorporated into the mainstream health care system, more informed decisions regarding the appropriateness of acupuncture for patients in varying situations will be made (NIH Consensus Panel, 1998). As health care professionals, it is important to guide patients from a perspective of evidence, not marketing.

More and more patients are seeking acupuncture treatments. Acupuncture is gaining more practitioners with Western medicine backgrounds and more general support from Western practitioners. Along with others, some nurses are going through extensive training to become licensed practitioners of acupuncture. Issues of training, licensure, and accreditation are in the process of being clarified. In the United States, educational standards have been developed for the training of physician and nonphysician practitioners. An agency recognized by the U.S. Department of Education has accredited many of the acupuncture educational programs. Physician acupuncturists can sit for a nationally recognized exam. Nonphysician acupuncturists can sit for an entry-level competency exam that is offered by a national credentialing

agency. Unfortunately, there is much variation from state to state. This includes differences in the requirements to obtain licensure
and in the titles conferred. This variation
leads to confusion and to less confidence in
the qualifications of acupuncture practitioners. It is important that nurses be aware
of the requirements and titles conferred in
the states in which they practice, in order to
guide patients who desire a TCM evaluation
for acupuncture to the most qualified, safe
practitioners (NIH Consensus Panel, 1998).

A more detailed discussion of acupressure and acupuncture is beyond the scope of
this text. Nurse educators desiring to include
more information of these techniques in the
nursing curriculum are encouraged to seek
out licensed practitioners of acupuncture for
collaboration. Some schools of nursing have
faculty who are also licensed acupuncturists.
At this time, most insurance policies do not
cover acupuncture or other integrative approaches, and most patients and families have
to pay out of pocket for these interventions.

Mind-Body Interventions

Music has been shown to be an effective intervention for pain control through a variety of physiological and psychological effects.
Affective, cognitive, and sensory processes can
be engaged, activated, and altered by music.
This is done by processes such as use of prior
skills, relaxation, distraction, alteration of
mood, and improved sense of control. Physical
effects include increasing or decreasing pulse
and blood pressure (Magill-Levreault, 1993;
Tuls Hallstead & Tuls Roscoe, 2002). Music
therapy, as defined by Spross and Wolff Burk
(1995), is "the scientific and systematic use of
music to effect beneficial changes in physiological and psychological processes that influence
experiences of pain and illness" (p. 175). The
use of music therapy in the medically ill can
reduce mood disturbance (Cassileth, Vickers,

& Magill, 2003) and affect the suffering and
total pain that a sick individual experiences.

In using music with an individual, one
needs to evaluate the patient's medical situation, general mood state, coping abilities,
degree of isolation, and prior musical experiences, in addition to the total pain experience.
People may be music listeners, music eventers, or music performers. By understanding
someone's prior musical experiences and integrating it into music therapy, the intervention
will provide opportunities to regain a sense of
identity and sense of control. As with distraction, the use of music can be a passive or an
active experience. The level of involvement often will be related to the energy status of the
individual (Magill-Levreault, 1993).

Music listeners can use audiotapes to promote distraction and relaxation and to alter
mood disturbances such as anxiety, depression, fear, anger, and sadness; and to promote
spiritual connecting and facilitate communication with others (Magill-Levreault, 1993;
Tuls Halstead & Tuls Roscoe, 2002). Music
eventers are those who may view music as a
backdrop to significant life events. Especially
for these individuals, the use of familiar songs
can assist in reminiscing, life review, and
opening communication between patients
and others. Music performers, depending
on their condition, can participate in music
by tapping out rhythms with their fingers,
conducting, or actually performing (Magill-Levreault, 1993). Tuls Halstead and Tuls
Roscoe (2002) offer nurses many concrete examples of how to use music to assist listeners,
eventers, and performers.

Music therapists are especially effective in
this type of work, facilitating personal growth
and enhanced self-expression. Often, they are
able to select and perform songs that initially
matches the mood and needs of a patient and
then use the music as a catalyst to mobilize
feelings and open communication (Magill-
Levreaul, 1993). Involvement of significant

others is encouraged, if the patient desires. In the clinical situation, one should be aware of a patient's personal music preference. Not all types of music are considered universally pleasant (Magill-Levreault, 1993; McCaffery & Pasero, 1999; Spross & Wolff Burke, 1995). A patient's needs may change daily. Because of this, the music selection is best done with the individual on a day-to-day basis. "The aim is always to promote comfort, healing, and a decreased sense of pain. Working in collaboration with other pain modification approaches, music therapy can help soothe pain as well as heal the suffering" (Magill-Levreault, 1993, p. 45). Schroeder-Sheker (1994) explores the use of music in the actively dying.

The cognitive interventions discussed earlier under the umbrella of psychological interventions, such as relaxation, guided imagery and hypnosis, also fall under the NCCAM category of mind-body methods that may be helpful to the individual with pain.

Manipulative and Body-Based Methods

The use of massage, a manipulative mind-body technique, is covered under the physiatric intervention section as a cutaneous stimulation technique. However, readers desiring to learn more about the use of massage may also find information from integrative or complementary and alternative medicine sources (Berenson, 2005; Deng et al., 2004).

Energy Therapies

Therapeutic touch (TT) is a complementary technique based on systems theory of the multidimensional nature of the individual and the homeostatic concepts of balance and wholeness, which work with energy fields in promoting relaxation states, reducing pain, and promoting healing. It was developed by Dolores Krieger, a nurse physiologist, in con-

junction with Dora Kunz, a healer (Owens & Ehrenreich, 1991a).

Despite its name, TT does not involve physical touching. It involves a conscious intention on the part of the healer to help the client (Spross & Wolff Burke, 1995). The practitioner of TT first centers himself or herself in the here and now. Then the practitioner does an assessment of the client's energy field for symmetry by placing his or her hands 4 to 6 inches from the body, starting at the head and moving towards the feet. The energy field is then "unruffled" by the practitioner's performing sweeping motions of the hands to smooth out the energy field. During the next phase, the treatment phase, the practitioner channels energy to areas of the field that the practitioner senses are imbalanced or void. Finally, in the last phase, reassessment, the energy field is reevaluated for repatterning of energy flow (Owens & Ehrenreich, 1991b).

Use of this technique for palliative patients who are interested may be useful because it involves no effort or expenditure of any energy on the part of the patient. Patients who are debilitated do not have to learn new skills at a time when they may be unable to do so. Also, there do not seem to be any adverse effects. It is thought to promote a profound relaxation response that alleviates the pain (Berenson, 2005). Anecdotal evidence suggests that TT can be a beneficial adjunct to traditional therapies (Kotora, 1997). A study that looked at the desire for serenity by persons nearing death and nursing interventions to facilitate this state found that pain control, TT, and assisting clients to build trust were the three highest ranked interventions both in the frequency of use and in effectiveness (Messenger & Roberts, 1994).

The research base to support the use of TT in clinical practice is not solid. A recent meta-analysis of TT research found that there are many approaches to TT and that the TT practices vary from study to study. These factors may lead to less convincing conclusions when evaluating the effectiveness of TT as a modality. Although a number of studies had mixed or negative results, most studies supported the hypotheses regarding the efficacy of TT (Winstead-Fry & Kijek, 1999). One study (Giasson & Bouchard, 1998) looked at the effect of TT on the well-being of individuals with terminal cancer, and the results showed a positive increase in the sensations of well-being following three TT treatments. Well-being was measured using the Well-Being scale, a visual analog scale that measures pain, nausea, depression, anxiety, shortness of breath, activity, appetite, relaxation, and inner peace (Giasson & Bouchard, 1998). Some of the proponents of TT feel that even if it is determined that TT is basically taking advantage of a placebo effect, this is still a beneficial adjuvant nursing intervention from a holistic nursing point of view. Meehan (1998) expresses the thought that "the potential of TT to enhance the placebo phenomenon requires further exploration but should not be discounted in seeking to relieve discomfort and distress and facilitate healing" (p. 117).

Therapeutic touch has been taught and researched since the 1970s. However, in recent years, its use has become more controversial. Some feel that TT should be treated as a religious practice. This would require new approaches to the practice and teaching of TT in nursing (Bullough & Bullough, 1998). Mainstream American medicine is unconvinced about the value of TT. In 1998, one study was published in the very major mainstream *Journal of the American Medical Association*. It concluded that because 21 experienced practitioners of TT were unable to detect the investigator's "energy field" at a rate greater than chance, there was unrefuted evidence that the "claims of TT were groundless and that further professional use is unjustified" (Rosa, Rosa, Sarner, & Barrett,

1998, p. 1005). Some question the validity of this study and the biases inherent in the peer review. However, because this was published in a leading peer-reviewed medical journal, many in mainstream Western medicine are unsupportive of the use of TT. Eskinazi and Muehsam (1999) point out that conventional journals may have difficulty evaluating integrative techniques fairly because some of the concepts implicit in these techniques are outside the current biomedical framework. Often, information and opinions presented by mainstream medicine may be misinformed or based on a misunderstanding of an area of alternative medicine. It is important to explore knowledge outside the existing dogmas to promote real progress (Eskinazi & Muehsam, 1999).

Reiki is another energy therapy. This therapy is currently being studied to evaluate its role in symptom management, including that of pain. Reiki is defined as a vibrational or subtle energy most commonly facilitated by light touch whose use is thought to balance the biofield and strengthen the body's ability to heal itself. Reiki practitioners gently place their hands on a fully clothed individual's head, back, front, and the site of discomfort (if the person desires) to promote relaxation and decrease pain (Berenson, 2005). A recent phase 2 study of Reiki in the management of pain in individuals with advanced cancer showed no overall reduction in opioid use, but did show improved pain control and improved quality of life using this safe, noninvasive intervention (Olson, Hanson, & Michaud, 2003).

Complementary services are being offered more frequently to patients at the end of life. A recent hospice survey found that 60% of 169 hospices offered complementary therapies to patients (Demmer, 2004). Massage therapy and music therapy, which are shown to have a positive effect on pain, were among the most popular. Barriers to providing integrative interventions were mostly limited to program constraints. These included lack of knowledge regarding these therapies, and how to offer them. Lack of qualified staff and funding problems also played a role.

HOW TO INTEGRATE NONDRUG INTERVENTIONS INTO A COMPREHENSIVE PAIN MANAGEMENT PLAN

A successful pain management plan is based on a comprehensive pain assessment and incorporates the components of treating underlying disease, pharmacologic interventions, psychological intervention, physiatric interventions, neurostimulatory interventions, invasive interventions, and integrative interventions. At the end of life, it may or may not be appropriate or feasible to treat underlying disease. Certainly, the patient with advanced disease may not be able to tolerate a surgery to remove a pain-producing tumor. Yet, some interventions aimed at treating underlying disease may be useful. For example, palliative radiation to areas of bony metastases may be well tolerated and decrease bone pain (Jacox et al., 1994). Pain caused by infection, such as pelvic abscess or occult infections from ulcerating tumors, may be relieved by treatment with appropriate antibiotics (Cherny & Portenoy, 1994b). The importance of pharmacological interventions, the mainstay of pain relief at the end of life, and how to integrate these interventions into the pain management plan have been well described in the previous chapter.

As part of the interdisciplinary team caring for a patient at the end of life, it is important for the nurse to understand how the nondrug interventions (psychological, physiatric, neurostimulatory, invasive, and integrative) are incorporated into the pain management plan. The availability of experienced consultants to perform certain interventions

also plays a role. If no one is available to perform a specific intervention, it cannot be offered as an option in the pain management plan for that individual at that point in time. A palliative care team may need to work on system issues to improve access to specialists that may be helpful to their patients. The use of any intervention is based upon the assessment of the patient. It is important to evaluate the individual carefully and apply what is appropriate for that individual in a particular situation. After the initiation of systemic analgesic therapy and treatment of underlying disease (if appropriate), the next step would be to consider the addition of psychological, physiatric, neurostimulatory, or integrative techniques to improve control and possibly improve the balance between analgesia and side effects (Cherny & Portenoy, 1994b; Rhiner et al., 1993). If these measures prove to be suboptimal, the consideration of the use of invasive techniques is appropriate (Cherny & Portenoy, 1994a; Miguel, 2000). Finally, if it is impossible to find the balance between pain relief and side effects, then sedation at the end of life (as described in chapter 12) must be considered. Figure 13.1 shows the flow of this process.

THE ROLE OF NURSES IN IMPLEMENTING NONDRUG INTERVENTIONS

Nurses caring for patients at the end of life have both collaborative and independent functions in implementing nondrug interventions. First, nurses must be aware of which interventions they are able to perform. Factors to consider when making this determination include education in the use of particular techniques, comfort in teaching or implementing a particular technique, patient and family educational materials available, availability and affordability of specific necessary devices

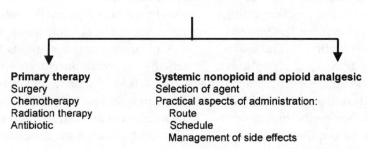

Comprehensive Assessment

Primary therapy
Surgery
Chemotherapy
Radiation therapy
Antibiotic

Systemic nonopioid and opioid analgesic
Selection of agent
Practical aspects of administration:
    Route
    Schedule
    Management of side effects

If balance between pain relief and side effects is suboptimal, consider . . .

Noninvasive strategies to improve balance between analgesia and side effects
Reduce opioid requirement:
    Appropriate primary therapy
    Addition of nonopioid analgesic
    Addition of adjuvant analgesic
    Use of cognitive or behavioral techniques
    Use of an orthotic device or other physical medicine approach
Switch to another opioid

If balance between pain relief and side effects is suboptimal, consider . . .

Invasive strategies to improve balance between analgesia and side effects
Regional analgesic techniques (spinal or intraventricular opioids)
Neural blockade
Neuroablative techniques

If balance between pain relief and side effects is suboptimal, consider . . .

Role of sedating pharmacotherapy

FIGURE 13.1   A strategy for the management of cancer pain.

From Cherney, N. I., & Portenoy, R. K. (1994). The management of cancer pain. *Ca: A Cancer Journal for Clinicians,* *44*(5), p. 263. (Reprinted with permission.)

and materials, and time available to an individual nurse to initiate a particular intervention. Psychological interventions that an individual nurse must be comfortable initiating include patient and family education, and ideally cognitive interventions such as distrac-tion, self-statements, brief-method relaxation techniques, and behavioral interventions such as a pain diary. Physiatric interventions that an individual nurse might initiate for an end-of-life patient's pain control could include positioning and movement, use of superficial heat or cooling, massage, or vibration. (Depending on the practice setting, the nurse may need to obtain orders for some of the physiatric interventions.) The use of music, an integrative technique, may also be initiated by an individual nurse. If the nurse has had additional training, he or she may consider the use of therapeutic touch, deep relaxation methods, or cognitive behavioral therapy. In addition, the nurse needs to know which members of the immediate primary team can perform nondrug interventions that may be useful as part of a comprehensive pain management plan. Also to be determined is the availability of special consultants, such as neurosurgeons, anesthesiologists, hypnotherapists, or acupuncturists, for consultation and intervention as necessary. The nurse may need to assist in making appropriate referrals to these consultants. Finally, as part of the team, it may be necessary to educate other team members about the efficacy of nondrug methods so that these techniques can be integrated more efficiently into the pain management plan (Rhiner et al., 1993).

Only after it is determined who is capable and available to teach or perform a particular nondrug intervention can the nurse and his or her team realistically consider its use for an individual patient based upon the pain assessment. As with the pharmacological interventions, the nondrug interventions need to be directed at etiologic factors. For example, when applied with moderate pressure, vibration, a physiatric modality can help to relieve pain by decreasing sensation to a painful area and may act to decrease tension in muscles (Rhiner, Ferrell, Ferrell, & Grant, 1993). This would make this approach a useful addition to the pharmacologic regimen already in place for an individual found to have pain from muscle spasm.

It is also important to consider whether a patient or the family has the physical, mental, or emotional energy necessary to participate in a particular intervention. Nondrug interventions that need a high level of patient involvement may not be possible when an individual is debilitated. Assessment needs to include a patient's ability to concentrate and follow directions, level of fatigue, and cognitive status (McCaffery & Pasero, 1999). Also include in the assessment an individual's previous experience and attitude towards nondrug interventions (McCaffery & Pasero, 1999; Rhiner et al., 1993). Determine which methods may be not useful because of religious or cultural issues or concerns or because they counter an individual's usual coping style (McCaffery & Pasero, 1999).

The next step is active collaboration by the nurse with the patient to choose a nondrug intervention that may be useful (Spross & Wolff Burke, 1995). As with CBT, it is useful to review with the patient the pain-related problems present, assign priorities to the problems, focus on the priority problems, set goals, and implement an intervention designed to address the priority problem (Fishman & Loscalzo, 1987). As part of this process, the nurse needs to be aware of what is realistically possible with the individual patient at that moment in time, given his or her medical condition (Loscalzo, 1996). Spross and Wolff Burke (1995) recommend focusing on only one or two nondrug interventions at a time. At this point, the patient's family, friends, and caregivers need to be asked if they wish to be involved in the nondrug intervention (McCaffery & Pasero, 1999; Spross & Wolff Burke, 1995). Some will want to be actively involved, and others will feel too overburdened (McCaffery & Pasero, 1999). Obstacles to the use of the selected nondrug intervention will need to be anticipated along with the development of strategies to overcome these obstacles (Spross & Wolff Burke, 1995).

Patient, family, and caregiver education follows. Even if the patient's family, friends, or caregivers are not actively involved, they will need information about the role of the nondrug intervention in the pain management plan (Spross & Wolff Burke, 1995). This helps to elicit their cooperation and promote successful use of the intervention (Rhiner et al., 1993). Written and audio materials that reinforce verbal information are useful (McCaffery & Pasero, 1999; Spross & Wolff Burke, 1995). It is important to emphasize that nondrug interventions are not a replacement for analgesics (McCaffery & Pasero, 1999). Patients and their families will need opportuni-

ties to develop skills using the nondrug intervention (Spross & Wolff Burke, 1995). Ideally, they actually will be able to use the intervention with the nurse present before utilizing it independently.

It is useful to debrief a patient and the caregiver following the use of a nondrug intervention. In this debriefing, the effect on pain and other outcomes and the need for more assistance should be assessed (Spross & Wolff Burke, 1995). If a nondrug intervention is assessed to be ineffective, then it should be modified or replaced (Spross & Wolff Burke, 1995).

EDUCATION PLAN 13.1   Plan for Achieving Competencies: Nondrug Management of Pain

Knowledge Needed	Attitudes	Skills	Undergraduate Behavioral Outcomes	Graduate Behavioral Outcomes	Teaching/Learning Strategies
Nondrug interventions for pain management: —Benefits —Development of scientific evidence regarding efficacy of nonpharmacological agents.	*Verify the use of nonpharmacological interventions as complementary therapies to the pharmacological management of pain. *Support the use of nonpharmacological interventions that have been empirically validated as effective in pain management.		*Critique scientific research to determine the value and appropriate utilization of nonpharmacological interventions in pain management.	*Participate in research studies to determine the efficacy of nonpharmacological interventions in the pain management, particularly related to palliative care.	*Conduct a review of the research literature to analyze the efficacy of various nonpharmacological interventions in pain management. Present the findings in a written paper or class presentation.

Nondrug Interventions for Pain Management: • Psychological; • Psychiatric; • Neurostimulatory; • Invasive; • Integrative.	*Respect patients' opinions, preferences, and desires/requests regarding nonpharmacological interventions for pain management.	*Demonstrate skill in the administration of select nonpharmacological interventions for pain management.	*Educate patients and families, and other health professionals about nonpharmocological approaches to pain management, including techniques, benefits, and contraindications. *Accurately and appropriately administer basic nonpharmacological interventions for effective pain management, such as education, distraction, self-statements, relaxation techniques, guided imagery, use of a pain diary,	*Accurately and appropriately administer advanced nonpharmacological interventions for effective pain management, such as hypnosis, cognitive behavioral therapy, and accupressure if educationally prepared. *Advocate for the availability of specialists who are prepared to administer selected nonpharmacological interventions for pain management.	*Invite a guest speaker to class to discuss and demonstrate selected nonpharmacological interventions for pain management. *Demonstrate selected nonpharmacological interventions with a return demonstration by students/nurses. Discuss the experience as the provider and recipient of the intervention.

(continued)

EDUCATION PLAN 13.1   *(continued)*

Knowledge Needed	Attitude	Skills	Undergraduate Behavioral Outcomes	Graduate Behavioral Outcomes	Teaching/Learning Strategies
			positioning, movement, supportive and assistive devices, heat and cold, massage, vibration, use of TENS unit, music therapy, and therapeutic touch. *Seek referral to appropriate specialists for nonpharmacological interventions for pain management.	*Develop a comprehensive plan of care that includes the use of pharmacological and non-pharmacological therapies for pain management.	*View the video series available through the Holistic Nurses Association, which discusses and demonstrates various nonpharmacological interventions. *Based on case studies, evaluate the appropriateness of a pain management plan utilizing nonpharmacological interventions based on type of illness, etiology of pain, pain history and assessment, patient preference, health status, and goals of care.

*In the clinical setting, implement a plan of care for pain management of a select patient utilizing nonpharmacological interventions. In postconference, discuss the barriers to the use of nonpharmacological interventions, the patient's response to the intervention, side effects experienced by the patient, and recommended changes, if needed, in the plan of care.

REFERENCES

Adelhardt, J., Byrnes, M., Derby, S., Holritz, K., Layman-Goldstein, M., Racolin, A., et al. (1995). *Care of the patient in pain: Standard of oncology nursing practice.* New York: Memorial Sloan-Kettering Cancer Center.

Arbit, E., & Bilsky, M. H. (1998). Neurosurgical approaches in palliative care. In D.

Doyle, G. W. C. Hanks, & N. MacDonald (Eds.), *Oxford textbook of palliative medicine* (2nd ed., pp. 414–420). Oxford, UK: Oxford University Press.

Baily, P. P. (1999)*Asthma.* In T.M. Buttaro, J. Trybulski, P. P. Bily, & J. SandbergCook (Eds.), Primary care: a collaborative practice (pp. 283–308). St Louis: Mosby.

Bauer, W. C., & Dracup, K. A. (1987). Physiological effects of back massage in patients with acute myocardial infarctions. *Focus Critical Care, 14*(6), 42– 46.

Benson, H. (1975). *The relaxation response.* New York: William Morrow.

Berenson, S. (2005). Complementary and alternative therapies in palliative care. In B. R. Ferrell & N. Coyle (Eds.). *Textbook of palliative care nursing.* New York: Mosby.

Bullough, V. L., & Bullough, B. (1998). Should nurses practice therapeutic touch? Should nursing schools teach therapeutic touch? *Journal of Professional Nursing, 14,* 254–257.

Cassileth, B. R., Vickers, A. J., & Magill, L. A. (2003). Music therapy for mood disturbance during hospitalization for autologous stem cell transplantation: A randomized controlled trial. *Cancer, 98,* 2723–2729.

Cassileth, B. R., & Vickers, A. J. (2004). Massage therapy for symptom control: Outcome study at a major cancer center. *Journal of Pain and Symptom Management, 28,* 244–249.

Cherny, N. I., Arbit, E., & Jain, S. (1996). Invasive techniques in the management of cancer pain. *Hematology/Oncology Clinics of North America, 10,* 121–137.

Cherny, N., & Portenoy, R. K. (1994a). Sedation in the management of refractory symptoms: Guidelines for evaluation and treatment. *Journal of Palliative Care, 10,* 31–38.

Cherny, N. I., & Portenoy, R. K. (1994b). The management of cancer pain. *Ca: Cancer Journal for Clinicians, 44,* 262–303.

Cheville, A. L. (1999). Cancer rehabilitation and palliative care. In Conference Course Syllabus Abstract of *Cancer rehabilitation in the new millennium: Opportunities and challenges* (pp. 125–128). R. Payne & A.L. Cheville, course directors. New York: Memorial Sloan-Kettering Cancer Center.

Cleeland, C. S. (1987). Nonpharmacological management of cancer pain. *Journal of Pain and Symptom Management, 2*(2), S23–S28.

Copley Cobb, S. (1984). Teaching relaxation techniques to cancer patients. *Cancer Nursing, 7,* 157–161.

Dalton, J. A., & Coyne, P. (2003). Cognitive-behavioral therapy: Tailored to the individual. *Nursing Clinics of North America, 38,* 465–476.

Dalton, J. A., Keefe, F. J., Carlson, J., & Youngblood, R. (2004). Tailoring cognitive-behavioral treatment for cancer pain. *Pain Management Nursing, 5*(1), 3–18.

De Conno, F., Panzeri, C., Brunelli, C., Saita, L., & Ripamonti, C. (2003). Palliative care in a national cancer center: Results in 1987 vs. 1993 vs.2000. *Journal of Pain and Symptom Management, 25,* 499–511.

de Leon-Casasola, O. A. (2000). Critical evaluation of chemical neurolysis of the sympathetic axis for cancer pain. *Cancer Control, 7,* 142–148.

Decker, G. M. (2000). An overview of complementary and alternative therapies. *Clinical Journal of Oncology Nursing, 4*(1), 49–52.

Demmer, C. (2004). A survey of complementary therapy services provided by hospices. *Journal of Palliative Medicine, 7,* 510–516.

Deng, G., Cassileth B. R., & Simon Yeung, K. (2004). Complementary therapies for cancer-related symptoms. *Supportive Oncology 2*, 419–429.

Devine, E. C. (2003). Meta-analysis of the effect of psychoeducational interventions on pain in adults with cancer. *Oncology Nursing Forum 30*(1), 75–89.

Dietz, H. (1982). *Rehabilitation oncology.* New York: Wiley.

Dunajcik, L. (1999). Chronic nonmalignant pain. In M. McCaffery & C. Pasero (Eds.), *Pain: Clinical manual* (2nd ed., pp. 467–521). St. Louis, MO: Mosby.

Eisenberg, E., Carr, D. B., & Chalmer, T. C. (1995). Neurolytic celiac plexus block for treatment of cancer pain: A meta-analysis. *Anesthesia and Analgesia, 80*, 290–295.

Esch, T., Guarna, M., Bianchi, E., Zhu, W., & Stefano, G. B. (2004). Commonalities in the central nervous system's involvement with complementary medical therapies: Limbic morphinergic processes. *Medical Science Monitor 10*(6), MS6–MS17.

Eskinazi, D., & Muehsam, D. (1999). Is the scientific publishing of complementary and alternative medicine objective? *Journal of Alternative and Complementary Medicine, 5*, 587–594.

Fanning, P. (1988). *Visualization for change.* Oakland, CA: New Harbinger.

Fernandez, E. (1986). A classification system of cognitive coping strategies for pain. *Pain, 26*, 141–151.

Ferrell, B. R., Grant, M., Chan, J., Ahn, C., & Ferrell, B. A. (1995). The impact of cancer pain education on family caregivers of elderly patients. *Oncology Nursing Forum, 22*, 1211–1218.

Fishman, B. (1992). The cognitive behavioral perspective of pain management in terminal illness. *Hospice Journal, 8*(1–2), 73–88.

Fishman, B., & Loscalzo, M. (1987). Cognitive-behavioral interventions in management of cancer pain: Principles and applications. *Medical Clinics of North America, 71*, 271–287.

Gaertner, J., Elsner, F., Pollmann-Dahmen, K., Radbruch, L., & Sabatowski, R. (2004). Electronic pain diary: A randomized crossover study. *Journal of Pain and Symptom Management, 28*, 259–267.

Giasson, M., & Bouchard, L. (1998). Effect of therapeutic touch on the well-being of persons with terminal cancer. *Journal of Holistic Nursing, 16*, 383–398.

Giller, C. A. (2003). The neurosurgical treatment of pain. *Archives of Neurology, 60*, 1537–1540.

Given, C., Given, B., Rahbar, M., Jeon, S., McCorkle, R., Cimprich, B., et al. (2004). Effect of a cognitive behavioral intervention on reducing symptom severity during chemotherapy. *Journal of Clinical Oncology, 22*, 507–516.

Goldberg, S. (1983). *Clinical neurology made ridiculously simple.* Miami, FL: MedMaster.

Grant, M. M., & Rivera, L. M. (1995). Pain education for nurses, patients, and families. In D. B. McGuire, C. Henke Yarbro, & B. R. Ferrell (Eds.), *Cancer pain management* (2nd Ed.) (pp. 289–319). Boston: Jones and Bartlett Publishers.

Jacox, A., Carr, D. B., Payne, R., Berde, C. B., Breithart, W., Cain, I. M., et al. (1994). *Management of cancer pain. Clinical Practice Guideline No. 9.* (AHCPR Publication No. 94–0592). Rockville, MD: Agency for Health Care Policy and Research, U.S. Department of Health and Human Services, Public Health Services.

Kotora, J. (1997). Therapeutic touch can augment traditional therapies. Oncology Nursing Forum, *24*(8), 1329–1330.

Labyak, S. E. & Metzger, B. L. (1997). The effects of effleurage back rub on the physiological components of relaxation: a meta-analysis. *Nursing Research, 46*(1), 59–62.

Layman-Goldstein, M., & Altilio, T. (1993). *Cancer pain: Cognitive and behavioral* approaches to cancer pain management-relaxation training [video script]. New York: Memorial Sloan-Kettering Cancer Center.

Loscalzo, M. (1996). Psychological approaches to the management of pain in patients with advanced cancer. *Hematology/Oncology Clinics of North America, 10,* 139–155.

Lundeberg, T., Nordeman, R., & Ottoson, D. (1984). Pain alleviation by vibratory stimulation. *Pain, 20*(1), 25–44.

Magill-Levreault, L. (1993). Music therapy in pain and symptom management. *Journal of Palliative Care, 9*(4), 42–48.

Marhofer, P., Greher, M., & Kapral, S. (2005). Ultrasound guidance in regional anaesthesia. *British Journal of Anaesthsiology, 94*(1), 7–17.

Marhofer, P., Sitzwohl, C., Greher, M., & Kapral, S. (2004) Ultrasound guidance for infraclavicular brachial plexus anaesthesia in children. *Anaesthesia, 59*(7), 42–46.

Mast, D., Meyers, J., & Urbanski, A. (1987a). Relaxation techniques: A self-learning module for nurses: Unit I. *Cancer Nursing, 10,* 141–147.

Mast, D., Meyers, J., & Urbanski, A. (1987b). Relaxation techniques: A self-learning module for nurses: Unit II. *Cancer Nursing, 10,* 217–225.

Mast, D., Meyers, J., & Urbanski, A. (1987c). Relaxation techniques: A self-learning module for nurses: Unit III. *Cancer Nursing, 10,* 279–285.

McCaffery, M., & Wolff, M. (1992). Pain relief using cutaneous modalities, positioning, and movement. *Hospice Journal, 8,* 121–154.

McCaffery, M. (1999). Pain management: Problems and progress. In M. Caffery & C. Pasero (Eds.), *Pain: Clinical manual* (2nd ed., pp. 1–14). St. Louis, MO: Mosby.

McCaffery, M., & Pasero, C. (1999a). *Pain: Clinical manual.* (2nd ed). St Louis, MO: Mosby.

McCaffery, M., & Pasero, C. (1999b). Practical nondrug approaches to pain. In M. McCaffery & C. Pasero (Eds.), *Pain:*

Clinical manual (2nd ed., pp. 399–427). St. Louis, MO: Mosby.

Meehan, T. C. (1998). Therapeutic touch as a nursing intervention. *Journal of Advanced Nursing, 28,* 117–225.

Meek, S. S. (1993). Effects of slow stroke back massage on relaxation in hospice clients. *Image: Journal of Nursing Scholarship, 25,*(1) 17–21.

Messenger, T., & Roberts, K. T. (1994). The terminally ill: Serenity nursing interventions for hospice clients. *Journal of Gerontological Nursing, 20*(11), 17–22.

Meyerson, B.A. (2001). Neurosurgical approaches to pain treatment. *Acta Anaesesiologica Scandinavica, 45,* 1108–1113.

Miaskowski, C., Dodd, M., West, C., Schumacher, K., Paul, S.M., Tripathy, D., & Koo, P. (2004). Randomized clinical trial of the effectiveness of a self-care intervention to improve cancer pain management. *Journal of Clinical Oncology, 22,* 1713–1720.

Miguel, R. (2000). Interventional treatment of cancer pain: The fourth step in the World Health Organization analgesic ladder? *Cancer Control 7,* 149–156.

Nagaro, T., Adachi, N., Tabo, E., Kimura, S., Arai, T., & Dote, K. (2001). New pain following cordotomy: Clinical features, mechanisms, and clinical importance. *Journal of Neurosurgery, 95,* 425–431.

National Comprehensive Cancer Network. (2005a). NCCN Clinical Practice Guidelines in Oncology: Adult Cancer Pain, Version 2. 2005. Retrieved from http://www.nccn.org on September 22, 2005.

National Comprehensive Cancer Network. (2005b). NCCN Clinical Practice Guidelines in Oncology: Pediatric Cancer Pain, Version 1. 2005. Retrieved from http://www.nccn.org on September 22, 2005.

National Institutes of Health Technology Assessment Panel on Integration of Behavioral and Relaxation Approaches into the Treatment of Chronic Pain and Insomnia.

(1996). Integration of behavioral and re-laxation approaches into the treatment of chronic pain and insomnia. *Journal of the American Medical Association, 276,* 313–318.

National Institutes of Health Consensus Conference. (1998). Acupuncture. *Journal of the American Medical Association, 280,* 1518–1524.

Oliver, J. W., Kravitz, R. L., Kaplan, S. H., & Meyers, F. J. (2001). Individualized patient education and coaching to improve pain control among cancer patients. *Journal of Clinical Oncology, 19,* 2206–2212.

Olson, K., Hanson, J., & Michaud, M. (2003). A phase II trial of Reiki for the manage-ment of pain in advanced cancer patients. *Journal of Pain and Symptom Management, (26)* 990–997.

Owens, M. K., & Ehrenreich, D. (1991a). Literature review of nonphamacologic methods for the treatment of chronic pain. *Holistic Nursing Practice, 6*(1), 24–31.

Owens, M. K., & Ehrenreich, D. (1991b). Ap-plication of nonphamacologic methods of managing chronic pain. *Holistic Nursing Practice, 6*(1), 32–40.

Rhiner, M., Ferrell, B. R., Ferrell, B. A. & Grant, M. M. (1993). A structured non-drug intervention program for cancer pain. *Cancer Practice, 1,* 137–143.

Rosa, L., Rosa, E., Sarner, L., & Barrett, S. (1998). A close look at therapeutic touch. *Journal of the American Medical Associa-tion, 279,* 1005–1010.

Saberski, L. R. (1998). Interventional ap-proaches in oncologic pain management. In A. Berger, R. K. Portenoy, & D. E. Weiss-man (Eds.), *Principles and practice of sup-portive oncology* (pp. 93–107). Philadel-phia: Lippincott-Raven.

Sanders, M., & Zuurmond, W. (1995). Safety of unilateral and bilateral percutaneous cervical cordotomy in 80 terminally ill cancer patients. *Journal of Clinical Oncol-ogy, 13,* 1509–1512.

Schaffer, S. D., & Yucha, C. B. (2004). Relax-ation and pain management: The relax-ation response can play a role in managing chronic and acute pain. *American Journal of Nursing, 104*(8), 75–82.

Schroeder, M. E. (1986). Neurolytic nerve block for cancer pain. *Journal of Pain and Symptom Management, 1*(2), 91–94.

Schroeder-Sheker, T. (1994). Music for the dying: A personal account of the new field of music thanatology history, theories, and clinical narratives. *Journal of Holistic Nurs-ing, 12*(1), 83–99.

Schumacher, K. L., Koresawa, S., West, C., Dodd, M., Paul, S. M., Tripathy, D., et al. (2002a). The usefulness of a daily pain man-agement diary for outpatients with cancer-related pain. *Oncology Nursing Forum, 29,* 1304–1313.

Schumacher, K. L., Koresawa, S., West, C., Hawkins, C., Johnson, D., Wais, E., et al. (2002b). Putting cancer pain management regimens into practice at home. *Journal of Pain and Symptom Management, 23,* 369–382.

Smith, M. C., Kemp, J., Hemphil, L., & Vojir, C. P. (2002). Outcomes of therapeutic mas-sage for hospitalized cancer patients. *Jour-nal of Nursing Scholarship, 34,* 257–262.

Spross, J. A., & Wolff Burke, M. (1995). Non-pharmacological management of cancer pain. In D. B. McGuire, C. H. Yarbro, & B. R. Ferrell (Eds.), *Cancer pain manage-ment* (2nd ed., pp. 159–205). Boston: Jones and Bartlett.

Stedman, T. L. (1995). *Stedman's medical dic-tionary* (26th ed.). Baltimore: Williams & Wilkins.

Stephens, R. L. (1993). Imagery: A strategic intervention to empower clients part II—A practical guide. *Clinical Nurse Specialist, 7,* 235–240.

Swarm, R. A., & Cousins, M. J. (1998). Anaesthetic techniques for pain control. In D. Doyle, G. W. C. Hanks, & N. MacDonald (Eds.), *Oxford textbook of palliative medicine* (2nd ed., pp. 390–414). Oxford, UK: Oxford University Press.

Syrjala, K. L., Donaldson, G. W., Davis, M. W., Kippes, M. E., & Carr, J. E. (1995). Relaxation and imagery and cognitive-behavioral training reduce pain during cancer treatment: A controlled clinical trial. *Pain, 63,* 189–198.

Thomas, E. M., & Weiss, S. M. (2000). Nonpharmacological interventions with chronic cancer pain in adults. *Cancer Control, 7,* 157–164.

Thompson, J. W., & Filshie, J. (1998). Transcutaneous electrical nerve stimulation (TENS) and acupuncture. In D. Doyle, G. W. C. Hanks, & N. MacDonald (Eds.), *Oxford textbook of palliative medicine* (2nd ed., pp. 421–437). Oxford, UK: Oxford University Press.

Tuls Halstead, M., & Tuls Roscoe, S. (2002). Restoring the spirit at the end of life: Music as an intervention for oncology nurses. *Clinical Journal of Oncology Nursing, 6,* 332–336.

Tunkel, R. S., & Lachmann, E. A. (1998). Rehabilitative medicine. In A. Berger, R. K. Portenoy, & D. E. Weissman (Eds.), *Principles and practice of supportive oncology* (pp. 681–690). Philadelphia: Lippincott-Raven.

Tyler, D. O., Winslow, E. H., Clark, A. P., & White, K. M. (1990). Effects of a 1 minute back rub on mixed venous oxygen saturation and heart rate in critically ill patients. *Heart Lung, 19,* 562–565.

Wells, N., Hepworth, J. T., Murphy, B. A., Wujcik, D., & Johnson, R. (2003). Improving cancer pain management through patient and family education. *Journal of Pain and Symptom Management, 25,* 344–356.

West, C. M., Dodd, M. J., Paul, S. M., Schumacher, K., Tripathy, D., Koo, P., et al. (2003). The PRO-SELF©: pain control program— An effective approach for cancer pain management. *Oncology Nursing Forum, 30*(1), 65–73.

Winstead-Fry, P., & Kijek, J. (1999). An integrative review and meta-analysis of therapeutic touch research. *Alternative Therapies in Health Medicine, 5*(6), 58–67.

Yegul, I., & Erhan, E. (2003). Bilateral CT-guided percutaneous cordotomy for cancer pain relief. *Clinical Radiology, 58,* 886–889.

14

Peri-Death Nursing Care

Marianne LaPorte Matzo

AACN Competencies

#7: Use scientifically based standardized tools to assess symptoms (e.g., dyspnea, constipation, anxiety, fatigue, nausea/vomiting, and altered cognition) experienced by patients at the end of life.

#8: Use data from symptom assessment to plan and intervene in symptom management using state-of-the-art and traditional approaches.

#9: Evaluate the impact of traditional, complementary, and technological therapies on patient-centered outcomes.

#10: Assess and treat multiple dimensions, including physical, psychological, social, and spiritual needs, to improve quality of care at the end of life.

> To everything there is a season, a time for
> every purpose under heaven:
> A time to be born, and a time to die . . .
> A time to weep, and a time to laugh; a time
> to mourn, and a time to dance.
> —Ecclesiastes 3

As an experiential process, dying and death for the individual, his or her family, and the health care practitioner can be one of the most profound and significant events experienced in one's lifetime. The last hours of life are conceptualized as the peri-death period, which specifically encompasses the symptoms and experiences right before death

occurs, the actual death, and the care of the body after death. This time requires intensive holistic nursing care.

The purpose of this chapter is to relate the role of the nurse during the peri-death period and convey the core knowledge necessary for nurses to help facilitate a "good" death. The information in this chapter should be considered a requirement for nurses educated at a basic level. The role of the advanced practice nurse regarding peri-death nursing includes mentoring and modeling appropriate behaviors for the novice nurse, as well as directing symptom management. Additionally the role includes supporting the novice nurse through the dying experience, and support of the family during the decision-making process regarding autopsy and funeral arrangements.

PERI-DEATH 1: SYMPTOMS AND EXPERIENCES BEFORE DEATH

The peri-death period begins with a preparation phase, the hallmark of which is the realization or acknowledgment that death is inevitable and temporally near. The patient and family members begin to prepare for the death. Similarly, the preparation phase for the terminally ill person is also a time when patients and families have many decisions to

443

make regarding home or hospital care, hospice referral, advance directives, and Do Not Resuscitate orders.

The patient may be so uncomfortable with the physical (e.g., pain, dyspnea, fatigue) and emotional (e.g., depression, dependency) aspects of dying that he or she may feel ready for life to end. This sense of readiness may be in tension with a reluctance to die based upon fear of the unknown and concern for how the family will cope after the death. Family members are confronted with their role in the dying process, the prospect of losing their loved one, and the conflicts that arise from these and other issues. The patient's role within the family may change as the family learns how to provide care.

Any, all, or none of the following symptoms may occur during the final stages of the dying process. In-depth nursing interventions for the person with advanced disease can be found in the previous chapters of this book. The focus here is on the physiological changes that occur as death is imminent and the nursing interventions that are appropriate at this time.

PAIN

As the body begins to shut down and die, the need for pain medication may change or decrease. Drugs most often used to manage pain at the end of life are MS Contin, Morphine Sulfate Instant Release (MSIR), OxyContin, and Oxycodone (Institutes of Medicine [IOM], 1997). The liver conjugates these drugs and active metabolites remain in the body, exerting a pharmacological effect until they are cleared by the kidneys. As the body is dying, renal and hepatic function is compromised and the drugs are cleared from the system very slowly. This results in an increase in serum opioid concentrations, which results in increased drowsiness or mild confusion. A nursing priority should be to keep the patient pain free and comfortable but with the understanding that the dosage to accomplish this may be considerably less than what had been previously needed for effective pain management.

Patients, health care providers, and family need an understanding of the importance and value of pain management during the dying process. The patient may seek pain relief or may view pain as a way to atone for sins and refuse to be medicated. Health care professionals may worry that using too high a dose of morphine will result in hastening or causing the death of the patient. Like the nurse, the family may fear being the person to give the "last dose" of morphine before the patient dies. Not adequately medicating for pain, though, can interfere with the memories that the family will carry with them for the rest of their lives. They will remember the death of their loved one as a time of agony and pain rather than a time that could have been used for conversations that are more meaningful and memorable.

The role of the nurse in pain management is to assess the level of pain the patient is having and the patient and family's attitudes toward pain, and to assure patients and families that comfort and alleviation of pain is a priority. Encouraging patients to report their pain before it becomes intense will prevent unbearable suffering. Determining the adequacy of the pain control and its duration are important assessment data so that those dosages can be appropriately adjusted. Pain relief is an attainable goal, but may require sedation in order to achieve adequate control (Panke, 2003).

Given that pain medications frequently cause constipation, nurses must be vigilant in assessing for constipation. Caregivers should be encouraged to continue prophylaxis bowel regimens to prevent or alleviate its associated discomfort. Other nonpharmacological interventions that alleviate pain are a calm environment, soothing music, and aromatherapy. Simple human touch or therapeutically intended touch, such as Reiki or therapeutic touch, can relieve stress, be a source of comfort or support, and overcome fear of abandonment.

Anorexia/Dehydration

As patients approach the end of life, they may say they are not hungry, which is a normal predeath finding. Decreased eating results in a metabolic imbalance whereby the energy a patient takes in does not cover the energy they expend, resulting in a state of dehydration. Although healthy people who are experiencing dehydration will report pain, abdominal cramps, nausea, vomiting, and dry mouth, patients who are terminally ill do not report such symptoms. At the end of life, patients typically only complain of having a dry mouth, which is often unrelated to hydration status and most often is the result of medication side effects, increased respiration, or mouth breathing.

Food represents more than nutrition to many families and can have a vital role in helping them to maintain hope and providing comfort to the patient. It is regrettable that attempts to feed the dying patient are not only frustrating for everyone involved, but can also add to the patient's suffering (Cimino, 2003). In many cases, artificial hydration and nutrition provide an opportunity to "do something" at a time when the mistaken perception is that there is little else the nurse can do for them.

Intravenous fluids given to a person who is actively dying increases urinary output, which may result in the necessity for a Foley catheter. It may increase respiratory secretions and increase cough as well as increasing gastrointestinal fluids, leading to abdominal distention, nausea, or vomiting. Increasing the intravascular volume in the presence of

decreasing renal function can further result in peripheral edema and increase the incidence of decubitus ulcers. Pain can result from the IV site and restraints may become necessary to prevent the patient from removing the tubing. The presence of the IV may act as a physical barrier to the family and may be a cause of anxiety to them. In essence, artificial nutrition and hydration at this stage may lead to symptoms of congestive heart failure, increased tracheal and bronchial secretions, nausea and vomiting, painful edema, and diarrhea (Gates & Fink, 1997), rather than improving symptoms or prolonging life (Craig, 2000).

In contrast, there are many benefits to the patient in withholding food and fluids as death nears. With calorie deprivation comes an increased production of ketones, which results in an elevation of naturally occurring opioid peptides or endorphins that provide analgesia. An electrolyte imbalance, if present, will also result in increased analgesia. Decreased fluid intake will result in fewer pulmonary fluids, which ease respiration, lessens coughing, and reduces drowning sensations. If a tumor is present, dehydration may make it smaller in size by reducing the edematous layer around the tumor resulting in less pressure and pain.

Nursing interventions focus on meticulous mouth care to alleviate mouth dryness and prevent sores, dental problems, and infections. Scrupulous cleaning and moistening of the mouth can be one of the most important interventions to prevent suffering in a patient nearing death (Field & Cassel, 1997). The mouth and teeth can be cleaned with a soft-bristled toothbrush or sponge-covered oral swabs. To maintain moisture in mucosal membranes, the mouth should be rinsed frequently with water. A spray bottle can be used to mist the mouth often; a room humidifier is also very helpful. Commercial salivary substitutes or supplements such as Salivart,

Oral Balance, Salagen, and MoiStir can also help keep the patient comfortable. Chamomile tea is also very soothing and can be used to clean the mouth or offered to the patient to sip on. Generously applying lip lubricant can prevent dry, chapped lips and alleviate associated discomfort. Family members should be shown how to give good mouth care and be supported by the nurse in their efforts. It is essential for everyone involved in the care of the patient to realize that not providing food and fluids is not the same as not caring for the patient, only that the concentration of care is on meeting the needs of the dying person and providing comprehensive symptom management (Soden, Hoy, Hoy, & Clelland 2002).

If the patient is experiencing oral pain, morphine or morphine elixir can be used if the pain is severe or during mouth care and meals. Topical agents for mouth pain include Viscous Xylocaine 2% solution, 5–15 ml, swish and spit every 2 to 4 hours as needed. KBX solution (Kaopectate, Benadryl, Xylocaine viscous in equal parts), 5–15 ml, swish for 1 minute, then spit or swallow every 2 to 4 hours as needed may also be ordered. The Xylocaine provides topical anesthesia; the Benadryl is a short-acting anesthetic; and the Kaopectate (Mylanta may be substituted) serves as an alkalizing agent (Gates & Fink, 1997).

If the patient is still sipping fluids, encourage those fluids that contain salt to help prevent electrolyte imbalance. Fluids such as bullion soup, tomato juice, or sport drinks like Gatorade may be well-tolerated. Avoid citrus juices or foods that may irritate the mouth, as well as temperature extremes of foods. It is important not to force food or fluids at this point and to support the family who may have a difficult time accepting the patient's refusal to eat or drink. Families can be reminded that even in the case of acute illness, such as the flu, food and fluids can create additional distress.

As death approaches patients often lose their ability to swallow due to weakness or a decrease in neurological function. The gag reflex may diminish and secretions will tend to accumulate in the tracheo-bronchial tree. Positioning is important to prevent the accumulation of secretions in the back of the throat and upper airways (Ferrell, Virani, & Grant, 1999). Scopolamine transdermal patches can be used to decrease secretion production and decrease the occurrence of the "death rattle," which although not distressing to the patient can be very upsetting to the family (Hoyal, Grant, Chamberlain, Cox, & Campbell, 2002).

Weakness and Fatigue

Fatigue is a primary complaint of patients in the last 4 weeks of life (Gorman, 1998). The tiredness may be a result of both the disease and the treatment for the disease, as well as malnutrition and disrupted sleep patterns. Fatigue may interfere with a person's ability to move, bathe, or toilet (Field & Cassel, 1997).

The nurse should be aware that while the patient is at high risk for a pressure ulcer, turning and positioning should be done as frequently as possible but only as often as comfort permits. Bony prominences should be padded and supported if this is comfortable for the patient. If any of these interventions result in increased pain or suffering, they should not be implemented. Initially, this may be difficult for the novice nurse to support, as it is contrary to the basic nursing skills they have been taught. When a patient is actively dying, intervention goals should focus on comfort; any intervention that compromises this goal should be discontinued.

Dyspnea

Dyspnea is a common symptom experienced at the end of life and results from the lungs' inability to function in proportion to the metabolic demands of the body (Field & Cassel, 1997). When a person has trouble breathing, there must be either an increase in ventilation or a decrease in activity. Terminal dyspnea occurs in as many as 75% of patients in the peri-death period (LaDuke, 2001). Changes in respiration are normal and should be anticipated prior to death. Physiologically increased carbon dioxide in the blood stimulates respiration. During the peri-death period increased pulmonary congestion and poor gas exchange results in a rise in carbon dioxide levels, but the brain is less responsive to this signal (Pitorak, 2003). The breathing pattern can become irregular and include shallow breathing altered with apnea lasting 5 to 60 seconds (Cheyne-Stokes breathing). Fluids can accumulate in the back of the throat resulting in what is known as a "death rattle" (Ferrell et al., 1999).

Families should be warned that dyspnea and loud respirations are a possibility during the peri-death period. Patients may fear they will suffocate while they are dying and families fear they will have to watch their loved one struggle to breathe. Nurses should educate the patient and family regarding what they can expect and give assurances that medications will be used to effectively palliate these symptoms (Tarzian, 2000).

Nursing interventions include positioning the patient with the head of the bed raised and/or turning the person on one side. For opioid naive patients, low-dose opiates, such as morphine 5mg PO every 4 hours, can alleviate the sensation of breathlessness. If morphine is already being used for pain, an increase of 2.5 mg times their regular dose is generally effective. Oxygen is typically only effective if the dyspnea is secondary to hypoxia (e.g., COPD, pulmonary fibrosis), although it may provide a placebo effect (Horn, 1992). A fan blowing a gentle breeze toward the patient's face can also be very effective. Suctioning is usually not recommended as it may incidentally increase secretion production. Emotion-focused interventions such as relaxation techniques, prayer and meditation,

and distraction may alleviate the anxiety often associated with dyspnea (Horn, 1992).

Multisystem Failure

As the body is shutting down, there is a decrease in blood perfusion and a resulting shutdown of the major organs (e.g., renal and hepatic). Decreased cardiac output and intravascular volume result in tachycardia and hypotension. Additionally, the body will conserve blood volume for vital organs, which results in peripheral cooling (as the body conserves heat) and peripheral and central cyanosis. The skin may therefore become mottled and discolored, which is normal before death and a sign that it is imminent. Mottling is typically seen on the earlobes and the soles of the feet before other areas.

Urine output is greatly diminished and there can be a loss of sphincter control resulting in urinary or fecal incontinence. It may be a good idea to insert a urinary catheter to reduce the need for frequent bedding changes and to prevent skin breakdown. The catheter also helps the continent patient conserve energy by removing the need to use a bedpan or urinal.

Neurological dysfunction is a result of multiple, concurrent, and nonreversible organ failure. Consequently, the patient may experience reduced cerebral perfusion, hypoxemia, metabolic imbalances, acidosis, accumulation of toxins from renal and hepatic failure, and sepsis (Ferrell et al., 1999). The net effect of these changes may be a decreased level of consciousness or terminal delirium.

Terminal Delirium

Terminal delirium can be manifested as confusion, anxiety, agitation, or restlessness; restlessness and delirium are typical symptoms that are indicative that the patient is close to death. These can be distressing symptoms for patients and their families and it is estimated that up to 80% of patients develop delirium (Macleod & Whitehead 1997). Confusion is a mental state in which a person reacts inappropriately to their environment because they are confounded or disoriented. It may be the side effect of medications or caused by the dying process itself (Field & Cassel, 1997). Anxiety is the biological and emotional reaction to stressful situations, including the approach of death.

The patient may experience dread, danger, or tension with somatic complaints that includes shortness of breath, nausea, or diarrhea (Field & Cassel, 1997). Moaning and grimacing can accompany agitation and restlessness and may be misinterpreted by the nurse as pain (Ferrell et al., 1999). The patient may be restless and make repetitive motions (e.g., pulling on clothing or the sheets). The underlying cause of the restlessness may be opioid toxicity, metabolic disorders and lowered seizure threshold, or full bladder or bowel (Heming & Colmer, 2003).

Nursing interventions to manage terminal delirium should focus on the treatment of the underlying physical cause if it is practical and possible. Antianxiety agents like benzodiazepines (lorazepam, diazepam, alprazolam) and neuroleptics (Haldol) for drug toxicity can help to quiet distressing symptoms. Methotrimeprazine can be effective if the patient's jerking movements are secondary to renal failure and it possesses anti-emetic characteristics (Kaye, 2003).

The family is in need of education and support regarding the cause and the irreversible nature of the behavior. Maintaining a calm environment, spiritual comfort, and emotional support are vital at this time. The family can be advised to continue to talk to the patient and calm the patient with their words. Light massage of the arms, back, or forehead can be very soothing. Soft music and low lights can also be effective. It may be suggested that the number of people in the room be decreased if there is a lot of activity. Refraining from asking the patient many questions can diminish agitation.

Eventually the patient's level of consciousness will decrease and they may even become unable to be aroused. This is a very upsetting time for families because the patient may seem unresponsive and withdrawn, but it is a normal aspect of the dying process. At this time the patient is starting to "let go" in preparation for death and is detaching from relationships and the physical environment. A patient may ask to be with only one person toward the end or seem distracted from the family. Reassure the family that this is not a personal rejection, only another aspect of the dying process. A dying person may talk about seeing people who have already died or talk about taking a trip with a long-deceased relative. Patients may describe feeling separate from their body. This is a normal experience and is not considered a hallucination.

Even if the patient is unresponsive, encourage family members to talk with him or her. Assume that the patient hears everything; this is the time for loved ones to say "Good-bye," "I'm sorry," "I love you," or "Thank you." The patient may have difficulty letting go and the nurse may need to encourage the family to give the patient permission to die. Encourage the family to show affection to the patient, touch them, and let them know they will be missed.

Affirming Life and Maintaining Hope

Two very important goals of palliative care nursing are to help patients live until they die, and to encourage hope. First, the nurse can help patients live until they die by encouraging socialization, listening, being honest, and helping them finish any unfinished business. By offering patients choices regarding routines, food, and activities, nurses promote continued independence and the ability to help maintain control over their lives. Of course, the degree of independence depends on patients' energy level and ability (Birchenall & Streight, 1997). Furthermore, patients' wishes should be respected even if those wishes are inconsistent with the family's or health care provider's values.

Second, hope is an important component of the emotional stages of dying and death. It has been a factor in helping the patient and family continue through the difficult months and years leading up to the death. Hope is what maintains a person's spirit and helps the person to go on; as the person is dying *what* he or she hopes for may change, but it does not go away. There may be hope for the "miracle" of a complete cure; it is not acceptable for the nurse to take this hope away or to tell the patient and family to be "realistic."

Their hopes may change from that of cure to the hope for a full night's sleep, a visit from an important person, or for less pain. Persons with hope have been found to live longer and have a greater quality of life than those who are hopeless (Birchenall & Streight, 1997). What is important is for the nurse to be present for the patient and family wherever they are in this process and support the feelings that are experienced. The rights of the dying can be found in Table 14.1. Listening and caring for their needs are important nursing functions at this time of life.

Family Support During the Last Hours of Life

Supporting the family during the last hours of the patient's life is an important nursing

TABLE 14.1   The Dying Person's Bill of Rights

- I have the right to be treated as a living human being until I die.
- I have the right to maintain a sense of hopefulness, however changing its focus may be.
- I have the right to be cared for by those who can maintain a sense of hopefulness, however challenging this might be.
- I have the right to express my feelings and emotions about my approaching death, in my own way.
- I have the right to participate in decisions concerning my care.
- I have the right to expect continuing medical and nursing attention even though "cure" goals must be changed to "comfort" goals.
- I have the right not to die alone.
- I have the right to be free from pain.
- I have the right to have my questions answered honestly.
- I have the right not to be deceived.
- I have the right to have help from and for my family accepting my death.
- I have the right to die in peace and dignity.
- I have the right to retain my individuality and not be judged for my decisions, which may be contrary to the beliefs of others.
- I have the right to discuss and enlarge my religious and/or spiritual experiences, regardless of what they may mean to others.
- I have the right to expect that the sanctity of the human body will be respected after death.
- I have the right to be cared for by caring, sensitive, knowledgeable people who will attempt to understand my needs and will be able to gain some satisfaction in helping me face my death.

Source: From S. A. Sorrentino, *Assisting with Patient Care* (p. 843). St. Louis, MO: Mosby, 1999. Used with permission.

role. When possible, one nurse should be assigned to be with the family through the last phase of life. Enough time with the dying person should be given to the family so that they have the opportunity to resolve any final interpersonal issues. If the death is occurring at home the family should have access to a Symptom Relief Kit with detailed, easy to understand instructions for its use (Appendix A). Depending on cultural and religious considerations, the family should be afforded privacy and clergy support. The primary nurse should communicate with the family regarding what they can expect the dying process to be like and how they will know when the person has died.

Many people have not been with someone who is actively dying and do not know what to expect. Even though no two deaths are alike, it helps to give significant others an idea of what the final stage of life may be like and the symptoms they may see during this period. Table 14.2, which shows the final stages of dying, is an information sheet written for the general population regarding the dying process and is a good handout for students.

TABLE 14.2   VNA Hospice Manchester, NH. FINAL STAGES—DYING PROCESS

When a person enters the final stage of the dying process, two different dynamics are at work. On the physical plane, the body begins the final process of shutting down, which will end when all the physical systems cease to function. Usually this is an orderly, progressive series of physical changes that are not medical emergencies. These physical changes are the natural way in which the body prepares itself to stop. The most appropriate kinds of responses are comfort-enhancing measures.

The other dynamic of the dying process is emotional and spiritual in nature. The "spirit" of the dying person begins the final process of release from the body, its immediate environment and all attachments. This release also tends to follow its own priorities, which may include the resolution of whatever is *unfinished* of a practical nature and exercising permission from family members to "let go." The most appropriate kinds of responses to the emotional/spiritual changes are those that support and encourage this release and transition.

When a person's body is ready and wanting to stop, but the person is still unresolved or is not reconciled about some important issue or relationship, the person may tend to linger in order to finish whatever needs finishing. On the other hand, when a person is emotionally/spiritually resolved and ready for this release, but his/her body has not completed its final physical process, the person will continue to live until the physical shutdown is completed.

The experience we call "death" occurs when the body and the spirit complete the natural process of shutting down, reconciling, and finishing. These processes need to happen in a way appropriate and unique to the values, beliefs, and lifestyle of the dying person.

The physical and emotional/spiritual signs and symptoms of impending death that follow are offered to help you understand the natural kinds of things that may happen and how you can respond appropriately. Not all these signs and symptoms will occur with every person, nor will they occur in this particular sequence. Each person is unique and needs your full acceptance, support, and comfort.

The following signs and symptoms are indicative of how the body prepares itself for the final stage of life:

Coolness: The person's hands, arms, feet and legs may be increasingly cool. At the same time, the color of the skin may change. The underside of the body may become darker and the skin mottled or discolored. This is a normal indication that the circulation of blood is decreasing to the body's extremities and being reserved for the most vital organs. Keep the person warm with a nonelectric blanket.

TABLE 14.2   *(continued)*

Sleeping: The person may spend an increasing amount of time sleeping and appear to be uncommunicative or unresponsive, at times difficult to arouse. This normal change is due in part to changes in the metabolism of the body. Sit with your loved one, speak softly and naturally. Plan to spend time when the person seems most alert and awake. Try not to talk as if the person were not there. Speak directly as you normally would, even though there may be no response. Never assume the person cannot hear; hearing is the last of the senses to be lost.

Fluid and Food Decrease: The person may have a decrease in appetite and thirst, wanting little or no food or fluid. The body will naturally begin to conserve energy that would be expended on these tasks. Do not try to force food or drink into the person. To use guilt or manipulation only makes the person more uncomfortable. Small chips of ice, frozen Gatorade or juice may be refreshing in the mouth. If the person is able to swallow, fluids may be given in small amounts by syringe (ask the hospice nurse for guidance). Glycerin swabs may help keep the mouth and lips moist and comfortable. A cool, moist washcloth on the forehead may also increase physical comfort.

Incontinence: Control of urine and/or bowels may be lost as the muscles in that area begin to relax. Discuss with your hospice nurse what can be done to protect the bed and keep your loved one clean and comfortable. If it would make the person more comfortable, the nurse may suggest a catheter to drain the bladder into a collection bag. The person's normal urine output may decrease and become dark due to the decrease in circulation through the kidneys.

Congestion: The person may have gurgling sounds coming from the chest as though marbles were rolling around inside. These sounds may become very loud. This normal change is due to the decrease of fluid intake and the inability to cough up normal secretions. The sound of the congestion does not indicate the onset of severe or new pain. Suctioning usually increases the secretions. The nurse or home health aide can show you how to keep the mouth clean with "touthettes."

Breathing Pattern Change: The person's regular breathing pattern may change and become irregular, e.g., shallow breaths with periods of no breathing for 5 to 30 seconds and up to a full minute. This is called Cheyne-Stokes breathing. The person may also experience periods of rapid shallow panting. Elevating the head and/or turning the person on one side may bring comfort. Use your hands to touch and soothe. Speak gently.

Disorientation: The person may seem to be confused about the time, place, and identity of people, including those close and familiar. This is due in part to metabolism changes. Identify yourself by name before you speak rather than asking the person to guess who you are. Speak softly, clearly, and truthfully when you need to communicate something important, such as, "It's time to take your medication," and explain the reason for the communication, such as, "So you won't begin to hurt." Never use this method to try to manipulate the person to meet your own needs or values. It may be difficult to make this distinction.

Restlessness: The person may make restless and repetitive motions, such as pulling at bed linen or clothing. This often happens and is due to the decrease in oxygen circulation to the brain and to metabolism changes. Do not interfere with or try to restrain such motions. Occasionally the person may twitch or make jerking motions. This may have to do with medication or the disease itself. Sometimes other medication helps decrease this twitching.

(continued)

TABLE 14.2   *(continued)*

To have a calming effect, speak in a quiet, natural way; lightly massage the forehead, back, or arms; read to the person, or play some soothing music. Try to decrease the number of people around the person. Asking a lot of questions may increase the person's agitation.

EMOTIONAL SYMPTOMS AND RESPONSES

Withdrawal: The person may seem unresponsive, withdrawn, or in a comatose-like state. This indicates preparation for release, a detaching from surroundings and relationships and a beginning of letting go. Because hearing remains almost all the way to the end, now is the time to say whatever you need to say that will help the person let go. The person may only want to be with a very few or even just one person. This is another sign of preparation for release. If you are not part of this inner circle at the end, it does not mean you are not loved or are unimportant. It means you have already fulfilled your tasks, and it is time for you to say good-bye.

Vision-like experiences: The person may speak or claim to have spoken to persons who have already died, or to see places not presently accessible or visible to you. This does not indicate hallucinations or a drug reaction. The person is beginning to detach from this life and is preparing for the transition. Do not contradict, explain, belittle, or argue about what the person claims to have seen or heard. Affirm the experiences. They are normal and natural.

Letting Go: The person may continue to perform repetitive and restless tasks. This may indicate that something is still unresolved or unfinished and preventing the letting go. The hospice team can assist you in identifying what may be happening and help the person find release from tension or fear. As hard as it might be, you need to give the person permission to let go.

Saying Good-Bye: When the person is ready to die, and you are able to let go, saying good-bye is your final gift of love. It achieves closure and makes the final release possible. It may be helpful to hold or touch and say the things you want to say. It may be as simple (or as complicated) as saying "I love you." It may include recounting favorite memories, places, and activities you shared. It may include saying "I'm sorry for whatever I've done to cause any tensions or difficulty." You may also want to say "Thank you." Tears are a normal and natural part of saying good-bye. You don't need to apologize for them or try to hide them. They are a natural expression of your sadness and loss. It is all right to say "I will miss you so much."

How will you know when death has occurred?

Although you may be prepared for the dying process, you may not be prepared for the actual moment. It may be helpful for you and your family to think about and discuss what you would do if you were alone when the death occurs. The death of a hospice patient is expected and is not an emergency. Nothing must be done immediately. The signs of death include such things as:

- No heartbeat
- Release of bowel and bladder
- No response
- Eyelids slightly open
- Pupils enlarged
- Eyes fixed on a certain spot
- No blinking
- Jaw relaxed and mouth slightly open

TABLE 14.2   (continued)

You may now notify a hospice nurse or the on-call nurse as you have been instructed. The nurse will make the pronouncement and notify your physician. The body does not have to be moved until you are ready. The nurse can call the funeral home, but you or a member of your family will probably need to speak with the funeral director.

Later On

Hospice staff and volunteers continue to be available to support you and your family through the Bereavement Program. We will contact you a week or so after the death has occurred, after all the "busyness" is over and the visitors have gone. If you need or want to communicate with us before then, please do not hesitate to call. Even if you just need a place to go for comfort and support, call or stop in.

We salute you for all you have done during this difficult time. We know it has been an enormous commitment and a true act of love. We feel honored to have shared this experience with you in spite of your pain. You accompanied someone you love as far as you could on life's final journey. We hope you feel good about what you've done. We hope this feeling will sustain you, give you courage, and allow you eventually to go on with your life.

PERI-DEATH 2: DEATH

Signs of Death

Signs of death include cessation of a heartbeat and respiration, release of bowel and bladder, eyelids slightly open and not blinking, pupils fixed and dilated, drop in body temperature; as the blood settles, body color turns to a waxen pallor, jaw is relaxed and slightly open, and there is no response from the patient. These signs do not occur in sequence and it may take a few minutes for the body to completely stop (Ferrell et al., 1999). If the death occurs at home the family should be told that it is not considered an emergency but be given a number to call to inform hospice staff or their physician of the death. The body does not have to be moved immediately so the family should not feel rushed or pressured to act.

When Death Has Occurred

Postdeath nursing care involves preparing the body for the morgue or funeral home and helping the family through decisions regarding autopsy and burial. When death has occurred, the blood will begin to pool in the areas of the body closest to the ground; if the corpse was supine this would be the back and buttocks. A purple-red discoloration of the skin is evident and results from the blood accumulating in the dependent vessels; this is called *livor mortis*. The body begins to cool and this fall in body temperature after death is called *algor mortis* (Kastenbaum & Kastenbaum, 1989). Initially, at the time of death, the muscles in the body relax, but within 2 to 6 hours *rigor mortis* begins. Rigor mortis is the stiffening of all muscle groups beginning with the eyelids, neck, and jaw. During the next 4 to 6 hours, it will spread to the other muscles including the internal organs. Rigor mortis will usually last between 24 and 48 hours depending on the ambient temperature after this time the muscles relax and secondary flaccidity develops (Iserson, 2001).

Care of the body by the nurse should include closing the eyes, inserting dentures and closing the mouth, and elevating the head of the bed so that the blood does not drain into the face and discolor it. Any IV or catheter can be removed at this time, and the physical environment should be straightened. Removal of tubes and equipment is dependent on institutional protocol. Follow the agency protocol regarding jewelry; if there is a wedding ring, secure it on the finger with tape. The body should be bathed in plain water and dried; a bed protector should be placed under the body. If there are dressings on wounds, they should be replaced with clean ones. The hair should be combed, the extremities straightened, and the right great toe tied with an identification tag (Sorrentino, 1999).

If the family wants to participate in the preparation of the deceased for the funeral home, they should be encouraged to do so. The family should also be offered the opportunity to bathe and dress the body if they wish. Some people find comfort in giving the last bath and it helps them to believe that no one else will touch the body in this way again.

When the body and the room have been prepared, family and those close to the patient can be encouraged to say a final good-bye. Within the confines of cultural, personal, and religious practices, the family can be invited to touch or hold the person's body and to take the time they need. This time spent with the deceased can help to promote the transition from acute grief to a new stage of the grieving process (Ferrell et al., 1999). Accepting the reality of the death is considered one of the first tasks of mourning necessary for working through the grief (Worden, 1992). Seeing the dead body helps the bereaved see the reality of the death and to say good-bye. The body should not be transported to the morgue or mortuary until the family is prepared and they have given their permission. The family's wishes should be respected regarding their presence during the removal of the body.

When the family has given permission for the body to be moved, the nurse should follow the institutional protocol regarding shrouding the body. If a person has died at home and it is an expected death, the undertaker is called and they remove the body as it is. In a hospital or nursing home setting, the body is wrapped in a shroud or body bag. The shroud should be secured with safety pins or ties and a second identification tag attached to the shroud or body bag. The body is then taken to the morgue (Sorrentino, 1999).

The nurse can offer help with making personal phone calls to give the family time to become accustomed to the immediate loss. The physician should be notified of the death and the nurse should be certain to follow agency protocol regarding the removal of medications and equipment. If the family wishes, support from their clergy or bereavement professionals can be offered.

In many states, the nurse can sign the death certificate if the death occurs in the hospital or nursing home or at the family home if hospice is involved. Once the death certificate is signed, the family can contact the mortuary and the body can be transported to the funeral home or crematorium. If the nurse or physician is unwilling to sign the death certificate because of a suspicious nature of the death, the medical examiner is called and assumes responsibility for the body (Iserson, 2001). If the death is sudden and unexpected or if it occurs at home, the medical examiner must be notified and he or she will decide if an autopsy is required. The family has no authority to stop an officially mandated autopsy (Lynn & Harrold, 1999).

The next of kin may request an autopsy even if the medical examiner declines to do one. The nurse should be available to educate the family about the autopsy and assist them in their decision-making process. An autopsy will help determine the cause of death but

TABLE 14.3   The Uses of Autopsies

Benefits to Medical Practice and Science
Discover or elucidate new diseases
Explain unknown or unanticipated medical complications
Assist in the development/quality assurance of new technology, procedures, and therapy
Educate medical students
Continue physician education

Benefits to the Judicial System
Classify and explain sudden, unexpected, and/or unnatural deaths

Benefits to Public Welfare
Identify infectious and contagious diseases
Identify and monitor occupational and environmental health hazards
Quality control and risk assessment in hospital practices
Provide a source of organs and tissues for medical and scientific purposes
Provide materials and hypotheses for research
Improve accuracy, and therefore usefulness, of vital statistics

Benefits to the Deceased's Family
Assist in the grief process
Provide a vehicle for contribution
Discover contagious diseases within the family
Assist in genetic counseling and identification of family health risks
Provide information for insurance/death benefits

From K.V. Iserson. K. V. *Death to Dust.* Tucson, AZ: Galen Press, Ltd., 2001. Used with permission.

the family may be charged a fee for this service (as much as $2,000). Autopsies also serve other purposes, as shown in Table 14.3.

The word autopsy comes from the Greek *autopsia,* which means seeing with one's own eyes. Pathologists, who are physicians who have specialized in human anatomy, perform them. Organs are removed and inspected, and body fluids are analyzed. There are three degrees of autopsy: complete, limited, and selective. A complete autopsy exposes all body cavities (including the head) for examination; limited autopsy usually excludes the head; and selective autopsy involves examination of only one or more organs specific to the nature of the illness (Iserson, 2001).

If the deceased has requested that his or her organs be donated, the nurse is often the person responsible for notifying the proper agencies for organ and tissue harvesting. Organ donation is the practice of giving a part of the deceased body for transplantation into another person. Persons designate this wish to donate organs by signing the back of their driver's license, indicating their preferences; by specifying organ donation in an advance directive; or by filling out an organ donor card. Organ donor cards can be ordered from the United Network for Organ Sharing (UNOS) (804–782–4800 or http://www.unos. org). Persons younger than 18 years of age must have the consent of parents or guardians to sign an organ donor card. Some states will record the intent to donate an organ in a donor registry, which is a central repository of information regarding the intent to donate. When a potential donor is identified, the donor registry is contacted to determine the person's intent (Office of the Inspector General, 2002).

Even with the proper documentation, the family may refuse to allow a relative's organs to be donated. In the United States, at least 5,000 human organs are buried because relatives refuse donation. Unless the deceased has specified that he or she does not want his or her organs donated, the senior next of kin may donate all or part of a relative's body (Iserson, 2001).

Depending on what organ is being donated, the time for organ removal varies. Eyes must be removed within 4 hours of the death but once they are in a preservative they can wait 10 to 14 days to be transplanted. Tissue (e.g., bone, skin, and tendons) can wait 12 to 24 hours to be removed from the deceased and can be preserved (depending on the method of preservation) for 3 to 5 years. If the body has been refrigerated within 4 hours of the death, saphenous veins can be harvested in the following 10 hours and heart valves within 24 hours (Iserson, 2001).

Once the organs are removed from the body, it is ready for embalming or cremation. Embalming is the process by which the corpse is preserved and prepared for viewing; it is common for health reasons and protects mourners from being in the presence of a decaying body (Quested, 2003). "Basically, the embalmer is a creator of illusions—of pleasant illusions which banish the traces of suffering and death and present the deceased in an attitude of normal, restful sleep. In the practice of embalming this illusion is called a 'memory picture'" (Strub & Frederick, 1967, p. 133). There is no legal requirement that the body be embalmed, even if it is going to be viewed. The average cost for embalming is about $500 (Iserson, 2001).

There are four embalming methods that all involve the injection of chemicals to pre-serve the body. Arterial embalming injects the chemicals into the blood vessels; cavity embalming injects the chest and abdomen; hypodermic embalming injects under the skin; and surface embalming is the application of chemicals in gel or liquid form to the body surface (Iserson, 2001). The size of the body, age, water content, temperature, decomposition, condition of the body's blood vessels, and premortem medication regime (e.g., gentamycin inactivates embalming fluid) will dictate the types, solution strengths, and injection rates of the embalming chemicals.

Primarily formaldehyde and methyl alcohol are used as preservative chemicals because they change the cell proteins to prevent putrefaction. Embalmers inject these chemicals into the body using a centrifugal pump that pushes the fluids into the body with 5–10 psi of pressure. At the same time, blood and fluid are drained from the body by gravity or electrical aspirators. The embalmer will look for evidence that the chemicals have reached the hands and face and facilitate this process by massaging and repositioning the corpse. When the embalming fluid reaches the hands, they are placed in their final position over the chest or abdomen and the fingers are held together by using cyanoacrylate (e.g., superglue). The muscles will gradually harden over the 8- to 12-hour period following the embalming; once they are set, the body's position will not be able to be moved.

If there is going to be a viewing at the funeral home the body is prepared with the use of cosmetics. The hair is styled and the deceased is dressed. The body is then "casketed" in the coffin; typically, the right shoulder is lower than the left so the body does not look like it is flat on its back.

Cremation is an increasingly popular alternative to embalming and burial. Cremation is a process to reduce the "corpse and its container to ashes and small bone fragments" (Iserson, 2001, p. 236). Intensive heat is used to burn the body, which evaporates water (70% to 80% of non-bone tissue), burns soft tissue, and reduces the average-sized adult to 4 to 8 pounds of ash (cremains). It takes about an hour and a half to cremate a body and what is left are grey ash and bone fragments. The cremains are then processed through an electric grinder to pulverize the bone fragments into an even consistency. The costs for this service ranges between $1,000 and $2,500.

Prosthetic devices do not burn (e.g., dental gold, metal plates, and screws) and are removed with a magnet from the ashes. Pacemakers with lithium batteries will explode when burned and are removed before cremation. The body does not have to be embalmed before cremation nor does the family need to purchase a coffin. The only requirement is that the body be burned in a combustible container (e.g., cardboard or particleboard). Typically, there is a 24- to 48-hour waiting period after the death before cremation can legally take place.

Crematories are the facilities that contain the oven or retorts where the cremation will take place. It is becoming increasingly common for funeral homes to build crematories on the site and to offer a wide range of disposal options. Some cemeteries will have a columbarium for the interment of the urn containing the cremains. Memorial gardens are also available for the ashes to be scattered or buried and give visitors a place to visit or place a marker. Some people will divide the cremains to bury, scatter, keep in an urn, share among family members, or even wear in specially designed jewelry.

Burning the body as a way of disposal dates back to prehistoric times. Our primitive ancestors believed they could return to their bodies and harm the living and therefore feared the dead; destroying the corpse removed that danger. Ancient civilizations believed that cremation would provide the dead with heat and warmth in the next world and protected the body from mutilation by animals or other humans. Native Americans believe that souls are conveyed to paradise by means of fire.

PERI-DEATH RELIGIOUS AND CULTURAL RITUALS

Nursing care does not stop when a patient dies. There is tremendous variability around the world regarding the care of dead bodies and funeral practices. In India, there are funeral pyres; there are second burial rites by Indonesian hill tribes; and the pervasiveness of embalming practices in the United States (Quested, 2003). Throughout the dying process, and particularly at the very end of life, the nurse must be aware of cultural and religious values, practices, and traditions of the patient and the family. Customs and rituals have tremendous significance in the healing process following death, and the grief response is often structured by these rituals. The nurse's role is to help the family carry out the rites and practices that provide solace and support. The nurse should be open-minded and understanding of the physical, psychosocial, and spiritual needs of the dying patient and his or her family and offer them respect and privacy (Purnell & Paulanka, 1998).

Rituals and customs vary based on a person's faith background or culture. For those of the Roman Catholic faith, priests will offer the Sacrament of the Anointing of the Sick, which in the past was called Extreme Unction or the Last Rites. The sacrament is for those who are seriously ill; the family, friends, and priest gather at the bedside to pray for healing. If it is God's will that the person not recover from their illness, then the prayer is that God will accompany the dying person toward the rewards of heaven (Miller, 1993). The nurse can ask the family if they would like the priest to be called. The priest would hear the patient's confession of sins, absolve the individual, and offer the Sacrament of the Sick. The comfort this ritual can bring to the dying Catholic and his or her family cannot be underestimated.

The preference of the Catholic Church is that the body of the deceased be present for the funeral rites; Masses with cremated remains present can be performed. When cremated remains are present they must be contained in a "worthy vessel," placed on a table, or in the place normally occupied by the casket, and must be covered with a pall, that is, a heavy drape or cloth. The prayer of committal would read "earthly remains" in place of "body" (Archdiocese of San Antonio, 2002).

Out of respect for the human body, the cremains should to be treated with regard and buried in a grave or entombed in a mausoleum or columbarium. Scattering at sea, from the air or ground, or keeping the cremains at home are not considered reverent disposition. The Church still recommends burial or inurnment (placing the cremains in an urn) in a Catholic cemetery. Throughout the history of the Church, the Catholic cemetery has served as a visible sign of the faith community, attesting to the dignity of the baptized and the promise of the Resurrection (Archdiocese of San Antonio, 2002). Mourning traditionally has been expected to be kept to a minimum with the view that people should "get on with their lives" (Bhungalia & Kemp, 2002).

In the Church of Jesus Christ of Latter-Day Saints (Mormons), church members of the same gender who have permission to be admitted into the temple are the ones who dress deceased members. The body is dressed in white undergarments that are covered by a robe, cap, and apron. Prior to burial, a white cap is placed on a deceased man, and a deceased woman's face is veiled (Iserson, 2001).

A Hindu who is dying may also request holy rites before death; readings and hymns from holy books are also comforting. Some may wish to lie on the floor to symbolize their closeness to the earth. A Hindu priest would administer the holy rites, which may include tying a thread around the wrists or neck of the dying person, sprinkling blessed water from the Ganges, of placing a sacred tulsi leaf in the dying person's mouth. Some Hindus may wish to return to India to die, especially to the holy city of Banaras. Many believe that to die in Banaras insures a rebirth in heaven or even a release from continued rebirth. At a minimum, a Hindu will request to die at home because death in the hospital is very distressing. Only another Hindu should touch the dead body; if it is necessary for a non-Hindu to touch it, disposable gloves should be worn. Sacred threads, jewelry, and other religious objects should not be removed. The body should not be washed but only wrapped in a plain sheet. Washing of the body is a part of the funeral rite and is typically carried out only by family members; a mixture of milk and yogurt is used to cleanse the body. In India, a funeral would take place within 24 hours; adult Hindus are cremated although young children and infants may be buried (Green, 1989a, 1989b, 1989c).

The dying person of the Muslim faith may wish to lie or sit facing Mecca. If it is possible, the bed should be positioned to accommodate this wish. Those of Islamic faith believe that the body belongs to God, and therefore autopsies are forbidden unless ordered by the coroner. Likewise, organ donation and cremation are not acceptable. In Iran, a person is immediately placed in a casket if he or she has died during the day. If death occurs at night, a copy of the Koran should be placed on the chest of the deceased and a lighted candle at the head (Iserson, 2001); the body is watched during the night by a person reading the Koran.

Following the death, non-Muslims should wear gloves when touching the body. If there is no family available to carry out postmortem care, the nurse should wear gloves in administering care of the body. However, the body is not washed and hair and nails are not cut; the eyes are closed. According to Green (1989d),

> the normal Muslim procedure is that the body is straightened immediately after death. This is done by flexing the elbows, shoulders, knees and hips first, before straightening them. This is thought to ensure that the body does not stiffen, thus facilitating its washing and shrouding. Turn the head towards the right shoulder. This is so the body can be buried with the face towards Mecca. (p. 57)

The body is then covered with a sheet that cloaks the whole body until a Muslim is available to perform the ritual bath.

The ritual bath includes washing the body three times, first with lotus water, and then camphor water, and last with plain water (Iserson, 2001). This bathing is done from head to toe and front to back. All body orifices are closed and packed with cotton (to prevent body-fluid leakage that is considered unclean). Prayers from the Qu'ran are read (especially verses of hope and acceptance) and the body is wrapped in a special cotton shroud. This shroud is made from three pieces of white unsewn cloth, 9 yards long, that are wrapped above, below, and around the midsection. Muslims are buried in a brick- or cement-lined grave with the head facing east toward Mecca. In Iran, the body is buried directly in the earth with the shroud removed from the face and one side of the face turned to be in contact with the earth (Purnell & Paulanka, 1998).

When those of the Jewish faith are dying, they may want to hear or recite special prayers, such as the Shema, which confirms one's belief in one God; or psalms, in particular Psalm 23 ("The Lord is my Shepherd").

The person may also wish to hold the written prayer in his or her hand (Green, 1989e). A relative remains with the dying person to ensure that the soul does not leave the body when she or he is alone; it is a sign of disrespect to leave the body alone. Even after death, the body is not left alone until the funeral, so that the body is not left defenseless (Purnell & Paulanka, 1998). The eyes should be closed after death, preferably by a child of the deceased; the body should be covered and left untouched (Green, 1989e). Autopsies are not permitted, although organ transplants are. The body should be handled as little as possible by non-Jews, and burial should take place within 24 hours. Burial is usually only delayed for the Sabbath. Embalming and cosmetics are not part of traditional practice. Orthodox Jews are always buried, although Jews who are more liberal may select cremation. The body is wrapped in a shroud and a prayer shawl. The casket is made of wood, so that the body and the casket decay at the same rate. There is no wake or viewing of the body. At the funeral, the *Kaddish,* the *prayer* for the dead is said, which praises God and reaffirms faith (Purnell & Paulanka, 1998).

For those who are Buddhist, an important consideration is the state of mind at the time of death; dying thoughts and desires are crucial in determining the next rebirth of the deceased. A Buddhist monk or minister should be notified at the time of death. The length of time between death and burial can vary between 3 and 7 days depending on the Buddhist tradition. Family members plan the burial; the tradition is to wear white to the funeral.

In terms of differences based on cultural backgrounds, Cuban Americans who are dying are usually attended by large groups of family and friends. Depending on their religious affiliation, a Catholic priest, Protestant minister, rabbi, or *santero* may be called to perform death rites. For followers of *santero,* these rites may include animal sacrifice, ceremonial displays, and chants (Purnell & Paulanka, 1998). After the death, candles are lit to light the path of the spirit to the afterlife. Burial is the common custom although there is no restriction to cremation.

African Americans generally prefer to have people with terminal illness cared for in the home, but prefer death to occur in the hospital for fear of bad luck being brought to the home. Grief is expressed openly and publicly. Autopsy is acceptable, although organ donation is not.

Mexican Americans may take turns sitting vigil over the dying person; dying in a hospital is not desirable because the spirit may become lost. Spiritual amulets, rosary beads, or other religious artifacts are kept near the patient. Typically, organ donation or autopsy is not allowed. When death occurs, family and friends will often come long distances for the funeral. A *velorio* is a festive watch of the deceased body before burial. Traditional families may exhibit hyperkinetic shaking and seizurelike activity called *ataque de nervios,* which is a way to release emotions related to grieving. The family may erect altars in their homes in honor of the anniversary of their relative's death and may include candles, decorations, and having the deceased's favorite meal at a graveside picnic (Purnell & Paulanka, 1998).

Native Americans have different traditions in each tribe. There is a belief that the spirit of the deceased remains where the person has died; therefore family may not want the person to die at home. At the same time, it is considered inappropriate for the person to die alone. If the person dies at home, the house must be abandoned or a ceremony is held to cleanse it. Families gather together at the time of death and material possessions are dispersed. When a person dies, a cleansing ceremony is performed or else the spirit of the deceased may try to take over someone else's spirit. Those who work with the dead also must have a ceremonial cleansing to protect themselves from the dead person's spirit. No embalming is done; the deceased are buried in sacred ground with their shoes on the wrong feet, rings on their index fingers, and with many gifts surrounding them; or the body is cremated (Purnell & Paulanka, 1998).

For Appalachians, a death is an important event, even for extended family. The funeral is a significant social occasion and family and friends will come great distances to attend. The body is displayed for long periods of time so that all can see the body who wish to. The deceased is buried in his or her best clothes and some people have custom-made clothes for burial (Purnell & Paulanka, 1998). At the funeral home, personal possessions are displayed and it is common to bury these items with the person. Gravesites are typically on hillsides because of the fear they will be flooded out in low-lying areas (Purnell & Paulanka, 1998).

Subgroups from China, Vietnam, Laos, Thailand, and Burma together are called the Hmong. The Hmong believe that proper burial and worship of the dead and other ancestors directly affects the safety, health, and prosperity of the family. The belief is that the spiritual world coexists with the physical world and that the spirits are able to influence human life. The preference is to die at home because they believe their soul will wander for all of eternity without a resting place if they were to die elsewhere. Some groups believe that death should take place in the hospital so as not to bring bad luck into the home. Autopsy and cremation are acceptable practices to some families. For these groups, burial occurs in the afternoon.

The Chinese will place a coin in the deceased's mouth so that the deceased has money to pay anyone who interferes in the journey. In northern China, the body is placed in burial clothes, and an unpadded quilt is used as a shroud. The face is covered with cloth or paper and the feet are tied with colored string. The wife or oldest son wipes the eyes of the deceased with cotton floss before the coffin is closed. Instead of being buried immediately after the funeral, the body may be stored so that a husband and wife can be buried together (Iserson, 2001).

The Japanese bathe their dead, shave some of the hair, and dress the person in white. The deceased wears a ceremonial hat or triangular piece of white paper tied to the forehead. Koreans use perfume to wash the body and dress the body in silk or hemp clothes tied in seven places that correlate with the seven stars in the Ursa Major constellation (Iserson, 2001).

PERI-DEATH 3: FUNERALS AS A CEREMONY OF DEATH

Across cultures, people accept a responsibility to care for, respect, and honor their dead. For most ethnic groups and religious groups, the process of physically preparing the body for the funeral and burial are handled by persons outside the family. The undertaker—a person who "undertook" the responsibility to keep the body safe and make the funeral arrangements—has been a part of society since ancient times. The general public interchangeably refers to the person who prepares the body for burial and conducts all aspects of the funeral service as the undertaker, mortician, embalmer, or funeral director (Iserson, 2001).

In modern society, funeral directors coordinate all the details of the funeral for the family. They supervise preparation of the body for viewing or burial, oversee embalming procedures if embalming is desired, coordinate cremation planning, instruct and support the pallbearers, arrange the transportation of the family and the deceased to the cemetery, place death notices in the newspaper, and otherwise facilitate the family's burial decisions. Most funeral directors in the United States have at least a bachelor's degree and about 85% of all funeral homes are family operated (Iserson, 2001). Funeral homes employ embalmers, cosmetologists, hairdressers, and hearse and limousine drivers.

The funeral director therefore orchestrates all aspects of the funeral. Those who work in the funeral industry know that the funeral must be perfectly organized and executed because they will not get a second chance to make things right. It was originally believed that the funeral held merely theological value, but for many people the funeral is one of the first steps of successful grieving. The funeral is "*of* the person who has died. . . . It is *for* those who survive" (Raether, 1993, p. 211).

For families that have a wake, this is the first component of postdeath ritual. It may be one of the few times the entire family will reassemble for an event. It is a time for family and friends to view the dead body and to pay their final respects. Seeing the dead body emphasizes the fact that the person is dead; declining to see the body may delay grieving.

> I was recently again reminded of how valuable and legitimate a funeral service can be. I accompanied a friend to the funeral of his mother. She had died of a chronic and wasting illness and I had been present at her deathbed. My friend experienced a deep and profound consolation seeing his mother with the lines of suffering erased from her face and lying at peace. (Raether, 1993, p. 211)

The second component of postdeath rituals is the funeral. It is a ceremonial service typically consisting of music, prayers, poetry, eulogies, and it may be part of a funeral Mass where Communion is celebrated. Some people will plan their funerals before they die, which can be comforting to those who are dying as well as their families (Raether, 1993).

The committal service is the concluding funeral rite. It is the final act of caring for the deceased and is celebrated at the grave, tomb, or crematorium. This service is a "symbolic demonstration that the kind of relationship which has existed between the mourner and the deceased is now at an end" (Raether, 1993, p. 212).

Eight specific therapeutic values have been assigned to the funeral process as delineated by Raether (1993, p. 209). First, the "therapy of direct expression" denotes that the funeral furnishes the setting and opportunity for the bereaved to express their grief physically. Funerals offer "therapy of language" by providing the bereaved an opportunity to talk about what has happened, voice their feelings, and begin to feel relief in the telling.

The "therapy of sharing" is the coming together of the family and significant others to provide emotional and physical support to each other. Time spent with the bereaved is an important aspect of burying the dead. Immersion in the many aspects of the funeral process also encompasses the "therapy of activity." The routine of greeting mourners at the funeral home or interacting with those who offer their sympathy prevents the bereaved from withdrawing and focuses their energy in the immediate postdeath period. The funeral also provides the "therapy of ceremony" that is both glorifying and ennobling. The liturgical aspect of the funeral ceremony encompasses the views of the meaning of life and the nature of life hereafter. Given that accepting the reality of the death is difficult for many people, the "therapy of viewing" establishes a final and amended view of the deceased. This revised image replaces those

composed during the illness or at the time of death and may bring comfort to the mourner. Finally, the "therapy of suffering" addresses the guilt that mourners may be experiencing and provides the occasion to verbalize what had been left unsaid previously.

Another important aspect of the postdeath experience for the bereaved is the formation of a new identity within their community. The role of widow, of no longer having a child, or of one who has lost a parent brings with it a change in how the bereaved interact and correspond to society at large. Social groups may shrink, volunteer opportunities may be lost, and favorite activities may be forfeited due to the loss of the deceased. Nurses need to be aware of the difficulties inherent in these role shifts and offer alternatives and community-support referrals during this transitional stage.

When the nurse is providing end-of-life care, the unit of care is the dying person and that person's family. When the death occurs, the family is still in need of nursing care and interventions. The goal of postdeath nursing care is to promote optimal adjustment and to help the family and significant others with the tasks of bereavement. Bereavement is an important developmental stage; the nurse should provide interventions that offer the opportunity for healing and growth, a re-definition of self, and opportunities to make new plans. Follow-up is important during the bereavement period, as well as encouraging memorial rituals to commemorate the deceased's life and death. Unique opportunities exist in peri-death nursing to support the dying patient and the patient's family in making what is a painful and difficult process one that is also priceless.

EDUCATION PLAN 14.1   Plan for Achieving Competencies : Peri-Death Nursing Care

Knowledge Needed	Attitude	Skills	Undergraduate Behavioral Outcomes	Graduate Behavioral Outcomes	Teaching/Learning Strategies
In the last hours of life: —Symptom assessment and management; —Spiritual goals; —Family support; —Signs of death.	*Value patient and family comfort as a priority. *Appreciate the importance of presence during the active phase of dying. *Emphasize the value of complementary therapies.		*Facilitate a peaceful, comfortable, and dignified death.	*Implement interventions in collaboration with members of the interdisciplinary team to address unrelieved symptoms that may necessitate palliative/terminal sedation. *Identify situations of complicated mourning or acute spiritual distress and make appropriate referrals.	*Assign students to the care of the patient who is actively dying in an institutional, hospice, home-care or long-term-care setting, and to the patient's family. *Develop a plan of care for the patient who is actively dying, and for the family, using the nursing process.

(continued)

EDUCATION PLAN 14.1   *(continued)*

Knowledge Needed	Attitude	Skills	Undergraduate Behavioral Outcomes	Graduate Behavioral Outcomes	Teaching/Learning Strategies
					*Interview a family member regarding the death of a significant other, documenting the symptoms experienced in the last hours of life, spiritual perceptions, paranormal experiences, immediate family needs, and apparent signs of death.
Culturally specific peri-death rituals and customs	*Develop cultural awareness, sensitivity, and responsiveness regarding peri-death rituals. *Accept cultural and spiritual diversity.		*Provide culturally competent care during the peri-death period.	*Coordinate institutional and/or community resources in addressing cultural needs at the end of life.	*Develop a case study and plan of care for a dying person from a culture other than students'/nurses' own culture.

| Post-Death Nursing Care: Expected physiological changes and related nursing care
—Care of the body
—Family support
—Pronouncing death
—Autopsy | *Develop emotional and spiritual comfort in caring for the deceased and their family. | *Perform respectful postmortem care. | *Administer respectful care of the deceased and support of the family | *Pronounce death and/or request an autopsy. | *Interview a clergy member or community elder to discuss death rituals and customs specific to that culture. Report findings in post-conference or write a paper comparing and contrasting their findings with their own religion or culture.

*Have senior staff nurses serve as preceptors in assisting students in the physical care of the deceased patient and support of the family. |

(continued)

EDUCATION PLAN 14.1   *(continued)*

Knowledge Needed	Attitude	Skills	Undergraduate Behavioral Outcomes	Graduate Behavioral Outcomes	Teaching/Learning Strategies
					*Conduct a post-conference or seminar to explore feelings and fears related to care of the deceased and their family.
Funerals as ceremonies of death: —Components of funerals —Therapeutic value —Personal grief in response to a patient's death	*Appreciate the therapeutic value of ceremonies of death.		*Participate in death-related ceremonies or rituals.	*Coordinate and/or conduct bereavement rituals or support groups for colleagues.	*Visit a funeral home or invite a funeral director to class to discuss burial/cremation options, components of a funeral, and responsibilities of the funeral director as a member of the interdisciplinary team.

Write a reaction paper that addresses students'/nurses' perceptions and experiences related to this experience. *During a post-conference or seminar. Have the students/nurses brainstorm strategies that would support health professionals in coping with a patients' death.

REFERENCES

Archdiocese of San Antonio. (2002). Cremation for Catholics? *Catholic cemeteries and mausoleums.* Retrieved July 15, 2004, from http://www.catholiccemeteriesofsa.org/index.htm

Birchenall, J., & Streight, E. (1997). *Home care aide.* St. Louis, MO: Mosby.

Craig, G. (2000). On withholding nutrition and hydration in the terminally ill. In D. Dickenson (Ed.), *Death, dying and bereavement.* London: Open University Press/Sage.

Bhungalia, S., & Kemp, C. (2002). (Asian) Indian health beliefs and practices related to end of life. *Journal of Hospice and Palliative Nursing, 4*(1), 54–58.

Cimino, J. (2003). The role of nutrition in hospice and palliative care of the cancer patient. *Topics in Clinical Nutrition, 18,* 154–161.

Ferrell, B. R., Virani, R., & Grant, M. (1999). Analysis of end of life content in nursing textbooks. *Oncology Nursing Forum, 26,* 869–876.

Field, M., & Cassel, C. (1997). *Approaching death: Improving care at the end of life.* Washington, DC: National Academy Press.

Gorman, L. M. (1998). In R. M. Carroll-Johnson, L. M. Gorman, & N. J. Bush (Eds.), *Psychosocial nursing care along the cancer continuum* (pp. 3–25). Pittsburgh, PA: Oncology Nursing Press.

Gates, R. A., & Fink, R. M. (1997). *Oncology nursing secrets.* St. Louis, MO: Mosby.

Green, J. (1989a). Death with dignity: Baha'i Faith. *Nursing Times, 85*(10), 50–51.

Green, J. (1989b). Death with dignity: Buddhism. *Nursing Times, 85*(9), 40–41.

Green, J. (1989c). Death with dignity: Hinduism. *Nursing Times, 85*(6), 50–51.

Green, J. (1989d). Death with dignity: Islam. *Nursing Times, 85*(5), 56–57.

Green, J. (1989e). Death with dignity: Judaism. *Nursing Times, 85*(8), 65–65.

Heming, D., & Colmer, A. (2003). Care of dying patients. *Nursing Standard, 8*(10), 47–56.

Horn, L. W. (1992, March/April). Terminal dyspnea: A hospice approach. *American Journal of Hospice and Palliative Care,* 24–32.

Hoyal, C., Grant, J., Chamberlain, F., Cox, R., & Campbell, T. (2002) Improving the management of breathlessness using a clinical effectiveness programme. *International Journal of Palliative Nursing, 8*(2), 78–87.

Iserson, K. V. (2001). *Death to dust: What happens to dead bodies?* Tucson, AZ: Galen Press.

Kastenbaum, R., & Kastenbaum, B. (Eds.) (1989). *Encyclopedia of death.* Phoenix, AZ: Oryx Press.

Kaye, P. (2003) *A–Z pocket book of symptom control.* Northampton, MA: EBL.

LaDuke, S. (2001). Terminal dyspnea and palliative care. *American Journal of Nursing, 101*(11), 26–31.

Lynn, J., & Harrold, J. (1999). *Handbook for mortals: Guidance for people facing serious illness.* New York: Oxford University Press.

Macleod, A., & Whitehead, L. (1997) Dysgraphia and terminal delirium. *Palliative Medicine, 11*(2), 127–132.

Miller, E. J. (1993). A Roman Catholic view of death. In K. Doka & J. D. Morgan (Eds.), *Death and spirituality* (pp. 33–50). Amityville, NY: Baywood.

Office of the Inspector General. (2002). *Organ donor registries executive report # OEI-01–01–00350.* Retrieved July 15, 2004, from http://oig.hhs.gov/oei

Panke, J. (2003). Difficulties in managing pain at the end of life. *Journal of Hospice and Palliative Nursing, 5*(2), 83–90.

Pitorak, E. F. (2003). Care at the time of death: How nurses can make the last hours of life a richer, more comfortable experience. *American Journal of Nursing, 103*(7), 42–52.

Purnell, L. D., & Paulanka, B. J. (1998). *Transcultural heal care: A culturally competent approach.* Philadelphia: Davis.

Quested, B. (2003). Nursing care of dead bodies: A discursive analysis of last offices. *Journal of Advanced Nursing, 41,* 553–560.

Raether, H. C. (1993). Rituals, beliefs, and grief. In K. Doka & J. D. Morgan (Eds.), *Death and spirituality* (pp. 207–216). Amityville, NY: Baywood.

Soden, K., Hoy, A., Hoy, W., & Clelland, S. (2002) Artificial hydration during the last week of life in patients dying in a district general hospital. *Palliative Medicine, 16,* 542–543.

Sorrentino, S. A. (1999). *Assisting with patient care.* St. Louis, MO: Mosby.

Strub, C. G., & Frederick, L. G. (1967). *The principles and practice of embalming.* Dallas, TX: Frederick.

Tarzian, A. J. (2000). Caring for dying patients who have air hunger. *Journal of Nursing Scholarship, 32,* 137–143.

Transition rituals: A faith-by-faith guide to rites for the deceased. Retrieved December 22, 2002, from http://www.beliefnet.com/story/78/story_7894.html

Worden, W. (1992). *Grief counseling and grief therapy* (2nd ed.). London: Routledge.

Index

Page numbers followed by f or t indicate figures and tables, respectively.